Principles
and Practice
of
ORAL
MEDICINE

2nd Edition

Principles and Practice of ORAL MEDICINE

2nd Edition

Stephen T. Sonis, D.M.D., D.M.Sc.
Chief, Division of Oral Medicine and Dentistry
Brigham and Women's Hospital
Boston, Massachusetts
Professor of Oral Medicine and Chairman
Department of Oral Medicine and Diagnostic Sciences
Harvard School of Dental Medicine
Boston, Massachusetts
Associate Physician
Dana-Farber Cancer Institute
Boston, Massachusetts

Robert C. Fazio, D.M.D.
Associate Clinical Professor of Surgery
Yale University School of Medicine
New Haven, Connecticut
Attending Periodontist
Yale-New Haven Hospital
New Haven, Connecticut
Attending Periodontist
Norwalk Hospital
Norwalk, Connecticut

Leslie Fang, M.D.
Chief, Walter Bauer Firm
  Medical Services
Massachusetts General Hospital
Boston, Massachusetts
Assistant Professor of Medicine
Harvard Medical School
Boston, Massachusetts

W.B. SAUNDERS COMPANY
A Division of Harcourt Brace & Company
Philadelphia ■ London ■ Toronto ■ Montreal ■ Sydney ■ Tokyo

W.B. SAUNDERS COMPANY
A Division of
Harcourt Brace & Company

The Curtis Center
Independence Square West
Philadelphia, Pennsylvania 19106

Library of Congress Cataloging-in-Publication Data

Sonis, Stephen T.

Principles and practice of oral medicine / Stephen T. Sonis,
Robert C. Fazio, Leslie Fang.—2nd ed.

   p.   cm.

Includes bibliographical references and index.

ISBN 0–7216–8449–1

1. Oral medicine.   I. Fazio, Robert C.   II. Fang, Leslie S. T.
   III. Title.   [DNLM: 1. Mouth Diseases—complications.
   2. Mouth Diseases—therapy.   3. Tooth Diseases—
   complications.   4. Tooth Diseases—therapy.
   5. Dental Care for Chronically Ill.   6. Dental Care for
   Disabled.   WU 140 S698p 1995]
RC815.S66 1995   616'.00246176—dc20

DNLM/DLC   94–12256

Principles and Practice of Oral Medicine, 2nd ed.   ISBN 0–7216–8449–1

Printed in the United States of America.

Last digit is the print number: 9   8   7   6   5   4   3   2   1

FOR
Trudy, Amanda, and Jonathan,
Barbara, Danielle, and Alexandra,
Barbara and Caitlin

Preface

It is hard to believe that 10 years have passed since the first edition of *Principles and Practice of Oral Medicine* was completed. We noted at that time that dentists were treating medically compromised patients at an increasing rate. In fact, dental management of the medically compromised patient is becoming a routine and increasingly important part of dental practice. A number of factors are contributing to this phenomenon. First, the population continues to age, and many older patients have multiple medical conditions. Second, as medical care becomes more effective and cost issues are emphasized, many patients are being treated on an ambulatory basis to avoid hospitalization. Consequently, these individuals are in the community and readily seek dental care. Third, the sophistication of medical treatment is prolonging life. And fourth, the level of and access to available dental care has improved, which has resulted in more patients, regardless of medical status, wanting dental treatment.

There have been significant advances in the practice of medicine since the first edition was published. HIV infection was still relatively new 10 years ago, and health reform was largely limited to academic discussion. Bone marrow transplants were considered an experimental therapy. A large number of medications currently used were yet to be introduced. We have tried to identify and address these items in this edition.

As with the first edition, we have maintained as our major objective providing the reader with the essentials of assessment and management of patients. We have purposefully avoided the esoteric and have focused on the practical. The use of management-related risk categories, which was so successful in the first edition, remains.

Chapters dealing with the diagnosis and management of oral diseases have been updated.

We hope that this edition will be a frequently and easily used reference for the practitioner and will produce a foundation from which the student can integrate medicine with the practice of dentistry.

We are grateful to the editorial staff at Saunders for their help in the preparation of this edition.

STS
RCF
LF

Contents

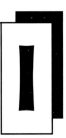

Patient Assessment

History, Physical, and Laboratory Evaluation

OBJECTIVES

In the past, the simple question "Are you generally in good health?" provided all the information necessary to proceed with dental treatment. Such cursory inquiries are no longer acceptable. Today, dentists and physicians need to know more about past and present medical conditions because of the increasing number of geriatric patients who require dental services, the proliferation of medications that may be significant in a stress-inducing situation, the use of inhalation and intravenous sedation techniques, and a general improvement in the standards of medical and dental practice.

The major objectives of pretreatment patient evaluation are the following: (1) establishing the diagnosis; (2) determining pre-existent medical conditions; (3) discovering concomitant disease; (4) managing emergencies; and (5) patient management.

Establishing the Diagnosis

The establishment of oral diagnosis is frequently not difficult, particularly when the pathology involves grossly recognizable chronic tooth or periodontal disease. However, the complexity of primary oral pathology compels the dentist to approach the diagnosis of less obvious conditions with care. The diagnostic problem is compounded by the fact that oral lesions requiring identification are frequently not of the primary variety and not locally restricted; sometimes they represent systemic disease with local manifestations. Because the delineation between local and systemic disease is often blurred, complete patient evaluation is required for accurate diagnosis.

Even if a carefully administered evaluation does not reveal the precise diagnosis of a lesion, it usually provides indications for additional studies, such as bacteriologic cultures, laboratory tests, biopsies, or consultations. It should be recognized that most difficult diagnoses, whether in the oral-facial region or elsewhere, are the result not of flashes of brilliance but of a meticulous and systematic assimilation of a complex body of patient information. An approach to oral diagnosis is discussed in Chapter 2.

Medical Conditions

The dentist should routinely check the history of each patient for an event, condition, or medication that might significantly affect a projected oral treatment plan. Discovery of a history of allergic reactions to a drug may avoid a rash, at least, and possibly a catastrophe. Furthermore, significant past illnesses, such as rheumatic fever, may require the use of prophylactic antibiotics. Current illnesses may be suspected when a patient is regularly seeing the physician or using a specific medication. If the patient is being treated for concomitant disease by a physician, the dentist should not hesitate to consult with him or her.

It should be emphasized that an evaluation for pre-existing medical conditions must be performed prior to any therapeutic measures. This is particularly true for the patient who is seeking emergency care, when the tendency is to treat the acute situation and to attend to the formalities of a medical history later. With some exceptions, time must be allowed to determine the presence of significant present or past illness. The discovery of a serious concurrent medical condition after complications have arisen benefits neither the dentist nor the patient.

Discovery of Concomitant Disease

A significant proportion of the population regularly seeks the services of a dentist and only rarely visits the family physician for physical examinations. This situation provides dentists with opportunities to contribute to the general health of their patients. The presence of previously undiagnosed concomitant systemic disease may be suggested either by significant physical findings (e.g., hypertension), which are routinely reviewed during the evaluation, or by a carefully scrutinized history (e.g., diabetes mellitus). When a significant condition is incidentally encountered, it is not the responsibility of the dentist to treat the disease. The patient should be informed of the suspicion and promptly referred to the family physician or an appropriate specialist. Thus, the patient receives treatment for a disease that otherwise would have proceeded undiagnosed, and the dentist earns the respect of both the patient and the physician.

Medical Emergencies

The pretreatment evaluation aids the practitioner in the management of office emergencies in three ways. First, and most important, the performance of a complete evaluation prior to treatment prevents most office emergencies. The medical history informs dentists of any pre-existing medical conditions and allows them to alter the patient's treatment to avoid complications. For example, the diabetic patient may require modifications in diet, medications, and the time or length of appointments when a dental procedure is anticipated. Second, a knowledge of the patient's past history saves valuable time when making an emergency diagnosis and alerts the clinician to have appropriate medications available. Many office emergencies are actually acute exacerbations of chronic or long-standing diseases. Finally, routine diagnostic procedures used during the physical evaluation, such as taking blood pressure may, in an emergency, be quickly converted into therapeutic measures for monitoring vital signs and delivering crucial medications.

Patient Management

It must be assumed that dental procedures are stressful situations, regardless of whether local anesthesia, local anesthesia with sedation, or general anesthesia is employed. The stress induced, however, is frequently not commensurate with the complexity or duration of the anticipated operation; the patient's response is often prompted by preconceived anticipations and anxieties. For many patients, the anxiety induced by a simple examination and prophylaxis exceeds that experienced by others undergoing relatively extensive procedures. Thus, the physical evaluation presents an important opportunity for the dentist to establish rapport with patients and to minimize their anxiety.

Diagnosis and appropriate treatment depend on a sound and comprehensive data base obtained through patient assessment, which includes the history, the examination, radiographs, and laboratory tests.

HISTORY

The backbone of the diagnosis is the history. The good clinician is a studious listener. Careful, thorough questioning of a patient without prodding always yields significant information.

The taking of the history is usually the first opportunity for communication between the dentist and the patient. The way in which this interview is conducted frequently provides the patient with an image of the clinician that can color the future relationship between the two. An unsatisfactory impression made at this point is extremely difficult to remedy in the future. Thus, the initial interview should do everything possible to establish a rapport between the patient and the clinician.

There are numerous intangible factors involved in developing a good dentist-patient relationship. These include the general appearance of the clinician, an ability to empathize with the patient's complaints and, most important, a sincere concern and interest in each patient as an individual. Clinicians who are disheveled and ungroomed may suggest to patients that they are equally careless in attending to the details of diagnosis and treatment. In taking the history, the clinician must proceed with self-confidence; hesitation or embarrassment is often met with incomplete or inaccurate responses.

Usually, a well-intentioned attempt to establish rapport is rewarded with spontaneous and uninhibited responses. Occasionally, however, the most sincere efforts produce only apathy, indifference, or frank hostility. The query "What does that question have to do with cavities?" is not uncommon. In this situation, the patient should be informed of the potential significance of apparently obscure and unrelated events in the diagnosis and dental management.

Adherence to a definite order of inquiry and

categorization of information is required to ensure completeness and to help the clinician reach accurate conclusions. The source of the history is, however, the patient, and people vary in their ability to observe and describe symptoms, depending on their intelligence, education, emotional status, and degree of confidence they have in the examiner. For this reason, the clinician must be prepared to modify the interview to suit individual patients. At no time should history taking be reduced to a mechanical and impersonal recitation of routine questions.

There are five basic categories of information to be obtained in the course of every formal history:

1. Identification of the problem (chief complaint)
2. Clarification of the circumstances surrounding the onset and development of the problem (history of the present illness)
3. Documentation of diseases or conditions in the past (past medical history)
4. Investigation into possible genetic, social, or environmental factors influencing the problem (family health, personal and social history)
5. Summary of additional symptoms by organ system (review of systems)

The source of the history may be the patient, members of the family, friends, a referring doctor or, in the case of the hospitalized patient, an old record from a previous admission. When an individual other than the patient serves as the informant, the name, address, and telephone number should be recorded in the event that clarification of data becomes a necessity. Each source of information must be evaluated for its reliability and recorded accordingly. For example, when the patient is demented, senile, or an infant, it is obvious that other sources of information must be sought.

Elements of the History

Chief Complaint. The primary reason the patient originally consults the dentist constitutes the chief complaint. The complaint should be stated as briefly as possible in the patient's own words and from their perspective. The recording of a precise diagnosis (e.g., periapical abscess) or the use of vague terminology (e.g., tooth trouble) is to be discouraged, because this does not contribute to an understanding of the complaint.

History of the Present Illness. The history of the present illness is an elaboration of all the circumstances surrounding the onset and progression of the patient's symptoms. During the interview, the patient should be allowed to proceed with the story, emphasizing those incidents considered to be significant. The facts should be ordered chronologically, but frequent interruptions should be avoided so that the patient is not discouraged from relating all the relevant events. At the conclusion of the patient's narrative, the examiner should briefly summarize for the patient all the essential facts to ensure that an accurate exchange of information has taken place. The synopsis usually includes data pertinent to the location, duration, progress, and character of the disease, its relation to function, and the effect of previous treatment.

Past Medical History. In the dental office, the past medical history is usually obtained by both a written questionnaire and a verbal interview, and is divided into a history of past illnesses and a review of systems.

History of Past Illnesses. A summarization of past medical events or conditions should cover allergies, diseases, medication, and hospitalizations.

Allergies. The importance of documenting allergic manifestations, particularly when drugs are the offending agents, is obvious. When present in the history, allergens should be identified along with the types of reactions encountered. It is essential that notices of allergy be prominently displayed on patients' records and hospital order sheets.

Diseases. Although all people have experienced disease of some sort, it is important for the clinician to establish a history of certain significant diseases, such as rheumatic fever or diabetes mellitus, recording each illness along with the date it was contracted. In addition to asking patients broad questions such as "Do you have or have you had any pulmonary disease?" the clinician should inquire specifically about a number of diseases listed in Table 1–1, either verbally or in a written questionnaire.

Medications. It is imperative for the dentist to establish the patient's medication history. Drugs may be responsible for oral lesions (e.g., phenytoin or Dilantin), or may reflect an underlying condition that could seriously alter a proposed treatment plan (e.g., warfarin or Coumadin). It is important to determine past as well as current medications. A patient who

Table 1–1. DISEASES OR DISORDERS ABOUT WHICH PATIENTS SHOULD BE SPECIFICALLY QUERIED

Cardiovascular: rheumatic fever, murmurs or click, prolapsed mitral valve, congenital anomalies, hypertension, arrhythmias, myocardial infarction, angina or chest pain, cardiac surgery
Respiratory: asthma, chronic obstructive lung disease, tobacco use, tuberculosis
Gastrointestinal: colitis, ulcers, liver disease
Genitourinary: urinary tract infection, renal disease
Endocrine: diabetes mellitus, adrenal gland disorders, thyroid dysfunction, pregnancy
Neurologic: stroke, seizures, headaches
Hematologic: anemia, bleeding disorders, recurrent infections
Psychiatric: substance abuse, depression, anxiety, eating disorders
Infectious: hepatitis, herpes simplex, HIV infection, STDs

took steroids 6 months prior to dental treatment requires additional management considerations. When a history of the routine use of a medication is obtained, the generic name of the drug, the dosage regimen, and the route of administration should be documented.

Hospitalizations. A prior hospitalization may also reveal a condition or event that could influence a diagnosis or treatment plan. All previous hospitalizations are recorded chronologically with the names of the hospitals, the dates, the diagnoses, and any surgical procedures performed.

Review of Systems. The system review is a thorough report of specific symptoms related to individual organ systems. The review is conducted, first, to ensure against the inadvertent deletion of data that may help establish a diagnosis and, second, to account for the status of each individual organ system in relation to possible concomitant disease or projected treatment protocols.

The inquiry proceeds from head to toe and determines the presence or absence of specific symptoms relative to each system. A knowledge of the patient's chief complaint and the history of the illness may guide the clinician into investigating areas of particular interest in greater depth, but preconceived diagnoses should not cut short a thorough inquiry. It should be emphasized that the absence of one symptom often contributes as much to the solution of a diagnostic problem as the presence of another, so that complete documentation of "significant negatives" becomes mandatory. Furthermore, the clinician must exercise care in the construction and wording of questions commensurate with the patient's understanding.

Social History. The personal history of the patient reflects the influence the living environment or life style may have on disease. Moreover, an understanding of the patient's social relationships may help to anticipate emotional response to serious disease. Three areas are routinely investigated: present and past occupations and occupational hazards, smoking and chronic alcohol or drug abuse, and marital status.

Family History. The family history aids in determining genetic transmission of disease or a predisposition for disease. Conditions that appear to involve predisposing hereditary features include certain hemorrhagic disorders, allergic conditions, migraine, diabetes mellitus, hypertension, and certain types of malignant disease. The family history is also used to discover communicable diseases within the immediate family that may infect members of that household. The history should record the ages and health of all members of the immediate family, the ages and causes of death of any deceased members, and the presence of any of the more common genetically associated illnesses (Table 1–2).

Medical Questionnaire

The easiest and hence most widely used technique for obtaining a medical history in the dental office is the medical questionnaire. It enjoys excellent patient acceptance and is usually self-administered, thereby saving the dentist time. However, serious deficiencies in the reliability of the medical questionnaire have been noted.

To appreciate the limitations of the technique, one should analyze the data provided by the medical questionnaire. Although many adaptations of the form are in use, they never go beyond identification of the patient and the history of past illness. These data usually include past diseases, allergies, hospitalizations,

Table 1–2. DISEASES IN WHICH GENETICS MAY BE SIGNIFICANT

Diabetes mellitus
Hypertension
Myocardial infarction
Allergies, asthma
Bleeding disorders
Malignancies

operations, and medications, but exclude a detailed present complaint, a history of the present illness, and a review of systems. This limited information is usually sufficient to identify a medical condition that may interfere with a proposed, otherwise routine, treatment plan. However, in a complex diagnostic situation, the medical questionnaire does not provide sufficient data, and the clinician should proceed with a formal medical history.

The length and content of the medical questionnaire are subjects of some controversy. The questionnaire must be long enough to provide all potentially significant data, but should not be so long that it bores and discourages the patient who is filling it out. Individual clinicians must choose the questionnaire that, in their view, best satisfies these criteria. The form reproduced has generally proven adequate (Fig. 1–1).

If the patient's responses on the questionnaire are incoherent, the clinician should restate appropriate questions or seek a more reliable information source. Invariably, the information provided by a self-administered medical questionnaire must be supplemented by a verbal history.

Verbal History

After the medical questionnaire has been completed in private, the clinician should interview the patient. The objectives of the interview are the following: (1) to supplement the questionnaire with the chief complaint and history of the present illness; (2) to determine whether the health questionnaire is adequate for the requirements of the clinical situation; (3) to discuss salient features of the questionnaire that require amplification; and (4) to establish a personal rapport with the patient.

The verbal history should begin with an inquiry into the patient's complaint, because the complaint and history of the illness usually determine whether the facts provided by the health form are sufficient to deal with the clinical situation. Moreover, this approach makes the patient aware of the clinician's concern with the immediate problem and establishes the sympathy and rapport essential to a good patient-dentist relationship. Once it has been established that the questionnaire is sufficient, every significant response is further investigated with appropriate questioning. If the examiner suspects that the patient has failed to comprehend portions of the questionnaire, the questions should be rephrased to ensure reliability.

EXAMINATION

The physical examination collects data relevant to the signs of disease. The documentation of signs appears relatively simple when compared with the problem of dealing with subjective symptoms, because signs are observable phenomena amenable to objective description and quantification. However, accurate information is forthcoming only when the clinician adheres to proper techniques of observation.

Examination of the dental patient should include an overall assessment of the patient, recording of vital signs, and a complete head and neck examination (Chap. 2). Each patient should receive a thorough facial, oral, nasal, aural, and neck examination in addition to recording of blood pressure, pulse, and respiration. These observations are used not only to detect subclinical disease, but also to establish baseline values of vital signs should an emergency occur.

The examination involves the routine application of four methods of observation, inspection, palpation, percussion, and auscultation. It should be recognized that these techniques are not equally effective in evaluating all anatomic regions, and that some are less useful to the dentist than others.

Inspection. The visual observation of signs generally contributes more information pertinent to a potential diagnosis than any other physical technique, particularly in oral examinations. Inspection provides both the quantitative data of measurement and the qualitative data of description, such as color and symmetry. While taking the patient's medical history, the clinician can observe general characteristics such as body development, nutrition, gait, speech patterns, and skin color.

Palpation. After inspection, the patient should be touched and felt. Palpation reveals the consistency, mobility, and character of structures. The examination of the neck depends almost exclusively on palpation.

Percussion. Percussion involves the differential transmission of sound by various structures. The sound is produced by the striking finger of the examiner and is differentiated by either the ear or the vibratory sense in the examiner's hand. Whereas the application of percussion in the examination of the head and neck is limited, the technique is extremely valuable in the investigation of the chest and abdomen.

THE
WABAN
DENTAL
GROUP

1180 Beacon Street
Newton Highlands, MA 02161

DATE:_____

NAME:_____   HOME PHONE #_____   BUSINESS PHONE #_____

ADDRESS:_____   ZIP CODE:_____

SOCIAL SECURITY:_____   HEIGHT:_____ WEIGHT:_____ D.O.B._____

OCCUPATION:_____   EMPLOYER:_____

EMPLOYER'S ADDRESS:_____

NAME OF FAMILY PHYSICIAN:_____   PHONE #_____

PHYSICIAN'S ADDRESS:_____

DATE OF LAST PHYSICAL EXAMINATION:_____

INDIVIDUAL RESPONSIBLE FOR PAYMENT   NAME:_____

(IF DIFFERENT FROM ABOVE)   ADDRESS:_____

PHONE: Work_____

Home_____

DENTAL INSURANCE INFORMATION

PRIMARY CARRIER	POLICY HOLDER	DATE OF BIRTH	PROVIDER NUMBER (MAY DIFFER FROM SS#)	GROUP NUMBER
_____	_____	__/__/__	_____	_____

ADDRESS OF CARRIER'S OFFICE: _____

SECONDARY CARRIER	POLICY HOLDER	DATE OF BIRTH	PROVIDER NUMBER (MAY DIFFER FROM SS#)	GROUP NUMBER
_____	_____	__/__/__	_____	_____

ADDRESS OF CARRIER'S OFFICE: _____

Figure 1–1. Health questionnaire. (Courtesy of the Waban Dental Group, Newton Highlands, MA.)

HEALTH QUESTIONNAIRE

Please answer "YES" or "NO" to the Following Questions
Answers to the following questions are for <u>our records only</u> and will be considered confidential.

Yes..No 1. Are you in good health? _____

Yes..No 2. Has there been any change in your general health within the past year? _____

Yes..No 3. Are you under the care of a physician for any problem? _____

Yes..No 4. Have you ever had any serious illness or operations? _____

Yes..No 5. Do you have, or have you had any of the following: _____

Yes..No —Rheumatic fever	Yes..No —Hepatitis or liver disease
Yes..No —Mitral valve prolapse	Yes..No —Asthma
Yes..No —High blood pressure	Yes..No —Diabetes
Yes..No —Stroke	Yes..No —Seizures
Yes..No —Heart murmur or click	Yes..No —Cancer
Yes..No —Heart attack or disease	Yes..No —Frequent headaches
Yes..No —Chest pain or angina	Yes..No —Thyroid condition
Yes..No —Artificial joint or valve	Yes..No —Chronic illnesses
Yes..No —Bleeding or blood disorder	Yes..No —Herpes virus (Cold Sores)
Yes..No —Venereal disease	Yes..No —AIDS or HIV+ infection
Yes..No —Tuberculosis	Yes..No —Radiation or chemotherapy

Yes..No 6. Have you ever had surgery or x-ray treatment for a tumor or growth, or other condition of your mouth or face? _____

Yes..No 7. Are you now taking any drug or medicine (including aspirin) for any reason? If yes, please list: _____

Yes..No 8. Have you ever had abnormal bleeding from previous extractions, surgery, or when cut? _____

9. Are you allergic or sensitive to any of the following:

Yes..No —Local anesthetics ("novocaine")	Yes..No —Aspirin, codeine, or other drugs for pain
Yes..No —Penicillin or other antibiotics	Yes..No —Others (<u>please specify</u>) _____

WOMEN ONLY

Yes..No 10. Are you pregnant? _____

Date of Last Menstrual Period _____

SUMMATION

Allergies and reactions _____
_____
_____

Medications _____
_____
_____
_____
_____
_____

Figure 1–1. *Continued*

Illustration continued on following page

DENTAL QUESTIONNAIRE

Reason for this visit:_____

Date of last dental treatment:_____ Date of last dental x-rays: _____

Please Answer "YES" or "NO" to the Following Questions

Yes..No 1. Have you ever had any serious problems with previous dental treatment? _____

Yes..No 2. Are you presently in pain? _____

Yes..No 3. Are there any areas in your mouth you avoid or have difficulty chewing on? _____

Yes..No 4. Have you ever been told that you grind your teeth at night?_____

Yes..No 5. Do you experience any pain or fatigue in your jaws or face?_____

Yes..No 6. Do you experience frequent headaches? _____

Do any of the following stimuli bring on tooth pain?

Yes..No Cold

Yes..No Hot

Yes..No Sweet

Yes..No Biting Pressure

Yes..No Brushing

Yes..No Flossing

FOR
OFFICE
USE
_____
_____
_____
_____
_____
_____
_____
_____
_____

Yes..No 7. Have you had orthodontic therapy? _____

Yes..No 8. Have you had your wisdom teeth removed?_____

Yes..No 9. Do you wear dentures? _____

Yes..No 10. Do you gag easily?_____

Yes..No 11. Do you use a soft bristled toothbrush? _____

FOR
OFFICE
USE
_____
_____
_____

Yes..No 12. Are you pleased with the appearance of your teeth? _____

FOR
OFFICE
USE
_____
_____
_____
_____

Patient Signature   Interviewer Signature

Figure 1–1. *Continued*

Auscultation. The technique of auscultation also depends on the differential transmission of sounds. The stethoscope is generally used to appreciate such sounds and is most routinely used by the dentist for blood pressure determination.

Blood Pressure

The auscultatory determination of blood pressure is based on the vibrations of the blood as it passes through the arteries (Korotkoff sounds). Minimal equipment is required: a stethoscope (either a diaphragm or bell type is acceptable), and a blood pressure cuff (sphygmomanometer), or a mercury gravity manometer.

The technique for measuring blood pressure is straightforward and easily accomplished by the dentist or an assistant. The patient should be seated in a dental chair with the arm horizontal and at the level of the heart. The blood pressure cuff should be placed securely over the patient's upper arm above the antecubital fossa (Fig. 1–2). Most cuffs have Velcro material to ease fastening. The orientation of the cuff is usually indicated by arrows on the cuff that show its relationship to the brachial artery. The top of the cuff is the side free of tubing. It is important that the cuff be placed properly and that it be of correct size to avoid a false reading. If there is a gauge connected to the cuff, it is put in place with clips. The bell or diaphragm of the stethoscope is placed lightly over the brachial artery. The tubing of the stethoscope should be as short as practically possible to minimize distortion of sounds, and the earpieces should be oriented in the direction of the auditory canals.

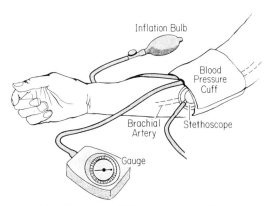

Figure 1–2. Placement of blood pressure cuff and stethoscope. The cuff should be applied approximately 1 inch above the antecubital fossa, with the bell or diaphragm of the stethoscope placed lightly over the brachial artery.

The patient should be as relaxed as possible. The valve on the bulb is closed. With the right hand feeling the radial pulse, the cuff is inflated to about 30 mm Hg after the pulse disappears, using a steady and regular force. Excessively rapid pumping is to be avoided. The cuff is then gradually deflated, with the operator noting the point at which the first sound is heard (the systolic pressure) and the point at which the sounds disappear (diastolic pressure). The sounds usually increase after the systolic point is heard and then become muffled before disappearing. The operator should continue listening until 0 mm Hg of mercury is reached, because the sounds may return after they are lost. This auscultatory gap can result in an inaccurate determination of the diastolic pressure if it is not noted. The points at which the first and last sounds are heard are recorded as a fraction, such as 120/80. Pressure in each arm is different. It is therefore important to record which arm was measured. Evaluation of blood pressure is discussed in Chapter 4.

Pulse

The pulse is a peripheral measurement of heart rate and rhythm. The dentist should learn how to take the pulse from both the radial and carotid areas. The radial pulse is located by having the patient rotate the hand in a palm-up position. The pulse can be felt by resting the fingers just above the wrist and behind the thumb. The carotid pulse is located just anterior to the sternocleidomastoid muscle at the level of the thyroid cartilage.

When examining the pulse, note first the rate of the heart. This is best accomplished by leaving the fingers in place for a period of 60 seconds. Inaccuracies result if one measures for less time and then multiplies by a factor to yield the rate per minute. The normal resting rate is about 72 beats per minute, bpm (range, 60 to 100 bpm). Next, the rhythm of the pulse should be assessed to ascertain its consistency and regularity. Abnormalities may indicate an arrhythmia (Chaps. 9 and 10). Finally, the strength or weakness of the pulse should be noted.

Respiratory Rate

The respiratory rate is easily determined by counting the rise and fall of the patient's chest over a 1-minute period. It is best not to inform the patient that the respiratory rate is being measured, because the patient may then try to change the breathing pattern. It is also important to note any signs of altered respiratory quality, such as wheezing, stridor, or straining.

Temperature

Any patient suspected of having an infection should have his or her temperature taken. This is most conveniently accomplished using an oral thermometer. The normal oral temperature is 37° C or 98.6° F. A temperature of 100° F or more is considered significant.

LABORATORY EXAMINATION

Use of the Clinical Laboratory

A relatively small number of laboratory tests are frequently used by the dentist (see Summary Table 1–I). Generally, these include examinations to determine or rule out anemia, white cell disorders, bleeding problems, diabetes mellitus, and hepatitis. In addition, bacteriologic culturing and antibiotic sensitivity testing may be used (Chap. 46). Unfortunately, many dental students rarely have significant contact with laboratory medicine during their undergraduate dental education. The clinical laboratory may seem foreign and intimidating to them. In fact, laboratories want to satisfy the people who supply them with patients and usually bend over backward to make their use as easy as possible.

There are two major types of clinical laboratories. Some are associated with and located in hospitals. These laboratories usually offer a full range of services. A dentist does not need to be on the hospital staff to refer a patient for a laboratory test. The second group of laboratories is commercially owned and independent. Some of them provide a more limited range of tests than hospital laboratories. Because they are commercial, however, these laboratories may offer additional services, such as specimen pickup at the office or house calls to obtain samples from housebound patients. It is incumbent on the dentist to become familiar with the local clinical laboratories. The College of American Pathologists has a surveillance program for quality control, and laboratory participation in this program usually indicates a commitment to accuracy. Dentists may also ask physicians in the area to recommend laboratories.

Ordering a laboratory test for a patient is as easy as writing a prescription and may be done over the telephone. The dentist simply calls the laboratory (if calling a hospital, contact the department of pathology) and gives the secretary or technician the patient's name, the test requested, and the dentist's name, address, and telephone number. To avoid any confusion, it is helpful to give the patient a request form to bring to the laboratory. These are usually provided on request by the laboratory and should be kept in the office until needed. Usually, the laboratory sends written results of the test 3 or 4 days after it is performed. If the dentist needs the result more quickly, the laboratory should be so informed and asked to call or fax the information as soon as it is available.

Specific Laboratory Tests and Their Interpretation

Although there are a staggering number of tests that can be performed on fluids from the body, only a few are of interest to the dentist. The discussion that follows is divided into three sections: tests that are frequently used by the dentist (Table 1–3); tests that are occasionally used by the dentist (Table 1–4); and tests that are rarely used by the dentist but are frequently used by physicians in patient assessment or may be used as adjuncts in the diagnosis of oral disease (Table 1–5).

Tests Frequently Used by the Dentist

Complete Blood Count (CBC). The CBC is one of the most useful and inexpensive labo-

Table 1–3. LABORATORY TESTS FREQUENTLY USED BY DENTISTS

Complete blood count (CBC)*
  Hemoglobin (Hgb)
  Hematocrit (Hct)
  White blood count (WBC)
  Differential white blood cell count

Bleeding studies
  Prothrombin time (PT)
  Partial thromboplastin time (PTT)
  Bleeding time (BT)
  Platelet count

Fasting blood sugar

Hepatitis screening: Australia antigen

*Most laboratories include mean corpuscular volume (MCV), mean corpuscular hemoglobin (MCH), mean corpuscular hemoglobin concentration (MCHC), and red blood cell count (RBC).

Table 1–4. LABORATORY TESTS OCCASIONALLY USED BY DENTISTS

Tests for disturbance in bone
    Calcium
    Phosphorus
    Alkaline phosphatase

Erythrocyte sedimentation rate

Urinalysis—used routinely in hospitalized patients

Syphilis screening

ratory tests available. It measures the patient's hemoglobin, hematocrit, and white blood cell count. A differential white blood cell count may be included, but in some cases must be specifically requested. Hemoglobin is found uniquely in red blood cells (RBCs). Decreases in the hemoglobin level are associated with anemia; increases are seen in polycythemia. The hematocrit measures the percentage of formed elements in blood. Hence, changes in the hematocrit are associated with the same conditions as for hemoglobin. Routinely, laboratories include calculations of RBC volume (mean corpuscular volume, MCV) and hemoglobin concentrations (mean corpuscular hemoglobin, MHC, or mean corpuscular hemoglobin concentration, MCHC) as part of the CBC. Such information is helpful in defining anemias (Chap. 25). The white blood count (WBC) is a measure of the absolute number of white cells per cubic millimeter of whole blood. The WBC is elevated (leukocytosis) in a number of conditions of importance to the dentist, including infection, inflammation, leukemia, and tissue destruction. A reduction in the WBC (leukopenia) is seen in aplastic anemia, drug toxicity, and some viral infections. Whereas the WBC supplies valuable information, a differential white blood cell count done simultaneously significantly augments it.

In a conventional differential white blood cell count, a smear of peripheral blood is stained (Fig. 1–3) and the percentage of each type of white cell determined. Current flow cytometry technology permits differential white blood cell counts to be done mechanically. The most common white blood cell is the neutrophil (PMN). It plays an important role in the phagocytosis of bacteria, and the number of PMNs is increased by infection and inflammation. Decreases in neutrophils may be caused by aplastic anemia, cyclic neutropenia, or drug-induced myelosuppression. Lymphocytes are cells that mediate many cellular functions of the immune system. Two major types of lymphocytes have been identified, T cells and B cells. In addition, subpopulations of T cells are known that have both functional and regulatory functions. The numbers and ratios of these cells may be affected in a number of diseases, including HIV infection and viral infections in which lymphocytosis is noted. Monocytosis is relatively unusual and is seen in tuberculosis and subacute bacterial endocarditis. Eosinophils have an undefined role but are affected by diseases that have some involvement with the immune system. An increased number of eosinophils is noted in allergies, parasitic infections, scarlet fever, brucellosis, and a number of hematologic malignant diseases, including Hodgkin's disease and some forms of leukemia. A reduced number

Table 1–5. TESTS RARELY ORDERED BY BUT SIGNIFICANT TO DENTISTS

Enzymes
    Creatinine phosphokinase (CPK)
    Serum glutamic-oxaloacetic
      transaminase (SGOT)
    Serum glutamic-pyruvic
      transaminase (SGPT)
    Lactic dehydrogenase (LDH)

Bilirubin

Reticulocyte count

Creatinine

Blood urea nitrogen

Acid phosphatase

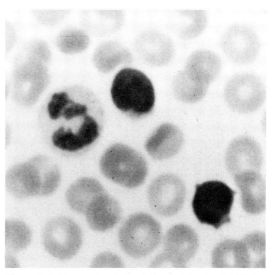

Figure 1–3. Smear of peripheral blood stained with Wright's stain and demonstrating the presence of red blood cells, two lymphocytes, and one polymorphonuclear leukocyte (neutrophil).

of eosinophils is observed in Cushing's syndrome.

Measurements of Clotting Factors. Four laboratory tests can be used to screen patients for potential bleeding disorders, platelet count, bleeding time, prothrombin time (PT), and partial thromboplastin time (PTT). The disorders associated with bleeding dyscrasias are discussed in Chapter 26.

Bleeding problems are the result of too few platelets, abnormal platelet function, or defects in the intrinsic, extrinsic, or common clotting pathways. Thrombocytopenia is easily detected by a platelet count, an estimate of which is usually included in a differential white blood cell count. Platelet function is assessed by the determination of a bleeding time in which small wounds are made on the patient's forearm and the time required for coagulation is measured. Deficiencies in Factors I, II, V, VIII, and X prolong the PT, as does anticoagulant therapy, liver disease, and aspirin. The PTT measures the intrinsic and common pathways and is prolonged by defects in Factors VIII, IX, XI, and XII and in common pathway–required Factors I, II, V, and X. Anticoagulant therapy with heparin also results in an increased PTT.

Tests for Diabetes Mellitus. The dentist may want to rule out diabetes mellitus in a number of situations. Patients at high risk for diabetes mellitus (Chap. 14) should be screened if such a procedure has not been performed within 6 to 12 months. Patients with recurrent oral infections, periodontal disease in excess of observed local factors, or a symptomatic history of polyuria, polyphagia, or polydipsia should be evaluated. Finally, it may be advisable to determine the level of control in patients receiving treatment for diabetes mellitus. A number of laboratory tests are available for such determinations. In addition, diabetics themselves may routinely monitor the adequacy of their treatment.

Patients with diabetes mellitus cannot metabolize a glucose load appropriately. Thus, a reasonable screening test for diabetes is the determination of a fasting blood sugar level.

Occasionally, abnormalities in glucose metabolism can only be uncovered after glucose loading in an oral glucose tolerance test (Chap. 14), in which serial determinations of blood glucose levels are made after the ingestion of 100 g of glucose. In the normal patient, one observes a transient increase in glucose levels, which then return to normal within 2 hours after the loading dose. In the patient

with diabetes, the increased glucose level lingers and is slow to return to baseline levels (Fig. 1–4).

Many patients who are being treated for diabetes mellitus test their urine daily for the presence of glucose. Because the renal threshold for glucose is about 180 mg/dl and may be lowered by pregnancy and other conditions, urine determination of glucose is not a sensitive screening test for the disease. Some tests for urine glucose, in which copper sulfate is reduced (Benedict test, Clinitest strips), also measure other reducing substances such as lactose, galactose, xylose, and fructose. Some glucose-specific methods are available (Clinistix). The test is performed by noting colorimetric changes of a tablet or a dipstick, which is then matched to a standard color chart (Fig. 1–5). Quantitative measurement of blood glucose is now available for patients using a glucometer and has widely replaced colorimetric methods.

Tests for Hepatitis. Although the risk of hepatitis B for dentists and dental staff has been markedly reduced with the advent of vaccine, there are instances in which it is important for dentists to determine the infectivity of patients with a history of the disease. Radioimmunoassays are available for both the viral surface and core antigens. In addition, because vaccination does not confer lifelong immunity, the titer of antibody to the virus might also be a test requested by the dentist.

Tests for Human Immunodeficiency Virus (HIV). As noted in Chapter 47, a number of

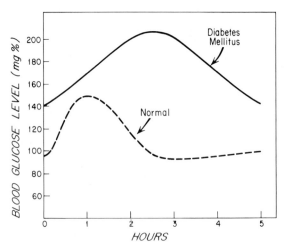

Figure 1–4. Glucose tolerance curve in a normal patient and in a patient with diabetes mellitus. In the normal patient there is a transient increase in blood glucose levels, which then return to normal within 2 hours after the glucose loading dose. In the patient with diabetes mellitus, the increased blood glucose level lingers and is slow to return to baseline levels.

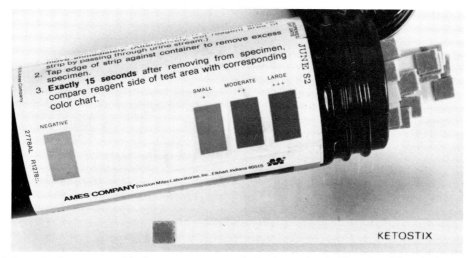

Figure 1–5. Example of test tape used for home measurement of urine ketone levels. The color of the strip is compared to a color chart. Similar strips are available to measure glucose, protein, pH, and blood levels.

oral findings are associated with HIV infection. Often, the dentist is the practitioner who makes the initial diagnosis of HIV infection. Clearly, sensitivity, confidentiality, and access to comprehensive medical care are prerequisites in dealing with the discovery of this infection.

In general, the laboratory diagnosis of HIV infection involves a two-step approach. Initially, the patient's serum is screened for antibodies to the protein components of the virus using an enzyme-linked immunosorbent assay (ELISA). If this test is positive, it is confirmed using a more specific method that detects individual viral proteins. This technique is called the Western blot method.

Before tests for HIV infection are obtained, a written consent is required. If the dentist orders the test, he or she must be prepared to refer the HIV-positive patient to an appropriate physician for treatment.

Tests Occasionally Used by the Dentist

Tests for Disturbances in Bone. Generally, the dentist has radiographic or clinical evidence of some form of bone pathology that prompts the ordering of one of these tests, which are used primarily to diagnose hyperparathyroidism, Paget's disease, metastatic diseases of bone, and disturbances in absorption. The three most common tests are for calcium, phosphorus, and alkaline phosphatase levels.

Increases in serum calcium levels usually result from the mobilization of bone calcium into the blood and are seen in hyperparathyroidism, dietary and absorption disturbances,

metastatic bone disease, and vitamin D toxicity. Decreased calcium levels are associated with hypoparathyroidism, renal failure, and vitamin D deficiency.

Patients with parathyroid dysfunction frequently exhibit changes in phosphorus levels, because one of the major actions of parathyroid hormone is the regulation of phosphate excretion by the kidneys. Rickets may cause low phosphorus levels, as does hyperparathyroidism. Increases in phosphorus levels may be caused by hypoparathyroidism, renal disease, and Cushing's syndrome.

Alkaline phosphatase is an enzyme found in many organs but especially in liver and bone, and diseases of these organs may produce changes in alkaline phosphatase levels. Hyperparathyroidism, Paget's disease, metastases, and obstructive liver disease all produce increases.

Erythrocyte Sedimentation Rate (ESR). The ESR is a nonspecific test for evidence of tissue destruction caused by infection, infarction, trauma, or malignancy. The test measures the rate of sedimentation of red blood cells in a tube of fixed volume, which is prolonged in the conditions noted.

Urinalysis. Urinalysis is performed by examining the gross and microscopic appearance of urine and performing a limited chemical analysis. The test is a routine part of the laboratory workups for patients admitted to hospitals. As a screening test for dental patients in other settings it is of limited value, because other tests offer more specific information.

Data from the urinalysis may provide information with respect to diabetes, liver disease, the state of patient's hydration, hemolytic anemia, and infection. Specific interpretations of urinalysis are found in Summary Table 1–II.

Screening Tests for Syphilis. Although identification of *Treponema pallidum* by darkfield microscopic examination is the only way to diagnosis syphilis definitively, screening tests for dental patients are best performed by serologic testing, which demonstrates the presence of antibodies to the invading organism or to other antibodies called syphilis reagin, which have the capability to combine with lipids. Tests for the former antibodies are more expensive and less accurate than tests for syphilis reagin, which are either flocculation tests or complement fixation tests. Flocculation tests include the VDRL (Venereal Disease Research Laboratories) and RPR (rapid plasma reagin) tests, which are inexpensive and easy to perform. The antigen used is not specific for syphilis reagin; false-positive readings can be produced by malaria, mononucleosis, leprosy, collagen diseases, and immunization with DPT and tetanus. The Wassermann test is the most common complement fixation test.

Tests become positive within 2 to 3 weeks after chancre formation. Before then, the only way to diagnose the disease is by darkfield microscopy. In the secondary stage of the disease (Chap. 30) all tests are positive, with 85% remaining positive subsequently.

Tests Rarely Used by the Dentist

Serum Enzyme Levels. Serum enzyme levels are used mainly as indicators of tissue inflammation and necrosis. Serum glutamic-pyruvic transaminase (SGPT) is specifically associated with the liver and thus is significantly elevated in diseases involving liver cell injury. Serum glutamic-oxaloacetic transaminase (SGOT) is distributed in a variety of tissues, including the brain, liver, and heart, and is elevated by cell death in any of these organs. Like SGOT, lactate dehydrogenase (LDH) is nonspecific in origin. Elevations in this enzyme may signal damage to the heart or liver. However, the electrophoretic separation of LDH into five distinct isoenzymes provides more specific information, because the fastest migrating fraction (LDH_1) is associated with myocardial damage and the slowest migrating fraction (LDH_5) is associated with liver cell necrosis. Creatine phosphokinase (CPK) is another nonspecific intracellular enzyme, which when released because of tissue damage is a helpful clinical indicator. In myocardial injury, it is the first enzyme level to rise.

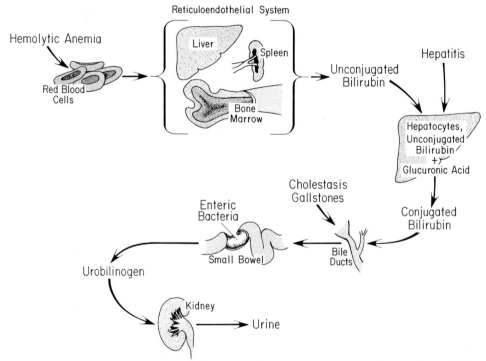

Figure 1–6. Bilirubin metabolism demonstrating the causes of increases in unconjugated or conjugated bilirubin. The increases depend on whether the pathology occurs before or after the conjugation of bilirubin with glucuronic acid in the liver.

From the dentist's perspective, the major importance of serum enzymes is in assessing a patient's liver status following hepatitis or other hepatic diseases.

Bilirubin. Bilirubin is a bile pigment that is derived from erythrocytes as they are broken down in the reticuloendothelial system. Increases in bilirubin levels are responsible for the clinical manifestations of jaundice and may occur as a result of increased formation due to hemolysis, reduced uptake by the liver, decreased formation of conjugated bilirubin (so that it cannot be excreted), and blockage of the excretion of conjugated bilirubin (Fig. 1–6).

Reticulocyte Count. Reticulocytes represent an intermediate stage of red blood cell development between the nucleated forming cell and the non-nucleated mature form. Normally, a small percentage (0.5 to 1.5%) of circulating red blood cells retains staining characteristics associated with this morphologic state. Because of their interim role, reticulo-cytes are a good measure of the number of erythrocytes being put into the circulation. The number is increased when red blood cell production is increased, as in such disorders as the hemolytic anemias.

Blood Tests for Renal Function. Blood tests for renal function determine the levels of urea and creatinine, two substances that are uniquely excreted by the kidney. Of the two, measurements of creatinine are more meaningful, because it is excreted at a fairly constant rate and is not subject to fluctuation.

Creatinine is formed by the breakdown of phosphocreatine and creatine in muscle and body mass. Free creatinine is not neutralized and is excreted by the kidney at a constant rate. Renal failure or impairment increases the level of creatinine.

Blood urea nitrogen (BUN) is one of the nonprotein nitrogenous compounds. Increases in BUN are associated with changes in plasma volume, protein catabolism, hemorrhage, and shock, as well as renal failure. Increases in the BUN level are called azotemia.

SUMMARY TABLE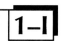

Laboratory Tests and Their Significance

TEST	NORMAL VALUE	SIGNIFICANCE
Complete Blood Count (CBC)		
Hemoglobin (g/dl)	♂, 14–18; ♀, 12–16; newborn, 16–19; children, 11–16	May indicate anemia if reduced, polycythemia if increased
Hematocrit (%)	♂, 40–54; ♀, 37–47; newborn, 49–54; children, 35–49	Reduced in anemia; increased in polycythemia
White blood cell count	5,000–10,000 cells/mm³	Increased in bacterial infection, tissue-destructive disease, and some leukemias; reduced in aplastic anemia, drug-induced myelosuppression, viral infection, and overwhelming bacterial sepsis
Differential White Cell Count		
Neutrophils (polymorphonuclear leukocytes, PMNs)	50–70%	Increased in bacterial infection, steroid therapy, following acute hemorrhage; reduced in aplastic anemia, cyclic neutropenia, cancer chemotherapy, and viral infections
Lymphocytes	30–40%	Increased in certain viral infections, such as mononucleosis
Monocytes	3–7%	Increased in some bacterial infections, such as subacute bacterial endocarditis, tuberculosis, and typhoid fever

Table continued on following page

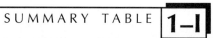
Laboratory Tests and Their Significance

TEST	NORMAL VALUE	SIGNIFICANCE
Differential White Cell Count *(continued)*		
Eosinophils	0–5%	Increased in allergy, parasitic infections, Hodgkin's disease, sarcoidosis, metastatic carcinoma, and chronic skin (autoimmune) diseases
Basophils	0–1%	
Tests for Bleeding Disorders		
Platelet count	150,000–400,000 cells/mm³	See reduction in thrombocytopenia
Bleeding time, Ivy method; template (min)	<4; 3–9	Increased in thrombocytopenia or qualitative platelet disorders, such as prolonged aspirin intake and von Willebrand's disease
Prothrombin time, PT (sec)	11 (Depends on laboratory control. Result expressed as ratio of test/control)	Measures extrinsic and common pathways; prolonged in deficiencies of Factors I, II, VI, VII, and X in anticoagulant therapy and liver disease
Partial thromboplastin time (sec)	35 (depends on laboratory control result expressed as ratio of test to control)	Prolonged with deficiencies in Factors VIII, X, XI, and XII (intrinsic) and in common pathway; also increased in heparin therapy
Other Hematologic Tests		
Red blood cell (RBC) count	4–5 million cells/mm³	Reduced in some anemias; increased in polycythemia
Sedimentation rate (mm/hr)	♂, <10; ♀, <20	Increased in tissue-destructive disorders such as trauma, infections, and malignancies
Mean corpuscular volume, MCV*	82–98 fl	Volume of average red blood cell; reduced in microcytic anemia, increased in macrocytic anemia
Mean corpuscular hemoglobin, MCH†	30 μμg	Hemoglobin (Hgb) content of individual RBC; reduced in microcytic anemia; increased in macrocytic anemia
Mean corpuscular hemoglobin concentration, MCHC‡	35/dl	Average amount of Hgb in 100 ml of packed red blood cells; reduced in hereditary spherocytosis; decreased in microcytic anemia
Blood Chemistry		
Glucose	80–120 mg/dl	Increased in diabetes mellitus, Cushing's disease, acromegaly, stress, and increased epinephrine output; decreased in pancreatic tumors of islet cells, metabolic defects, advanced cirrhosis, hepatitis, and insulin overdose
2 hr postprandial glucose	Normal levels 2 hr after standard glucose load	Increased in diabetes mellitus

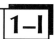

Laboratory Tests and Their Significance

TEST	NORMAL VALUE	SIGNIFICANCE
Blood Chemistry (continued)		
Glucose tolerance test	Periodic sampling for 2 hr after glucose load	Should not exceed twice the fasting level and should return to normal within 2 hr
Calcium	8.5–10.5 mg/dl	Increased in hyperparathyroidism and bone malignancies
Phosphorus	2.5–4.5 mg/dl	Increased in hypoparathyroidism; decreased in hyperparathyroidism, vitamin D deficiency, and malabsorption syndromes
Alkaline phosphatase	1.5–4.5 Bodansky units	Increased in hyperparathyroidism, Paget's disease, hepatic disease, tumors of bone, and osteogenesis imperfecta; reduced in hypophosphatasia, hypothyroidism, and malnutrition
Serum glutamic-oxaloacetic transaminase, SGOT	10–150 mU/ml	Found in brain, liver, heart, skeletal muscle, and pancreas; tissue destruction causes increase, especially in myocardial infarction and hepatitis
Serum glutamic-pyruvic transaminase, SGPT	6–36 mU/ml	Intracellular enzyme of hepatocytes; increased in liver disease (hepatitis)
Lactate dehydrogenase, LDH	90–200 mU/ml	Intracellular enzyme found in many tissues including heart, skeletal muscle, liver, kidney, blood cells, and skin; increased in tissue-destructive diseases
Bilirubin	0.8 mg/dl	Breakdown product of bilirubin; increased in liver disease, increased production, and inability to excrete
Amylase	60–150 Somogyi units/dl	Increased in pancreatic and salivary gland disease and bowel obstruction
Creatinine	0.7–1.4 mg/dl	Increased in kidney failure and breakdown of muscle
Blood urea nitrogen, BUN	10–20 mg/ml	Increased in renal failure; affected by metabolic abnormalities and diet
Creatine phosphokinase, CPK	5–50 I mU/ml	Intracellular enzyme in hair, liver, and heart; increased in myocardial infarction
Screening Tests for Hepatitis		
Hepatitis B surface antibody (anti-HBs)	Normally not present (see comments)	Antibodies to hepatitis B surface antigen are present in individuals who have been successfully immunized for hepatitis B and in individuals who have been clinically exposed to the virus and then develop immunity; the presence of anti-HBs implies that the patient is not infectious

Table continued on following page

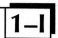
Laboratory Tests and Their Significance

TEST	NORMAL VALUE	SIGNIFICANCE
Blood Chemistry (continued)		
Hepatitis B surface antigen (HBsAg)	Normally not present	Present in patients who are actively infected with hepatitis B or are chronic carriers of the virus
Australia antigen (hepatitis B surface antigen, HBsAg)	Normally not present	Present in patients with active hepatitis B and in patients who are carriers
Screening Tests for Syphilis		
Direct demonstration of *Treponema pallidum* by smear; darkfield microscopy		Present in primary and secondary stages
Flocculation tests—Venereal Disease Research Laboratory test, VDRL		Positive 2–3 wk after chancre formation; 100% positive in secondary stage, 80% in later stages; can yield false-positive results

$$*MCV = \frac{\text{hematocrit (Hct)} \times 10}{RBC}$$

$$\dagger MCH = \frac{\text{hemoglobin (Hgb)} \times 10}{RBC}$$

$$\ddagger MCHC = \frac{Hgb \times 100}{Hct}$$

 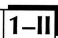
Urinalysis

EXAMINATION	NORMAL	SIGNIFICANCE
Gross Examination		
Color	Yellowish amber	Changes may indicate presence of endogenous (bile, hemoglobin) or exogenous (food, drugs) pigments
Appearance	Clear	Cloudiness may indicate increased protein, white cells, bacteria, red cells, or crystals
Specific gravity	1.003–1.030	Measurement of level of hydration; changes seen in diabetes insipidus (reduced), overhydration (reduced), dehydration (increased), and uncontrolled diabetes mellitus (increased)
Chemical Examination		
pH	4.8–7.5	Measures ability of renal tubules to exchange H^+ for Na^+

Urinalysis

EXAMINATION	NORMAL	SIGNIFICANCE
Chemical Examination (continued)		
Protein	2–8 mg/dl	Proteinuria; may be transient and physiologic as in pregnancy, fever, stress, and exercise; persistent proteinuria may be caused by renal damage or lower urinary tract hemorrhage
Glucose	Threshold, 180 mg/100 ml	Glucose is seen in urine if level exceeds blood threshold, as in diabetes mellitus, Cushing's disease, pheochromocytoma, high glucose intake, stress, and increased intracranial pressure
Ketones	None	Result from incomplete combustion of carbohydrates; are the basis for the presence of insufficient glucose or a reduced ability to use glucose; seen in ketoacidosis caused by diabetes mellitus and in fever, starvation, certain diets, and dehydration
Hemoglobin	None	Hemolysis of red cells, as in hemolytic anemia, renal disease, trauma, and glucose-6-phosphate dehydrogenase deficiency
Bilirubin	None	Liver disease
Bence Jones protein	None	Light chains seen in multiple myeloma (20–50% of patients)
Microscopic Examination		
White blood cells	0–5/hpf*	Urinary tract infection
Red blood cells	0–1/hpf	Renal disease, blood dyscrasia, excessive exertion, and trauma
Epithelial cells		
Renal origin	None	Renal damage
Transitional cells	None	Lower urinary tract damage
Casts (protein material that conforms to anatomy of renal tubules)		Different types; may indicate renal or cardiac disease, infection, shock, or fever
Crystals		Little significance

*High-power field.

Diagnosis of Oral Disease

The diagnosis and management of oral lesions are two of the most challenging and rewarding services a dentist can provide. Although the diagnosis of oral lesions may seem intimidating when one contemplates the myriad lumps, bumps, and sores that dot textbooks of oral pathology, the dentist who develops an organized and systemic approach to these lesions can actually enjoy the process of diagnosis.

Before proceeding, a few facts may help dispel the sense of anxiety and inadequacy that all dentists have felt in dealing with oral lesions. First, there are a finite number of diseases that affect the mouth, and most lesions fall into a small number of diagnostic categories such as white lesions, ulcerations, vesicles, tumors, or pigmented lesions. The others are rare and stump even the most expert diagnostician. Second, almost all oral lesions can be diagnosed by histologic examination; the biopsy is probably the most effective laboratory test leading to diagnosis. Third, there is no sin in being wrong. The only individuals who never make errors in diagnoses are those who never see an oral lesion.

EVALUATION OF ORAL LESIONS

History

As noted in Chapter 1, a complete history is the cornerstone on which the successful diagnostician relies (Fig. 2–1). In some instances, a diagnosis can be made on the basis of a history alone, as in the case of traumatic ulceration or amalgam tattoo. In dealing with oral lesions, there are six elements in the history crucial to an accurate diagnosis—symptoms, type of onset, duration, distribution of lesions, clinical course, and exogenous modifiers.

It is best to let patients describe their symptoms with as little leading or probing as possible. Probably the symptom that most frequently leads a patient to seek professional care is pain. Patients may also complain of swelling, pigmentation, roughness of the mucosa, bleeding, or a variety of other symptoms. It is not uncommon for oral lesions to be asymptomatic and to be noted by the clinician as an incidental finding during routine soft tissue examination.

The nature of onset of oral lesions may be acute or chronic. Lesions with an acute onset are absent one day and present the next. Generally, these lesions are inflammatory and are rarely neoplastic. In contrast, lesions with a chronic onset develop slowly and progress over periods of weeks or months. The duration of the lesion and its clinical course are also important. Is the lesion healing, getting worse, or not changing? Are there signs of systemic involvement, such as fever or lymphadenopathy? All this information should give the diagnostician a reasonable idea of the status of the lesion.

The distribution of lesions is often important in differentiating local from systemic problems. The clinician should ascertain whether skin lesions are present, as well as whether there are any systemic signs associated with the oral lesions (fever, malaise, lymphadenopathy). Oral manifestations of diseases of systemic cause, such as allergy or viral infections, tend to be bilateral, whereas local diseases tend to be unilateral.

Finally, the dentist should determine whether there are exogenous factors that may have caused or modified the oral lesion. Smoking, alcohol intake, drug intake, family members with oral lesions, recent contact with a sick individual, foreign travel, and recent dental care may all be pertinent in the diagnosis of an oral lesion.

Clinical Examination

In clinically evaluating an oral lesion, a complete head and neck examination is critical. It

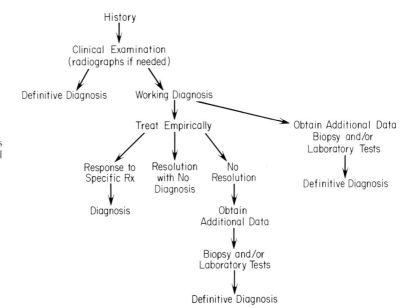

```
                          History
                            ↓
                 Clinical Examination
                 (radiographs if needed)
                    ↙              ↘
     Definitive Diagnosis      Working Diagnosis
                                   ↓        ↘
                            Treat Empirically    Obtain Additional Data
                          ↙      ↓      ↘              Biopsy and/or
               Response to  Resolution   No            Laboratory Tests
               Specific Rx  with No    Resolution           ↓
                    ↓       Diagnosis     ↓          Definitive Diagnosis
               Diagnosis               Obtain
                                    Additional Data
                                         ↓
                                  Biopsy and/or
                                 Laboratory Tests
                                         ↓
                                Definitive Diagnosis
```

Figure 2–1. Possible sequences leading to the diagnosis of an oral lesion.

should be performed at the patient's first visit to the dentist's office and at subsequent recall visits. Although the patient may be aware of one specific area of disease, other areas of the mouth are frequently involved. The clinician who approaches an oral lesion with tunnel vision is at a tremendous disadvantage in gathering a complete clinical picture of the patient's problem. To ensure that no area is overlooked, an orderly approach to examination should be undertaken. In addition to the head and neck examination, the overall appearance of the patient, pulse, blood pressure, and temperature should be observed (Chap. 1).

The examination should be performed in a comfortable environment with adequate lighting. An orderly, step-by-step routine minimizes the chances of forgetting some aspect of the examination. One should consider performing the intraoral phase of the examination before the extraoral phase simply because some patients do not like the "taste" of their skin. Following an examination of the lips, buccal and labial mucosa, and hard and soft palates, the oral pharynx is examined (Fig. 2–2). This is most easily accomplished by having the patient relax the tongue and having the operator pull it forward and then push it down with a tongue blade. Such a technique offers the best view of the oropharynx and minimizes the likelihood of the patient's gagging.

The tongue and floor of the mouth are best examined by grasping the tongue with a 2- × 2-inch gauze sponge and pulling it gently forward, upward and laterally. Both areas should also be palpated bimanually by placing one hand within the mouth while the other hand provides opposing pressure. The salivary glands should be palpated and the ducts observed for clear, copious, painless salivary flow. Breath odor should be noted.

The extraoral examination should include observation of the facial symmetry and of the ears, nose, and eyes. The examiner should note any rashes or lesions. The submental, submandibular, and cervical areas should be palpated for lymphadenopathy. This can be done easily from the front or rear of the patient's head (Fig. 2–3). The thyroid area should be palpated.

After the entire mouth has been examined,

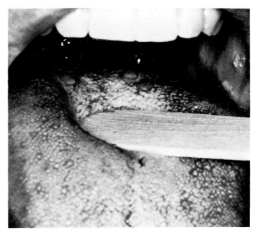

Figure 2–2. Technique for examining the oropharynx. The tongue is gently pulled forward and then pushed down with a tongue blade.

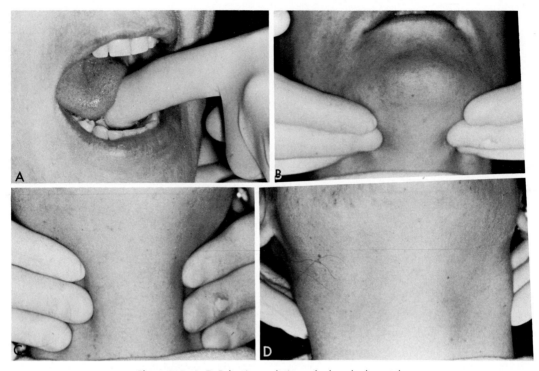

Figure 2–3. *A–D,* Palpation techniques for lymphadenopathy.

a detailed evaluation of the oral lesion may begin. If possible, the tissue should be dried with a 2- × 2-inch sponge. The lesion should be assessed for color, texture, size, consistency, and location. The overall classification of a lesion (e.g., white lesion, ulceration) should be noted. In the case of a white lesion, the ability of a lesion to be scraped from the underlying mucosa is important. If a vesiculobullous lesion is noted, it may also be scraped. All information must be meticulously recorded.

ADJUNCTIVE TECHNIQUES FOR A DIAGNOSIS

Biopsy

Most oral lesions can be definitively diagnosed by histologic examination. This is a requirement in dealing with suspected malignancies. The oral pathologist's expertise is also of value in diagnosing vesiculobullous diseases, specific infections, and white and pigmented lesions. With few exceptions, the biopsy of an oral lesion is a safe, easy, and reliable way to assist in making a definitive diagnosis. The risks of biopsy are minimal and far outweigh the consequences of an incorrect or inadequate diagnosis. Almost all diagnostic biopsies

are technically within the realm of the general dental practitioner, although it may be prudent to refer the patient to a specialist for biopsies of lesions involving the floor of the mouth or the salivary duct.

There are two major types of biopsy—excisional biopsies, in which the lesion is totally removed, and incisional or diagnostic biopsies, in which a segment of the lesion is removed (Fig. 2–4). There has been a great deal of discussion as to whether a suspected malignancy should be excised by an individual other than the one who is prepared to treat the malignancy. In view of this controversy, the safe course is to do an incisional biopsy for any lesions suspected of being malignant and reserve excisional biopsies for small, benign lesions.

The biopsy is a relatively simple procedure. The instruments required include a scalpel handle and blade (no. 15), forceps (a rat-tooth or small Allis forceps is ideal), a needle holder, sutures, and a local anesthetic. The biopsy is performed following the placement of a few drops of local anesthetic at the periphery of the lesion. It is important not to inject directly into the lesion, because this can result in tissue damage and prevent adequate histologic diagnosis. An elliptic or wedge incision is then made that includes both normal and abnormal

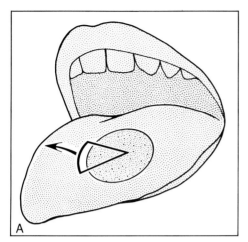
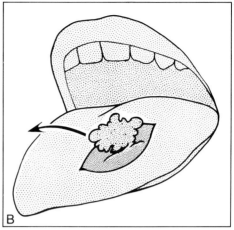

Figure 2–4. Fundamental biopsy techniques applied to an oral lesion. *A,* Incisional biopsy technique. A wedge of the lesion along with a portion of normal tissue is removed. *B,* Excisional technique. The lesion is removed in its entirety.

tissue within the lesion. The biopsy does not have to be exceptionally wide or deep, but the operator must remember that the pathologist needs an adequate amount of tissue. A helpful technique for obtaining an adequate tissue sample is to grasp the tissue with the forceps and then circumscribe the area while under tension. A suture can be used for the same purpose (Fig. 2–5). Once the sample is removed, it is placed in fixative (10% formalin), which is usually supplied by a biopsy service. The sample, along with a description, is then sent for histologic examination.

Hemostasis can be accomplished by direct pressure, suture, or the placement of a periodontal pack. Postoperative infection is rare, and there is generally no need to place the patient on antibiotic coverage unless the medical condition makes it necessary.

Most dental schools provide biopsy services through their departments of oral pathology. Usually, specimen containers and mailers (Fig.

2–6), along with specimen reports (Fig. 2–7), can be obtained at no charge simply by writing to the department. In areas that are not readily accessible to dental schools, the department of pathology at a local hospital can supply containers and solutions for biopsies on request.

Usually, the biopsy report accompanying the specimen is self-explanatory. The clinician should remember that the pathologist's task is much easier if there is an accurate clinical description of the lesion and a concise clinical history, including symptoms, duration, relevant habits (smoking, alcohol intake), location, radiographic appearance, and shape, texture, color, and consistency of the lesion. Also include the time and date of the fixation of the specimen and the age and sex of the patient.

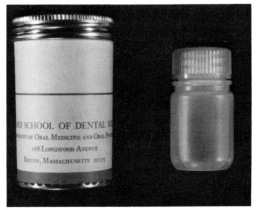

Figure 2–6. Specimen container of 10% formalin and a mailer of the type supplied by departments of oral pathology for the submission of a biopsy.

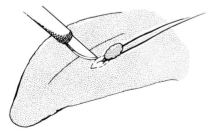

Figure 2–5. Use of a suture to expedite biopsy. The suture is pushed through the lesion and then pulled with gentle tension to raise the area of biopsy.

BIOPSY RECORD AND PATHOLOGICAL REPORT

DEPARTMENT OF ORAL MEDICINE AND ORAL PATHOLOGY

HARVARD SCHOOL OF DENTAL MEDICINE
188 LONGWOOD AVE.
BOSTON, MASSACHUSETTS 02115

(please print)

PATIENT: S—

ADDRESS: FROM:

DATE OF BIRTH: SEX: ADDRESS:

Clinical Record No.:   DATE:

Organ or Tissue Involved:

Clinical Description

1. Location and extent:

2. Color:

3. Size:

4. Shape:

5. Consistency:

6. Texture:

7. Lymphadenopathy:

Duration and Course:

Radiographic Findings:

Pertinent History:

Clinical Impressions:

Submitted by:

Fixation:

Solution:

Date and Time Placed in Fixation

PATIENT: S—

REFERRED BY: Clinical Record No.:

GROSS DESCRIPTION OF SPECIMEN:

MICROSCOPIC DESCRIPTION:

MICROSCOPIC DIAGNOSIS:

COMMENT:

EXAMINED BY:

DATE:

Figure 2–7. Biopsy record and pathologic report, as supplied by departments of oral pathology or commercial laboratories. The practitioner completes the patient identification and clinical description side of the form and submits it with the biopsy specimen. The biopsy service then provides a gross and microscopic description of the specimen and a histologic diagnosis.

Exfoliative Cytology

Cytologic smears are of limited value in the diagnosis of oral lesions. If a lesion is suspicious enough to smear, it should be biopsied. A study by Guinta and colleagues demonstrated a 15% false-negative rate of smears of patients with malignancies proved by biopsy. Histologic examinations were, in contrast, 100% accurate. Cytologic smears can be used in oral diagnosis as a screening device in situations in which many patients are examined over a short period of time, as in health fairs or community cancer screening clinics. The smear may also be helpful in the diagnosis of viral or fungal infections and certain vesiculobullous diseases, such as pemphigus vulgaris, by demonstrating changes in cell morphology, nuclear-cytoplasmic ratio, or the presence of infecting organisms.

The technique for performing a smear is simple (Fig. 2–8). The lesion is stroked gently but firmly with the tip of a wet wooden tongue blade. The cellular debris is spread evenly on a glass microscope slide and placed in a fixa-tive of alcohol and ether. If it is anticipated that many smears are to be performed, a spray-type fixative may be used. Hair spray may be substituted for commercial fixative sprays. The smear is sent to a laboratory with the appropriate clinical information for interpretation.

Immunofluorescence

Immunofluorescence testing, using sera or biopsies, may play a significant role in the diagnosis and assessment of autoimmune diseases, including pemphigus vulgaris, pemphigoid, systemic lupus erythematosus, and lichen planus. These tests are frequently an important adjunct to histologic studies of tissue. Immunofluorescence testing demonstrates diseases in which antitissue antibodies are suspected. Coombs first demonstrated that fluorescent dyes could be coupled to antibodies without destroying their specificity. Therefore, if conjugates of antibody and fluorescein are reacted with tissue that contains antigen with which the antibody reacted, the complex can

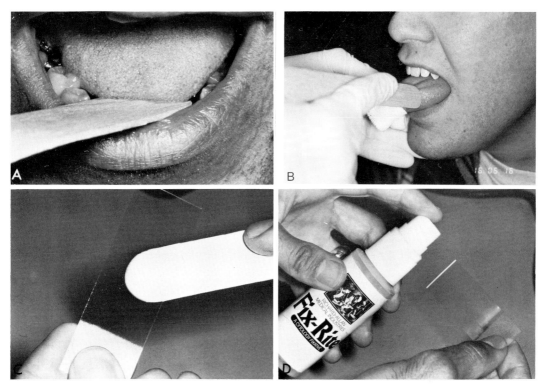

Figure 2–8. Technique for obtaining a smear for cytologic analysis of an oral lesion. The tongue blade is placed under the tongue *(A)* to moisten it and then stroked firmly over the lesion *(B)*. Cellular debris is spread evenly on a glass microscope slide *(C)*, which is then placed in or sprayed with a fixative *(D)*.

be visualized with the use of an ultraviolet microscope. Immunofluorescence techniques are of two types, direct and indirect (Fig. 2–9).

Direct Test. In the direct test, the antibody is conjugated with fluorescein and applied directly to the tissue substrate. For example, in tests for pemphigus or pemphigoid, IgG isolated from the patient's serum is labeled with fluorescein and incubated with a biopsy specimen of the patient's oral mucosa. In pemphigus, the fluorescence is found in the intercellular spaces of the stratified squamous epithelium. In pemphigoid, the fluorescence is seen at the basement membrane zone between the epithelium and the connective tissue. In both these diseases, the autoantibodies localize at the major sites of pathology—the intercellular cement or desmosomal spaces of epithelium in pemphigus and the basal lamina in pemphigoid.

Indirect Test. Indirect immunofluorescence is used to test for the presence of antitissue antibody in a tissue sample. The test is performed by reacting the patient's tissue (thought to contain antitissue antibody) with

animal antihuman antibody. The antihuman antibody is conjugated with fluorescein and is usually produced in goats or rabbits by immunization with human immunoglobulin. Thus, the antihuman antibody binds to any human immunoglobulin present in the tissue sample with which it is reacted. As with other forms of immunofluorescence, the reaction is observed microscopically. Because the antihuman antibody used in the test reacts with multiple antigenic sites on the human immunoglobulin, indirect immunofluorescence often highlights the presence of antibody tissue.

A variation of the indirect test is sometimes used. The oral mucosa of a rhesus monkey, or the oral or esophageal mucosa of some other animal species, is incubated with the patient's serum to attach the antibodies to the animal tissue specimen. The tissue is then incubated with fluoresceinated rabbit or goat antihuman IgG serum. The indirect test is not as reliable as the direct test for the demonstration of antibodies in cases of pemphigus or pemphigoid, when lesions are limited to the oral cavity. It may be postulated that the antibody levels in some of these cases of localized disease are not

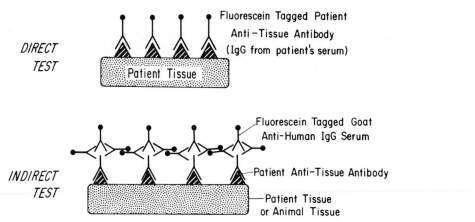

Figure 2–9. Immunofluorescence tests. (From Shaw, J. H., Sweeney, E. A., Cappuccino, C. C., and Meller, S. M. (eds.): Textbook of Oral Biology. Philadelphia, W. B. Saunders, 1978.)

sufficiently high for adequate demonstration by indirect techniques, in which the antibody must first be attached to animal mucosal tissue. One advantage of this technique is its ease, because a single fluoresceinated reagent (the anti-immunoglobulin) can be used to screen many sera. Immunofluorescence has been used in systemic lupus erythematosus to demonstrate autoantinuclear antibodies (ANAs) reacting to nuclear components in cells close to the basement membrane zone. Indirect immunofluorescence has also been used to demonstrate specific antibodies in Sjögren's syndrome, in which antibodies react with salivary gland excretory duct antigens but not with acinar antigens.

Logistics of Immunofluorescence Testing

There are currently available a number of immunofluorescence testing services that the dentist can use. These services provide, at no charge, containers for biopsies of mucosa to be sent for immunofluorescence testing and containers for serum. Both these materials can be sent by mail and require no special handling procedures. Mailing containers for serum specimens, kits with tubes for serum samples, containers for holding solution for immunofluorescence studies of biopsies, and tubes of fixative for routine hematoxylin and eosin histologic studies are available to the dentist at no cost. Serum samples are obtained from whole blood; the patient should go to a commercial laboratory or hospital and have the blood drawn, and the serum obtained and mailed directly. Biopsy specimens obtained in the usual fashion can be placed in fixative and sent directly to the laboratory.

DIAGNOSIS OF LESIONS

The diagnostic process is simply the result of an orderly series of decisions based on clinical, historical, and laboratory data. Although there are many diseases that affect the oral cavity they can, fortunately, be divided into a relatively small number of categories based on their gross morphologic appearance. The five major categories of lesions affecting the soft tissues of the mouth are white lesions, ulcers, vesiculobullous lesions, pigmented lesions, and raised lesions.

White lesions on the oral mucosa arise as a consequence of surface necrosis or hyperkeratosis (Chap. 36). The simplest way to differentiate the two clinically is to scrape the lesion with a moist tongue blade. Whereas necrotic lesions are removed by scraping, usually leaving a raw, bleeding surface, keratotic lesions are undisturbed by such manipulation. In general, necrotic lesions tend to be more symptomatic than hyperkeratotic areas.

Necrotic white lesions are a result of trauma or infection. Chemical or electrical burns are frequent examples of the former. It is not uncommon to see mucosal burns in the ill-informed patient who has tried to palliate a painful tooth topically with aspirin (Fig. 2–10). Candidiasis is the most common oral infection producing white surface necrosis (Fig. 2–11). These lesions readily scrape off. If the scraped debris is placed on a slide and observed microscopically, the offending organism can be identified.

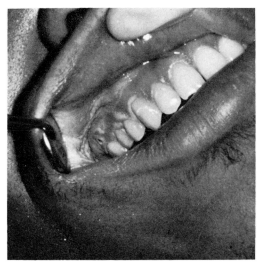

Figure 2–10. Mucosal burn in a patient who tried to treat a painful tooth topically with aspirin.

Keratotic lesions of the oral mucosa may result from chronic irritation, systemic disease, hereditary conditions, or carcinoma. Frequently, these lesions appear as confluent raised plaques (Fig. 2–12) or as collections of papules (Fig. 2–13). Because 10% of hyperkeratotic lesions are malignant or premalignant, biopsy should be considered for any persistent white lesion that cannot be scraped from the oral mucosa.

Ulcers of the oral mucosa are frequent and may result from trauma or a number of local or systemic disorders (Chap. 35). Ulcers associated with underlying pathology, such as aphthae or carcinomas, are usually circular breaks in the mucosa with smooth or raised

(indurated) borders (Fig. 2–14). The floor of the lesion may be composed of whitish or yellowish necrotic material. Because of the varied causes of nontraumatic ulcers, biopsy is mandatory in any lesion that fails to heal spontaneously within 14 days of onset. In contrast, ulcers that are traumatic in origin usually follow the shape of the source of the trauma and may therefore be linear.

Vesiculobullous lesions result from a collection of fluid beneath the epithelial surface that forms a blister (Fig. 2–15). Vesicles and bullae are distinguished by size, with bullae being 5 mm or larger. The clinician does not often observe intact vesicles, because they frequently rupture before the patient presents for diagnosis, leaving ulcerative or erosive lesions with ragged borders.

Vesiculobullous lesions are most frequently the result of viral infections in which crop-like vesicular eruptions are observed (Chap. 48). The diagnosis of viral diseases can usually be made on the basis of the history, symptomatology, and clinical appearance. Cytologic smears of lesions may be helpful in identifying cellular changes consistent with viral infection. Serologic tests for antiviral antibodies may be of use in retrospectively establishing the fact that the patient had a specific viral infection. For example, if one obtains a serum sample when a patient is symptomatic for what is suspected to be a herpes simplex infection and there is no evidence of neutralizing antibody, and a subsequent sample taken 6 weeks later demonstrates antibody, the diagnosis is confirmed.

Autoimmune diseases and drug eruptions account for the remainder of the vesiculobul-

Figure 2–11. Oral candidiasis.

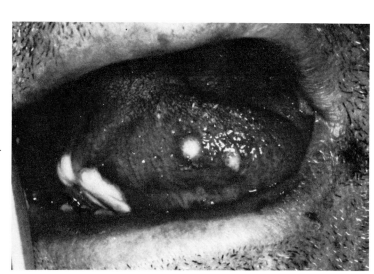

Plaque

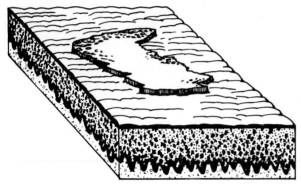

Figure 2–12. Configuration of an oral keratotic plaque.

Papules

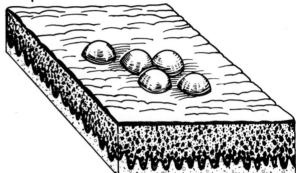

Figure 2–13. Configuration of a papillary oral lesion.

Ulcer

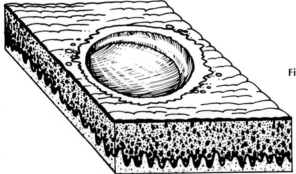

Figure 2–14. Configuration of a mucosal ulcer.

Bulla

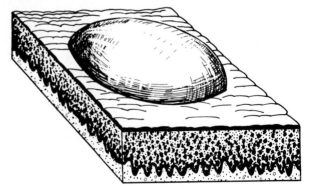

Figure 2–15. Configuration of a vesiculobullous lesion.

lous diseases seen in the mouth (Chaps. 37 and 48). In these diseases biopsy and, at times, immunofluorescence testing are required for definitive diagnosis. Cytologic smears of cells at the base of a vesicle or bulla may provide evidence suggestive of a specific diagnosis.

Pigmented areas in the mouth may result from endogenous or exogenous pigmentation and may be diffuse or localized (Chap. 38). They are generally not raised and may present a color different from that of normal oral mucosa. This type of lesion is often the first sign of systemic illness, such as Addison's disease.

Diagnosis is based on the history, clinical examination, biopsy, and laboratory tests.

There are many raised lesions affecting the mouth. Although most are benign, a number are not. Hence, biopsy is mandatory. Although clinical diagnosis may be highly suggestive, a definitive diagnosis requires microscopic tissue examination (Chaps. 40 and 41).

This discussion is meant only as an introduction to help the reader in categorizing lesions for diagnosis. More information on specific lesions, diagnosis, and treatment is to be found in subsequent chapters.

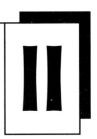
Evaluation and Management of the Patient with Cardiovascular Disease

Atherosclerosis

Atherosclerosis is a disease of unknown origin, but it represents the most common pathophysiologic cause for cardiovascular, cerebrovascular, and peripheral vascular diseases. These diseases account for more than 50% of all deaths in the United States.

At the tissue level, atherosclerosis is caused by an abnormal accumulation of lipids on the walls of the arteries. These accumulations, or atherosclerotic plaques, are raised lesions that encroach on the vascular lumen (Fig. 3–1). As the vessel narrows, the distal blood supply is compromised and oxygen deprivation or ischemia results. The plaques are subject to fibrosis, calcification, internal hemorrhage, and ulceration, and they act as seeding areas for thrombosis or local blood clot formation. The resultant thrombosis may completely obstruct the vessel, causing a distal infarction of the related organ systems. Thrombi may also produce circulating blood clots, or emboli, which can cause infarctions in other parts of the body. Atherosclerotic changes may weaken the arterial wall, creating a bulge, or aneurysm, that can rupture and cause hemorrhage into the tissues or, when major arteries such as the aorta are involved, even death. Atherosclerotic changes of vessels supplying the brain lead to transient cerebral ischemic attacks and strokes. Atherosclerosis of the smaller arteries of the extremities results in peripheral vascular occlusion and can manifest clinically as severe muscle cramping or intermittent claudication (Fig. 3–2).

The most important vessels affected by atherosclerosis are the coronary arteries (Fig. 3–3). It is evident that most men and many women above the age of 50 in the United States have moderately advanced coronary atherosclerosis, even though they have no symptoms. After a variable presymptomatic period of atherosclerosis, various clinical manifestations of atherosclerotic heart disease may appear, such as angina pectoris, acute myocardial infarction, arrhythmia, heart failure, or sudden death. When a coronary artery is sufficiently narrow, the resultant ischemia of the heart muscle may produce angina pectoris (Chap. 5) with symptoms of chest pressure, tightness, or pain. When the narrowing progresses to occlusion, myocardial infarction or death of heart muscle may result (Chap. 6). Ischemia to the heart muscle can also affect the normal function of the conduction pathways in the heart and lead to abnormalities in heart rhythm, called arrhythmias (Chaps. 9 and 10). Arrhythmias can progress to a stage of cardiac arrest in which the heart stops functioning and sudden death ensues. Another sequela of progressive myocardial injury and damage is heart failure as a result of inadequate myocardial function (Chap. 6). Atherosclerosis is, therefore, a major cause of morbidity and mortality in patients above the age of 50.

DENTAL EVALUATION

For the dentist, the importance of detailed evaluation of patients with histories of angina pectoris, myocardial infarction, heart failure, arrhythmia, or stroke is obvious. Equally important, however, is the recognition by the dentist that some patients may be at high risk for atherosclerosis. Although these patients may be asymptomatic at presentation, symptoms can develop while they are under the care of the dentist and complicate dental management. One must, therefore, be aware of the risk factors believed to contribute to atherosclerosis.

One study showed that 75% of soldiers in their early twenties killed in action demonstrated pathologic evidence of atherosclerosis at autopsy. However, clinically important disease usually occurs later in life. For the dentist, the population of concern consists of men over the age of 50 and postmenopausal women. The presence of certain risk factors in this group of patients should alert the dentist to possible problems with atherosclerosis that may complicate dental therapy.

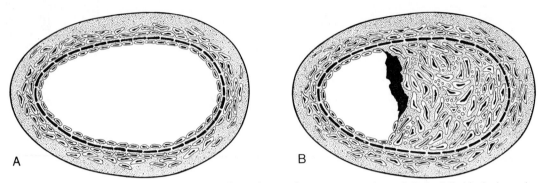

A   B

Figure 3–1. Occlusion of vascular lumen with atherosclerotic plaques. *A,* Normal vessel. *B,* Partially blocked vessel.

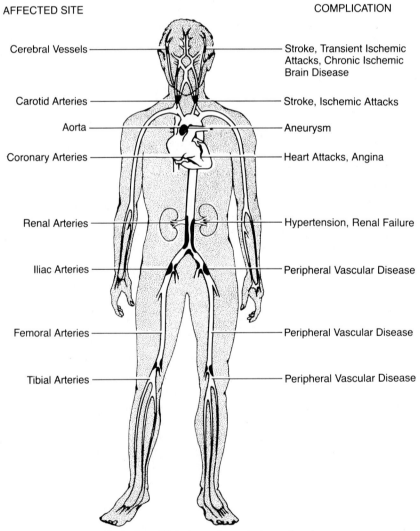

AFFECTED SITE

COMPLICATION

Cerebral Vessels —— Stroke, Transient Ischemic Attacks, Chronic Ischemic Brain Disease

Carotid Arteries —— Stroke, Ischemic Attacks

Aorta —— Aneurysm

Coronary Arteries —— Heart Attacks, Angina

Renal Arteries —— Hypertension, Renal Failure

Iliac Arteries —— Peripheral Vascular Disease

Femoral Arteries —— Peripheral Vascular Disease

Tibial Arteries —— Peripheral Vascular Disease

Figure 3–2. Clinical correlates of atherosclerosis.

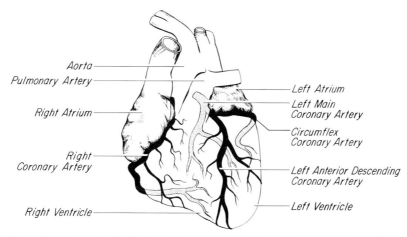

Figure 3–3. Anatomic distribution of the coronary arteries and the anatomy of the heart.

Some risk factors are definitely associated with the development of coronary heart disease, peripheral vascular disease, and cerebral vascular disease. These include hypertension, cigarette smoking, and high concentration of blood cholesterol, particularly low-density lipoproteins. Other risk factors—including diabetes mellitus, impaired glucose tolerance, stress, family history, genetic factors, postmenopausal state, and the use of contraceptive pills—are thought to be important, but their associations with atherosclerosis have not been so convincingly demonstrated. The association of obesity and physical inactivity with atherosclerosis is uncertain.

Over 75% of patients who die suddenly with no previous symptomatic heart disease have a history of two or more of the following four risk factors: hypertension, cigarette smoking, hypercholesterolemia, and diabetes mellitus. Therefore, all patients in the target population (men above the age of 50 and postmenopausal women) should be asked about a history of these and other risk factors, including a family history of atherosclerotic heart disease. In the female patient, the use of contraceptive pills and the state of the menses should be noted. On inspection, weight problems should be noted. On examination, the blood pressure and pulse rate should be recorded. This rapid assessment should provide reasonable guidelines for dental management.

DENTAL MANAGEMENT

A patient with multiple risk factors should have had a medical evaluation within the past 18 months, including a physical examination and an electrocardiogram, to rule out clini-

cally silent atherosclerotic disease. Patients with risk factors such as smoking or obesity who have not had a recent medical evaluation can have nonsurgical dental procedures (types I, II, and III) and simple surgical procedures (type IV) carried out using normal dental operating procedures, but more advanced surgical procedures (types V and VI) should be deferred until after medical evaluation. However, *a number of risk factors, such as diabetes and hypertension, carry specific dental procedural recommendations (Chaps. 4 and 14).*

ORAL FINDINGS

There are no specific intraoral findings related to atherosclerosis. There are, however, findings related to certain of the risk factors contributing to atherosclerosis (e.g., diabetes mellitus). These are discussed in detail in subsequent chapters.

■ Examples of Dental Evaluation and Management

EVALUATION

Four patients present for treatment who have no past medical history of ischemic heart disease. All have a history of multiple high-risk factors for atherosclerosis. All have normal blood pressures at initial examination. All are in the target population of men over 50 years of age or postmenopausal women.

Patient 1. The patient smokes two packs of cigarettes a day and is overweight. She has a 3-

year history of hypertension controlled by HydroDIURIL (hydrochlorothiazide, a diuretic). Her last physical examination was 6 months ago. Her dental needs include generally advanced operative, nonsurgical procedures (type III).

Patient 2. The patient has a past medical history identical to that of Patient 1. His dental needs, however, are far more extensive, requiring significant operative and prosthetic dentistry (type III), minor to moderate periodontal surgical procedures (types IV and V), and possible extensive surgical procedures (type VI).

Patient 3. The patient smokes two packs of cigarettes each day and is overweight. He has a history of diabetes and is taking oral agents for hyperglycemia. His last physical examination was over 2 years ago. He requires the same extensive dental procedures (types III through VI) required by Patient 2.

Patient 4. The patient smokes two packs of cigarettes each day and is overweight. He has mild hypertension, currently under control by HydroDIURIL. His last physical examination was over 2 years ago. He presents with asymmetric facial swelling, with progressive pain over the last 24 hours. On examination, he has a temperature of 100° F and a nonrestorable maxillary molar.

MANAGEMENT

Patient 1. The patient's smoking, hypertension, and obesity are high-risk factors for atherosclerosis. Her medical evaluation is recent, and her blood pressure is under excellent control. Her dental requirements are all nonsurgical. Normal operative procedures are appropriate for her dental management.

Patient 2. The patient has the same risk factors as Patient 1, but his dental needs include moderate surgical procedures (type V). The patient has had a normal recent medical evaluation. Therefore, normal dental protocol with appropriate adjunctive sedation techniques would be appropriate (Chap. 51).

Patient 3. The patient has the same risk factors as Patients 1 and 2, with the addition of diabetes. He has not had a recent physical examination, and he requires extensive nonsurgical and surgical dental therapy. For these reasons, the patient should be referred to his physician for a medical evaluation. An unremarkable medical evaluation would allow the dentist to treat Patient 3 as he would Patient 2, using normal protocol. On the other hand, previously undiagnosed ischemic heart disease that requires specific dental management (e.g., arrhythmia) may be discovered. The dentist, therefore, should defer the more advanced procedures (types V and VI) until after the medical evaluation.

Patient 4. This patient has multiple risk factors for atherosclerosis, but his dental needs are of an emergent nature, and he requires attention to a nonrestorable maxillary molar. The physical examination revealed normal blood pressure and, despite the fact that he has not seen a physician for the past 2 years, the extraction (type IV procedure) can be performed.

SUMMARY TABLE **3–1**

Atherosclerosis: General Information

DEFINITION
Atherosclerosis is a disease of blood vessels involving the abnormal accumulation of lipids on the walls of the arteries.

CAUSE
The cause is unknown.

IMPACT
Accumulations of "atheromatous plaques" encroach on the vascular lumen, limiting the blood flow to the affected organs. The atheromatous plaques also act as a potential site for thrombosis (blood clot formation) and embolism.

CLINICAL MANIFESTATIONS
1. Arteriosclerotic heart disease (ASHD)
2. Cerebrovascular disease
3. Peripheral vascular disease

Ischemic Heart Disease*

DEFINITION

Ischemic heart disease refers to those cardiac diseases resulting from an imbalance of limited myocardial oxygen supply and excessive oxygen demand.

CAUSE

It is caused by arteriosclerotic constriction of the coronary arteries (ASHD, arteriosclerotic heart disease).

CLINICAL ENTITIES (See specific chapters)

1. Angina
2. Myocardial infarction
3. Arrhythmias
4. Congestive heart failure
5. Sudden death

CLINICAL IMPLICATIONS

All ischemic heart disease implies advanced atherosclerosis and a higher risk of mortality.

*Coronary heart disease.

Asymptomatic Ischemic Heart Disease (Suspected ASHD)

DEFINITION

Asymptomatic ischemic heart disease refers to arteriosclerotic heart disease (ASHD) suspected in patients in the target population (men over 50 and postmenopausal women) because of the presence of multiple risk factors. (See Summary Table 3–IV)

CLINICAL IMPORTANCE

1. Dental patients in the target age population with multiple high-risk ASHD factors are those patients most likely to develop symptomatic ischemic heart disease (angina, myocardial infarction, arrhythmias, congestive heart failure) while under the dentist's care.
2. More than 75% of patients who die suddenly from ischemic heart disease have two or more of the four high-risk factors (hypertension, diabetes mellitus, smoking, hypercholesterolemia).

Risk Factors for Developing Atherosclerosis*

ESTABLISHED RISK FACTORS

Hyperlipidemia

Hypertension

Cigarette smoking

PROBABLE RISK FACTORS

Diabetes

Stress

Family history

Postmenopausal state

Contraceptive pills

SUSPECTED RISK FACTORS

Obesity

Sedentary life style

*As defined by the National Heart and Lung Institute Task Force on Arteriosclerosis.

Dental Evaluation of and Approach to the Patient with Asymptomatic ASHD (Suspected ASHD)

1. Identify the target population—men over 50 years and postmenopausal women.
2. Determine the date of the patient's last comprehensive medical physical examination.
3. Determine the history of multiple risk factors contributing to ASHD.
4. Record the blood pressure and pulse at the initial visit.
5. The patient in the target population with multiple high-risk factors should be suspected of having clinically silent atherosclerosis. This tentative diagnosis has dental implications if moderate to advanced dental surgical procedures (types V and VI) are planned.

Dental Management of the Patient with Asymptomatic ASHD (Suspected ASHD)

GENERAL PRINCIPLES

If there is a positive history of high-risk factors for ASHD in an asymptomatic individual in the target population,

1. A recent comprehensive medical physical examination is advisable.
2. Physician examination and consultation are recommended prior to advanced dental surgical procedures (types V and VI).*

Presumed ASHD Asymptomatic	*Dental Procedures*	*Management**
1. Multiple risk factors	I–V	Normal protocol
Medical evaluation within 18 months	VI	Physician consultation and clearance, sedation techniques (Chap. 51)
2. Multiple risk factors	I–IV	Normal protocol
No recent medical evaluation	V–VI	Refer to physician for evaluation and clearance, sedation techniques

*Note that certain risk factors, such as diabetes and hypertension, require specific dental management considerations (see appropriate chapters).

Hypertension

Hypertension is the abnormal elevation of the resting arterial systolic blood pressure above 140 mm Hg and/or the elevation of the diastolic blood pressure above 90 mm Hg. Approximately 10 to 20% of the dentist's adult population is affected by the disease. Although more emphasis is sometimes placed on diastolic elevations, systolic hypertension has been shown to be a significant risk factor for subsequent cardiovascular complications. A 35-year-old with an untreated blood pressure of 150/100 can expect a life span that is 17 years shorter than the general average.

Hypertension adversely affects the host by accelerating atherosclerosis. Epidemiologic studies have demonstrated that untreated moderate hypertension is associated with increased morbidity and mortality from cerebrovascular disease, peripheral vascular disease, renal disease, and cardiovascular disease (Chap. 3). Prospective studies have also shown that the control of hypertension is effective in the prevention of cerebrovascular accidents, congestive heart failure and, to a lesser extent, coronary atherosclerosis. Controversy has surrounded the therapy for mild hypertension, but evidence is accumulating that untreated mild hypertension is also associated with progressive end-organ compromises. Because hypertension is usually asymptomatic, routine screening is important in the detection of the disease and in the prevention of its long-term sequelae.

Physiologically, arterial blood pressure is a function of cardiac output, intravascular fluid volume, and the resistance of the peripheral vasculature. Of patients with hypertension, 90% have essential (primary or idiopathic) hypertension. Simply stated, this diagnosis implies an unknown cause for the disruption of the balance of the above three physiologic variables. The remaining 10% of patients have secondary hypertension, which is most often the result of primary renal disease, although renovascular disease and adrenal gland lesions (e.g., Cushing's disease, primary aldosteronism, and pheochromocytoma) may also contribute to this condition. Whereas some forms of secondary hypertension can be surgically approached and cured, management of essential hypertension requires long-term use of medications that may affect dental therapy.

MEDICAL EVALUATION AND MANAGEMENT

The physician's evaluation of a patient with hypertension starts with a detailed history and physical examination. Laboratory evaluation usually includes a hemogram, urinalysis, serum potassium and blood urea nitrogen (BUN) determinations, a chest x-ray, and an electrocardiogram. When clinically indicated, other diagnostic procedures such as an intravenous pyelogram and special blood and urinary tests (e.g., plasma renin activity, urinary metanephrine, 17-hydroxysteroids, 17-ketosteroids) may also be performed. These tests are important in ruling out the 10% of cases with known cause (secondary hypertension).

Antihypertensive drugs are the most important means of therapy. All other measures should be considered ancillary. It is preferable to emphasize the role of antihypertensive drugs and to interfere as little as possible with the patient's lifestyle. Undue emphasis on diet, salt restriction, and smoking to the exclusion of drug treatment is probably unwarranted.

Patients with mild hypertension are usually managed with a single drug, and many drugs are regarded as reasonable first-line medications for the management of hypertension. Diuretics (Summary Table 4–III) are still used frequently but are less popular because of concerns over side effects, which range from volume depletion and hypokalemia to a mild degree of hyperlipidemia. Beta blockers (Summary Table 4–III) are also reasonable first-line drugs, but may also raise serum lipid levels slightly. Converting enzyme inhibitors (Summary Table 4–III) are now used as first-line medications with increasing frequency. These drugs are effective and have few side effects (Summary Table 4–IV). Calcium channel blockers (Summary Table 4–III) are effective antihypertensive agents with few side effects. In general, medications are started at a low dose, which is increased according to the level of blood pressure control.

Patients with moderate hypertension often require a combination of drugs to obtain adequate control. Diuretics can be added to converting enzyme inhibitors or calcium channel blockers to augment their effectiveness. If diuretics are to be avoided, converting enzyme inhibitors in combination with calcium channel blockers are effective. Beta blockers in combination with vasodilators such as hydralazine or prazosin are also effective.

Alpha blockers such as methyldopa (Summary Table 4–III) are less frequently used because of side effects such as sedation, depression, and impotence. However, an alpha- and beta-blocking agent, labetalol (Summary Table 4–III), is gaining popularity and appears to be effective, with fewer side effects than the alpha- or beta-blocking agent alone.

Clonidine is a central-acting alpha-adrenergic drug that is effective in blood pressure control. Clonidine, however, can cause xerostomia and can therefore aggravate periodontal conditions. More importantly, clonidine cannot be withdrawn abruptly, because severe rebound hypertension has been reported.

Patients with severe hypertension may require multiple drugs for control. Potent diuretics (Summary Table 4–III) are often added to other medications. Minoxidil (Summary Table 4–III) is a potent vasodilator usually reserved for patients with severe hypertension. The drug is often used in combination with a diuretic, because it causes fluid retention. Ganglionic blockers (Summary Table 4–III) are infrequently used because of their side effects (Summary Table 4–IV).

A number of symptomatic side effects such as dehydration, orthostatic hypotension, sedation, impotence, xerostomia, and depression are associated with some of the medications commonly prescribed for hypertension. The physician's choice of drug combination and dosage must therefore strike a delicate balance between effectiveness in controlling blood pressure and side effects that may adversely affect patient compliance. Ideal blood pressure control requires long-term interaction between a concerned physician and a cooperative patient.

DENTAL EVALUATION

Dentists should play a major role in the detection of hypertension, because they routinely see patients for multiple visits and semiannual checkups. Monitoring a patient's blood pressure is an easy task and an important aspect of comprehensive dental-medical care, because patients with hypertension are often asymptomatic (Chap. 1).

In addition to playing a critical role in the screening process for hypertension, the dentist should also know how hypertension can complicate dental therapy. Poorly controlled hypertension may acutely elevate blood pressure during stressful situations and precipitate angina, congestive heart failure or, rarely, a cerebrovascular event (e.g., stroke, hemorrhage). Careful attention to the blood pressure prior to dental procedures minimizes the risk of developing these problems.

A dentist can assess the severity of a patient's hypertension by means of a medical history, a physical examination, and consultation with the patient's physician. Patients often record a history of hypertension in the dentist's medical questionnaire. The dentist should then determine the time of the diagnosis, past and present treatment (Summary Table 4–III), and complications (Summary Table 4–I). Most importantly, the dentist should ask about the types and dosages of current medications and especially note recent changes in regimen.

A list of the patient's medications can provide some idea of the severity of the patient's hypertension and can alert the dentist to the possible side effects that may complicate dental therapy (Summary Table 4–IV). Patients on diuretics may have significant volume depletion and mild orthostatic changes in blood pressure. Diuretics can also lead to a decreased serum potassium level, which is usually asymptomatic but may aggravate arrhythmias in patients with underlying heart diseases (Chap. 9). Patients on potent vasodilators such as hydralazine, prazosin, minoxidil, or guanethidine may have significant orthostatic changes in their blood pressure. A patient who is brought from a supine to an upright position may feel light-headed and dizzy and actually faint. It is therefore important to monitor the patient's blood pressure in a supine position and avoid abrupt positional changes. Patients should be instructed to sit up slowly and to dangle their legs before assuming an upright position after dental procedures. Some patients on propranolol may develop congestive heart failure or wheezing. A withdrawal syndrome following the sudden cessation of therapy with clonidine has occasionally been reported. Headache, palpitations, sweating, and a rise in blood pressure may develop after the last dose. Patients requiring large dosages of clonidine (e.g., greater than 0.6 mg daily) for blood pressure control may have to have other antihypertensive drugs substituted if they undergo extensive dental surgical treatment (e.g., type VI procedures in a hospital setting) and are not expected to be able to take oral medications for longer than 24 hours.

During the initial examination in the dentist's office, each new patient should have the blood pressure recorded (Chap. 1). All recordings in excess of 140/90 (systolic or diastolic or both) should be repeated at subsequent visits. If the patient's pressure is below 140/90, a yearly repeat determination should suffice. The patient diagnosed as having hypertension should have frequent repeat determinations. The anxiety of being examined in a dental office can account for a temporary elevation of blood pressure in an otherwise normal individual. However, repeated measurements in excess of 150/100 in any patient warrant referral to the patient's physician for evaluation.

The following categories are reasonable guidelines for the dentist:

Normal	120/80 mm Hg
Controlled	Up to 140/up to 90
Mild hypertension	140–160/90–105
Moderate hypertension	160–170/105–115
Severe hypertension	170–190/115–125
Malignant hypertension	Severe hypertension (often 190+/125+) associated with central nervous system symptoms such as blurring of vision, headache, or changes in mental status.

From the standpoint of dental management, certain guidelines can be established according to the degree of control of hypertension.

DENTAL MANAGEMENT

Once the severity of hypertension is established, the dentist may formulate the dental treatment plan (Fig. 4–1). There is no substitute for proper long-term medical management. Without proper control, ideal dental treatment planning may be compromised.

The control of anxiety is an important therapeutic adjunct in the management of the hypertensive dental patient. Patient rapport is therefore crucial. As the difficulty of dental procedures increases, so does the patient's anxiety level. Certain patients may be especially anxious, and a transient increase in blood pressure may occur in the dental office. The dentist should repeat blood pressure recordings before performing anxiety-inducing dental procedures to better assess the patient's status at the time of the appointment. Additional blood pressure measurements may assist in assessing the patient's response to stressful treatment. Poorly controlled hypertension may require rescheduling of dental procedures or necessitate the use of adjunctive sedation techniques.

After due consideration of the effect of the individual's anxiety on the specific dental procedure planned, the following guidelines should be observed.

Controlled or Mild Hypertension. The patient with controlled or mild hypertension can tolerate all nonsurgical and simple surgical procedures (types I–IV) using normal operative protocol. Multiple extractions or quadrant or full-arch periodontal and oral surgery (types V and VI procedures) may require the use of various sedation techniques (Chap. 51), including N_2O-O_2 inhalation analgesia or additional augmentation by oral sedatives or tranquilizers such as diazepam (Valium) some time prior to the appointment.

Moderate Hypertension. The patient with undiagnosed moderate hypertension should be referred to a physician for evaluation. The patient with diagnosed, treated, but still moderate hypertension should be referred back to a physician for a review of the medical management and possibly more aggressive medical therapy. The dentist should consult the physician early in dental treatment planning to allow for integrated medical and dental care. Patients with moderate hypertension can undergo nonsurgical procedures (types I and II and most type III) using normal operating methods. Advanced crown and bridge (some type III) and all simple surgical procedures (type IV) should use adjunctive sedation techniques. Intermediate and advanced surgical procedures (types V and VI) should generally not be performed in the office for a patient with moderate hypertension. Vigorous bleeding may accompany dentosurgical procedures in patients with poorly controlled hypertension. Accompanied by proper sedation or gen-

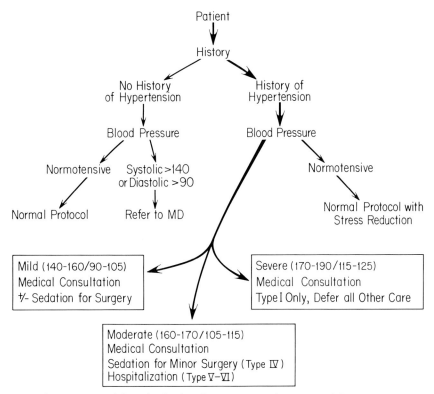

Figure 4–1. Guidelines for the dental management of patients with hypertension.

eral anesthesia, these procedures are best completed in a hospital surgical setting, where proper medical support for the management of acute hypertension is available. Significant operator training and experience, in an office well equipped for emergency procedures, may justify the outpatient care of some patients requiring moderately complicated surgical procedures (type V).

Severe Hypertension. The patient with severe hypertension should receive examination (type I procedures) only and be referred to a physician for further medical management prior to additional dental care.

Malignant Hypertension. Malignant hypertension is a medical emergency, and the patient should be immediately referred to a physician for acute intervention.

PATIENTS TAKING CALCIUM CHANNEL BLOCKERS

Oral Findings

Calcium channel blockers are a relatively frequent cause of gingival hyperplasia. Clinically, patients commonly present with enlarge-

ment of the marginal and papillary gingivae, which mimics the presentation of hyperplasia induced by Dilantin. Interestingly, the histologic evaluations of tissue from both forms of hyperplastic tissue are indistinguishable. Because hyperplastic changes in the gingiva often predispose to plaque accumulation and limit oral hygiene, a superimposed inflammatory process is often present.

Preliminary data have suggested an incidence of gingival hyperplasia as high as 15 to 20% for nifedipine (Procardia). Gingival changes reportedly have occurred as soon as 2 months after the initiation of therapy. Gingival hyperplasia has also been reported to be associated with most other calcium channel blockers. Specific data relative to the incidence and clinical course are not yet available. Additionally, it is difficult to predict a patient's individual risk of developing the condition because epidemiologic data, such as age, sex, duration of treatment, dosage, and oral hygiene, are not available.

Considerations for the Dentist

The major dental consideration for patients taking calcium channel blockers is maintenance of periodontal health in view of the risk of drug-induced gingival hyperplasia. Because inflammation is likely to exacerbate gingival changes, aggressive oral hygiene and frequent professional maintenance are critical. When possible, margins of fixed restorations should be placed supragingivally. Gingival resection may be required to eliminate overgrown tissue. In severe, recurrent cases, or in patients who have difficulty with home care, physician consultation concerning alternative medications is recommended.

■ Examples of Dental Evaluation and Management

EVALUATION

Three patients present to the dental office for extensive dental care. All three are found to have blood pressures (BP) of 165/105. The histories obtained from these patients reveal the following:

Patient 1. This patient (BP 165/105) has never been told that he has hypertension, is currently not on medication, and has not been seen by a physician in 2 years.

Patient 2. This patient (BP 165/105) was diagnosed as having hypertension 3 years ago. He is currently on 50 mg of hydrochlorothiazide (Hydrodiuril) and 0.2 mg of clonidine daily. The patient has not seen his physician in over a year.

Patient 3. This patient (BP 165/105) was diagnosed as having hypertension 2 years ago. He is currently on 10 mg of minoxidil and 80 mg of furosemide (Lasix) daily. He has been followed by his physician closely and has had monthly adjustments of his medications.

MANAGEMENT

Although all three patients currently have moderate hypertension, the nature of their diseases is different, as is the proper dental management.

Patient 1. This patient has moderate hypertension that was previously undiagnosed and should be referred to his physician for evaluation. It is 90% probable that the evaluation will reveal essential hypertension. Unlike secondary forms of hypertension, which can be surgically approached, essential hypertension requires long-term management. The physician can try to control the blood pressure with a single drug,

such as a converting enzyme inhibitor or calcium channel blocker. If the patient is placed on a calcium channel blocker, the dentist must be aware of its potential to cause gingival hyperplasia. Dental procedures for this patient should be routine for all nonsurgical procedures (types I, II, and III). As the patient's hypertension becomes reasonably controlled, more advanced dental procedures can be undertaken using simple sedation techniques such as N_2O-O_2 inhalation or oral diazepam (Valium).

Patient 2. This patient also has moderate hypertension and has been started on an antihypertensive regimen. However, low doses of diuretics and clonidine have not brought his blood pressure under sufficient control. Furthermore, he has not seen his physician in a year. The dentist should consult the physician for re-evaluation of the patient's status and should anticipate modifications of the drug regimen designed to bring the patient's blood pressure under better control. More complex dental procedures should be deferred until a "controlled" blood pressure level is attained. At the patient's present blood pressure, however, the dentist can undertake examination and simple operative procedures (types I and II) using normal protocol. Simple sedation techniques such as the use of oral diazepam or N_2O-O_2 inhalation, may be necessary for some advanced restorative procedures (type III). More aggressive sedation techniques such as the use of intravenous diazepam may be necessary for simple surgical procedures (type IV). Hospitalization for close patient monitoring and sedation is advised for advanced surgical procedures (types V and VI). Outpatient management with appropriate sedation for some advanced surgical procedures (type V) may be undertaken by an operator with the appropriate expertise.

The dosage of clonidine administered to this patient is low, and "rebound hypertension" following the withdrawal of clonidine is not a serious concern. In patients on high dosages of clonidine who are expected not to be able to take oral medications for more than 24 hours, medical consultation should be sought, and alternate antihypertensive agents may have to be used perioperatively.

Patient 3. This patient has moderate hypertension in the presence of reasonably potent antihypertensive agents (minoxidil and furosemide). Even with aggressive medical management and close monitoring by his physician, this patient's blood pressure is not well controlled, and improvement in blood pressure cannot be anticipated. The patient's physician should be consulted to discuss the optimal mode of management of the patient during the required dental procedures. Examination and simple operative procedures (types I and II) may be accomplished by normal operative protocol, but mild adjunctive sedation with oral diazepam or N_2O-O_2 may be necessary. Frequent blood pressure measurements should be obtained during the operative procedures. Advanced nonsurgical and simple surgical procedures (types III and IV) require adjunctive sedation. Advanced periodontal and oral surgical procedures (types V and VI) are best accomplished in a hospital setting with advanced sedation techniques or general anesthesia. Because this patient is taking minoxidil and furosemide, orthostatic changes in blood pressure are a significant concern. The patient should be instructed to sit up slowly after dental procedures and to dangle his legs for a minute or two before standing to avoid problems with orthostatic hypotension.

These examples serve to illustrate that although presenting blood pressures may be identical, the medical and dental management and the possible complications from medications are distinctly different.

SUMMARY TABLE

Hypertension: General Information

DEFINITION
Hypertension is a resting blood pressure in excess of 140 systolic or 90 diastolic, or both.

INCIDENCE
It affects 10–20% of adult patients.

SYMPTOMS
It is asymptomatic in the majority of the patients, but may occasionally present with headache, visual blurring, or changes in mental status.

COMPLICATIONS
Common sequelae of long-term untreated hypertension include the following:
1. Cerebrovascular disease
2. Renal disease
3. Coronary artery disease

CAUSE
Hypertension is essential (primary or idiopathic) in 90% of cases, but can be secondary to renal parenchymal, renovascular, or adrenal diseases in 10% of cases.

GUIDELINES FOR CLINICAL STATUS OF BLOOD PRESSURE

Normal	120/80 mm Hg
Controlled	Up to 140/up to 90
Mild hypertension	140–160/90–105
Moderate hypertension	160–170/105–115
Severe hypertension	170–190/115–125
Malignant hypertension	Severe hypertension (often 190+/125+) associated with central nervous system symptoms such as blurring of vision, headache, or changes in mental status

SUMMARY TABLE 4–II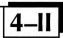

Hypertension: Medical Management

GOAL OF MEDICAL EXAMINATION AND STUDIES
Rule out secondary forms of hypertension.

MEDICAL MANAGEMENT
Essential hypertension: drug therapy

Secondary hypertension: in selected instances, can be surgically approached and cured

PROBLEMS FOR THE PHYSICIAN
Rule out secondary hypertension.

Attempt to attain a balance of effective drugs with minimal side effects.

SUMMARY TABLE 4–III

Commonly Used Antihypertensive Drugs

	TRADE NAME	GENERIC NAME
Thiazide Diuretics	Diuril	Chlorothiazide
	Esidrix	Hydrochlorothiazide
	Hydrodiuril	Hydrochlorothiazide
Long-Acting Thiazides	Enduron	Methyclothiazide
	Hygroton	Chlorthalidone
	Zaroxolyn	Metolazone
	Diulo	Metolazone
Potassium-Sparing Diuretics	Aldactone	Spironolactone
	Dyrenium	Triamterene
	Midamor	Amiloride
Loop Diuretics	Lasix	Furosemide
	Edecrine	Ethacrynic acid
	Bumex	Bumetanide
Combination Diuretics	Aldactazide	Hydrochlorothiazide and spironolactone
	Dyazide	Hydrochlorothiazide and triamterene
	Maxzide	Hydrochlorothiazide and triamterene
	Moduretic	Hydrochlorothiazide and amiloride
Beta-Adrenergic Blockers	Inderal	Propranolol
	Lopressor	Metoprolol
	Tenormin	Atenolol
	Blocadren	Timolol
	Corgard	Nadolol
	Sectral	Acebutolol
	Visken	Pindolol
	Kerlone	Betaxolol
	Levatol	Penbutolol
Alpha-Beta Blockers	Normodyne	Labetalol
	Trandate	Labetalol

Commonly Used Antihypertensive Drugs *Continued*

	TRADE NAME	GENERIC NAME
Alpha-Adrenergic Blockers	Minipress	Prazosin
	Hytrin	Terazosin
	Cardura	Doxazosin
Calcium Channel Blockers	Procardia	Nifedipine
	Cardizem	Diltiazem
	Dilacor	Diltiazem
	Calan	Verapamil
	Verelan	Verapamil
	Isoptin	Verapamil
	Norvasc	Amlodipine
	Plendil	Felodipine
	Cardene	Nicardipine
Angiotensin-Converting Enzyme (ACE) Inhibitors	Capoten	Captopril
	Vasotec	Enalapril
	Prinivil	Lisinopril
	Zestril	Lisinopril
	Altace	Ramipril
	Monopril	Fosinopril
	Lotensin	Benazepril
	Accupril	Quinapril
Other Drugs	Ismelin	Guanethidine
	Serpasil	Reserpine
	Apresoline	Hydralazine
	Loniten	Minoxidil
	Catapres	Clonidine
	Aldomet	Methyldopa
	Tenex	Guanfacine
Combination Drugs		
DRUGS WITH CLONIDINE (CATAPRES)	Combipres	Clonidine and chlorthalidone
DRUGS WITH ATENOLOL (TENORMIN)	Tenoretic	Atenolol and chlorthalidone
DRUGS WITH NADOLOL (CORGARD)	Corzide	Nadolol and bendroflumethiazide
DRUGS WITH HYDRALAZINE (APRESOLINE)	Apresazide	Hydralazine and hydrochlorothiazide
	Ser-Ap-Es	Reserpine, hydralazine, and hydrochlorothiazide
DRUGS WITH METHYLDOPA (ALDOMET)	Aldoclor	Methyldopa and chlorothiazide
	Aldoril	Methyldopa and hydrochlorothiazide
DRUGS WITH RESERPINE (SERPASIL)	Diupres	Reserpine and chlorothiazide
	Hydropres	Reserpine and hydrochlorothiazide
	Ser-Ap-Es	Reserpine, hydralazine, and hydrochlorothiazide

SUMMARY TABLE **4–IV**

Common Side Effects of Antihypertensive Medications

MEDICATIONS	SIDE EFFECTS
Diuretics	Dehydration, hypokalemia
Methyldopa	Drowsiness, impotence
Propranolol	Bronchospasm and congestive heart failure in some patients
Clonidine	Xerostomia, rebound hypertension (rare)
Reserpine	Sedation, depression
Guanethidine	Postural hypotension, diarrhea
Calcium channel blockers	Gingival hyperplasia
Converting enzyme inhibitors	Chronic cough

SUMMARY TABLE **4–V**

Dental Evaluation of the Patient with Hypertension

HISTORY (TO ASSESS SEVERITY)

Time of discovery of hypertension

Medication regimen—present and recent changes, dosage and drug combinations

Presence of end-organ complications—stroke, renal disease, coronary artery disease

EXAMINATION (RECORDING THE BLOOD PRESSURE)

Blood pressure at initial examination and yearly for all patients

Blood pressure at each visit for patients with initial reading of 140/90 or higher

Blood pressure prior to all types IV–VI surgical procedures for all patients

Blood pressure during lengthy dental procedures in the diagnosed or suspected hypertensive patient

SUMMARY TABLE **4–VI**

Dental Management for Specific Dental Procedures*

BLOOD PRESSURE	TYPE(S) OF PROCEDURES	PROTOCOL
Controlled (BP, 140/90) and mild (BP, 140–160/90–105)	I, II, III, (IV)	Normal protocol ±† physician referral
	(IV), V, VI	Above ± "sedation techniques" (Chap. 51)
Moderate (BP, 160–170/105–115)	I, II, (III)	Physician referral or review of medical management with physician
	(III), IV	Above plus "sedation techniques"
	V, VI	Hospitalization
Severe (BP, 170–190/115–125)	I only	Referral to physician; other procedures should be deferred until appropriate medical management is instituted; if blood pressure correction is impossible, less complex dental treatment plans are recommended
Malignant hypertension		*Medical emergency*: contact physician immediately

*The primary consideration in proper dental management of the hypertensive patient is appropriate long-term care instituted and monitored by the physician. "Sedation techniques" (Chap. 51) are only valuable short-term adjuncts to allow completion of certain dental procedures and to adequately control anxiety, both of which may adversely affect blood pressure.

†±, with or without.

Angina Pectoris

Angina pectoris is a form of symptomatic ischemic heart disease. The underlying pathophysiology is a transient myocardial oxygen demand in excess of the available oxygen supply for the coronary vessels. In the majority of cases, arteriosclerotic heart disease or the atherosclerotic obstruction of one or more of the three major coronary arteries is the causative factor (Fig. 5–1). Less frequently, angina can result from excess oxygen demand, limited oxygen-carrying capacity of the blood (e.g., anemia), or inadequate perfusion of the coronary arteries (e.g., hypotension).

Angina pectoris literally means "compression of the chest." A classic case of angina is precipitated by emotional stress or physical exertion and is relieved by rest. Poorly localized retrosternal pain of moderate intensity is characteristic (Summary Table 5–I and Fig. 5–2). During an anginal attack, the typical patient shows signs of anxiety. He or she is unable to point exactly to the source of the discomfort but often closes the fist over the sternum in an attempt to describe the pain. The pain is often described as a heavy sensation over the precordial area and can radiate to the shoulders, arms, or mandible. It is usually of brief duration, lasting 3 to 5 minutes if the precipitating

factor is removed. In contrast, the pain associated with myocardial infarction is usually more severe. It is often described by the patient as crushing in nature, and is poorly and incompletely relieved by sublingual nitroglycerin.

MEDICAL EVALUATION
(Summary Table 5–II)

In evaluating a patient with chest pain, especially if the history is not classic for angina, other causes of chest pain should be considered. Musculoskeletal diseases, hiatal hernia, reflux esophagitis, gastritis, gallbladder disease, and psychogenic pain must all be ruled out.

The diagnosis of angina is usually made on the basis of the history. Cardiovascular examinations between attacks are usually unrevealing, and the resting electrocardiogram usually shows only nonspecific changes (Chap. 8). If the diagnosis remains in doubt after the initial evaluation, an exercise test may be performed to demonstrate ischemic changes. During the stress test, the patient is asked to perform a graded amount of exercise, usually on a tread-

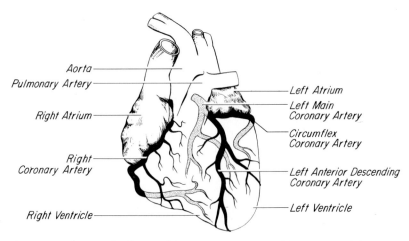

Figure 5–1. Anatomic distribution of the coronary arteries and the anatomy of the heart.

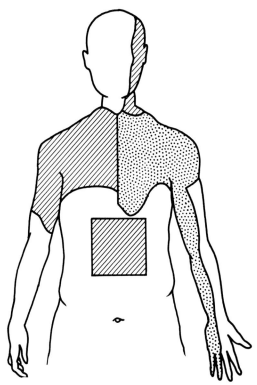

Figure 5–2. Patterns of radiating chest pain. The dotted areas represent the most common distribution of pain of cardiac origin; the slashed areas are those that are less frequently symptomatic. (Adapted from Jastak, J. T., and Cowan, F. F., Jr.: Patients at risk. Dent. Clin. North Am., 17:363, 1973.)

mill, while under constant electrocardiographic monitoring. The test examines the patient's electrocardiogram for ischemic changes under defined amounts of stress. It is particularly helpful for diagnosing a patient who has a normal resting electrocardiogram.

The injection of thallium-201 considerably enhances the sensitivity of the conventional exercise test. In this test, the patient is given an injection of radioactive thallium prior to the exercise period. The distributions of thallium-201 during exercise and at rest are compared. Because thallium distributes in the myocardium according to the pattern of blood perfusion, it does not enter areas of ischemia, and a "cold spot" is seen when the myocardium is scanned (Fig. 5–3). This test is particularly useful for patients with abnormal resting electrocardiograms.

If noninvasive tests are not diagnostic, coronary arteriograms may have to be performed. Coronary arteriography is a procedure involving the cannulation of a peripheral artery with a catheter, the retrograde feeding of the catheter to the origin of the coronary arteries, and the injection of contrast medium selectively into each of the coronary arteries (Fig. 5–4). The procedure is done under fluoroscopy, and the coronary anatomy can be recorded on film for future reference. Coronary angiograms provide evidence of hemodynamically significant obstruction in the coronary vessels in the majority of patients with angina pectoris associated with arteriosclerotic heart disease. The procedure carries a small risk and should be reserved for the patient deemed a candidate for coronary artery bypass surgery.

Once the diagnosis of angina is established, the severity of the disease must be assessed. The frequency, pattern, and severity of attacks, the stability of the episodes, the medications required to control the symptoms, and the associated risk factors should all be carefully evaluated. A detailed history provides a reasonable estimate of the severity of the disease. For the purposes of dental management, angina can be classified as mild, moderate, or severe and unstable (Summary Table 5–III). The patient with mild angina has predictable and infrequent attacks that are usually precipitated by excessive physical exertion or emotional stress and are promptly relieved by rest. The patient with moderately severe angina reports more frequent episodes precipitated by moderate exertion and stress, and may have angina after a large meal or during sexual intercourse. The patient with severe angina has frequent attacks, often in the absence of excessive exertion or stress. The pain is more severe and may last for longer periods.

MEDICAL MANAGEMENT

The medical management of angina pectoris includes a modification of the patient's life style as well as the use of medications (Summary Table 5–IV). The patient is encouraged to lose weight, discontinue smoking, reduce anxiety and tension, and avoid situations that provoke stress. A controlled exercise program may also be initiated. For immediate relief of chest pain, nitroglycerin, a short-acting nitrate, is prescribed in doses ranging from 0.3 to 0.6 mg, given sublingually. If the angina is moderate in severity, long-acting nitrates such as isosorbide dinitrate (Isordil) may be given. The medication can be given sublingually or orally in doses ranging from 5 to 40 mg every 4 to 8 hours. It can also be given prophylactically in anticipation of increased physical activity or stress. For patients with moderate or severe angina, propranolol in dosages ranging from

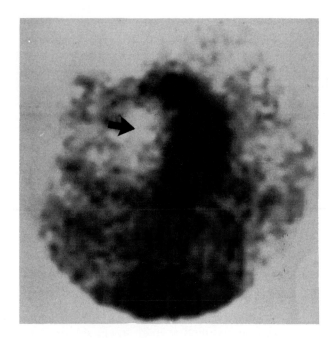

Figure 5–3. Thallium-201 scan demonstrating areas of cardiac ischemia. (From Braunwald, E. [ed.]: Heart Disease: A Textbook of Cardiovascular Medicine. Philadelphia, W. B. Saunders, 1980.)

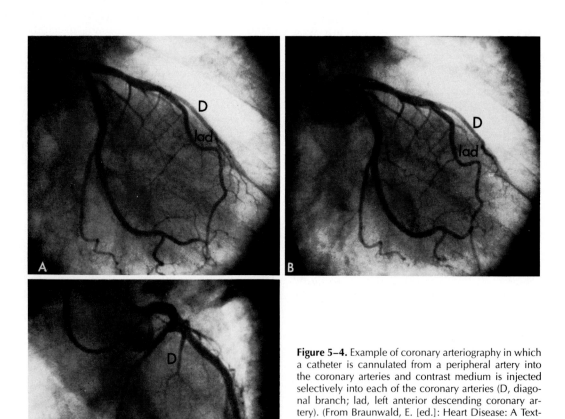

Figure 5–4. Example of coronary arteriography in which a catheter is cannulated from a peripheral artery into the coronary arteries and contrast medium is injected selectively into each of the coronary arteries (D, diagonal branch; lad, left anterior descending coronary artery). (From Braunwald, E. [ed.]: Heart Disease: A Textbook of Cardiovascular Medicine. Philadelphia, W. B. Saunders, 1980.)

40 to 320 mg daily may be added. This agent is thought to be effective in the control of angina because it reduces myocardial contractility and hence myocardial oxygen requirements. Calcium channel blockers are also extremely useful in the management of patients with angina pectoris. These agents cause dilation of the coronary arteries and optimize blood flow to the myocardium. Four calcium channel blockers are now in clinical use, nifedipine (Procardia), verapamil (Calan, Isoptin), diltiazem (Cardizem), and amlodipine (Norvasc) (Summary Table 5–III).

Occasionally, a patient may experience a change in the pattern of angina. With an increase of the frequency and severity of the pain or with the appearance of angina at rest, the patient is said to have unstable angina. A significant fraction of patients with unstable angina progress to myocardial infarction within a short time. These patients are therefore treated aggressively. Prospective randomized studies have demonstrated that patient survival is equivalent whether the patient is treated with medical therapy or with coronary artery bypass surgery. Coronary artery bypass surgery, however, is more effective in alleviating anginal symptoms. Currently, bypass surgery is reserved for patients with intractable angina despite maximal medical therapy and for patients with high-grade obstruction of the left main coronary artery (who, as a group, have a high mortality when managed medically). Percutaneous transluminal coronary angioplasty has now been used to dilate critically stenosed coronary arteries. In this procedure, a catheter with an inflatable balloon at its tip is positioned in the stenotic area during cardiac catheterization. The balloon is then inflated rapidly to dilate the affected area of the coronary artery. The procedure has obviated coronary bypass surgery in appropriate candidates and can provide an option for patients deemed to be unsuitable candidates for undergoing coronary artery surgery.

Prognostically, the mortality of patients with angina depends partly on other concurrent medical problems. The average mortality rate for all patients surviving the initial anginal attack is 4% per year. Concurrent medical conditions including hypertension, diabetes, hypercholesterolemia, and a smoking habit significantly increase the mortality risk. The concurrent presence of two of these factors increases the mortality risk to three times that for the angina patient without any of the risk factors. The presence of hypertension and an abnormal resting electrocardiogram, for instance, increases the mortality risk of the patient to 8%/year. The extent of coronary artery disease as defined by the arteriogram also correlates with mortality risk. The patient with disease involving a single coronary vessel has a 2%/year risk, two-vessel disease involves a 4% risk, and triple-vessel involvement is associated with a 7% annual mortality. Patients with congestive heart failure have a markedly increased mortality, approaching 50% over 5 years.

DENTAL EVALUATION

For the dentist, an assessment of the severity of the patient's angina greatly facilitates optimal patient management. The major concern of the dentist in the management of the patient with angina is the possibility of precipitating an anginal attack during dental procedures.

The dental evaluation of the patient can be accomplished by taking a chairside history (Summary Table 5–VII). The frequency of attacks, the daily dosage of nitroglycerin, and the relationship of the anginal episodes to exertion or stress should be noted. Based on the history, the dentist should be able to categorize the angina as mild, moderate, or severe (Summary Table 5–III). Because of the stress a dental visit can generate, the dentist should particularly note a history of anginal attacks related to emotional stress.

After determining the severity of the disease, the dentist should try to assess the stability of the patient's angina. The patient with a history of increasing frequency and severity of pain or a history of recent onset of pain at rest is most likely to have problems. For this patient, elective dental procedures should be deferred until medical therapy is optimized.

In the evaluation, the patient's medications, dosages, and dose schedules should be noted. The patient with mild angina commonly uses sublingual nitroglycerin as needed. Patients with moderate or severe angina may require both long-acting nitrates, calcium channel blockers, and beta blockers. The dentist should be particularly concerned if large doses of nitrates and propranolol fail to control the patient's symptoms, and the physician should be consulted prior to extensive dental procedures.

The dentist should also be aware of some of the side effects of the commonly used antianginal medications (Summary Table 5–V).

Nitroglycerin and long-acting nitrates can produce headaches and orthostatic hypotension. Propranolol can cause excessive bradycardia, precipitate congestive heart failure in patients with borderline ventricular function, and induce wheezing in patients with asthma. Nifedipine can cause peripheral edema in some patients. Diltiazem can cause bradycardia. All the calcium channel blockers can cause mild gastrointestinal distress. Awareness of these potential problems is important in the dental management of the patient with angina.

During the evaluation, the dentist should determine whether a medical consultation is necessary. In general, extensive dental procedures should not be performed on patients with severe or unstable angina without close collaboration with the patient's physician.

DENTAL MANAGEMENT

The dentist should be familiar with the treatment of angina (Summary Table 5–VIII). Nitroglycerin tablets (0.3 to 0.4 mg) in an airtight amber bottle that are replaced every 6 months should be available in the emergency kit. If the patient reports the onset of angina during a procedure, the dental treatment should be stopped immediately. The patient should be reassured and allowed to remain at a 45° incline. Nitroglycerin should be administered sublingually, and oxygen should be administered at a rate of 4 to 6 liters/minute. Nitroglycerin can be readministered at 5-minute intervals with careful monitoring of the patient's blood pressure. The blood pressure should be monitored because transient hypotension can occur after sublingual nitroglycerin. If the systolic blood pressure falls below 100, the patient should be allowed to lie flat with the feet elevated. If pain is not relieved within 8 to 10 minutes with the use of nitrates, the patient's physician should be alerted and the patient transported to a hospital by ambulance.

It is important to know how to treat an acute episode of angina, but the first priority is to anticipate and avoid attacks. Careful assessment of the patient's angina permits the development of an integrated medical and dental treatment plan. In general, good patient rapport and short appointments minimize the risk of precipitating angina.

Patients with mild stable angina tolerate most nonsurgical dental procedures (types I to III) using normal dental protocol. Some advanced restorative dentistry (type III) and minor surgery (type IV) may require mild sedation with N_2O-O_2, which may be supplemented with oral diazepam (Valium). More advanced dental surgery (types V to VI) should be performed using appropriate sedation techniques (Chap. 51). It should be stressed that patients with mild angina develop symptoms infrequently, and appropriate sedation is usually the only intervention necessary for dental procedures. Prophylactic nitroglycerin is not recommended for these patients.

For patients with moderate angina, examination (type I) and most simple operative procedures (type II) can be accomplished using normal protocol. Prior to advanced operative or simple surgical tasks (type III or IV), the patient should take prophylactic nitroglycerin. Nitroglycerin (0.3 to 0.4 mg) or long-acting nitrates (e.g., isosorbide dinitrate, Isordil, 5 mg) are given sublingually just prior to the dental procedure. Appropriate sedation techniques are also employed. Prophylactic nitrates and adjunctive sedation techniques should be used as well for more advanced surgical procedures (types V and VI). In selected patients, the controlled environment of the hospital setting should be considered for extensive surgical procedures.

For patients with severe angina, only the examination (type I procedures) should be completed using a normal protocol. A medical consultation should be sought before planning additional dental treatment. Simple operative dentistry (type II procedures) can be performed with the use of prophylactic nitrates and mild sedation. Advanced operative and simple surgical procedures (types III and IV) must include adjunctive sedation techniques and are best accomplished in a hospital setting. All moderate to advanced dental surgery (types V and VI procedures) should be performed in a controlled hospital environment. With patients requiring large dosages of propranolol (more than 160 mg daily) for control of angina, special care has to be taken during the perioperative period. If the patient is expected not to be able to take oral medication for more than 12 to 24 hours, medical consultation is essential to guide the perioperative use of intravenous propranolol. Abrupt withdrawal of propranolol therapy has been reported to precipitate severe angina and myocardial infarction.

Patients with unstable angina should have their dental procedures deferred until their symptoms have been stabilized.

PATIENTS TAKING CALCIUM CHANNEL BLOCKERS

Oral Findings

Calcium channel blockers are a relatively frequent cause of gingival hyperplasia. Clinically, patients commonly present with enlargement of the marginal and papillary gingivae, which mimics the presentation of hyperplasia induced by Dilantin. Interestingly, the histologic evaluations of tissue from both forms of hyperplastic tissue are indistinguishable. Because hyperplastic changes in the gingiva often predispose to plaque accumulation and limit oral hygiene, a superimposed inflammatory process is often present.

Preliminary data have suggested an incidence of gingival hyperplasia as high as 15 to 20% for nifedipine (Procardia). Gingival changes reportedly have occurred as soon as 2 months after the initiation of therapy. Gingival hyperplasia has also been reported to be associated with most other calcium channel blockers. Specific data relative to the incidence and clinical course are not yet available. Additionally, it is difficult to predict a patient's individual risk of developing the condition because epidemiologic data, such as age, sex, duration of treatment, dosage, and oral hygiene, are not available.

Considerations for the Dentist

The major dental consideration for patients taking calcium channel blockers is maintenance of periodontal health in view of the risk of drug-induced gingival hyperplasia. Because inflammation is likely to exacerbate gingival changes, aggressive oral hygiene and frequent professional maintenance are critical. When possible, margins of fixed restorations should be placed supragingivally. Gingival resection may be required to eliminate overgrown tissue. In severe, recurrent cases or in patients who have difficulty with home care, physician consultation concerning alternative medications is recommended.

■ Examples of Evaluation and Dental Management

EVALUATION

Patient 1. A 64-year-old male patient has mild angina and reports fewer than six episodes of chest pain a year. He has been involved in a bitter divorce proceeding, and the chest pain usually occurs when he argues with his wife. The pain is promptly relieved by nitroglycerin, which the patient has been instructed to carry with him at all times, but he frequently forgets to do so. He smokes two packs of cigarettes a day, and his blood pressure was normal at the initial examination. Medical consultation with his physician reveals that the patient's general physical examination, electrocardiogram, and chest film are all normal. The dental needs of the patient include an examination, simple and advanced operative procedures (types I to III), a gingivectomy (type IV) around the abutments for an anticipated bridge, and the removal of a partially erupted and impacted mandibular third molar (type V).

Patient 2. A 55-year-old male patient has moderate angina and reports chest pain on a weekly basis associated with activities such as mowing the lawn or shoveling snow. He occasionally has angina after a big holiday meal. The patient is a factory foreman, and arguments with his workers and his boss have precipitated angina. He currently takes 10 mg of oral Isordil three times a day. The episodes have had "about the same frequency" over the past 2 years. The patient smokes two packs of cigarettes a day and has been told that his blood pressure is occasionally "a little high." On the initial examination, his blood pressure is 150/90, and he appears anxious. The patient's physician has followed his blood pressure closely and feels that antihypertensive therapy is not indicated at this time. The patient's electrocardiogram and chest x-ray are normal. He requires advanced periodontal therapy (type V), advanced caries control, and multiple units of crown and bridge (type III).

Patient 3. A 62-year-old male patient has severe angina and has daily chest pain precipitated by minimal exertion, such as walking short distances or climbing a short flight of stairs. He has been taking nitroglycerin and long-acting nitrates for 3 years. In the past month, propranolol 80 mg four times a day has been added to control angina at rest. The patient does not smoke and does not have diabetes, hypertension, or lipid abnormalities. His blood pressure at the time of the initial evaluation is 130/78. Consultation with his physician reveals that his electrocardiogram demonstrates an old myocardial infarction. His chest x-ray reveals mild enlargement of the heart (cardiomegaly). His dental needs are identical to those of Patient 2.

MANAGEMENT

Patient 1. The examination and simple and advanced operative procedures (types I to III) can be done using normal protocol. For the gingivectomy (type IV procedure) the dentist may use N_2O-O_2 analgesia. The removal of the impacted third molar may require more advanced sedation techniques. N_2O-O_2 sedation with an augmented dose of oral diazepam may be employed. Intravenous diazepam may have to be administered to the patient with a high degree of anxiety, but prophylactic nitroglycerin is probably not necessary.

Patient 2. The dental examination is completed using normal protocol. If the patient had only simple prophylactic and isolated operative needs (type II procedures), normal protocol and shorter appointments would have been sufficient. However, the rampant caries require quadrant caries control, and subgingival scaling must be part of the periodontal therapy (both type III procedures). To keep each appointment reasonably short, multiple quadrant or half-quadrant scaling visits rather than full-arch or full-mouth scaling should be scheduled. The same applies to the caries control aspect of therapy.

The dentist effectively simplifies the scheduled operative appointments by performing two short "simple" operative procedures (type II) instead of one "advanced" operative procedure (type III). For all procedures, the patient should stay on his usual regimen of oral Isordil. Prophylactic sublingual nitroglycerin should be used for all advanced operative (type III) and all surgical (types IV to VI) procedures. Mild sedation using N_2O-O_2 inhalation may be necessary if the patient demonstrates limited tolerance for advanced operative procedures (type III). Moderate to advanced sedation techniques (Chap. 51) may be required for advanced operative (type III) and simple surgical procedures (type IV). Such sedation is definitely required for moderate to advanced surgical procedures (types V and VI). Hospitalization should also be considered for these latter procedures.

Patient 3. Only a dental examination can be performed using normal protocol. The patient should be on his usual medical regimen, and prophylactic nitroglycerin should be taken prior to any dental procedures (types II to VI). The patient's physician must be consulted before the initiation of therapy. The patient's medical problems are severe enough that even substantive treatment planning may have to be altered. Full periodontal therapy and ideal prosthetic management are difficult under these circumstances; caries control, the hygiene phase of periodontal care, extraction of symptomatic teeth, and the use of simple removable prostheses may be more appropriate. Each office appointment should be kept as short as possible. For advanced operative procedures (type III), elective admission to the hospital has to be considered. Many surgical procedures (type IV) and all types V and VI procedures are best done in a controlled hospital setting. Medical consultation for the perioperative management of this complicated case is essential. If the patient is expected to be unable to take oral medication for longer than 12 to 24 hours, judicious use of intravenous propranolol under careful medical monitoring is necessary to minimize the problems associated with the abrupt withdrawal of propranolol.

SUMMARY TABLE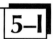

Angina Pectoris

DEFINITION
Angina pectoris is a symptom complex highlighted by chest pain.

It is transient, symptomatic, ischemic heart disease.

CHEST PAIN CHARACTERISTICS
Moderate intensity

Poorly localized retrosternal pain

Radiation of the pain to left arm and shoulder or neck and mandible

Brief duration (2–10 min)

Relieved by nitroglycerin (noticeably within 2 min)

STABLE ANGINA
Pain on exertion, relief with rest

UNSTABLE ANGINA
Pain at rest or markedly changing frequency of attacks

CAUSE
Most commonly, atherosclerotic narrowing of one or more coronary vessels

SUMMARY TABLE

Medical Evaluation of the Patient with Angina

History

Physical examination

Resting electrocardiogram

Exercise stress test

Thallium-201 stress test

Angiography

Dental Classification of the Patient with Angina Pectoris

	MILD ANGINA	MODERATE ANGINA	SEVERE ANGINA
Frequency of Attacks	Up to 1/mo	Up to 1/wk	Daily episodes
Stability	Stable	Stable	Unstable
Changing Frequency	None	Slight increase over previous year or more distant past	Change in last 6 months
Onset	Following severe exertion or emotion	Following moderate exertion or emotion or (infrequently) meals	Following rest, decreasing or mild emotion or exertion, and meals (frequently)
Medications	Nitroglycerin (symptomatically)	Nitroglycerin; long-acting nitrates; beta blockers; calcium channel blockers	Nitroglycerin; long-acting nitrates; beta blockers; calcium channel blockers
Medical Consultation			Left ventricular compromise (clinical congestive heart failure, radiographic cardiac enlargement), ECG abnormalities (premature ventricular contractions, arrhythmias)

Medical Regimens for Angina Pectoris

SEVERITY	TREATMENT
Mild	Nitroglycerin (symptomatically), 0.3-, 0.4-, and 0.6-mg doses; some ancillary measures: weight reduction, anxiety and tension reduction, controlled exercise program, discontinuing smoking, control of blood lipid and cholesterol levels
Moderate	Long-acting nitrates (Isordil), with or without beta blockers or calcium channel blockers
Severe (successful medical drug management)	Long-acting nitrates, beta blockers, and calcium channel blockers
Severe (unsuccessful medical drug management)	Percutaneous transluminal coronary angioplasty, coronary artery bypass surgery

SUMMARY TABLE

Common Side Effects of Angina Pectoris Medications

NITROGLYCERIN (WITHIN MINUTES OF ADMINISTRATION)
Headache

Postural hypotension

Tachycardia

Tolerance (develops at more than 10 doses/day)

LONG-ACTING NITRATES
Headache

Hypotension

BETA BLOCKERS
Bradycardia (heart rate, 55–65/min, is therapeutic range)

Precipitation of congestive heart failure in patients with borderline ventricular function

Aggravation of bronchospasm in patients with mild asthma

Rapid propranolol therapy withdrawal (exacerbation of angina, precipitation of myocardial infarction)

CALCIUM CHANNEL BLOCKERS
Nifedipine can cause peripheral edema; diltiazem can cause bradycardia

All calcium channel blockers but especially nifedipine can cause gingival hyperplasia

SUMMARY TABLE **5–VI**

Selected Brand Names and Dosage Range for Angina Pectoris Medications

GENERIC NAME	TRADE NAME	DOSAGE
Nitroglycerin		0.3, 0.4, 0.6 mg/dose; onset of action: 1–5 min
Isosorbide dinitrate (long-acting nitrate)	Isordil, Iso-Bid, Laserdil, Sorbitrate	5–40 mg sublingual or oral dose; onset of action: 5–15 min
Long-acting nitroglycerin	Nitro-Bid, Nitrong	
Beta blockers		
Propranolol	Inderal	160–320 mg/day
Metoprolol	Lopressor	50–100 mg/day
Atenolol	Tenormin	25–100 mg/day
Timolol	Blocadren	10–20 mg/day
Nadolol	Corgard	40–240 mg/day
Acebutolol	Sectral	400–1200 mg/day
Pindolol	Visken	10–60 mg/day
Calcium channel blockers		
Nifedipine	Procardia	40–120 mg/day
Verapamil	Calan, Isoptin	40–120 mg/day
Diltiazem	Cardizem	30–120 mg/day
Amlodipine	Norvasc	5–10 mg/day

Dental Evaluation of Angina: Information Requirements

CHAIRSIDE HISTORY

General information—presence of these factors must be determined:
1. Obesity
2. Sedentary life style
3. Psychosocial tension
4. Family history of premature myocardial infarction

Specific information:
1. Frequency of angina attacks (daily, weekly, monthly)
2. Stability: frequency or severity of attacks changing? precipitating events less stressful?
3. Medications: nitroglycerin, long-acting nitrates, beta blockers, and calcium channel blockers
4. Use of medications: recent changes in dosage
5. Presence of other risk factors for ischemic heart disease—smoking, hypertension, hyperlipidemia (especially increased low-density lipoproteins), diabetes

MEDICAL CONSULTATION

Additional high-risk factors determined by physician's examination:
1. Left ventricular compromise (clinical evidence of congestive heart failure, radiographic evidence of cardiac enlargement)
2. ECG abnormalities (e.g., premature ventricular contractions, arrhythmias)

SUMMARY TABLE **5–VIII**

Treatment of an Acute Anginal Attack in the Dental Office

DIFFERENTIAL DIAGNOSIS OF MODERATE CHEST PAIN
1. Musculoskeletal disease
2. Angina
3. Myocardial infarction
4. Hiatus hernia
5. Gastritis
6. Gallbladder disease

SIGNS AND SYMPTOMS
1. Chest pain ±* radiation (Summary Table 5–I)
2. Weakness
3. ± dyspnea (shortness of breath)
4. Apprehension
5. Increased blood pressure and pulse rate
6. ± sweating

TREATMENT
1. Stop dental treatment.
2. Recline patient to 45° angle; lower head position if systolic BP < 100.
3. Reassure patient.
4. Administer nitroglycerin (sublingually, 0.3–0.4 mg):
   a. Anginal pain is relieved in 3–5 min.
   b. May be repeated twice at 5-min intervals.
   c. Mild headache suggests a therapeutic dose has been given.
   d. Failure to relieve pain suggests evidence of myocardial infarction or preinfarction angina.
5. O_2 administration (this alone does not relieve angina distress)
6. If pain persists after the above therapy
   a. Transport the patient to a hospital by ambulance.
   b. Monitor blood pressure and pulse every 5 min.
   c. Be prepared to administer cardiopulmonary resuscitation in the event of an arrest.

*±, with or without.

SUMMARY TABLE  **5–IX**

General Principles of Dental Management of the Patient with Angina Pectoris

Good patient rapport

Shorter appointments

Prophylactic nitroglycerin

Sedation techniques (Chap. 51)

Hospitalization

Dental treatment plan modification

SUMMARY TABLE **5–X**

Dental Management for the Patient with Angina Pectoris

RISK CATEGORY	PROCEDURES	PROTOCOL
Mild risk	I, II, (III, IV)	Normal protocol
	(III, IV), V, VI	± * sedation techniques
Moderate risk	I, (II)	Normal protocol + medical consultation
	(II), III, IV	Prophylactic nitroglycerin ± sedation techniques
	V, VI	Prophylactic nitroglycerin; sedation techniques, ± hospitalization
Severe risk	I	Normal protocol + medical consultation
	II	Prophylactic nitroglycerin ± sedation techniques
	III, IV	Prophylactic nitroglycerin ± sedation techniques ± hospitalization
	V, VI	Hospitalization; less complex dental treatment plans recommended

* ±, with or without.

Myocardial Infarction

Myocardial infarction is not an uncommon problem. In one prospective study, 1.3% of patients above age 30 and 10% of patients above age 40 undergoing noncardiac surgery gave a history of previous myocardial infarction. A significant proportion of the dentist's population therefore has had an infarction. It is important to be able to recognize the symptoms of ongoing myocardial injury (Chap. 5) and to determine any past history of myocardial injuries. This chapter deals primarily with the risks of dental therapy among patients with previous myocardial infarctions.

Myocardial infarction is the result of prolonged ischemic injury to the heart. The most common reason for having a myocardial infarction is progressive coronary artery disease secondary to atherosclerosis (Chap. 3; Fig. 6–1). Other clinical syndromes that can lead to myocardial ischemia and infarction include spasms of the coronary arteries, vasculitic involvement of the coronary arteries, and on rare occasions, trauma to either the myocardium or the coronary arteries. Regardless of the causative factors, the clinical presentation and consequences of myocardial infarction are the same.

The patient usually presents with severe chest pain in the substernal or left precordial area. The pain may radiate to the left arm or to the jaw and may be associated with shortness of breath, palpitations, nausea, or vomiting. The pain is often described as being similar to that of angina (Chap. 5) but is more severe and protracted. A patient with ongoing myocardial injury often appears diaphoretic and in acute distress. The diagnosis is usually made on the basis of the clinical history, but confirmatory evidence can be obtained from an electrocardiogram during the episode.

The complications of myocardial infarction include arrhythmias and congestive heart failure and depend in part on the extent of injury. Patients with minimal myocardial injury usually recover without significant morbidity, whereas patients with large areas of injury are more likely to suffer heart failure and life-threatening arrhythmias. Regardless of the extent of injury, a history of myocardial infarction indicates significant compromises in the coronary arteries. Consequently, patients with recent myocardial infarctions have higher morbidity and mortality, even with elective surgery.

MEDICAL EVALUATION

The patient with a previous myocardial infarction can have some of the complications of atherosclerotic cardiovascular diseases such as angina, congestive heart failure, arrhythmia, or conduction abnormality. (The management of these cardiovascular complications is discussed in detail in Chs. 5, 7, and 9.)

A recent myocardial infarction is perhaps the most important risk factor to consider for patients with cardiac diseases prior to any surgical therapy. There is an increased likelihood of arrhythmia during anesthesia and stress, as well as possible myocardial suppression secondary to anesthesia. Reports have indicated that the first 6 months after a myocardial infarction is the period of highest risk for a recurrence. Surgery during this period carried a 50 to 80% risk of recurrent myocardial infarction, with an extremely high mortality. More recent studies have placed the incidence at 18 to 22%, undoubtedly the result of improved anesthetic and surgical techniques and better perioperative monitoring of patients. The mortality of patients with perioperative myocardial infarction has remained high, even in the more recent studies. The mortality is especially high if the new infarct occurs in the same area as the previous infarction. Because about half of perioperative myocardial infarctions are clinically silent, with no symptoms of chest pain, careful perioperative monitoring and serial cardiac evaluations are necessary to minimize unexpected complications.

After the 6-month period, the incidence of

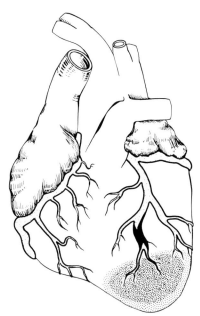

Figure 6–1. Schematic representation of a myocardial infarction demonstrating blockage of a coronary artery and subsequent myocardial ischemia and necrosis.

perioperative myocardial infarction decreases progressively. After the first 12 months, the incidence stabilizes at approximately 5%.

The data available are mostly derived from patients undergoing major surgical procedures, and it is difficult to extrapolate these data to dental stress. It is probably best to err on the side of safety in these instances to avoid unnecessary morbidity and mortality.

DENTAL EVALUATION

Dental evaluation should include a detailed history listing the dates of all of the myocardial infarctions the patient may have had. The most recent infarction is of particular interest, because it largely dictates the feasibility of elective dental therapy. The dentist should be particularly alerted to myocardial infarctions within the past year because they increase the danger of surgical procedures.

The history should also list complications after myocardial infarctions. A history of substernal chest pain should alert the dentist to the possibility of angina. Dyspnea, orthopnea, paroxysmal nocturnal dyspnea, and peripheral edema may indicate congestive heart failure. Palpitations or syncope should suggest possible arrhythmias or conduction abnormalities.

The dental evaluation should also include a brief discussion with the patient's physician, when necessary, to define the medical status of the patient. The most recent physical examination, electrocardiogram, and chest roentgenogram are all important sources of information to have prior to the initiation of dental therapy. Any abnormalities should be appropriately addressed.

DENTAL MANAGEMENT

The dental management of the patient with a previous myocardial infarction depends on the severity and course of the infarction. Patients who have undergone an uncomplicated acute myocardial infarction are able to tolerate procedures (types I to IV) of short duration at any time following the event. More stressful procedures are best postponed until 6 months after the infarct. Physician consultation is suggested. There appears to be no contraindication to the use of epinephrine in concentrations of 1:100,000 in local anesthesia in these patients. However, protocols to minimize the use of vasoconstrictors should be employed. Good patient-dentist communication, stress reduction, and monitoring are essential for the safe management of the postinfarction patient.

Patients who have undergone a complicated myocardial infarction or whose recovery is unstable require a more conservative approach for the first 6 months after the infarction. These patients can undergo dental examinations without special protocol (type I procedures) and urgent, simple operative procedures (type II) after consultation with the patient's physician. All other dental treatment should be deferred until the patient has been stable for at least 6 months. Patients in this group with a dental emergency should be treated as conservatively as possible. However, if extraction or surgery is required, the patient's physician should be consulted. Stress minimization protocols should be used. If possible, the procedures are best performed in a hospital setting, with constant monitoring.

Patients Who Have Had Myocardial Infarctions 6 to 12 Months Before Proposed Dental Treatment

These patients can undergo dental examinations (type I procedures) without special protocols. Nonsurgical procedures (types II to III) and simple surgical procedures (type IV) can be carried out after consultation with the patient's physician. With these patients, care should be taken to minimize stress. Longer procedures should be divided into several shorter ones, and adjunctive sedation techniques should be used. Early morning appointments may be desirable.

Although no data specific for dentistry are available, morbidity and mortality associated with nondental surgery are still increased during this period. Therefore, it may be prudent to defer moderate to advanced dental surgical procedures (types V to VI) until the patient has been stable for at least 12 months after the myocardial infarction.

Patients Who Have Had Their Most Recent Myocardial Infarctions More Than a Year Ago

It is important to remember that these patients still have significant coronary artery disease despite their stability during the past year. They can, however, more readily tolerate nondental surgical procedures than patients with more recent myocardial infarctions. They can undergo dental examinations (type I procedures) and nonsurgical and simple surgical procedures (types II to IV), with appropriate attention to sedation techniques and minimization of stress. Moderate and advanced surgical procedures (types V to VI) should be undertaken only after careful consultation with their physicians.

Elective hospitalization to permit adequate monitoring should be considered for all advanced dental surgery (type VI procedures) and is mandatory if general anesthesia is required.

■ Examples of Dental Evaluation and Management

EVALUATION

Patient 1. A 42-year-old man who has had a "heart attack" presents for dental treatment. He has a history of hypertension dating back to age 26 and had a myocardial infarction at age 40. He has been stable ever since, with no symptoms of angina, congestive heart failure, or arrhythmia. He has been working full time and has been active in a cardiac rehabilitation program. He was last seen by his physician 4

months ago and had an electrocardiogram that was described as "unchanged." He is on nifedipine, 30 mg qid, for hypertension. His dental needs include a full range of restorative procedures (types I to III), simple extractions, periodontal surgery, and the removal of a third molar vertical bony impaction.

On examination, he has a blood pressure of 130/84 and a regular pulse of 80 bpm.

Patient 2. A 58-year-old man with two prior myocardial infarctions presents for dental treatment. He has a history of adult-onset diabetes mellitus but has been stable on diet alone. His most recent myocardial infarction occurred 8 months ago. He saw his physician 3 months ago and had a normal examination and a normal electrocardiogram. He is asymptomatic and is on no medications. His dental needs are similar to those of Patient 1.

On examination, his blood pressure is 110/80, and he has a regular pulse at 80 bpm.

Patient 3. A 60-year-old man with a history of three myocardial infarctions presents for dental therapy. He has a long history of hypertension and has had myocardial infarctions in the past 4 years. His most recent infarction was 4 months ago. He was last examined by his physician 2 weeks ago. His last electrocardiogram was taken a month ago and was described as "basically unchanged." He is on digoxin, 0.25 mg daily, furosemide (Lasix), 40 mg bid, and diltiazem, 10 mg qid. His dental needs are similar to those of Patients 1 and 2.

On examination, he has a blood pressure of 160/94 and a regular pulse of 92 bpm.

MANAGEMENT

Patient 1. This patient falls into the low-risk category. It has been more than a year since the myocardial infarction. He has no major complications from the infarction, and his hypertension is under good control. Routine dental care (types I to III nonsurgical procedures) can be performed using normal protocol. Because of the underlying ischemic heart disease, stress should be minimized. Long sessions should be divided into shorter sessions. When appropriate, sedation techniques should be used (Chap. 51). Simple and moderately advanced surgical procedures (types IV and V) can be performed in an outpatient setting after appropriate medical consultation. Hospitalization should be considered for advanced surgical procedures (type VI), such as the removal of the difficult impaction. For the anxious patient, hospitalization may be necessary for extensive periodontal procedures (type V surgery).

Patient 2. This patient has had no major complications after the myocardial infarction. A pre-existing medical condition, diabetes mellitus, is under good control. He is at slightly increased risk because the myocardial infarction is fairly recent. Following a thorough dental examination using normal protocol, the dentist should consult with the patient's physician before the initiation of therapy. Advanced surgical procedures and nonemergency dental care should be deferred until 1 year after the myocardial infarction. A reasonable dental therapeutic plan would therefore include the excavation of all deep carious lesions, the institution of endodontic therapy for devitalized teeth, and the completion of the hygienic phase of periodontal therapy (oral hygiene instruction, prophylaxis, scaling, and root planing). Stress should be minimized by resorting to short sessions and appropriate sedation techniques (Chap. 51). If local anesthetics are necessary, a preparation without a vasoconstrictor is pre-

ferred. If simple extractions (type IV procedures) have to be done, a medical consultation should be obtained. Moderately advanced and advanced surgical procedures (types V and VI), when absolutely indicated, should be performed in a hospital. One year after the infarct the deferred prosthetic and surgical procedures can be completed.

The patient also has diabetes mellitus, and appropriate attention should be paid to the management of this underlying disease (Chap. 14).

Patient 3. This patient is within 6 months of his most recent myocardial infarction. He has hypertension that is poorly controlled and has occasional angina. All surgical and advanced restorative procedures are contraindicated. Palliative therapy should be carried out after consultation with the patient's physician. Any emergency surgery should be performed in a hospital setting with close medical monitoring. Choices for local anesthetics, analgesics, and sedation techniques should be discussed with the patient's physician.

SUMMARY TABLE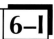

Myocardial Infarction: General Information

DEFINITION

A myocardial infarction (MI) is irreversible myocardial damage as the result of prolonged ischemic injury.

CAUSE

It is most commonly the result of progressive coronary artery disease secondary to atherosclerosis.

PREVALENCE

It affects 1.3% of all patients above age 30 and 10% of all patients above age 40.

CLINICAL PRESENTATION

Severe chest pain is present in the substernal or left precordial area, ±* left arm or jaw radiation.

Dyspnea, palpitations, nausea, and vomiting may also be part of the presentation.

DIAGNOSIS

This includes the clinical presentation, electrocardiographic evidence, and cardiac enzyme studies.

COMPLICATIONS

These include arrhythmias, congestive heart failure, and angina.

---

*±, with or without.

SUMMARY TABLE  6–II

Medical Evaluation of the Patient with Past Myocardial Infarction Undergoing Elective Surgery

Presence of other significant cardiovascular pathology and increased surgical risk:
  Congestive heart failure
  Arrhythmias
  Angina
  Hypertension

Time interval from myocardial infarction (MI) as a predictor of surgical risk:
  <6 mo post-MI   18–22% overall mortality with surgery and general anesthesia
  6–12 mo post-MI   10% overall mortality with surgery and general anesthesia
  >12 mo post-MI   5% overall mortality with surgery and general anesthesia

Individual assessment of the cardiovascular stability of the patient

Other risk factors:
  Diabetes mellitus
  Smoking
  Hypercholesterolemia and hyperlipidemia

SUMMARY TABLE 6–III

Dental Evaluation of the Patient with Previous Myocardial Infarction

History of past myocardial infarction and time elapsed since this event

Presence of other cardiovascular pathology:
  Congestive heart failure
  Arrhythmia
  Angina
  Hypertension

Presence of other risk factors:
  Hyperlipidemia
  Hypercholesterolemia

Medical consultation

Dental Management of the Patient with a Previous Myocardial Infarction

TIME INTERVAL	PROCEDURES	MANAGEMENT
≤6 mo post-MI	I	Normal protocol
	II	Defer if possible, medical consultation, minimization of stress, ±* adjunctive sedation techniques
	III–VI	Contraindicated—palliative therapy, if possible, all emergency surgery should be performed in hospital setting
6 mo–1 yr post-MI	I	Normal protocol
	II, III, IV	Defer if possible, medical consultation, minimization of stress, adjunctive sedation techniques
	V, VI	Defer if possible; hospitalization recommended
>1 yr post-MI	I	Normal protocol
	II–IV	Minimization of stress, sedation techniques
	V–VI	Medical consultation, ± hospitalization; hospitalization mandatory for general anesthesia

For specific management of other cardiovascular problems, see appropriate chapters.

*±, with or without.

7

Congestive Heart Failure

Heart failure is the result of the inability of the heart to deliver an adequate supply of oxygenated blood to meet the metabolic demands of the body. Congestive heart failure indicates significant cardiac dysfunction. Surgical procedures among heart patients, including dental procedures, are associated with high morbidity and mortality; the increase in risk depends on the severity of the congestive heart failure. The dentist should therefore be familiar with the clinical signs and symptoms of congestive heart failure and the possible precipitating factors.

The medications used in the treatment of congestive heart failure can also complicate dental management of the patient. It is therefore important to have an integrated plan prior to the initiation of dental therapy.

MEDICAL EVALUATION

Medical evaluation of the patient with congestive heart failure involves recognition of the clinical symptoms, evaluation of the precipitating factors, and treatment of the correctable causes of congestive heart failure. Patients with congestive heart failure often complain of shortness of breath or dyspnea (Summary Table 7–I), particularly with exertion. This may severely limit the patient's activities and is often worse when the patient lies flat (orthopnea). Patients may therefore give a history of having to sleep on several pillows. Shortness of breath can cause the patient to awaken at night (paroxysmal nocturnal dyspnea). Dyspnea is primarily a consequence of pulmonary congestion resulting from failure of the left side of the heart. Patients may also have symptoms associated with failure of the right side of the heart. These symptoms result from elevation of pressures in the right ventricle and right atrium and cause discomfort in the right upper abdomen because of hepatic congestion and enlargement. Similarly, the patient may notice swelling and fluid accumulation in the ankles (peripheral edema) and in the abdomen (ascites).

Heart failure can result from many disorders (Summary Table 7–II). In general, the imbalance between metabolic demands and the ability of the heart to deliver oxygenated blood results in symptoms of heart failure. Such an imbalance can be the result of decreased myocardial function, increased resistance to cardiac output, increased volume load, or increased metabolic demands.

Poor myocardial function is most commonly the result of ischemic heart disease. Coronary artery disease with myocardial infarction can result in significant compromises in myocardial function. Infiltrative diseases such as amyloidosis and metabolic disorders such as severe hypothyroidism are only rarely associated with myocardial dysfunction. Pharmacologic agents such as beta-blocking agents can lead to suppression of myocardial contractility and heart failure.

Increased resistance to cardiac output may also compromise cardiac performance. Uncontrolled and persistent hypertension accounts for up to 75% of the identifiable causes of congestive heart failure. Other causes include significant aortic stenosis and, rarely, coarctation of the aorta.

An increase in the volume of blood that the heart has to pump greatly increases the workload of the heart and can result in compromised cardiac performance. Patients with mitral or aortic regurgitation or atrial or ventricular septal defects with significant shunts may not be able to handle the increased volume load and can progress to congestive heart failure. Patients with chronic renal failure and excessive fluid retention can also present with congestive heart failure.

Less commonly, heart failure may be the result of the inability of the heart to meet excessive metabolic demands. This is encountered in patients with severe anemia and thyrotoxicosis.

The medical evaluation of the patient with

congestive heart failure emphasizes the identification of correctable causes of the disease and an assessment of the severity of the condition (Summary Table 7–III). The severity of the heart failure is usually assessed on the basis of presenting symptoms, physical examination, an electrocardiogram, and a chest roentgenogram. Physical findings consistent with congestive heart failure include cardiac enlargement, elevated neck veins, rales, and a third heart sound. Electrocardiographic findings reveal abnormalities in cardiac rhythm and evidence of old infarctions or ongoing ischemia (Chap. 5). The chest roentgenogram is useful in determining heart size and the presence of pulmonary congestion (Fig. 7–1). These examinations provide invaluable information about the heart failure and allow the physician to initiate necessary therapy.

MEDICAL MANAGEMENT

In the management of patients with congestive heart failure, factors that can precipitate or aggravate failure are eliminated (Summary Table 7–IV). Disorders such as anemia, thyrotoxicosis, hypertension, and arrhythmias should be corrected. Patients with valvular stenoses or regurgitations should have the lesions surgically corrected when appropriate. After the correction of reversible lesions, treatment of congestive heart failure can begin.

Patients with mild congestive heart failure are managed with bed rest and salt-restricted diets. Bed rest improves venous return and heart function and is an effective first step in therapy. Salt restriction is designed to minimize salt and volume overload in patients with marginal cardiac reserve. Whereas 8 to 10 g of salt are included in the normal American diet, patients with congestive heart failure should be brought down to about 4 to 5 g daily by eliminating added salt.

A variety of diuretics of varying potency can be used for patients with congestive heart failure to reduce excess extracellular fluid and salt. Patients with mild to moderate failure are often treated with a mild diuretic such as a thiazide. Numerous thiazide preparations are available and differ mostly in duration of action: chlorothiazide and hydrochlorothiazide are short-acting, whereas trichlormethiazide and chlorthalidone are longer acting and can usually be administered once daily. Patients with moderate to severe failure may not respond adequately to thiazides and may therefore require more potent diuretics such as furosemide (Lasix), ethacrynic acid (Edecrine), or bumetanide (Bumex). Potassium-sparing diuretics such as spironolactone (Aldactone) and triamterene (Dyrenium) may be used either singly or in combination with other diuretics. These agents are not potent diuretics but do conserve potassium. The recommended dosages of the diuretics commonly used in the treatment of congestive heart failure are listed in Summary Table 7–V.

In addition to diuretics, cardiac glycosides such as digoxin (Lanoxin) are often used to

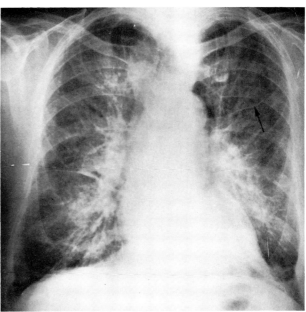

Figure 7–1. Chest roentgenogram demonstrating the presence of pulmonary congestion (note lack of clarity) and enlargement of the heart. (From Rabin, C. B., and Baron, M. G.: Radiology of the chest. Baltimore, Williams & Wilkins, 1979.)

improve myocardial contractility. Digoxin is the most commonly prescribed cardiac glycoside and is given in dosages ranging from 0.125 to 0.5 mg daily. Digitoxin and digitalis leaf are less frequently used because their absorption and excretion are more variable (Summary Table 7–VI).

Afterload reducing agents (Summary Table 7–VIII) are also important for the management of patients with severe congestive heart failure. Converting enzyme inhibitors (captopril, enalapril, or lisinopril) are frequently used. Vasodilators, agents used primarily for control of hypertension, have been found useful in the treatment of refractory congestive heart failure. The most commonly used vasodilators are hydralazine (Apresoline) and prazosin (Minipress), which are used primarily in cases of moderate to severe congestive heart failure.

The medications used in the treatment of congestive heart failure all have side effects that can complicate patient management (Summary Table 7–VIII). Diuretics such as thiazides, furosemide, and ethacrynic acid can lead to dehydration and hypokalemia. Hypokalemia is particularly a concern with patients on digitalis preparations, because it markedly enhances arrhythmias associated with digitalis excess. The potassium-sparing diuretics are usually not potent enough to cause dehydration, but their use can result in excessive retention of potassium and cardiac arrhythmia. Cardiac glycosides such as digoxin can cause significant toxicity with early symptoms of anorexia, nausea, vomiting, and visual disturbances. These symptoms of toxicity are important to recognize, because life-threatening arrhythmias can be associated with excessive levels of cardiac glycosides. Vasodilators can cause orthostatic hypotension; patients may complain of light-headedness and dizziness or may actually faint with abrupt changes of position. These patients should be instructed not to stand up from a sitting or lying position too abruptly.

The dentist should be aware of these potential complications and tailor dental management appropriately.

DENTAL EVALUATION

Patients can have varying degrees of congestive heart failure and can be grouped into the following risk categories (Summary Table 7–IX).

Patients at Low Risk

The patient with a history of mild congestive heart failure who is asymptomatic on therapy is at low risk for complications during dental therapy if there are no other complicating factors. The patient is probably on a mild diuretic such as a thiazide with or without digitalis. Prior to the start of dental treatment, the dentist should establish that the patient has had a medical evaluation within the past 12 months, is on a stable medical regimen, and has normal blood pressure, pulse rate, and rhythm. Complicating cardiac factors such as recent myocardial infarction, angina, arrhythmia, or persistent hypertension place these patients in higher risk categories (Chaps. 4 through 9). Other complicating factors such as valvular heart disease (Chap. 11), hyperthyroidism (Chap. 16), or severe anemia (Chap. 25) should be addressed separately.

Patients at Moderate Risk

Patients with moderately severe congestive heart failure have intermittent symptoms despite medical therapy. Although they are usually asymptomatic at rest, these individuals may develop dyspnea with significant exertion, are usually on potent diuretics and digitalis, and may be on an afterload reducing agent. A detailed history is crucial, and any other complicating cardiovascular factors should be attended to accordingly. It is important to determine the serum potassium level in patients on potent diuretics, especially if they are on digitalis, to minimize the likelihood of precipitating arrhythmias. Concern should also be raised if patients have symptoms suggesting digitalis toxicity, such as nausea, vomiting, visual disturbances, or palpitations.

Patients at High Risk

Patients with severe congestive heart failure have symptoms in spite of escalating doses of medications. They are usually on large doses of potent diuretics such as furosemide, ethacrynic acid, or bumetanide. They are often on an afterload reducing agent or digoxin, and may also be on vasodilators such as hydralazine or prazosin. They have frequent episodes of dyspnea, orthopnea, paroxysmal nocturnal dyspnea, and peripheral edema. On examination, they may be visibly tachypneic. Clubbing of the fingers and cyanosis of the nail beds may be evident (Fig. 7–2). These patients often have other complicating factors such as

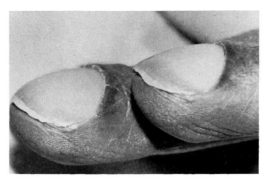

Figure 7–2. Clubbing of the fingers and cyanosis of the nail beds evident in a patient with congestive heart failure.

hypertension (Chap. 3), recent or multiple myocardial infarctions (Chap. 6), arrhythmias (Chap. 9), conduction abnormalities (Chaps. 8, 9, and 10), or valvular heart disease (Chap. 11), and are at high risk for complications during dental procedures.

DENTAL MANAGEMENT

General Guidelines

Certain general principles are applicable to the management of all patients with congestive heart failure (Summary Table 7–X). After carefully assessing the cardiac history of the patient, efforts should be made to minimize stress, limit the use of cardiac stimulants, and improve the medical status.

Whenever possible, lengthy procedures should be spread over several shorter appointments. Adjunctive sedation techniques should be considered, when appropriate (Chap. 51).

In general, the use of epinephrine should be minimized among patients with underlying cardiac compromises, because arrhythmia may become a significant problem.

Specific Guidelines

Patients at Low Risk

An asymptomatic patient with a past history of mild congestive heart failure and no other complicating factors can undergo nonsurgical procedures (types I to III) and simple surgical procedures (type IV) using normal protocols. Prior to moderate and advanced surgical procedures (types V and VI), the patient's physician should be consulted, and adjunctive sedation techniques may be used.

Patients at Moderate Risk

A medical consultation should be obtained prior to elective dental treatment among these patients to ensure that their medical status is optimal. Hypokalemia or digitalis excess should be corrected. Nonsurgical and simple surgical procedures (types I to IV) can be performed with normal protocol, using adjunctive sedation techniques, when appropriate. For moderate to advanced surgical procedures (types V and VI), hospitalization is recommended for optimal monitoring during the perioperative period.

Patients at High Risk

The patient's physician must be consulted prior to dental treatment. The patient should have a recent medical evaluation and a serum potassium determination to ensure optimal medical management. Nonsurgical and simple surgical procedures should be performed with attention to minimizing stress and limiting the use of epinephrine. Adjunctive sedation technique can be used when appropriate. Hospitalization is required for moderate and advanced surgical procedures (types V and VI). For patients with intractable congestive heart failure, it is prudent to avoid moderate to advanced elective surgical procedures when possible.

Substantive changes in the dental treatment plan must be considered. Advanced periodontal surgery and complex fixed prosthetics are generally contraindicated. Palliative cure, including possible extraction of questionable teeth and removable prosthetic management, may be advisable.

■ Examples of Dental Evaluation and Management

EVALUATION

Patient 1. A 55-year-old man with a history of mild hypertension for 18 years gives a history of having been on digoxin and furosemide since his myocardial infarction 3 years ago. He has been totally asymptomatic since and is not aware of the indications for the medications. He was last seen by his physician 4 months ago. On examination, his blood pressure is 130/88 and his pulse rate is 64 bpm and regular. He denies dyspnea, orthopnea, paroxysmal nocturnal dyspnea, or peripheral edema in the past year. He has advanced periodontal disease and requires multiple extractions, periodontal surgery, and a prosthesis.

Patient 2. A 61-year-old woman gives a history of angina and two myocardial infarctions in the past 5 years. Her last myocardial infarction was 14 months ago, and she had a long hospitalization. She was started on digoxin, quinidine, and furosemide for reasons not clear to the patient. She has been having intermittent episodes of ankle edema and dyspnea on exertion but denies orthopnea, paroxysmal nocturnal dyspnea, or palpitations. She has rare episodes of angina with exertion that respond to sublingual nitroglycerin. Her dental needs are the same as those of Patient 1.

Consultation with her physician reveals that she had multifocal ventricular premature contractions and pulmonary edema complicating her last myocardial infarction. She was last examined 3 months ago, when she was clinically doing well. Her electrocardiogram and chest x-ray were stable. Her electrolytes showed a potassium level of 2.1 mEq/liter. Her physician believes that her clinical status is stable and that she can undergo elective dental treatment that does not require general anesthesia.

Examination reveals a blood pressure of 120/76 and a regular pulse of 64 bpm.

Patient 3. A 41-year-old woman with a history of rheumatic heart disease has had increasing difficulties with dyspnea, orthopnea, paroxysmal nocturnal dyspnea, and peripheral edema over the past 4 months. Despite digoxin and increasing doses of furosemide and captopril, she has had progressive symptoms. She has had atrial fibrillation for the past 10 years and has been on sodium warfarin (Coumadin). She is scheduled for mitral valvular replacement and is referred to the dentist because of extensive periodontal disease. Her dental needs are the same as those of the previous two patients.

Consultation with her physician reveals that the patient was last examined a week previously and was found to have moderately severe congestive heart failure resulting from critical mitral stenosis. Her electrocardiogram showed atrial fibrillation, and her chest x-ray confirmed the clinical impression of congestive heart failure. Her electrolyte levels were normal at that time, and her prothrombin time was 19 seconds, with a control of 11 seconds.

Patient 4. A 50-year-old man who has had a large anterior myocardial infarction gives a history of progressive shortness of breath over the past year. He is currently on digoxin, large doses of ethacrynic acid, and prazosin but has

continued to have orthopnea, progressive peripheral edema, and dyspnea, even at rest. He is referred because of severe periodontal disease, and his dental needs are the same as those of the previous patients.

Consultation with his physician confirms that he has severe congestive heart failure. His last examination took place 2 months ago, when he was found to have moderately severe heart failure. His electrocardiogram and his chest x-ray were unchanged from his previous studies. His electrolyte levels were normal.

On examination, his blood pressure is 106/70 and his pulse is regular at 94 bpm. He is tachypneic at rest.

MANAGEMENT

Patient 1. This patient is at low risk for complications during dental therapy. He has been totally asymptomatic since his myocardial infarction 3 years ago and does not have other active cardiac problems. He can undergo all nonsurgical and simple surgical procedures (types I to IV)—including caries control, simple extractions, bridge placement, prophylaxis, scaling, and curettage—using normal protocols. Multiple extractions and periodontal surgery (types V and VI) may be accomplished using adjunctive sedation techniques.

Patient 2. This patient has intermittent symptoms of congestive heart failure secondary to coronary artery disease. She has angina and is on quinidine for ventricular arrhythmia, but both conditions appear to be quiescent at this time. Of some importance is the fact that she has had a low serum potassium level in the past. It is important to determine her serum potassium concentration again prior to elective dental treatment. Hypokalemia should be treated, because it may precipitate arrhythmia, especially in a patient on digoxin. The patient is at moderate risk for complications during therapy.

Lengthy procedures should be spread over several shorter appointments. Adjunctive sedation techniques should be used when appropriate.

Caries control, simple extractions, bridge placement, prophylaxis, scaling, and curettage may be performed using N_2O_2-O_2 inhalation sedation or oral diazepam (Chap. 51). Moderate to advanced surgical procedures, including multiple extractions and periodontal surgery, should be performed in a hospital to provide optimal monitoring.

Patient 3. This complicated case involves severe congestive heart failure and many other factors that would modify dental management. In many ways, congestive heart failure in this patient is the least complicated aspect of her management. Of great importance is the recognition that she needs prophylactic antibiotics prior to *any* dental procedures. In view of her extensive periodontal disease and the anticipated need for mitral valve replacement, full-mouth extraction is the appropriate dental treatment. The standard regimen is a convenient way of providing antibiotic prophylaxis, but an alternate regimen should be considered (Chap. 11) in view of the extensive periodontal disease and the anticipated trauma involved in full-mouth extraction (type VI procedure).

The patient should be hospitalized for the procedure. Medical consultation is mandatory. Her coagulopathy from Coumadin therapy needs to be corrected prior to surgery. Coumadin should be discontinued 2 days prior to the procedure, and the prothrombin time should be determined on the day of the procedure. The prothrombin time should be less than 1.5 times the control value. Rapid correction of the anticoagulation can be accomplished by the use of fresh-frozen plasma. The oral anticoagulant can be resumed the evening after surgery (Chap. 26).

Patient 4. This patient has severe congestive heart failure that partly limits the dental therapeutic options. Medical consultation should be obtained, and stress should be minimized.

Conservative caries control, prophylaxis, scaling, and curettage (types I to IV procedures) should be performed using adjunctive sedation techniques. Complex prosthetic treatment plans, multiple extractions, and periodontal surgery should be avoided if possible. All moderate and advanced surgical procedures (types V and VI) require hospitalization.

SUMMARY TABLE

General Information on Congestive Heart Failure

DEFINITION
Congestive heart failure is the inability of the heart to deliver an adequate supply of blood to meet metabolic demands.

SIGNIFICANCE
It indicates significant cardiac dysfunction; stressful procedures are associated with increased morbidity and mortality.

SYMPTOMS
Left-sided heart failure:
  Dyspnea (shortness of breath), especially on exertion
  Orthopnea (shortness of breath with recumbency)
  Paroxysmal nocturnal dyspnea

Right-sided heart failure:
  Peripheral edema
  Hepatic congestion
  Ascites

GOALS OF THERAPY
Identify and correct reversible causes.

Avoid possible precipitating factors.

Control symptoms with medical therapy.

Causes of Congestive Heart Failure

DECREASED MYOCARDIAL FUNCTION
Ischemic heart disease
Infiltrative diseases (e.g., amyloidosis)
Metabolic disorders (e.g., hypothyroidism)
Pharmacologic suppression (e.g., propranolol)

INCREASED VASCULAR RESISTANCE
Hypertension (75% of cases)
Aortic stenosis
Coarctation of the aorta

INCREASED BLOOD VOLUME
Valvular insufficiency (e.g., aortic or mitral insufficiency)
Atrial or ventricular septal defect
Chronic renal failure with fluid retention

EXCESSIVE METABOLIC DEMAND
Severe anemia
Thyrotoxicosis

Medical Evaluation of the Patient with Congestive Heart Failure

Identification of cause of congestive heart failure (Summary Table 7–II)

Assess severity of congestive heart failure:
   Symptoms
   Electrocardiogram (to assess rhythm and evidence of ischemia or infarction)
   Chest x-ray (to assess heart size and pulmonary congestion)

Medical Management of the Patient with Congestive Heart Failure

Correct reversible causes of congestive heart failure.

Management of the patient with mild congestive heart failure:
   Bed rest
   Salt restriction to 4 g/day
   Mild diuretic (Summary Table 7–V)

Management of the patient with moderate congestive heart failure:
   More potent diuretics (Summary Table 7–V)
   Digitalis preparations (Summary Table 7–VI)

Management of the patient with severe congestive heart failure:
   All of the above
   Addition of afterload-reducing agents (Summary Table 7–VII), converting enzyme inhibitors, or vasodilators

Diuretics Commonly Used in the Management of Congestive Heart Failure

PREPARATION	TRADE NAME	DAILY DOSAGE (mg)
Mild Diuretics		
Hydrochlorothiazide	HydroDiuril, Esidrix	50–100
Chlorothiazide	Diuril	500–1000
Longer-acting Diuretics		
Methyclothiazide	Enduron	2.5–100
Chlorthalidone	Hygroton	50–100
Metolazone	Zaroxolyn, Diulo	5–10
Trichlormethiazide	Naqua, Metahydrin	2–4
Potent Diuretics		
Furosemide	Lasix	20–80
Ethacrynic acid	Edecrin	50–200
Bumetanide	Bumex	1–5
Potassium-sparing Diuretics		
Spironolactone	Aldactone	25–200
Triamterene	Dyrenium	50–200
Amiloride		
Combination Diuretics		
Spironolactone and hydrochlorothiazide	Aldactazide	600–1600
Triamterene and hydrochlorothiazide	Dyazide	75–300
Amiloride and hydrochlorothiazide	Moduretic	1–4

Cardiac Glycosides Commonly Used in the Treatment of Congestive Heart Failure

PREPARATION	TRADE NAME	DAILY DOSAGE (mg)
Digoxin	Lanoxin	0.125–0.5
Digitoxin	Crystodigin	0.05–0.3
Digitalis		100–200

SUMMARY TABLE **7–VII**

Afterload-Reducing Agents in the Treatment of Congestive Heart Failure

PREPARATION	TRADE NAME	DAILY DOSAGE (mg)
Converting Enzyme Inhibitor		
Captopril	Capoten	25–200
Enalopril	Vasotec	5–20
Lisinopril	Zestril, Prinivil	5–20
Vasodilator		
Hydralazine	Apresoline	100–200
Prazosin	Minipress	3–15
Terazosin	Hytrin	1–5

SUMMARY TABLE **7–VIII**

Complications of Drugs Commonly Used to Treat Congestive Heart Failure

DIURETICS

Hypokalemia: can be induced by thiazides, furosemide, and ethacrynic acid.

Dehydration: can be induced by all diuretics

Hyperkalemia: can be induced by potassium-sparing diuretics

Hyperuricemia: can be induced by all diuretics

CARDIAC GLYCOSIDE OVERDOSE

Gastrointestinal symptoms: anorexia, nausea, vomiting

Visual disturbances: blurring of vision and green or yellow tinging of images

Cardiac complications: life-threatening arrhythmia

VASODILATORS

Orthostatic hypotension: dizziness, light-headedness, or fainting with abrupt changes in position

SUMMARY TABLE

Dental Evaluation of the Patient with Congestive Heart Failure

PATIENT AT LOW RISK
History of mild congestive heart failure

Asymptomatic on therapy

Usually on mild diuretics, with or without cardiac glycosides

PATIENT AT MODERATE RISK
History of moderately severe congestive heart failure

Asymptomatic at rest, but may have symptoms with exertion

Usually on more potent diuretics and cardiac glycosides

PATIENT AT HIGH RISK
Symptomatic despite therapy

Often on escalating doses of medications, including vasodilators

SUMMARY TABLE

Dental Management of the Patient with Congestive Heart Failure

GENERAL GUIDELINES
Minimization of stress (shorter appointments, adjunctive sedation)
Limit use of epinephrine

SPECIFIC GUIDELINES

Risk Category	Procedures	Protocol
Low risk	I–IV	Normal protocol
	V–VI	Medical consultation ±* sedation (Chap. 51)
Moderate risk		Medical consultation; check potassium level of patients on diuretics
	I–IV	Normal protocol ± sedation ± hospitalization
High risk	V–VI	Medical consultation; recent medical evaluation; check potassium level of patients on diuretics
	I–IV	Sedation
	V–VI	Hospitalization
		Less complex dental treatment plans recommended

*±, with or without.

The Electrocardiogram

The electrocardiogram is a record of the electrical activities of the heart that provides significant information about the functioning of the heart. Although the subtleties of the interpretation of the electrocardiogram may not be important in the daily practice of dentistry, it is important to understand the information that can be generated by electrocardiograms.

THE NORMAL ELECTROCARDIOGRAM

Normal heart cells are charged, or "polarized," in the resting state. When stimulated, the cells "depolarize" and contract. The electrocardiogram records the electrical activities of the heart, as detected by electrodes on the skin (Summary Table 8–I). The normal sequence of electrical conduction begins in a part of the atrium called the sinoatrial node (Fig. 8–1). The electrical activity then reaches an area at the junction of the atria and ventricles called the atrioventricular node before traveling down the conducting system located in the interventricular septum (right and left bundle branches). The electrical impulse starting in the sinoatrial node causes depolarization of the atria (Fig. 8–2A) and produces the P wave. The electrical impulse then reaches the atrioventricular node, where there is a delay of about 0.10 seconds in the conduction, a delay represented in the electrocardiogram by the PR interval (Fig. 8–2B). The impulse then

travels down the conduction system in the interventricular septum and causes depolarization of the ventricles, which is represented by the QRS complex on the electrocardiogram (Fig. 8–2C). After the ventricular contraction, the myocardial cells repolarize, as reflected in the electrocardiogram by the T wave (Fig. 8–2D). Normally, the PR interval is less than 0.20 seconds, the QRS complex is less than 0.12 seconds, and the QT interval is less than 0.40 seconds (Summary Table 8–II).

A number of abnormalities of the heart function can be detected by changes in the electrocardiogram, including atrial arrhythmia; ventricular arrhythmia; myocardial ischemia, injury, or infarction; and conduction abnormalities.

ATRIAL ARRHYTHMIA

Atrial Premature Contraction (APC). A focus in the atrium other than the sinoatrial node may depolarize prematurely and result in an atrial premature contraction (Fig. 8–3A).

Paroxysmal Atrial Tachycardia (PAT). A focus in the atrium other than the sinoatrial node may also give rise to a series of rapid heartbeats at a regular rate of between 150 and 220 beats per minute (bpm) (Fig. 8–3B). This rapid heart rate is called paroxysmal atrial tachycardia.

Atrial Flutter. Electrical activity in the atrium in some instances can result in a rapid depo-

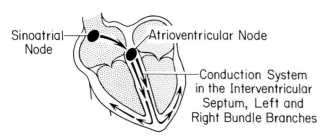

Figure 8–1. Conduction system in the normal heart.

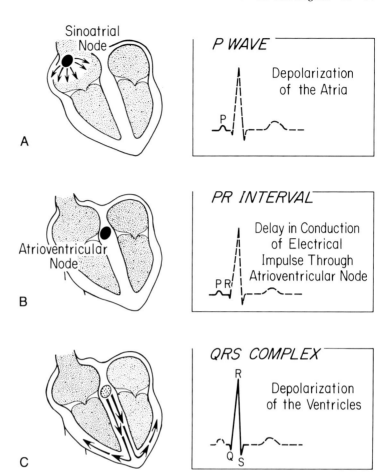

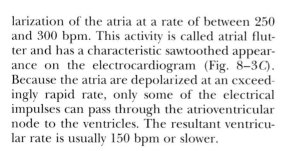

Figure 8–2. Components of the normal electrocardiogram.

larization of the atria at a rate of between 250 and 300 bpm. This activity is called atrial flutter and has a characteristic sawtoothed appearance on the electrocardiogram (Fig. 8–3C). Because the atria are depolarized at an exceedingly rapid rate, only some of the electrical impulses can pass through the atrioventricular node to the ventricles. The resultant ventricular rate is usually 150 bpm or slower.

Atrial Fibrillation (AF). In some disease states, the atria contract chaotically at a rate in excess of 300 bpm. This atrial fibrillation results in constant bombardment of the atrioventricular node, and only a small fraction of the impulses can pass through, producing a characteristic irregular ventricular rhythm (Fig. 8–3D).

VENTRICULAR ARRHYTHMIA

It is important to document abnormalities of ventricular rhythm, because they may lead to life-threatening arrhythmias. These rhythm disturbances can be detected on the electrocardiogram.

Ventricular Premature Contraction (VPC or PVC). In some disease states, electrical impul-

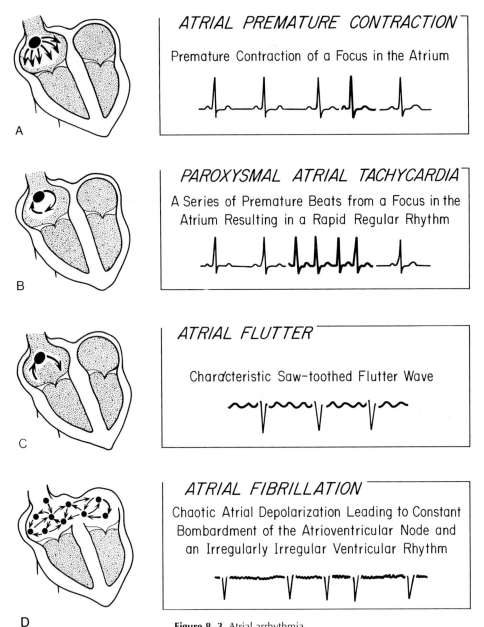

Figure 8–3. Atrial arrhythmia.

ses may originate from the ventricle prematurely, resulting in ventricular premature contractions. These can be differentiated from atrial premature contractions on the electrocardiogram. Because ventricular premature contractions arise from a ventricular focus, the electrical impulses do not travel down the normal conduction pathway. Therefore, on the electrocardiogram, a ventricular premature contraction is characterized by the absence of atrial activity (P wave) and a wide, bizarre-looking QRS complex (Fig. 8–4A).

Ventricular premature contractions may arise from one ventricular focus or from multiple foci. The latter gives rise to *multifocal ventricular premature contractions* (Fig. 8–4B). This is an important rhythm to recognize, because it often deteriorates into life-threatening ventricular arrhythmias.

Ventricular Tachycardia. In some disease states, salvos of ventricular premature contractions may occur. When three or more consecutive ventricular premature contractions occur at a rate of greater than 120/minute, the rhythm is termed "ventricular tachycardia"

(Fig. 8–4C). Ventricular tachycardia is generally considered the most serious of all tachycardias and may present with hypotension and syncope. On the electrocardiogram, it is characterized by wide ventricular complexes at a rate of between 120 to 200 bpm.

Ventricular Fibrillation. Chaotic electrical impulses originating from the ventricles produce ventricular fibrillation (Fig. 8–4D). Ventricular fibrillation is fatal unless it reverts spontaneously or is converted by a chest thump or cardioversion. On the electrocardiogram, it is characterized by chaotic ventricular rhythm.

ISCHEMIC HEART DISEASE

Myocardial Ischemia. When the heart muscle is receiving an inadequate blood supply,

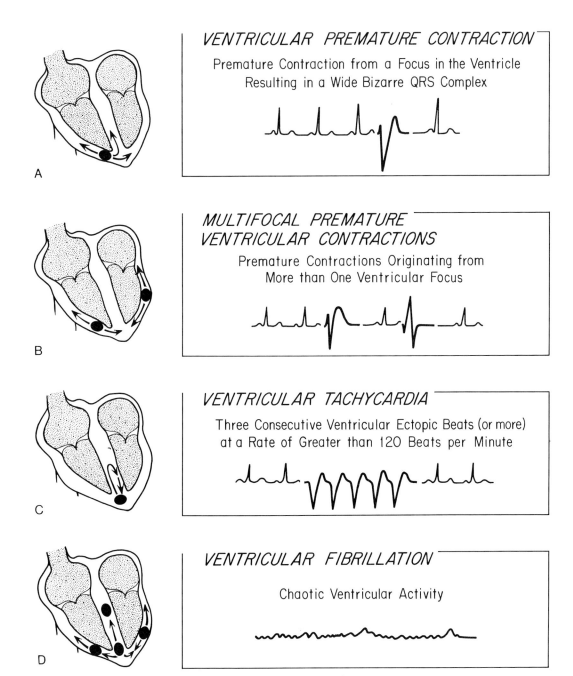

Figure 8–4. Ventricular arrhythmia.

ischemic changes can be detected on the electrocardiogram. Depression of the ST segment (Fig. 8–5A) and inversion of the T wave (Fig. 8–5B) are the most common manifestations of ischemic changes.

Myocardial Injury. In a patient with ongoing chest pain, the electrocardiogram can detect possible injury to the myocardial cells, which is most commonly represented by elevation of the ST segment and peaking of the T wave (Fig. 8–5C).

Myocardial Infarction. If the injury is significant, some myocardial cells die, and a myocardial infarction is said to have taken place. On the electrocardiogram, myocardial infarction is represented by the development of a Q wave (Fig. 8–5D).

CONDUCTION ABNORMALITIES

The electrocardiogram can also detect abnormalities in the conduction system of the heart and provide information about heart blocks.

First-Degree Heart Block. First-degree heart block reflects delays in the transmission of electrical impulses from the atria to the ventricles. On the electrocardiogram, it is character-

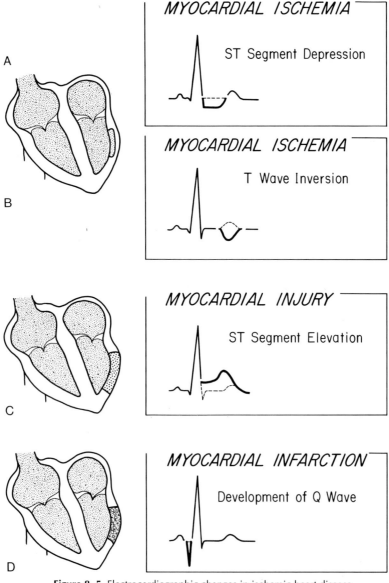

Figure 8–5. Electrocardiographic changes in ischemic heart disease.

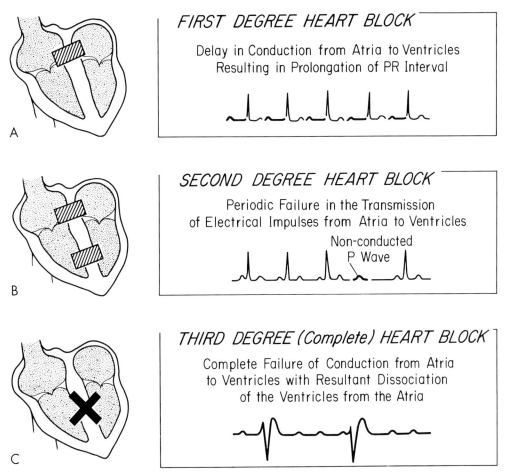

Figure 8–6. Conduction abnormalities.

ized by a prolongation of the PR interval to beyond 0.20 second (Fig. 8–6*A*). Despite the delay, all the electrical impulses from the atria are conducted to the ventricles.

Second-Degree Heart Block. Second-degree heart block is characterized by a periodic failure to transmit electrical impulses from the atria to the ventricles. It may be a result of diseases involving the atrioventricular node (type I, or Wenckebach heart block) or diseases affecting the conduction system (type II heart block). On the electrocardiogram, second-degree heart block is characterized by

the absence of a ventricular complex following some of the P waves (Fig. 8–6*B*).

Third-Degree (Complete) Heart Block. With complete heart block, none of the atrial electrical activities are transmitted to the ventricles, which contract at an exceedingly slow rate (between 20 and 40 bpm). On the electrocardiogram, there is evidence that the ventricles are contracting at a rate independent of the atrial rate (Fig. 8–6*C*). Patients with third-degree heart block may have significant hemodynamic compromise and often require the aid of a pacemaker.

SUMMARY TABLE **8–I**

Information Provided by the Electrocardiogram

NORMAL ELECTRICAL ACTIVITY OF THE HEART
ATRIAL TACHYARRHYTHMIAS
Atrial premature contraction (APC)

Paroxysmal atrial tachycardia (PAT)

Atrial flutter

Atrial fibrillation

VENTRICULAR TACHYARRHYTHMIAS
Ventricular premature contraction (VPC or PVC)

Ventricular tachycardia

Ventricular fibrillation

CONDUCTION ABNORMALITIES (BRADYARRHYTHMIAS)
First-, second-, and third-degree (complete) heart block

ISCHEMIC HEART DISEASE
Myocardial ischemia

Myocardial injury (acute)

Myocardial infarction

SUMMARY TABLE **8–II**

Normal Electrocardiographic Findings

P WAVE
Depolarization of the atria

PR INTERVAL
Delay of conduction through the atrioventricular node

QRS COMPLEX
Depolarization of the ventricles

T WAVE
Repolarization of the ventricles

Arrhythmia

A disturbance of the normal rhythm of the heart is called an arrhythmia. The abnormality may arise from disturbances in either the atria (resulting in atrial arrhythmias) or the ventricles (resulting in ventricular arrhythmia). Arrhythmias may be asymptomatic, detected only by routine examination and electrocardiograms, or the patient may have symptoms ranging from palpitations to syncope. Arrhythmias are often manifestations of underlying arteriosclerotic heart disease (Chap. 3).

Arrhythmias may be exacerbated by the stress and anxiety experienced during dental therapy. Significant arrhythmias increase the risk of angina, myocardial infarction, congestive heart failure, transient ischemic attacks, and cerebrovascular accidents. For the dentist, therefore, a knowledge of the types of arrhythmias and their associated risks, an understanding of the severity of a particular arrhythmia, and the ability to screen for potentially undiagnosed arrhythmias can greatly facilitate the management of patients.

Specific arrhythmias are defined in Chapter 8. This chapter focuses on the possible clinical presentations of various arrhythmias and the important warning signals that suggest specific dental management protocols.

MEDICAL EVALUATION AND MANAGEMENT

Sinus Tachycardia

A normal pulse rate should be regular and between 60 and 100 beats per minute, bpm. In response to stress, exercise, excitement, or anxiety, the pulse rate may exceed 100 bpm. This rapid regular rhythm is called sinus tachycardia. It is usually not associated with symptoms and does not require therapy.

Atrial Arrhythmias

As a general rule, atrial arrhythmias are seldom life-threatening but can occasionally cause symptoms and hemodynamic compromise.

The patient with atrial premature contractions (APC) may notice an occasional "skipped beat" but is usually asymptomatic and not compromised by the arrhythmia. Atrial premature contractions are the most common cause of an irregular pulse. They do not normally require therapy.

Patients with paroxysmal atrial tachycardia (PAT), atrial flutter, or atrial fibrillation have heart rates of 120 to 180 beats bpm. Healthy individuals can usually tolerate such rates, although they may complain of palpitations, dizziness, or lightheadedness. In patients with underlying heart disease, however, such arrhythmias can precipitate hypotension, chest pain, shortness of breath, or syncope. Patients with recurrent symptomatic atrial tachyarrhythmias are often on medications to prevent or control these arrhythmias when they occur. Digoxin, propranolol (Inderal), and quinidine (Quinaglute) are the most frequently used drugs. Occasionally, patients with atrial fibrillation are also placed on anticoagulants such as warfarin (Coumadin; Chap. 26) because of the complications of systemic emboli associated with this arrhythmia. Systemic emboli are particularly significant in patients with concurrent mitral stenosis.

Ventricular Arrhythmias

Ventricular arrhythmias are potentially life-threatening and often require chronic medical therapy.

The most common ventricular arrhythmia is the ventricular premature contraction (VPC or PVC). The patient may be asymptomatic or may only notice an occasional "skipping" or "fluttering sensation in the chest." Ventricular premature contractions occur rarely in normal individuals. Electrocardiographic evaluation usually reveals fewer than five premature contractions/minute from a single focus in the heart. Such contractions are benign and do not warrant medical intervention. However, frequent ventricular contractions (more than five to ten/minute) or ventricular premature contractions arising from several foci ("multifocal ventricular premature contractions") are more significant because they can degenerate into life-threatening ventricular tachycardia or ventricular fibrillations. Symptomatic patients with significant ventricular premature contractions are, therefore, treated medically on a chronic basis.

Clusters of three or more consecutive ventricular premature contractions at a rate of about 150 bpm produce a rhythm known as ventricular tachycardia. Patients with ventricular tachycardia often present with significant hemodynamic compromises. It is a life-threatening rhythm that frequently degenerates into ventricular fibrillation and is a medical emergency requiring in-hospital management.

Ventricular fibrillation is a totally chaotic ventricular rhythm that is always hemodynamically compromising. It may revert spontaneously but usually requires electrical cardioversion.

Patients with significant ventricular arrhythmias are usually on one or more antiarrhythmic agents, including quinidine sulfate (Quinaglute), propranolol (Inderal), procainamide (Pronestyl), phenytoin (Dilantin), mexiletene, or disopyramide (Norpace).

DENTAL EVALUATION

The evaluation should address the following issues:

1. Does the patient have symptoms of an ongoing arrhythmia?
2. Is the arrhythmia atrial or ventricular in origin?
3. What are the frequency and severity of the arrhythmia?
4. Is the patient currently receiving medications for the control of the arrhythmia?

The dental evaluation should include a detailed history and a careful determination of the patient's pulse rate and rhythm. The types of arrhythmias the patient has had, the frequency and severity of the arrhythmia, and the adequacy of control by therapy should all be carefully assessed.

Ideally, patients know their specific diagnosis and medications. More commonly, however, the patient merely reports symptoms such as "palpitations" or "skipped beats," which are common to several atrial and ventricular arrhythmias. In these instances, consultation with the patient's physician often clarifies the issue.

The physical examination should include a careful determination of the pulse rate and rhythm (Chap. 1). An anxious patient may have sinus tachycardia with a regular rhythm at a rate of more than 100 bpm. With rest, the pulse rate should slow to the normal range. Sustained sinus tachycardia at a rate in excess of 100 bpm is unusual in a patient at rest and may actually represent paroxysmal atrial tachycardia, atrial flutter, atrial fibrillation, or, rarely, ventricular tachycardia, all of which require immediate medical attention.

In addition to the rate, the regularity of the pulse should also be determined. The common causes of an irregular pulse include atrial premature contractions, ventricular premature contractions, and atrial fibrillation. In patients not known to have these arrhythmias, the detection of an irregular pulse warrants referral for medical evaluation and deferral of dental therapy. In patients known to have these arrhythmias, the detection of an irregular pulse is of less concern, but the physician should be consulted prior to dental treatment.

From a practical standpoint, patients with arrhythmias can be grouped into four categories, based on the risk of developing cardiovascular compromises.

Patients at Low Risk. Patients in this category have infrequent symptoms requiring no medications, such as atrial premature contractions, infrequent unifocal ventricular premature contractions, infrequent paroxysmal atrial tachycardia, infrequent paroxysmal flutter, or infrequent paroxysmal fibrillation.

Patients at Moderate Risk. These include patients with a history of atrial arrhythmias who are controlled and asymptomatic on medication. They may have a history of paroxysmal atrial tachycardia, paroxysmal atrial flutter, or paroxysmal atrial fibrillation, or atrial fibrillation with good rate control on medication. Although controlled, the pulse may continue to be irregular, even with the proper medication.

Patients at Significant Risk. These are patients with a history of ventricular arrhythmias who are controlled and asymptomatic on medications, including those with a history of significant ventricular premature contractions, ventricular tachycardia, or ventricular fibrillation.

Patients at High Risk. Patients with symptoms of palpitations, lightheadedness or syncope despite medications, undiagnosed arrhythmias, or heart rates in excess of 100 bpm at rest are at high risk and require immediate attention.

DENTAL MANAGEMENT

General Guidelines

In general, the major goals are to detect ongoing arrhythmias and to prevent exacerbations of underlying arrhythmias.

The stress associated with dental therapy can precipitate an arrhythmia, especially in patients with severe, pre-existing arrhythmias. Whenever feasible, lengthy procedures should be spread over several shorter appointments. Adjunctive sedation techniques should be considered when appropriate.

The use of epinephrine should be minimized in patients with significant underlying arrhythmias. Excessive amounts of epinephrine can precipitate life-threatening tachyarrhythmias.

The patient's physician should always be consulted to determine the nature of the arrhythmia and the adequacy of control.

Specific Guidelines

The dental management of the patient with arrhythmia differs according to the risk category.

Patients at Low Risk. In general, a normal dental operating protocol can be used for all nonsurgical and surgical procedures (types I to VI). The dentist may wish to use elective sedation techniques (Chap. 51) for moderate to advanced dental surgical procedures (types V and VI).

Patients at Moderate Risk. Patients with atrial arrhythmias who are asymptomatic on medications are at moderate risk. The dentist should check the pulse rate and rhythm. These patients can tolerate nonsurgical dental procedures (types I to III) using a normal protocol. Following medical consultation, sedation techniques may be considered for simple surgical procedures (type IV) and should be used for moderate to advanced surgical procedures (types V and VI). In addition, hospitalization should be considered for advanced dental surgical procedures (type VI).

Patients at Significant Risk. Patients with ventricular arrhythmias who are asymptomatic on medications are at significant risk. The dentist should check the pulse rate and rhythm. Oral examination (type I) can be performed using normal protocol. Following medical consultation, sedation techniques should be considered for nonsurgical and simple surgical dental procedures (types II to IV) and are mandatory for moderate and advanced surgical procedures (types V and VI). In addition, hospitalization for cardiac monitoring and advanced sedation techniques should be considered for moderate surgical procedures (type V) and is strongly recommended for advanced surgical procedures (type VI).

Patients at High Risk. These patients should be referred for medical evaluation prior to any dental therapy.

Finally, a patient may become symptomatic with a tachyarrhythmia during a dental procedure. The procedure should be stopped and the patient allowed to rest. The blood pressure (BP) and pulse rate should be closely followed. A patient with hemodynamic compromises or a sustained pulse rate of more than 150 bpm should receive immediate medical attention (Chap. 52). If the tachyarrhythmia resolves with rest, the ongoing dental procedure should be terminated as simply and as rapidly as possible. The patient should be referred for medical evaluation prior to the resumption of dental treatment.

ORAL FINDINGS

There are no oral findings associated with arrhythmias. Patients chronically on procainamide (Pronestyl) may rarely develop a lupus-like syndrome, with its associated oral findings (Chap. 36). Patients taking chronic doses of quinidine occasionally develop erythema multiforme (Fig. 9–1; Chap. 37). Xerostomia can be associated with disopyramide (Norpace), with an attendant increased risk for caries and periodontal disease.

■ Examples of Dental Evaluation and Management

EVALUATION

Patient 1. A 38-year-old woman with a history of "skipped beats" who was evaluated a year ago was told that she had a few "extra beats"

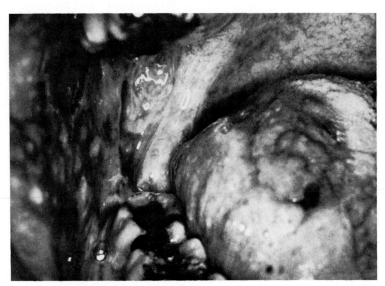

Figure 9–1. Erythema multiforme in a patient taking quinidine.

that should not cause problems. She was not started on medications. Her electrocardiogram shows rare unifocal ventricular premature contractions. Otherwise, her medical history is totally unremarkable. There is no past history of syncope. On examination, she has a pulse rate of 72 with a rare premature contraction causing slight irregularity of the pulse. Her BP is 110/70. She has extensive dental needs and requires moderate and advanced operative procedures, periodontal surgery, and several extractions.

Patient 2. A 48-year-old man who presented to his physician 2 years ago because of palpitations and dizziness was told that he had an irregular rhythm and was started on 0.25 mg of digoxin daily. Consultation with his physician reveals that he has atrial fibrillation. Cardiac evaluation failed to reveal any underlying lesions. He has been completely asymptomatic on the prescribed medical regimen and has no other medical problems. His most recent physical examination was 3 months ago, and his electrocardiogram at that time showed atrial fibrillation at a rate of 70 bpm. On examination now, he has an irregular pulse at a rate of 130 bpm. The pulse rate falls to 120 bpm after a period of rest. The patient is otherwise asymptomatic. His dental needs are the same as those of Patient 1.

Patient 3. A 58-year-old man with three previous myocardial infarctions, the last one 3 years ago, presents for dental therapy. Consultation with his physician reveals that he had recurrent ventricular tachycardia during his last myocardial infarction and has been on quinidine, 300 mg, qid. He has done well since and is followed closely by his physician. He was last examined 3 weeks ago and was found to be at his baseline state. His last electrocardiogram was taken 3 months ago and demonstrated normal sinus rhythm with rare ventricular premature contractions, in addition to evidence of old anteroseptal and inferior myocardial infarctions. He denies palpitations or syncope. On examination, he has a normal pulse at a rate of 80 bpm. His blood pressure is 140/84, and he is asymptomatic. His dental needs are the same as those for Patients 1 and 2.

MANAGEMENT

Patient 1. This patient has infrequent atrial premature contractions, is asymptomatic, and has not required medications. She is at low risk, and normal operating protocol can be used for all surgical and nonsurgical procedures (types I to VI). For moderate to advanced dental surgical procedures (types V and VI), elective sedation techniques may be employed.

Patient 2. This patient has atrial fibrillation and is under medical care. If his pulse rate were normal, he would be at moderate risk. However, he has an initial pulse rate of 130 bpm, and even at rest has an unacceptably high pulse rate. This places him in the high-risk category. He should be referred back to his physician, and dental therapy should be deferred until his atrial fibrillation is under better control.

Patient 3. This patient has a past history of significant ventricular arrhythmia and is currently well controlled by medication. He is at significant risk, and his physician should be consulted prior to the initiation of therapy. Oral examina-tion (type I procedure) can be performed fol-lowing normal operating protocol. Sedation techniques should be considered for nonsurgi-cal and simple surgical dental procedures (types II to IV). He should be hospitalized for moderate and advanced surgical procedures (types V and VI) to facilitate cardiac monitoring and advanced sedation techniques.

SUMMARY TABLE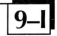

Arrhythmias: General Information

DEFINITION
Arrythmias show electrocardiographic evidence of abnormal atrial or ventricular electrical activity that can produce symptoms and frank cardiovascular compromise.

COMMON SYMPTOMS
"Skipped beats," "flutter," palpitations, dizziness, lightheadedness, dyspnea, hypotension, and syncope are commonly seen.

POTENTIAL COMPLICATIONS
Ischemic heart disease
   Angina
   Myocardial infarction
   Congestive heart failure
   Cardiac arrest

Transient ischemic attacks (TIA; Chap. 32) suggested by
   Blindness
   Irregular speech
   Partial face droop or hemiplegia
   Loss of limb sensation

Frank cerebrovascular accident

SUMMARY TABLE **9-II**

Commonly Used Antiarrhythmic Drugs

CHRONIC ORAL SUPPRESSIVE THERAPY

Atrial arrhythmias
    Digoxin
    Propranolol (Inderal)
    Quinidine (Quinaglute)

Ventricular arrhythmias
    Procainamide (Pronestyl)
    Disopyramide (Norpace)
    Phenytoin (Dilantin)
    Quinidine (Quinaglute)
    Propranolol (Inderal)

ACUTE (EMERGENCY) IV THERAPY

All arrhythmias
    Drugs (as above)
    IV lidocaine
    Cardioversion

SUMMARY TABLE **9-III**

Common Side Effects of Antiarrhythmic Agents

DRUG	SIDE EFFECTS
Digoxin	Digoxin excess results in toxicity: visual symptoms, nausea, vomiting, heart block, ventricular arrhythmias
Propranolol (Inderal)	Congestive heart failure in patients with borderline cardiac reserve; wheezing in patients with bronchospasm or bradycardia (Chap. 10).
Quinidine (Quinaglute)	Nausea, diarrhea, headache, visual symptoms, anorexia, stomatitis
Procainamide (Pronestyl)	Drug-induced lupus erythematosus
Disopyramide (Norpace)	Congestive heart failure, hypotension, urinary retention (especially in elderly men with prostatism), xerostomia
Mexiletene	Nausea, vomiting

Dental Evaluation of the Patient with Arrhythmia

PRESENCE

Past history

Pulse rate and rhythm examination

CHARACTER

Atrial

Ventricular

SEVERITY AND CONTROL

Medications and history of changes in medications

Frequency of symptoms (past and present)

Hospitalization

Pulse rate and rhythm (stat)

Drug side effects and toxicity

Dental Evaluation: Risk Categories for the Patient with Known Arrhythmias

RISK CATEGORY	FEATURES
Low risk	Atrial arrhythmia of unifocal premature ventricular contractions, no medication, infrequent symptoms
Moderate risk	Atrial arrhythmia, chronic medication, asymptomatic
Significant risk	Ventricular arrhythmia, chronic medication, asymptomatic
High risk	Symptomatic patient, pulse rate greater than 100 or less than 60, irregular pulse rhythm*

*An irregular pulse rhythm in a patient with a known arrhythmia and a normal pulse rate is of less concern than an irregular pulse in a patient with undiagnosed arrhythmia (i.e., an irregular pulse is not inconsistent with good medical control). Physician clearance for therapy to confirm medical control is in order prior to dental treatment.

General Guidelines for Dental Management of the Patient with Diagnosed Arrhythmia

Consult the patient's physician to ensure arrhythmia control.

Minimize stress ±* sedation techniques (Chap. 51).

Minimize use of epinephrine.

Consider hospitalization for more stressful procedures in the higher risk categories.

Consider less complex dental treatment plans in the higher risk categories.

*±, with or without.

Specific Guidelines for Dental Management of the Patient with Diagnosed Arrhythmia

RISK CATEGORY	PROCEDURES	PROTOCOL
Low risk	I–VI	Normal protocol
	V, VI	±* sedation techniques
Moderate risk	I–III	Normal protocol and medical consultation
	IV	± sedation techniques
	V, VI	Sedation techniques
	VI	± hospitalization
Significant risk	I	Normal protocol and medical consultation
	II–IV	± sedation techniques
	V, VI	Sedation techniques
	V	± hospitalization
	VI	Hospitalization
High risk	I only	Normal protocol
	II–VI	Contraindicated pending medical evaluation and consultation

*±, with or without.

Bradycardia

A pulse rate of less than 60 beats per minute (bpm) at rest in an adult is called bradycardia and should be investigated. Bradycardia can be found in normal patients, in patients with decreased excitability of the cardiac tissue, and in patients with abnormalities in the cardiac conduction system. Patients with bradycardias may be completely asymptomatic, or may have symptoms ranging from lightheadedness to frank syncope. Patients with symptomatic bradycardia are often managed with the placement of a pacemaker (Fig. 10–1). The dentist should be aware of the different causes of bradycardia and the medical implications of these disorders.

MEDICAL EVALUATION

The patient may come to medical attention either because of a slow pulse rate detected in a routine physical examination or because of symptoms associated with bradycardia. Symptoms arise from decreased blood supply to the brain resulting in dizziness, lightheadedness, or episodes of fainting. Bradycardia may be persistent or episodic. Medical evaluation is directed at determining the type of bradyarrhythmia and correcting the condition if the patient is having frequent symptoms.

Evaluation of the patient with bradyarrhythmias includes physical examination, an electrocardiogram and, in some cases, Holter monitoring. A Holter monitor is a recording device worn by the patient that continuously measures the patient's rhythm over an 8- to 12-hour period.

Bradycardia can be the result of conditions affecting the sinus node, the atrioventricular node, or the conduction system.

Sinus Bradycardia

Sinus bradycardia is defined as a resting heart rate of less than 60 bpm in an adult. The rhythm is usually regular. Electrocardiographic evaluation reveals that the electrical impulse originates normally from the sinus node.

Sinus bradycardia may be normal in young and physically active people, such as athletes. Other patients may have sinus bradycardia because of conditions that slow the discharge rate of the sinus node. Increased vagal tone, medications with parasympathetic effects (e.g., digoxin and phenothiazines), and medications suppressing the excitability of the heart (beta-adrenergic blocking agents, such as propranolol and metoprolol) can cause bradycardia. In most instances, a careful history and the review of the medications reveals the cause of the sinus bradycardia.

Sick Sinus Syndrome

Some patients have diseases affecting the sinus node and present with inappropriate sinus responses. These patients are usually elderly and may have symptoms of palpitations, lightheadedness, and syncope. An electrocardiogram may reveal abnormalities ranging from sinus bradycardia to sinus arrest. There may also be episodic supraventricular tachycardias such as atrial flutter, atrial fibrillation or, less frequently, paroxysmal atrial tachycardia.

Complete Heart Block

Degenerative, inflammatory, and infiltrative diseases affecting the atrioventricular node or the conduction system—including myocardial infarctions—can result in heart block and bradycardia. Drugs can similarly block conduction through the atrioventricular node and the most common culprit is excessive digoxin, which can produce bradycardia in patients with atrial fibrillation.

In most instances, the patient with complete heart block has significant bradycardia and is

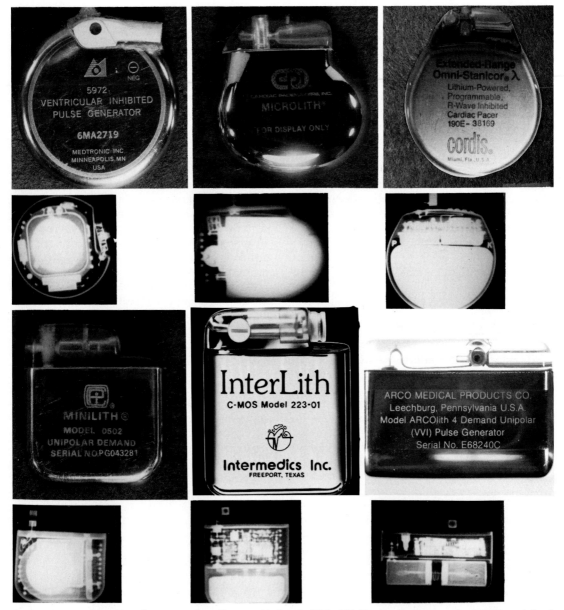

Figure 10–1. Examples of cardiac pacemakers. *Top row,* Medtronic 5972, CPI (Cardiac Pacemakers, Inc.) 0505, and Cordis 190E. *Bottom row,* CPI 0502, Intermedics 223, and Arco Li3D. (Courtesy of the manufacturers.)

symptomatic. The symptoms include dizziness, syncope (Stokes-Adams attacks), and congestive heart failure. The electrocardiogram indicates dissociation of the atrial and ventricular rhythms.

MEDICAL MANAGEMENT

The medical management is different for the different causes of bradyarrhythmia.

Sinus Bradycardia

Young, physically active people with sinus bradycardia require no further intervention. Conditions associated with increased vagal tone are usually obvious, and the medical therapy should be directed at the underlying conditions. Drugs causing sinus bradycardia are usually not a problem, and modification of the drug regimen is indicated only if symptomatic bradycardia results.

Sick Sinus Syndrome

Patients with sick sinus syndrome who are completely asymptomatic require no therapy. Patients with symptoms of bradycardia or tachycardia require intervention. Most commonly, a pacemaker is used to prevent bradycardic symptoms, and medications such as digoxin, quinidine, or propranolol are used to treat tachyarrhythmias (Chap. 9).

Complete Heart Block

Patients with transient dysfunction of the atrioventricular node or conduction system resulting from myocardial ischemia or drugs are usually managed conservatively until the difficulty resolves. Patients with permanent conduction difficulties and complete heart block are usually managed with ventricular pacemakers to avoid bradycardic symptoms.

DENTAL EVALUATION

The dentist may become involved in the management of a patient with bradycardia either by detecting a resting bradycardia during an examination or by treating a patient with a history of bradyarrhythmia.

A detailed history of cardiac arrhythmias and a list of all medications should be obtained. The patient should be asked specifically about symptoms of dizziness, lightheadedness, or syncope. When there is ambiguity, the patient's physician should be consulted.

The examination should determine the regularity and rate of the pulse. A resting pulse rate of less than 60 bpm in an adult should be investigated.

The patient with a pacemaker should have had a recent examination and electrocardiogram to determine the proper functioning of the pacemaker.

Based on the history, examination, and consultative advice from the patient's physician, the patient can be placed into one of the following risk categories.

Patients at Low Risk. A young, physically active patient with a slow regular pulse at a rate of 45 to 60 bpm and no symptoms probably has sinus bradycardia and is at low risk.

Patients at Moderate Risk. Patients who are asymptomatic on medications known to affect the function of the sinus node (e.g., propranolol) and have a regular pulse at a rate in excess of 50 bpm are at moderate risk, as are patients who are asymptomatic with normally functioning pacemakers.

Patients at High Risk. Patients with a pulse rate of less than 45 bpm or an irregular pulse of less than 60 bpm are at high risk. These patients may have complete heart blocks or atrial fibrillation with a slow ventricular response. The latter is associated with either excessive amounts of digoxin or intrinsic disease of the atrioventricular node. Patients with symptoms suggestive of bradyarrhythmias who are on medications capable of affecting the sinus node or the atrioventricular node are also at high risk. Patients with pacemakers and continuing symptoms of bradyarrhythmia may suffer intermittent failure of their pacemaker and are at high risk.

DENTAL MANAGEMENT

Based on dental evaluation, logical plans can be developed for the management of patients with bradyarrhythmias—plans that must take into account the fact that many patients with bradyarrhythmias also have underlying cardiac disease.

Patients at Low Risk. Asymptomatic young patients with sinus bradycardia can be managed using normal protocols.

Patients at Moderate Risk. Patients who are on medications capable of affecting the excitability of the heart may be unable to mount an adequate cardiac response under stress and are therefore at moderate risk. The patient's physician should be consulted, and the proposed dental treatment should be discussed. Dental therapy should proceed only when the medical condition of the patient has been optimized. Stress should be minimized by dividing long appointments into several shorter sessions.

Patients who have a pacemaker in place should have had a recent examination and evaluation to ensure proper functioning of the pacemaker. A patient with a cardiac pacemaker is at minimal risk for bacterial endocarditis (Chap. 11). Antibiotic prophylaxis for dental procedures is not required.

In general, a dental examination (type I procedure) and simple operative procedures (types II and III) can be performed using normal protocol. Adjunctive sedation techniques are recommended for all dental surgery. Patients who are at moderate risk and require extensive surgical intervention (type VI procedures) may be hospitalized for close monitoring.

Patients at High Risk. These patients should be referred to their physicians for evaluation, and dental treatment should be deferred.

■ Examples of Dental Evaluation and Management

EVALUATION

Patient 1. An 18-year-old long distance runner presents for dental treatment. He has no known medical problems and is on no medications. His dental needs include a full range of operative and surgical needs.

On examination, he has a resting pulse rate of 50 bpm. The pulse is regular, and he has no symptoms.

Patient 2. A 48-year-old man with mild hypertension presents for dental therapy. He has been known to have hypertension for 3 years and has been on propranolol for the past 6 months. He is asymptomatic and has no other known medical problems. His dental needs include a full range of operative and surgical procedures.

On examination, he has a resting pulse of 52 bpm. The pulse is regular, and he is asymptomatic. His blood pressure is 130/86.

Patient 3. A 34-year-old woman with a history of sick sinus syndrome presents for dental therapy. She had episodes of palpitations and fainting 4 years ago. A 24-hour Holter monitor recording at that time revealed periods of sinus bradycardia to less than 30 bpm and episodes of rapid atrial fibrillation. She had a pacemaker placed and was started on digoxin 0.25 mg each day. She has done exceedingly well since that time and has been completely asymptomatic. She had a medical examination 4 weeks ago and had a normal electrocardiogram at that time. Her dental needs are similar to those of the other two patients.

On examination, her blood pressure is 110/80 and she has a regular pulse at a rate of 64 bpm. She is asymptomatic.

Patient 4. A 55-year-old man had a myocardial infarction 3 years ago. The infarct was complicated by the development of complete heart block, which necessitated the placement of a pacemaker. He is on no medication and has not had recurrent angina. During the past 3 weeks, the patient has had episodes of lightheadedness and dizziness. His dental needs are similar to those of the other patients.

On examination, he has an irregular pulse at a rate of 43 bpm. He has no symptoms.

MANAGEMENT

Patient 1. This patient probably has sinus bradycardia, and normal dental protocols can be used.

Patient 2. This patient is on a medication known to cause sinus bradycardia. Because he is totally asymptomatic and has a regular pulse, he is in the moderate risk category. Normal protocol can be used for all operative dental care (types II and III procedures). Adjunctive sedation techniques should be used for surgical therapy (types IV to VI procedures), particularly in view of the patient's history of hypertension (Chap. 4).

Patient 3. This patient has a history of sick sinus syndrome, but has had appropriate medical management and has been asymptomatic. This places the patient in the moderate risk category, and the approach to dental therapy should be similar to that for patient 2. Patients with cardiac pacemakers are at minimal risk for bacterial endocarditis (Chap. 11) and do not require antibiotic prophylaxis.

Patient 4. The recent history of lightheadedness and dizziness, the significant bradycardia, and the irregular pulse place the patient in the high risk category. The symptoms and findings suggest that the pacemaker may be malfunctioning. All dental procedures should be deferred, and the patient should be referred for medical evaluation. Dental therapy may be initiated after correction of the pacemaker difficulties.

SUMMARY TABLE **10–I**

Bradycardia: General Information

DEFINITION

Bradycardia is a pulse rate of less than 60 bpm.

SYMPTOMS

May be completely asymptomatic

May have symptoms resulting from inadequate blood supply to the brain
    Dizziness
    Lightheadedness
    Syncope

Rarely, may have symptoms resulting from inadequate blood supply to the heart
    Angina
    Congestive heart failure

SUMMARY TABLE **10–II**

Medical Evaluation of the Patient with Bradycardia

HISTORY

Symptoms suggestive of bradycardia: dizziness, lightheadedness, or syncope

EXAMINATION

Pulse rate and regularity

LABORATORY EVALUATION

Electrocardiogram to differentiate among the various forms of bradycardia: sinus bradycardia, sick sinus syndrome, and complete heart block

Holter monitoring to detect the episodic occurrence of bradycardia

SUMMARY TABLE **10–III**

Pathogenesis of Bradycardia

SINUS BRADYCARDIA
Regular rhythm of less than 60 bpm

Usually in young and physically active adults

No associated symptoms

BRADYCARDIA SECONDARY TO INCREASED VAGAL TONE
Vomiting

Vasovagal episodes

Valsalva maneuver

Acute inferior myocardial infarction

BRADYCARDIA SECONDARY TO MEDICATIONS
Medications with parasympathetic effects (e.g., digoxin, phenothiazines)

Medications that suppress the excitability of the heart (beta-adrenergic blockers, such as propranolol and metoprolol)

SICK SINUS SYNDROME
Diseases affecting the sinus node (mostly ischemic diseases)

Usually in elderly patients

Symptoms: bradycardia (dizziness, lightheadedness, syncope); tachycardia (palpitations, dizziness, lightheadedness, syncope)

COMPLETE HEART BLOCK
Diseases affecting the atrioventricular node or conduction system

Causes include myocardial infarction and degenerative, inflammatory, and infiltrative diseases involving the conduction system (mostly ischemic diseases)

Drugs (e.g., digoxin) can cause heart block when given in excess

SUMMARY TABLE **10–IV**

Medical Management of the Patient with Bradycardia

SINUS BRADYCARDIA
Asymptomatic sinus bradycardia in young adults requires no intervention.

BRADYCARDIA SECONDARY TO INCREASED VAGAL TONE
Correct the cause of the increased vagal tone.

BRADYCARDIA SECONDARY TO MEDICATIONS
No treatment is necessary if the patient is asymptomatic.

Discontinue medications if the patient has significant symptoms.

SICK SINUS SYNDROME
No treatment is necessary if the patient is asymptomatic.

A pacemaker should be implanted for symptomatic bradycardia.

Digoxin, quinidine, or propranolol should be prescribed for symptomatic tachycardia.

COMPLETE HEART BLOCK
This is usually symptomatic and requires the placement of a pacemaker.

SUMMARY TABLE **10–V**

Dental Evaluation of the Patient with Bradycardia

HISTORY
Past history of bradycardia

Patient has pacemaker

Patient has symptoms of dizziness, lightheadedness, or syncope

EXAMINATION
Pulse rate

Regularity of the pulse

MEDICAL CONSULTATION
Refer all symptomatic patients for evaluation.

Inquire about the history of bradycardia and the function of the cardiac pacemaker.

A recent examination and electrocardiogram should be carried out in patients with a history of bradycardia, a pacemaker, and/or symptoms of bradycardia.

Risk Categories of Bradycardia

PATIENTS AT LOW RISK
Young, active patients with sinus bradycardia and no symptoms

PATIENTS AT MODERATE RISK
Asymptomatic patients on medications known to affect the function of the sinus node (e.g., propranolol)

Asymptomatic patients with cardiac pacemakers

PATIENTS AT HIGH RISK
Patients with a pulse rate of less than 45 bpm

Patients with irregular pulse and bradycardia
   Complete heart block
   Slow atrial fibrillation

Symptomatic patients with bradycardia

Bradycardia patients with cardiac pacemakers

Dental Management of the Patient with Bradycardia

RISK CATEGORY	PROCEDURES	PROTOCOL
Low risk	I–VI	Normal protocol
Moderate risk	I–III	Medical consultation, mimimize stress, otherwise normal protocol
	IV–VI	Medical consultation; adjunctive sedation techniques advisable
	VI	Consider hospitalization
High risk	I	Normal protocol
	II–VI	Deferred pending medical examination and evaluation

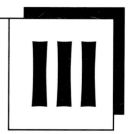

Evaluation and Management of the Patient at Risk for Bacterial Endocarditis

Bacterial Endocarditis

Bacterial endocarditis is a serious infection of the heart valves or the endothelial surfaces of the heart. Despite considerable progress in medical and surgical intervention, the mortality rate for bacterial endocarditis is still about 10%. Because dental manipulation is the leading identifiable cause of transient bacteremia that can result in infectious endocarditis, it is important for the dentist to understand the pathogenesis of the disease, to be able to identify the population at risk, and to be able to administer appropriate prophylactic antibiotic therapy.

RELATIONSHIP BETWEEN DENTAL PROCEDURES AND BACTERIAL ENDOCARDITIS

Underlying Cardiac Abnormalities

Bacterial endocarditis results from bacterial proliferation on altered cardiac surfaces. Damaged heart valves as a sequela of rheumatic fever or previous bacterial endocarditis, acquired valvular lesions, roughened cardiac surfaces as a result of a jet stream effect from blood crossing congenital cardiac lesions (such as ventricular septal defects), and prosthetic heart valves are the usual predisposing clinical conditions for bacterial endocarditis. Initially, a sterile platelet-fibrin clot or thrombus becomes implanted on the damaged surfaces. If bacteria are introduced, the thrombus can act as a nidus for bacterial proliferation (Fig. 11–1).

Clinical Consequences of Bacterial Endocarditis

The clinical consequences of bacterial endocarditis may be grouped into three major categories (see Fig. 11–1). First, local bacterial proliferation may inhibit valvular function, re-sulting in valvular insufficiency and, ultimately, congestive heart failure. Alternatively, the production of pus may cause the development of an abscess of the myocardium, with subsequent disruption of the normal conduction pathways of the heart. Second, pieces of infected valvular vegetation may break off and travel through the patient's body through the bloodstream. These infectious emboli may lodge in a number of organs and produce infection. Among the organs most commonly targeted by such emboli are the brain, kidney, and spleen. Finally, antibodies directed against the bacteria may bind to circulating bacterial antigens to form immune complexes. Deposition of these complexes may produce arthritis or glomerulonephritis or both by the activation of complement and other biologically active substances.

Treatment of bacterial endocarditis is dependent on the extent of valvular damage. When valvular damage is minimal, a 4- to 6-week antibiotic course is usually adequate to eradicate the infection. When valvular compromise is significant, as in valvular incompetence or ring abscesses, surgical replacement may be necessary after a full 4 to 6 weeks of antibiotic therapy.

Oral Flora and Bacterial Endocarditis

Organisms normally found in the oral cavity account for a sizeable proportion of the causative agents of bacterial endocarditis: alpha-hemolytic streptococci, enterococci *(Streptococcus faecalis)*, pneumococci, staphylococci, and group A streptococci. DeMoor and associates studied 500 patients suspected of having bacterial endocarditis and isolated *S. sanguis* from the blood of 208 patients and *S. mutans* from 35 patients. Serotyping the organisms, they found remarkable similarities between the blood isolates of these strains, of *S. viridans,*

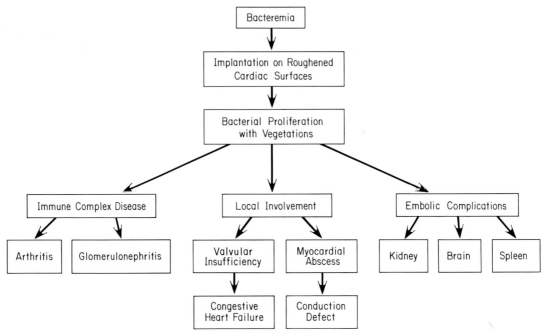

Figure 11–1. Possible clinical consequences of bacteremias induced by dental manipulation.

and of strains previously isolated from the dental plaques of the same patients.

Dental Manipulations Causing Bacterial Endocarditis

Dental procedures are the leading cause of transient bacteremia that can result in bacterial endocarditis. Burket and Burn swabbed cultures of *Serratia marcescens,* an organism not normally found in humans, at the tooth-gingival interface of patients undergoing extractions. The peripheral blood collected immediately after extraction demonstrated the growth of *S. marcescens* in 38% of patients studied.

The risks of such orally introduced bacteremias appear to depend on two important variables: the amount of soft tissue trauma induced by the dental procedure and the degree of pre-existing local inflammatory disease. The importance of soft tissue trauma is demonstrated by the high correlation between the frequency of bacteremia and the number of teeth extracted. A higher incidence of bacteremia is seen in patients with endodontic manipulation beyond the confines of the root canal as compared with less invasive manipulation limited to the root canal proper. The

importance of pre-existing inflammatory disease in inducing bacteremia is also well established. Okell and Elliot demonstrated that the incidence of bacteremia is six times higher if the patient has severe periodontal disease. Korn found that procedures that improve the health of the gingiva such as scaling and root planing significantly lower the risk of bacteremia during subsequent soft tissue surgery.

Although the incidence and the magnitude of bacteremia are related to the severity of pre-existing periodontal disease and the amount of soft tissue trauma, a large number of case reports have demonstrated that bacterial endocarditis can result from even simple dental manipulation. Transient bacteremias have been demonstrated following extraction, gingivectomy, curettage, prophylaxis, brushing, endodontic manipulation, chewing paraffin, and simple tooth rocking. There are even case reports of bacterial endocarditis attributed to transient bacteremia in edentulous patients with denture sores.

The dentist must assume that *any dental manipulation likely to result in gingival bleeding (even an intraoral examination with mirror, periodontal probe, and explorer) can lead to transient bacteremia.* Some form of antibiotic prophylaxis should therefore be used in any patient believed to be at risk for bacterial endocarditis.

RATIONALE FOR ANTIBIOTIC PROPHYLAXIS

Although there is no direct evidence that antibiotic prophylaxis is effective in preventing endocarditis in humans, there is adequate evidence that it decreases the incidence of bacteremia.

The choice of drugs for prophylaxis is largely empiric. From a theoretic standpoint, the drugs chosen should be bactericidal and directed at organisms commonly found in the oral cavity. The drugs should be administered at an appropriate interval prior to the procedure to ensure maximal blood level at the time of the procedure, and they should be continued for a period following the procedure to allow adequate time for tissue healing. Based on these considerations, clinical experience, and experimental models, the American Heart Association has recommended the regimens detailed in Summary Table 11–V.

In most cases, the standard regimen is used for dental prophylaxis. This regimen involves the use of oral amoxicillin. The standard regimen is clearly the most conveniently administered form of prophylaxis and is a reasonable treatment for most patients requiring antibiotic prophylaxis. An adult should receive a loading dose of 3.0 g of amoxicillin 1 hour before a procedure, followed by a 1.5 g of amoxicillin 6 hours after the initial dose. Amoxicillin is chosen because it is better absorbed from the gastrointestinal tract and provides higher and more sustained serum levels. However, the choice of penicillin V rather than amoxicillin is also acceptable.

Individuals who are allergic to penicillins (e.g., amoxicillin, ampicillin, or penicillin) should be treated with an alternative oral regimen. Erythromycin ethylsuccinate and erythromycin stearate are recommended because of more rapid and reliable absorption than other erythromycin formulations, resulting in higher serum levels. Erythromycin ethylsuccinate, 1600 mg, or erythromycin stearate, 1.0 g, can be administered orally 2 hours before a procedure, followed by half the dose in 6 hours. Erythromycin stearate must be administered in the fasting state or just prior to meals. The presence of food concurrently will adversely affect absorption. Most other erythromycins can be prescribed without regard to meals. Delayed-release-capsule erythromycin (e.g., ERYC) is slower to reach therapeutic blood levels but offers an alternative erythromycin for patients susceptible to the gastrointestinal

side effects of other formulations. Dosages are the same as for erythromycin stearate preparation, but the loading dose should be given 2½ to 3 hours prior to the appointment. For individuals who cannot tolerate penicillins or erythromycin, clindamycin hydrochloride is recommended. The dose for clindamycin is 300 mg 1 hour before the appointment, followed by 150 mg 6 hours later. Tetracyclines and sulfonamides, however, are not recommended for endocarditis prophylaxis.

Individuals who have prosthetic heart valves, a previous history of endocarditis, or surgically constructed systemic-pulmonary shunts or conduits are at high risk for developing endocarditis. In these individuals, bacterial endocarditis is associated with considerable morbidity and mortality. Therefore, previous recommendations emphasized the use of stringent prophylactic regimens, with a strong preference for the parenteral route of administration. In practice, there are substantial logistic and financial barriers to the use of parenteral regimens. Moreover, oral regimens have been used in individuals with prosthetic valves, and failures in prophylaxis have not been a problem. Consequently, it is often currently recommended that the standard regimen be used, even in high-risk patients. The anticipated soft tissue trauma of the dental procedure and the severity of the pre-existing periodontal disease must be evaluated in consultation with the patient's physician. It is recognized that some practitioners may prefer to use parenteral prophylaxis in these high-risk groups of patients. In such cases, ampicillin, gentamicin, or vancomycin can be administered parenterally.

MEDICAL EVALUATION

Although bacterial endocarditis can occur in patients without previously documented cardiac lesions, antibiotic prophylaxis for dental procedures is reasonable for patients with known underlying abnormalities.

In the majority of cases, patients come to medical evaluation because of a murmur found on physical examination. The murmur is created by turbulence in blood flow. Occasionally, the murmur may be "innocent" or "functional," especially in a person with a thin chest and/or a high velocity of blood flow. The innocent murmur does not reflect cardiac abnormalities and does not require intensive investigation. The most common clinical situations for such murmurs are the pregnant woman and the young child with a high fever. Such murmurs are not sustained.

Other murmurs usually result from valvular or other cardiac abnormalities and warrant further evaluation. A careful cardiac examination, a chest roentgenogram, and an electrocardiogram should provide information regarding the cause of the murmur. Other procedures can be performed to delineate the nature and significance of an underlying cardiac abnormality further, including a phonocardiogram, echocardiogram, and cardiac catheterization.

Cardiac abnormalities can be grouped into several major categories: rheumatic disease, other acquired valvular diseases, and congenital heart diseases (Summary Table 11–IV). Patients having these abnormalities—as well as patients with previous infectious endocarditis, prosthetic valves, or intravascular prostheses— should be considered for antibiotic prophylaxis.

Rheumatic Valvular Disease

Patients with rheumatic valvular diseases are at high risk for bacterial endocarditis. Before the introduction of antibiotics, the incidence of endocarditis in this group was estimated at 4 to 7% annually. The incidence has dramatically decreased with antibiotic prophylaxis.

For reasons that are not fully understood, the incidence of rheumatic fever is decreasing, and primary rheumatic fever is now a rare disease. Nonetheless, a small fraction of the dentist's patient population gives a history of having had rheumatic fever as a child. These patients may have had valvular disease and require antibiotic prophylaxis.

Patients with rheumatic valvular disease most commonly have involvement of the mitral valve. Aortic valve involvement is less common and seldom occurs in the absence of mitral valve involvement. Tricuspid valves are rarely involved. Some patients with a history of rheumatic fever have no demonstrable valvular lesions. Dental prophylaxis for these patients is rarely prescribed.

Other Acquired Valvular Diseases

Patients may have acquired valvular diseases that are not sequelae of rheumatic fever. Elderly patients may have calcium deposition in the area of the aortic valve, resulting in aortic stenosis. Aortic valve insufficiency can result from trauma or involvement of the aortic ring by syphilis. Although patients with nonrheu-

matic valvular diseases are also at risk for bacterial endocarditis, the exact incidence of endocarditis in this population is not known.

Mitral Valve Prolapse

Mitral valve prolapse (also called "click murmur syndrome" or Barlow's syndrome) is a common congenital condition that affects 5 to 10% of females. Loss of tone of the mitral valvular tendon results in prolapse of the mitral valve into the atrium, and may cause mitral regurgitation. Mitral valve prolapse can be suspected on clinical examination and is usually diagnosed by echocardiography. In the past 10 years, it has been concluded that, although patients with mitral valve prolapse and mitral regurgitation are at risk for endocarditis and require prophylaxis, patients with mitral valve prolapse and no regurgitation are not at risk and do not require prophylaxis. It is therefore important to consult with the patient's physician to assess the need for prophylaxis. If emergent dental treatment is required, the administration of a prophylactic antibiotic regimen is recommended.

"Innocent Murmur"

Not infrequently, patients may report a history of an "innocent murmur." Unfortunately, some of these patients actually have mitral valve prolapse. The true innocent murmur is a high-volume blood flow murmur across either the pulmonic valve or the aortic valve during times of high metabolic demand. A thinchested child may have a flow murmur during high fevers. A young woman may have a flow murmur during the third trimester of her pregnancy. The murmur is not present when the individual is otherwise not under stress. The dentist should be cautioned that a physician's assessment of an "innocent" or "not significant" murmur may refer only to the impact of the lesion on cardiovascular function and may not be pertinent to an assessment of the risk of bacterial endocarditis. It is recommended that the dentist consult with the physician when a patient acknowledges a murmur without a definitive diagnosis. If detailed inquiry of the patient and physician reveal that the murmur is indeed an innocent murmur, dental prophylaxis is not required.

Congenital Heart Disease

A number of congenital cardiac abnormalities have been associated with bacterial endocarditis. Infections have been reported in patients with ventricular septal defects, idiopathic hypertrophic subaortic stenosis, bicuspid aortic valves, tetralogy of Fallot, and complex cyanotic heart disease. Endocarditis has also been reported in patients with mitral valve prolapse and mitral insufficiency, but the incidence appears to be relatively low. All of the above patients require endocarditis prophylaxis. Patients with mitral valve prolapse without mitral regurgitation are not at significant risk and do not require endocarditis prophylaxis. Patients with atrial septal defects of the secundum type (anatomically high atrial septal defect) do not have an increased risk of developing bacterial endocarditis and do not require antibiotic prophylaxis.

Prosthetic Valves

Patients with prosthetic valves are at high risk of developing bacterial endocarditis. The incidence is estimated to be about 4% annually.

Previous Endocarditis

Patients with previous endocarditis have an exceedingly high incidence of recurrent endocarditis. In one series, patients with one previous episode of endocarditis were found to have a 10% risk annually of a second infection, and patients with two previous episodes of endocarditis were found to have a 25% risk of a third episode.

Vascular Anomalies or Intravascular Prostheses

Patients with vascular anomalies or intravascular prostheses should also be considered for antibiotic prophylaxis. Although they do not develop bacterial endocarditis, they are susceptible to intravascular infection, which presents with many of the same complications and requires the same intensive medical and surgical therapy.

Intravascular infections have been reported with congenital anomalies such as coarctation of the aorta, patent ductus arteriosus, and systemic-to-pulmonary artery shunts. Such infections are also seen in patients with intravascular prostheses such as aortoiliac bypass grafts, arteriovenous shunts or grafts used for dialysis, and ventriculoatrial shunts used for treatment of hydrocephalus. In addition, patients who

have had surgical corrections with Dacron grafts must be considered for antibiotic prophylaxis. Examples of such corrections include closure of a ventricular septal defect with a Dacron graft and similar repairs to aortic aneurysms or coarctation of the aorta. Data suggest that while most of the Dacron graft is epithelialized during healing, denuded areas persist. Therefore, a risk of infection, however small, remains. Because the risk of complications with antibiotic prophylaxis is low, such prophylaxis is recommended. Patients who have a permanent pacemaker or implanted defibrillator are at minimal risk of endocarditis and do not require prophylaxis.

It should be obvious from the preceding discussion that the risk of bacterial endocarditis and intravascular infections is different for the various underlying abnormalities. This should be taken into account when determining antibiotic regimens.

DENTAL EVALUATION
General Guidelines

The dental evaluation of patients depends on a detailed history and a medical consultation with the patient's physician. The history should include questions specifically inquiring about a history of heart murmur, congenital heart disease, rheumatic fever and associated rheumatic heart disease, valvular heart disease, previous infection of a heart valve, and cardiovascular surgery. Patients giving a positive history must be considered for prophylaxis. The dentist should consult the patient's physician and inquire into the nature of the underlying abnormalities and the need for prophylaxis. The most common problems for the dentist revolve around a history of a murmur, rheumatic fever, or cardiovascular surgery.

Heart Murmur

The patient known to have a heart murmur might not know the nature of the underlying cardiac lesion. In any case, it is important to consult the patient's physician and establish the nature and significance of the murmur. Patients with innocent murmurs—for example, mitral valve prolapse without regurgitation—or with atrial septal defects of a secundum type do not require antibiotic prophylaxis and can be managed with conventional protocol. All other cardiac lesions require antibiotic prophylaxis.

Rheumatic Fever

Rheumatic fever is a severe form of streptococcal infection characterized by hectic fever, rash, joint swelling and pain, chorea, and myocarditis. The most significant sequela of rheumatic fever is the development of valvular disease in about 50% of affected patients. A patient may give a history of having had rheumatic fever as a child. The patient's physician should be consulted to determine whether there are any cardiac sequelae of the illness.

Patients known to have rheumatic valvular disease require prophylaxis. Some patients may be maintained on low doses of continuous penicillin prophylaxis after a bout of rheumatic fever to prevent recurrence of the disease. The dosage of oral penicillin used in continuous prophylaxis is inadequate for endocarditis prophylaxis, and these patients need special consideration (see later, Dental Management: Specific Guidelines).

For patients with a history of rheumatic fever but no known valvular involvement, management is controversial. Theoretically, they should not need antibiotic prophylaxis, but prophylaxis may occasionally be recommended because of concern about occult valvular lesions. Medical consultation is essential to determine individual needs.

Cardiovascular Surgery

Patients who have had valvular surgery, correction of congenital heart lesions (except for primary repair of uncomplicated atrial septal defects of the secundum type), or placement of vascular grafts require prophylaxis. Patients who have a permanent pacemaker are not at an increased risk of endocarditis, and there is no need for prophylaxis. Patients who have undergone coronary artery bypass procedures are not at increased risk for endocarditis in the absence of other lesions, and do not require prophylaxis (Chap. 12).

Specific Guidelines

Once the nature of the underlying lesion is delineated, patients can be grouped according to relative risk for developing endocarditis.

Patients at High Risk. Patients are considered at high risk if they are particularly susceptible to intravascular infection or if infection carries a particularly bad prognosis. These include those with previous bacterial endocardi-

tis, prosthetic heart valves, and systemic-pulmonary shunts or conduits.

Patients at Significant Risk. Patients with rheumatic valvular disease, acquired valvular diseases, congenital heart disease, intravascular prostheses, or coarctation of the aorta are all at significant risk for developing endocarditis.

Patients at Low Risk. Patients with mitral valve prolapse without mitral regurgitation are at minimal risk and do not require prophylaxis. In some cases, however, the mitral valve may be thickened and is therefore at risk. Such individuals may require oral prophylaxis.

Patients Who Do Not Require Prophylaxis. Patients with innocent murmurs, patients with uncomplicated atrial septal defects, and patients who have undergone coronary artery bypass surgery have no increased risk for bacterial endocarditis and do not require antibiotic prophylaxis.

Patients with mitral valve prolapse without mitral regurgitation are at no increased risk and do not require prophylaxis. Patients with transvenous pacemakers or implanted defibrillators do not require prophylaxis. Patients with a history of rheumatic fever but no demonstrable associated valvular lesions do not require prophylaxis.

DENTAL MANAGEMENT

General Guidelines

Patients at high risk of developing infectious endocarditis should maintain the highest level of oral health to reduce potential sources of bacteremia. Even in the absence of dental procedures, poor dental hygiene or dental diseases such as periapical infections may induce bacteremia. The dentist should therefore provide meticulous oral hygiene instruction to these patients. Frequent re-evaluation of the periodontal status and diligent control are mandatory (Fig. 11–2).

The use of some hygiene aids is a subject of controversy. Electric toothbrushes and devices that use water under pressure to clean between teeth may improve dental hygiene, but they have also been shown to cause bacteremia, especially in the presence of significant inflammatory disease. Present data are insufficient for the American Heart Association to make firm recommendations with regard to their use in patients susceptible to endocardi-

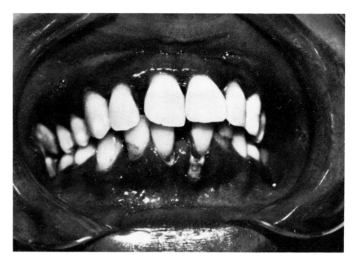

Figure 11–2. Periodontal disease with infection, calculus accumulation, and extrusion of teeth in a 21-year-old man with tetralogy of Fallot.

tis. However, caution is advised in their use by susceptible patients, especially if oral health is poor. The dentist must weigh the increased risk of bacteremia in the presence of ongoing periodontal disease against the risk of bacteremia created by the use of water jet or electric cleaning devices. *The dentist must control inflammatory tissue changes while the patient is receiving antibiotic prophylaxis before instituting aggressive at-home interproximal oral hygiene measures.*

Specific Guidelines

Patients at High Risk. Patients with prosthetic heart valves, systemic-pulmonary shunts or conduits, or previous episodes of bacterial endocarditis are particularly susceptible to intravascular infections, and the infection carries a particularly bad prognosis. These patients should receive dental prophylaxis. The American Heart Association's 1990 guidelines note that, based on international data, the standard regimen usually appears to be adequate. There are patients with prosthetic valves who have been managed successfully with oral endocarditis prophylaxis. However, in patients in whom excessive gingival bleeding is anticipated, parenteral antibiotics (alternate regimen) may provide more effective prophylaxis.

If infection is present or if there has been surgical intervention, the antibiotic should be continued during the healing period. In some patients, a series of dental procedures may be required. Continuous antibiotic prophylaxis would result in the emergence of resistant strains. Therefore, it is recommended that an interval of 7 to 14 days between the administration of antibiotic prophylaxis measures be observed.

Topical rinses such as chlorhexedine and povidone-iodine have been recommended as a means of degerming. Indeed, the current American Heart Association guidelines suggest that dentists consider this lavage. As a preoperative swab or rinse, the efficacy of these agents remains to be demonstrated.

Patients at Significant Risk. Patients at significant risk should receive the standard oral regimen for dental prophylaxis.

Patients on Continuous Oral Penicillin. Patients on continuous oral penicillin for the secondary prevention of rheumatic fever deserve special attention. The dose of penicillin used for continuous therapy is inadequate for the prevention of bacterial endocarditis. Although it is likely that the doses of amoxicillin recommended in the standard regimen are sufficient to control these organisms, the dentist may choose oral erythromycin or clindamycin, because these patients may have oral alpha-hemolytic streptococci that are relatively resistant to penicillin.

Patients at Low Risk. Patient with mitral valve prolapse without regurgitation do not need prophylaxis. The only exception is the patient who has a thickened mitral valve leaflet, as demonstrated on an echocardiogram. These patients are at slight risk for endocarditis and should receive the oral standard regimen for prophylaxis.

Patients at Minimal Risk. There is no evidence of increased risk of endocarditis in patients who have mitral valve prolapse with no clinical evidence of regurgitation, or in those with a coronary artery bypass graft, a transvenous pacemaker or implanted defibrillator, a history of rheumatic fever but with no demonstrable valvular dysfunction, or an innocent murmur. These patients do not need dental prophylaxis.

These guidelines have been proposed by the American Heart Association and take into consideration both the inherent risks of the underlying cardiac lesions and the risks of bacteremia involved in the dental procedures. With continuing research into the epidemiology, pathogenesis, prevention, and therapy of infectious endocarditis, the specific recommendations may change, but the basic guidelines and rationale should remain the same.

■ Examples of Dental Evaluation and Management

EVALUATION

Patient 1. This 36-year-old woman was found to have a murmur during a routine physical examination at age 22. She was told that it was "not significant" and has not had any physical limitations. Consultation with her physician reveals that she has mitral valve prolapse with regurgitation. Dental exam reveals multiple caries and moderately severe periodontal disease.

Patient 2. This 62-year-old woman had mitral valve replacement with a prosthetic valve 4 years ago. She has been asymptomatic since, and there has been no limitations of her activities. Consultation with her physician reveals that she is chronically in atrial fibrillation. Her last examination was 3 months ago, when she was found to be at her baseline state. Examination now reveals a blood pressure of 105/80 and a regular pulse at a rate of 70 beats per minute (bpm). She is on 5 mg of warfarin (Coumadin) and 0.25 mg of digoxin daily. She has severe periodontal disease and multiple caries and needs advanced dental care.

Patient 3. This 28-year-old man is a former drug addict and was hospitalized 3 years ago for bacterial endocarditis. He has had a murmur since but no symptoms or physical limitations. Consultation with his physician reveals that he had endocarditis involving his tricuspid valve. The infecting organism was *Staphylococcus aureus,* and he was treated for 6 weeks with large doses of nafcillin. He has had a murmur of tricuspid regurgitation since but is currently not on medication. On examination, he has a regular pulse at a rate of 80 bpm and a blood

pressure of 140/84. He has mild periodontal disease and caries.

Patient 4. This 35-year-old man had rheumatic fever as a child. He had a high fever and was on bed rest for a month, but made an uneventful recovery. He has had no residual problems, has been followed closely by his physician, and has no evidence of rheumatic heart disease. He was last examined a month ago and was in excellent health. He has multiple caries and severe periodontal disease.

MANAGEMENT

Patient 1. This patient has mitral valve prolapse with regurgitation and is therefore at significant risk for the development of bacterial endocarditis secondary to dental procedures. The patient's comment that the murmur is "not significant" refers to the physician's assessment of the impact of the lesion on cardiovascular function and is not pertinent to an assessment of the risk of bacterial endocarditis. She should therefore be covered with the standard regimen for all dental procedures.

Patient 2. This patient is at high risk for the development of bacterial endocarditis because of her prosthetic mitral valve. Antibiotic prophylaxis is mandatory for all dental procedures. In patients in whom excessive gingival bleeding is anticipated, parenteral antibiotics (alternate regimen) should be considered. Because the administration of parenteral antibiotics usually involves additional trips to the physician's office or to the hospital, multiple dental appointments should be consolidated into longer sessions. This patient has severe periodontal disease, which predisposes her to significant bacteremias. Most clinicians would opt for parenteral prophylaxis for all traumatic procedures.

The patient is also on Coumadin, and appropriate steps should be taken prior to dental surgical procedures and soft tissue manipulation. The management of patients on anticoagulants is discussed in Chapter 26.

From a long-term management standpoint, attention should be paid to preventive dental care. Frequent prophylaxis and re-examinations should be planned at the completion of active therapy.

Nonsurgical procedures (types I to III) could be performed using the standard regimen, but only under conditions of ideal gingival health and in consultation with the patient's cardiologist.

Patient 3. This patient is at high risk for the development of bacterial endocarditis because of his past history of bacterial endocarditis. The valvular surfaces are probably damaged and therefore susceptible to infection. He also required antibiotic coverage according to the standard regimen for all dental procedures. In patients in whom excessive gingival bleeding is anticipated, parenteral antibiotics (alternate regimen) should be considered.

Patient 4. This patient has had rheumatic fever, but there is no evidence of rheumatic heart dis-

ease (i.e., no history of cardiac murmur). It is therefore difficult to justify the use of antibiotic prophylaxis on theoretic grounds. The patient is at low risk for the development of bacterial endocarditis. The dentist should consult with the patient's physician and tailor the therapy to the patient's needs. In some instances, the physician may recommend standard regimen prophylaxis because of a concern about subclinical valvular involvement. Generally, however, this patient would not receive antibiotic prophylaxis.

SUMMARY TABLE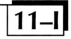

Bacterial Endocarditis: General Information

DEFINITION

Bacterial endocarditis is infection of the heart valves or the endothelial surfaces of the heart.

CLINICAL IMPORTANCE

Despite aggressive medical and surgical therapy, bacterial endocarditis still carries a 10% mortality rate.

Dental manipulation is the leading identifiable cause of transient bacteremia that can cause bacterial endocarditis.

PATHOGENESIS

A sterile platelet-fibrin clot becomes implanted on the damaged surfaces of the heart in susceptible patients. The thrombus acts as a nidus for bacterial proliferation if transient bacteremia occurs in these susceptible patients.

ORGANISMS CAUSING BACTERIAL ENDOCARDITIS

Oral organisms account for a sizeable proportion of causative agents of bacterial endocarditis.

Dental manipulations have been demonstrated to result in transient bacteremia.

The risks of dental manipulations in inducing bacteremia depend on the amount of soft tissue trauma induced by the procedure and pre-existing local inflammatory disease.

However, *any* dental manipulation likely to result in gingival bleeding can lead to transient bacteremia.

Complications of Bacterial Endocarditis

CARDIAC COMPLICATIONS

Valvular incompetence (aortic insufficiency, mitral insufficiency, tricuspid insufficiency)

Congestive heart failure, usually secondary to aortic insufficiency

Myocardial abscesses

Conduction abnormalities, usually as a result of myocardial abscesses invading the conduction pathway

Pericarditis (rarely)

EMBOLIC COMPLICATIONS

Cerebral embolic infarction

Renal infarction

Splenic infarction

Other systemic emboli

IMMUNE COMPLEX FORMATION

Arthritis

Glomerulonephritis

Considerations in the Choice of Drugs for Dental Prophylaxis

Drugs chosen should be directed at organisms commonly found in the oral cavity.

Drugs chosen should be bactericidal.

Drugs should be administered at an appropriate interval prior to the procedure to ensure maximal blood level at the time of surgery.

Drugs should not be administered for long periods before surgery to avoid the development of resistant organisms.

Antibiotics should be continued for a period of time following the procedure to allow for tissue healing.

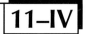

Patients at Risk for Bacterial Endocarditis

RHEUMATIC VALVULAR DISEASES
Incidence estimated at 4–7% annually before availability of antibiotics, significantly lower currently

OTHER ACQUIRED VALVULAR DISEASES
Calcific aortic stenosis in elderly patients

Aortic insufficiency secondary to trauma

Aortic insufficiency in syphilis

(The exact incidence of bacterial endocarditis in these patients is unknown.)

CONGENITAL HEART DISEASE
Mitral valve prolapse with regurgitation

Ventricular septal defect

Idiopathic hypertrophic subaortic stenosis

Bicuspid aortic valve

Tetralogy of Fallot

Other cyanotic heart disease

PROSTHETIC VALVES
Incidence estimated at 4% annually

PREVIOUS ENDOCARDITIS
Incidence estimated at 10% per year

VASCULAR ANOMALIES OR INTRAVASCULAR PROSTHESIS
Coarctation of the aorta

Patent ductus arteriosus

Systemic-pulmonary artery shunt

Vascular bypass graft

Arteriovenous shunt or graft

MINIMAL RISK PATIENTS WHO DO NOT REQUIRE ANTIBIOTIC PROPHYLAXIS
Innocent or functional murmurs

Uncomplicated atrial septal defect of the secundum type

Surgical repair without residua beyond 6 months of secundum atrial septal defect, ventricular septal defect (unless Dacron graft is used), or patent ductus arteriosus

Coronary artery bypass graft surgery

Mitral valve prolapse without valvular regurgitation

Previous rheumatic fever without valvular dysfunction

Cardiac pacemaker or implanted defibrillators

Kawasaki disease without valvular dysfunction

ENDOCARDITIS PROPHYLAXIS
Recommended for:
  Dental procedures known to induce gingival or mucosal bleeding, including professional cleaning and injection of intraligamentary anesthetic

Not recommended for:
  Dental procedures not likely to induce gingival bleeding—simple adjustment of orthodontic appliances, fillings above the gum line

  Injection of local intraoral anesthetic (except intraligamentary injections)

SUMMARY TABLE 11–V

Prophylaxis for Dental Procedures*

STANDARD REGIMEN†
Amoxicillin: 3.0 g orally 1 hr before procedure, then 1.5 g 6 hr after initial dose

Amoxicillin-Penicillin–Allergic Patients
Erythromycin: erythromycin ethylsuccinate, 1600 mg, or erythromycin stearate, 1.0 g, orally, 2 hr before procedure; then half the dose 6 hr after initial dose
  or
Clindamycin: 300 mg orally 1 hr before procedure; then 150 mg 6 hr after initial dose

Patients Unable to Take Oral Medications (i.e., Prior to General Anesthesia)
Ampicillin: IV or IM administration of ampicillin, 2.0 g, 30 min before procedure; then IV or IM ampicillin, 1.0 g or oral administration of amoxicillin, 1.5 g, 6 hr after initial dose

Ampicillin-Amoxicillin-Penicillin–Allergic Patients Unable to Take Oral Medications
Clindamycin: IV administration of 300 mg, 30 min before procedure; then IV or oral administration, 150 mg, 6 hr after the initial dose

PATIENTS CONSIDERED HIGH RISK AND NOT CANDIDATES FOR STANDARD REGIMEN
Ampicillin, gentamicin and amoxicillin: IV or IM administration of ampicillin, 2.0 g, plus gentamicin, 1.5 mg/kg (not to exceed 80 mg), 30 min before procedure; followed by amoxicillin, 1.5 g orally, 6 hr following initial dose; alternatively, parenteral regimen may be repeated 6 hr after initial dose

Ampicillin-Amoxicillin-Penicillin–Allergic Patients Considered High Risk
Vancomycin: IV administration of 1.0 g over 1 hr starting 1 hr before procedure; no repeat dose necessary

HIGH-RISK CANDIDATES
Prosthetic heart valve

Previous history of endocarditis

Surgically constructed systemic-pulmonary shunt or conduit

SPECIFIC SITUATIONS
Rheumatic fever: Low-dose penicillin antibiotic regimen used to prevent recurrence of acute rheumatic fever is inadequate for prevention of bacterial endocarditis; erythromycin or clindamycin regimens are recommended.

Anticoagulants: avoid IM injections; use IV or oral regimens

Renal dysfunction: adjust antibiotic dose, particularly gentamicin and vancomycin

Cardiac surgery (valvular or congenital heart disease): Preoperative dental evaluation; first-generation cephalosporin perioperatively; vancomycin perioperatively

*In the case of delayed healing or of a procedure that involves infected tissue, it may be necessary to provide additional doses of antibiotics.
†There are substantial logistic and financial barriers to the use of parenteral regimens. Moreover, oral regimens can be used in other countries in patients with prosthetic heart valves, and failures in prophylaxis have not been a problem.

Relative Risks of Bacterial Endocarditis Based on Underlying Cardiac Lesions

PATIENTS AT MINIMAL RISK WHO DO NOT REQUIRE ANTIBIOTIC PROPHYLAXIS

Innocent or functional murmur

Uncomplicated atrial septal defect of the secundum type

Surgical repair without residua beyond 6 months of secundum atrial septal defect, ventricular septal defect, or patent ductus arteriosus

Coronary artery bypass graft surgery

Mitral valve prolapse without valvular regurgitation

Previous rheumatic fever without valvular dysfunction

Cardiac pacemaker or implanted defibrillator

Kawasaki disease without valvular dysfunction

PATIENTS AT SIGNIFICANT RISK

Rheumatic valvular disease

Mitral valve prolapse and mitral regurgitation

Other acquired valvular disease

Congenital heart disease

Intravascular prosthesis

Coarctation of the aorta

PATIENTS AT HIGH RISK

Previous bacterial endocarditis

Prosthetic heart valve

Systemic-pulmonary shunt or conduit

Dental Mangement of Patients at Risk for Bacterial Endocarditis

GENERAL PRINCIPLE

The selection of the standard regimen or the more stringent alternate regimen depends on the risks associated with the particular cardiovascular defect and the risk of bacteremia for a particular procedure and oral health setting.

In general, standard regimen is sufficient. Alternate regimen should be considered in high-risk patients who are expected to have excessive gingival bleeding.

SPECIFIC GUIDELINES

Cardiovascular Defect	*Significant Soft Tissue Pathology or Surgical Trauma*	
	YES	*NO*
High risk	Alternate regimen	Standard regimen
Significant risk	Standard regimen	Standard regimen
Minimal risk	No prophylaxis	No prophylaxis

12

The Patient Undergoing Cardiac Surgery

The dentist may be consulted for an evaluation of the oral health of a patient who is scheduled to undergo cardiac surgery. The dentist should be integrally involved in the preoperative care of these patients. A number of cardiac surgical procedures can increase the risk of developing bacterial endocarditis. Because the primary source of transient bacteremia that can result in bacterial endocarditis is the oral cavity, the oral health of the patient should be optimized preoperatively, whenever feasible.

The most common cardiac surgical procedures are coronary artery bypass grafts, heart valve replacements, and the repair of congenital cardiovascular defects such as atrial septal defects, ventricular septal defects, tetralogy of Fallot, or coarctation of the aorta.

Coronary artery bypass surgery is usually performed in patients with angina refractory to medical management (Chap. 5). These patients have undergone coronary angiography and have been demonstrated to have surgically correctable coronary artery lesions. The procedure is usually performed by using the patient's own saphenous veins as grafts to bypass the diseased coronary arteries (Figs. 12–1 and 12–2). The procedure usually alleviates symptoms and may improve exercise tolerance.

Replacement of heart valves is usually done to correct a stenotic or leaky valve. The valvular lesions may be congenital or the result of rheumatic heart disease, trauma, or infective endocarditis. In surgery, the patient's defective valve is replaced by either an artificial valve (Fig. 12–3) or a porcine valve (Fig. 12–4).

Repairs of congenital cardiovascular defects are usually performed because of cardiac compromises. Grafts are often used in the repair. The congenital lesions requiring surgical corrections include atrial septal defects, ventricular septal defects, coarctation of the aorta, tetralogy of Fallot, and transposition of the great vessels.

The dentist should be aware of the risk that the patient may develop bacterial endocarditis

after various cardiac procedures and plan therapy accordingly.

MEDICAL EVALUATION

Some patients have significant medical compromises that limit dental therapeutic options and preclude extended and comprehensive dental care. This is particularly true of patients who have to undergo emergency cardiac surgery. In this instance, time constraints may dictate the extraction of teeth that might otherwise be salvageable given extended dental therapy. Similarly, dental therapeutic strategies for patients with unstable angina or severe congestive heart failure may have to be altered to minimize exacerbation of symptoms. (The dental evaluation and management of these patients are discussed in Chaps. 5 and 7.) The

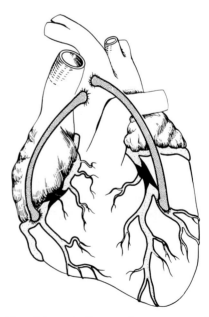

Figure 12–1. Schematic diagram of coronary artery bypass surgery demonstrating the use of vein grafts to bypass areas of diseased coronary arteries.

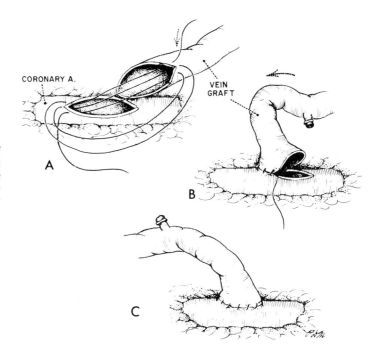

Figure 12-2. Example of technique of vein graft to a coronary artery. (From Cohn, L. H. [ed.]: The Treatment of Acute Myocardial Ischemia. An Integrated Medical-Surgical Approach. Mt. Kisco, NY, Futura Publishing, 1979.)

dentist has to be in close consultation with the patient's physician to determine the most appropriate dental therapy.

DENTAL EVALUATION

The dental evaluation should be directed primarily at assessing the risk of developing

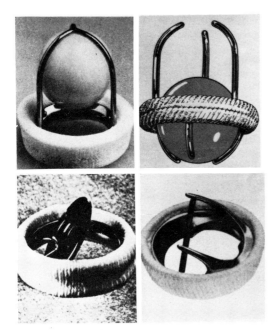

Figure 12-3. Artificial prosthetic valves. (From Braunwald, E. [ed.]: Heart Disease: A Textbook of Cardiovascular Medicine. Philadelphia, W. B. Saunders, 1980.)

bacterial endocarditis *after* cardiac surgical procedures. Patients who are at high risk for developing endocarditis postoperatively should have aggressive preoperative intervention to minimize the risk.

Different cardiac surgical procedures place the patient at varying risk for the development of postoperative bacterial endocarditis and require different dental therapeutic interventions.

Patients at Low Risk. Coronary artery bypass procedures and primary repair of an atrial septal defect of the secundum type involve no increased risk of developing bacterial endocarditis beyond the immediate postoperative period.

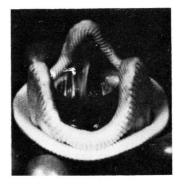

Figure 12-4. Porcine prosthetic valve. (From Braunwald, E. [ed.]: Heart Disease: A Textbook of Cardiovascular Medicine. Philadelphia, W. B. Saunders, 1980.)

Patients at Significant Risk. Patients requiring valvular replacement or repair of congenital lesions (other than uncomplicated atrial septal defects) are at significant risk for the subsequent development of bacterial endocarditis. They should have careful evaluation, and every attempt should be made to optimize oral health prior to cardiac surgery.

The dental examination should include extraoral and intraoral soft tissue inspection, occlusal, caries, and periodontal examination, and a complete current series of radiographs. The examination should be performed specifically to detect any acute or subacute infections that could compromise a patient's postoperative status. Active abscesses, fistulae, periapical disease, and active periodontal disease markedly increase the likelihood of transient bacteremia and can lead to bacterial endocarditis in the susceptible patient.

DENTAL MANAGEMENT

General Guidelines

Prior to any treatment in preoperative patients, the dentist should be aware of any underlying cardiac abnormalities and assess the need for antibiotic prophylaxis. Most patients undergoing valvular replacement or repair of congenital cardiovascular defects have significant underlying cardiac lesions. In contrast, patients undergoing coronary artery bypass surgery normally have coronary artery disease without other cardiac abnormalities. They are not at increased risk for the development of bacterial endocarditis and, in the absence of other indications, do not require antibiotic prophylaxis. (The various regimens commonly used for prophylaxis are discussed in detail in Chap. 11.)

Time constraints and the medical status of the patient may limit therapeutic options. Dental treatment should be tailored to the needs of the individual patient.

The dentist should try to minimize stress to the patient undergoing cardiac surgery. Whenever feasible, lengthy procedures should be spread over several shorter appointments. Adjunctive sedation techniques should be considered when appropriate.

In general, the use of epinephrine should be minimized in patients with significant underlying cardiac disease, especially if arrhythmia is a concern.

Because the majority of the patients undergoing cardiac surgery have significant underlying cardiac abnormalities, hospitalization should be considered for cardiac monitoring, especially if extensive dental therapy is necessary.

Specific Guidelines

The dental management of patients undergoing cardiac surgery depends on the risk of developing postoperative bacterial endocarditis.

Patients at Low Risk. Acute infections should be eliminated prior to cardiac surgery. Active abscesses, fistulae, periapical disease, and suppurative periodontal disease should be aggressively treated.

Patients at Significant Risk. The primary goal is to eliminate infection quickly before the operation to minimize the risk of *postoperative* bacterial endocarditis. In addition to the extraction of acutely infected teeth, any tooth with a questionable prognosis because of pulpal or periodontal disease should also be extracted.

■ Examples of Dental Evaluation and Management

EVALUATION

Patient 1. A 54-year-old man with critical aortic stenosis is referred for preoperative dental evaluation prior to aortic valve replacement. Dental examination reveals multiple caries and moderate to advanced periodontitis.

Patient 2. A 65-year-old man with severe angina is referred for preoperative evaluation prior to coronary artery bypass procedure. His dental needs are the same as those of Patient 1.

MANAGEMENT

Patient 1. The patient's underlying valvular disease places him at significant risk of developing bacterial endocarditis, and *all* dental manipulations should be carried out under antibiotic prophylaxis. Consultation with his physician reveals that the patient has symptoms and findings of congestive heart failure. These should be controlled medically prior to the initiation of dental treatment. The cardiac surgical procedure planned would place the patient at high risk for the development of bacterial endocarditis postoperatively, so dental treatment should optimize the patient's oral health preoperatively. If, after careful consultation with the patient's physician, it is decided that the patient can be managed as an outpatient, the following treatment plan is recommended:

1. Teeth with slight to moderate caries should be excavated and restored.
2. Teeth with deep caries, pulpal exposure, or near-pulpal exposure should be extracted.
3. Teeth with moderate to severe periodontal disease should be extracted.

If, in the opinion of his physician, the patient cannot tolerate extended preoperative dental therapy as an outpatient, the following treatment plan is recommended:

1. The patient should be admitted to the hospital for dental therapy. Ideally, the hospitalization should precede the planned valvular surgery by at least 10 to 14 days to permit adequate healing.

2. The patient's physician should be consulted to optimize the patient's cardiac status.
3. When the patient is clinically stable, the dentist should extract all teeth with questionable prognoses, moderate to severe periodontal disease, moderate or deep caries, or any evidence of pulpal disease.
4. Scaling and root planing of the remaining teeth should be performed.

Patient 2. The patient is not at increased risk for the development of bacterial endocarditis either preoperatively or postoperatively, so his dental management is largely dictated by the severity of the coronary disease. (The management of patients with severe angina was discussed in detail in Chap. 5.) Acutely infected teeth should be extracted preoperatively. If possible, preliminary periodontal therapy, deep caries excavation, and endodontic procedures can be completed as the medical condition allows.

SUMMARY TABLE **12–I**

Indications for Cardiac Surgery

CARDIAC SURGICAL PROCEDURES	INDICATIONS
Coronary artery bypass grafts	Coronary artery disease with angina or myocardial infarction
Valvular replacement	Valvular stenosis or insufficiency
Correction of congenital anomalies	Atrial septal defect, ventricular septal defect, tetralogy of Fallot, coarctation of the aorta

SUMMARY TABLE **12–II**

Risk Categories for Developing Bacterial Endocarditis After Cardiac Surgery

PATIENTS AT LOW RISK*
Paients with coronary artery bypass graft
Patients with repair of an atrial septal defect of the secundum type

PATIENTS AT SIGNIFICANT RISK*
Patients with correction of congenital anomalies (except for uncomplicated atrial septal defects)
Patients with valvular replacement

*See Chap. 11.

SUMMARY TABLE **12–III**

Dental Management of the Patient Undergoing Cardiac Surgery

GENERAL GUIDELINES

1. Antibiotic prophylaxis prior to treatment (Chap. 11):
    a. Coronary artery bypass graft—no prophylaxis
    b. Congenital anomalies—standard regimen
    c. Valvular lesions—standard regimen
2. Medical status of patient may limit therapeutic options
3. Minimize stress through shorter appointments and adjunctive sedation techniques
4. Limit use of epinephrine
5. Hospitalization

SPECIFIC GUIDELINES

1. Patients at low or significant risk for developing postoperative bacterial endocarditis: eliminate acute infections preoperatively
2. Patients at high risk for developing postoperative bacterial endocarditis: extract all acutely infected teeth and any tooth with a questionable prognosis caused by pulpal or periodontal disease

13

The Patient Who Has Undergone Cardiac Surgery

The patient who has undergone cardiac surgery requires special consideration prior to the initiation of dental therapy. The two major concerns are the risk of developing endocarditis and the risk of bleeding secondary to the administration of anticoagulants. Different cardiac surgical procedures place the patient at different risks for bacterial endocarditis, and the types of dental prophylaxis required differ accordingly. Furthermore, some patients may be placed on anticoagulants after the placement of prosthetic valves and therefore require special intervention.

MEDICAL EVALUATION

Because all patients who have undergone cardiac surgery have had some compromising cardiac lesions, it is important to be aware of the medical problems that can persist even after surgery.

Patients who have undergone coronary artery bypass procedures may have persistent angina or congestive heart failure (Chaps. 5 and 12).

Patients who have undergone prosthetic heart valve replacement may have residual heart failure. In some instances, leaking around the prosthetic valves (paravalvular leak) may aggravate the heart failure. Patients with prostheses are usually placed on anticoagulants to prevent clot formation on the prostheses. Patients with porcine valves, on the other hand, do not require prolonged anticoagulation.

Patients who have had correction of congenital heart lesions may have residual heart failure and may require medical intervention prior to dental therapy.

DENTAL EVALUATION

After assessing the patient's medical status, the dental evaluation should determine the need for antibiotic prophylaxis (Chap. 11) and the need for adjusting the dosage of anticoagulants (Chap. 26; Fig. 13–1).

In general, patients who have had coronary artery bypass grafts are not at increased risk for the development of bacterial endocarditis beyond the immediate postoperative period and do not need prophylaxis. Even during the first 6 months immediately after the operation, when there is ongoing healing of the suture sites, the risk of developing bacterial endocarditis is minimal and prophylaxis is optional.

Patients who have had primary repair of uncomplicated atrial septal defects of the secundum type, who have had a ventricular septal defect repaired without Dacron grafting, and who have had a patent ductus arteriosus repaired do not require subacute bacterial endocarditis prophylaxis for dental procedures 6 months or more after the cardiac surgery. All other patients who have undergone correction of congenital heart disease have a significant risk for developing bacterial endocarditis because of the synthetic graft and do require prophylaxis. In addition, vascular repairs with synthetic grafts (i.e., aortic aneurysm) also require prophylaxis. Data suggest that while most of the synthetic graft is epithelialized during healing, denuded areas persist. Therefore, a risk for infection, however small, remains. Because there is a very low risk of complications of antibiotic prophylaxis, it is recommended.

Patients with prosthetic heart valves are at high risk for the development of bacterial endocarditis and antibiotic prophylaxis is also

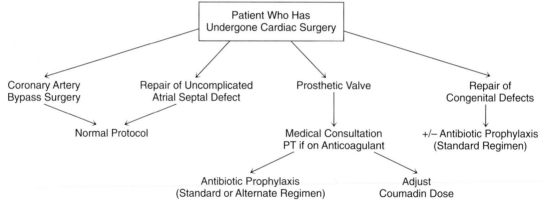

Figure 13–1. Dental evaluation and management of the patient who has undergone cardiac surgery.

mandatory. Some patients with prosthetic valves are also on chronic anticoagulation therapy, which may need to be modified (Chap. 26) when dental therapy is planned.

DENTAL MANAGEMENT

General Guidelines

A careful assessment of the patient's medical status and consultation with the physician are essential. Whenever feasible, the medical status should be optimized before the initiation of comprehensive dental therapy.

The dentist should try to minimize stress in patients with cardiac compromises. Whenever possible, lengthy procedures should be spread over several shorter appointments. Adjunctive sedation techniques should be considered when appropriate (Chap. 50).

In general, the use of epinephrine should be minimized in patients with underlying cardiac compromises, especially if arrhythmia is a significant problem.

Specific Guidelines

Coronary Artery Bypass Procedure. The patient does not require antibiotic prophylaxis except in the immediate postoperative period, when prophylaxis is optional.

Surgical Repairs Without Synthetic Grafts. Patients with primary repairs of uncomplicated atrial septal defects of the secundum type, ventricular septal defects repaired without Dacron grafting, and repaired patent ductus arteriosus do not require antibiotic prophylaxis 6 months or more after cardiac surgery.

Correction of Congenital Cardiac Lesions with Synthetic Grafts. These patients are at a significant risk for developing bacterial endocarditis. Patients with minimal inflammatory gingival changes undergoing simple dental procedures (types I to III) should receive the standard oral regimen. Patients with severe local inflammatory disease and patients requiring dental surgical procedures (types IV to VI) might need to receive alternate regimen coverage but usually can be treated with the standard protocol.

Prosthetic Heart Valve. Patients with prosthetic heart valves are at high risk for bacterial endocarditis and should receive antibiotic prophylaxis. The American Heart Association's 1990 guidelines note that, based on international data, the standard oral regimen usually appears to provide adequate prophylaxis. However, in patients with severe local gingival inflammatory disease and patients requiring dental surgical procedures (types IV to VI) when excessive gingival bleeding is anticipated, parenteral antibiotics (alternate regimen) may provide more effective prophylaxis. A consultation with the cardiologist is recommended.

Some patients may be on maintenance oral anticoagulants after the placement of prosthetic valves. These patients are obviously at high risk for excessive bleeding unless the anticoagulant is stopped prior to dental treatment. Because the cessation of anticoagulation may be associated with the formation of clots on prosthetic valves, the patient's physician should be involved in the adjustment of anticoagulant therapy (Chap. 26).

Cardiac Transplant. The success of cardiac transplants has improved remarkably over recent years, largely because of the use of cyclosporine, an effective antirejection drug that has fewer undesirable side effects than older immunosuppressive agents. Cardiac transplants are limited to patients with severe terminal disease, such as cardiomyopathy. The number of transplants performed each year is restricted by the availability of transplantable hearts, not by the number of potential recipients. The success rate for cardiac transplant is now over 80% after 1 year and 50% after 5 years.

The two major causes of death associated with the procedure are rejection and infection. The advent of cyslosporine has helped reduce the risk of rejection. However, because patients must be immunocompromised, their susceptibility to fungal, viral, and bacterial infections is high. As is the case with other immunocompromised patients, the mouth is a frequent site of infection, and is often a source of potential sepsis. Cardiac transplantation results in two clinical issues for dentists that are similar to those seen in patients receiving chemotherapy for cancer: (1), the need to identify and eliminate potential sources of infection prior to the transplant; and (2), considerations for dental therapy once the transplant has been successfully performed.

Patients being considered for a cardiac transplant should receive a complete dental evaluation prior to surgery consisting of a complete clinical examination, a full-mouth series of radiographs (those performed within 6 months are adequate), and a panoramic radiograph in patients with third molars. All areas of pathology should be eliminated as definitively as possible. Generally, extraction is preferable in cases of advanced periodontal disease or for teeth with pulpal involvement. The dentist must remember that the patient's cardiac status is exceptionally compromised, and long, involved treatment is to be avoided. More rigorous dental procedures (types III to VI) are best performed in the controlled environment of the hospital. Effective communication with the patient's cardiologist is mandatory, and adequate time must be allowed for healing. Many patients about to undergo cardiac transplant require prophylaxis for bacterial endocarditis prior to dental treatment.

Following the transplant, the patient should be more cardiodynamically stable. The major dental risk in the cardiac transplant recipient is infection. Antibiotic prophylaxis is recommended, as is aggressive treatment of dental infection. Patients should be instructed about the need for aggressive oral hygiene and

placed on frequent maintenance recall schedules. Cyclosporin therapy, particularly in higher doses, can cause gingival hyperplasia not unlike that caused by phenytoin therapy. Management of the hyperplasia involves rigorous oral hygiene and recall prophylaxis and surgical gingivectomy in some circumstances.

■ Examples of Dental Evaluation and Management

EVALUATION

Patient 1. This 48-year-old woman had mitral valve replacement with a prosthetic valve 3 years ago. She is currently completely asymptomatic. Consultation with her physician reveals that she underwent the cardiac surgical procedure because of severe mitral stenosis. She is currently on 0.25 mg of digoxin because of atrial fibrillation and 5 mg of warfarin (Coumadin) daily. She was last examined a week ago, when she was found to be at her baseline state with chronic atrial fibrillation. Her prothrombin time (PT) was 20 seconds, with a control value of 11 seconds. On examination now, her pulse is irregular, at a rate of 70 beats per minute (bpm) and her blood pressure is 110/60. She has moderate periodontal disease.

Patient 2. This 68-year-old man, 6 years after a coronary artery bypass procedure, is free of chest pain and does not have significant shortness of breath. He walks 2 miles daily without difficulty. On examination now, he has a regular pulse at a rate of 78 bpm and his blood pressure is 140/80. He has mild periodontal disease.

Patient 3. This 24-year-old woman had cardiac surgery to repair coarctation of the aorta at age 18. She is currently asymptomatic, has no limitation of her physical activities, and is on no medication. On examination, she has a regular pulse at a rate of 84 bpm and her blood pressure is 110/72. She has mild periodontitis.

MANAGEMENT

Patient 1. Oral examination reveals an intact dentition with moderate periodontitis and accumulation of subgingival calculus. The treatment plan includes deep scaling, root planing, and curettage. She has a prosthetic valve in place and is therefore at high risk for bacterial endocarditis. She needs antibiotic prophylaxis minimally with the standard regimen. Because of the inflammatory gingival changes and the anticipation of significant bleeding with curettage, the cardiologist might suggest the parenteral alternate reigmen. She has atrial fibrillation, but her rate appears to be under reasonable control on medication (Chap. 9). She is on oral anticoagulants, which create significant problems with bleeding. In consultation with her physician, Coumadin is stopped 2 days prior to the dental appointment. Her PT on the morning of the procedure is 15 seconds, with a control value of 11 seconds. Scaling and root planing are performed using adjunctive sedation techniques. Coumadin is resumed the evening after the dental procedure (Chap. 26).

Patient 2. The patient is at no increased risk for bacterial endocarditis after his coronary artery bypass procedure, and his dental procedures can be carried out using normal operating protocol with elective adjunctive sedation.

Patient 3. The patient requires scaling and root planing. She is at significant risk for the development of bacterial endocarditis and must receive antibiotic prophylaxis prior to all dental procedures. Usually such a patient would receive the oral standard regimen, but the alternate regimen might be used because of local tissue inflammation.

SUMMARY TABLE **13–I**

Medical Evaluation of the Patient After Cardiac Surgery

ASSESS CARDIAC STATUS

Angina

Congestive heart failure

Arrhythmia

Conduction abnormalities

ANTICOAGULANTS

Necessary for artificial prosthetic valves

Not necessary beyond the immediate postoperative period for porcine valves

---

SUMMARY TABLE **13–II**

Dental Evaluation of the Patient After Cardiac Surgery

Assess the patient's risk of developing endocarditis and the need for antibiotic prophylaxis:
    Coronary artery bypass graft—no increased risk
    Selected repairs of congenital lesions without synthetic grafts—no increased risk
    Correction of congenital anomaly with synthetic grafts—significant risk
    Valvular replacement—high risk

Assess the need for adjustment of the anticoagulant dosage (Chap. 26) and check the prothrombin time for patients with prosthetic valve replacement

SUMMARY TABLE **13–III**

Dental Management of the Patient After Cardiac Surgery

GENERAL GUIDELINES
Medical status:
  Should be optimized by a physician prior to elective dental therapy
  Medical consultation, when appropriate

Minimization of stress:
  Shorter appointments
  Adjunctive sedation techniques, when appropriate

Minimize the use of epinephrine

SPECIFIC GUIDELINES
Patients at No Increased Risk of Subacute Bacterial Endocarditis
No antibiotic prophylaxis

Patients at Significant Risk of Subacute Bacterial Endocarditis

GINGIVAL INFLAMMATION	PROCEDURES	PROTOCOL
Minimal	I–III	Standard regimen
	IV–VI	Standard or alternate regimen
Moderate to advanced	I–VI	Standard or alternate regimen

Patients at High Risk of Subacute Bacterial Endocarditis

GINGIVAL INFLAMMATION	PROCEDURES	PROTOCOL
Minimal	I–III	Standard regimen
	IV–VI	Standard or alternate regimen
Moderate to advanced	I–VI	Alternate or standard regimen

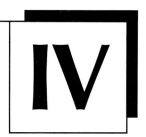

Evaluation and Management of the Patient with Endocrine Disease and of the Pregnant Patient

14

Diabetes Mellitus

Diabetes mellitus results from an absolute or relative insulin insufficiency caused either by a low output of insulin from the pancreas or by unresponsiveness of peripheral tissues to insulin. Diabetes is the third leading cause of death in the United States, the leading cause of blindness in adults, and the most common metabolic disorder. When the onset of diabetes is between the ages of 10 and 30, there is a 12- to 17-year decrease in life expectancy. The onset of diabetes after the age of 50 reduces life expectancy by 3 to 7 years. It is a common disease that affects approximately 200 million people in the world and 5 million people in the United States. Diabetes affects 17 people per thousand between the ages of 25 and 44 and 79 people per thousand over the age of 65. Thus, approximately 3 to 4% of the dentist's adult patients has diabetes.

The most important risk factor associated with the development of diabetes is heredity. Relatives of patients with diabetes are 2½ times more likely to develop the disease than the population at large. Obesity and old age are also risk factors.

The major symptoms of diabetes—polydipsia, polyuria, polyphagia, and weight loss—are the result of insulin deficiency. Insulin plays a crucial role in the regulation of carbohydrate, fat, and protein metabolism. Insufficient insulin results in decreased entry of blood glucose into tissues and an increase in the blood glucose level. An increase in blood glucose levels leads to increased delivery of glucose to the kidneys. The inability of the kidneys to reabsorb all this excess glucose results in glycosuria. This leads to osmotic diuresis and an increase in urine output (polyuria), which has to be compensated for by an increased oral intake of fluids (polydipsia). Continuous loss of glucose in the urine also results in weight loss, despite increases in dietary intake (polyphagia).

In addition to abnormalities in glucose utilization, insulin deficiency also leads to abnormal fat and protein metabolism. Increased breakdown of fat leads to increased generation of ketones. With severe insulin deficiency, ketone bodies can accumulate, resulting in ketoacidosis. Patients with ketoacidosis may give a history of increasing polydipsia and polyuria as well as systemic symptoms, such as nausea and vomiting. Clinically, they appear dehydrated, lethargic, and confused. They have exaggerated breathing (Kussmaul respiration) and a fruity acetone odor to their breath. Severe ketoacidosis results in alteration in mental status and cardiovascular instability. Coma and death can result if therapy is not instituted promptly.

In addition to the metabolic complications of diabetes, patients with the disease may develop vascular, neurologic, and infectious complications. Patients with diabetes have an increased incidence of large and small vessel diseases. Large vessel complications are manifested by accelerated coronary artery disease, cerebrovascular disease, and peripheral vascular disease. Small vessel diseases lead to diabetic retinopathy (which can result in blindness) and diabetic kidney disease (which can result in renal failure). Neurologic complications include peripheral neuropathy with prominent sensory losses. These can result in inadvertent trauma causing ulcerations or gangrenous changes in the digits, hands, and feet. Autonomic insufficiency is also observed in some patients, resulting in postural hypotension, sexual impotence, and abnormality in gastrointestinal motility. Diabetics are also more prone to infections because of compromised host responses. Skin and urinary tract infections occur frequently in such patients.

MEDICAL EVALUATION

The diagnosis of diabetes may occasionally be made during a routine test on an asymptomatic patient by the demonstration of an elevation of blood glucose (hyperglycemia) or glucose in the urine (glycosuria). Symptomatic patients with polyphagia, polydipsia, polyuria, and weight loss may have the diagnosis of diabetes confirmed by the demonstration of a fasting blood glucose level above 120 mg/dl. Because transient elevations in blood glucose occur after meals, elevations of blood glucose after fasting are more diagnostic of an abnormal state.

Occasionally, abnormalities in glucose metabolism can be uncovered only after glucose loading in an oral glucose tolerance test. In this test, serial determinations of blood glucose levels are made after the ingestion of 100 g of glucose. In the normal patient, there is a transient increase in glucose levels, which then return to normal within 2 hours after the glucose loading dose (Fig. 14–1). In a patient with diabetes, the increased glucose level lingers and is slow to return to baseline.

The clinical course of diabetes mellitus is variable. Some patients may continue to have only chemical evidence of glucose intolerance without symptoms and are often referred to as chemical diabetics. Others may have progressive metabolic, vascular, neurologic, and infectious complications.

Two forms of diabetes have been defined in terms of the patient's dependence on insulin: type I (insulin-dependent, ketosis-prone) and type II (non–insulin-dependent, non–ketosis-prone). Of patients with diabetes, 90% have type II diabetes, which usually develops after the age of 40. They tend to be obese and have glucose intolerance because of the resistance of peripheral tissues to the action of insulin. Ketoacidosis occurs less frequently in this group.

Type I diabetes occurs in 10% of diabetic patients, and they are dependent on insulin. These patients usually develop their disease before the age of 25. However, in many older patients, type II diabetes may also evolve to require insulin. Usually, this reflects diabetes secondary to an autoimmune disorder affecting the pancreas. Patients with this disorder have decreased endogenous secretion of insulin. Both groups of patients can have progressive cardiovascular, renal, and neurologic complications, but patients with diabetes mellitus are more likely to develop complications of the disease.

MEDICAL MANAGEMENT

Medical management of diabetes revolves around optimizing blood sugar control. Recent studies have demonstrated dramatically the importance of blood glucose control in the reduction of diabetic end-organ damage.

The medical management of diabetes is different for the two groups of diabetic patients.

Generally, the first therapeutic maneuver for patients with type II diabetes is an attempt to normalize the patient's weight to decrease the peripheral resistance to circulating insulin. Usually, returning the patient to an ideal body weight minimizes the problems associated with glucose intolerance. Patients may use reagent strips such as Dextrostix or Chemstrips for estimation of the blood glucose level (Fig. 14–2). Blood is usually obtained from a finger using a small lancet. Daily monitoring provides the patient and the physician with an estimate of the level of control of the disease.

Patients who continue to have significant hy-

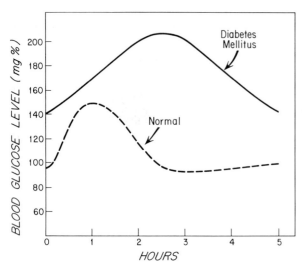

Figure 14–1. Glucose tolerance curve in a normal patient and in a patient with diabetes mellitus. In the normal patient there is a transient increase in blood glucose levels, which then return to normal within 2 hours after the glucose loading dose. In the patient with diabetes mellitus, the increased blood glucose level lingers and is slow to return to baseline levels.

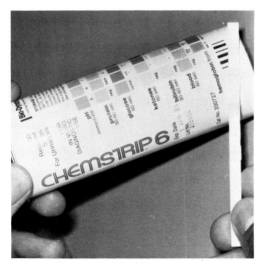

Figure 14–2. Example of Chemstrips, reagent strips used for the measurement of blood glucose levels.

perglycemia, despite attempts at weight control, can be managed either with oral hypoglycemic agents or with insulin. The long-term use of oral hypoglycemic agents is controversial because they have been associated with cardiovascular deaths. Many physicians limit the use of these agents to patients who are unable or unwilling to take insulin.

Two types of oral hypoglycemic agents are available: sulfonylureas and biguanides. The sulfonylureas—including medications such as acetohexamide (Dymelor), chlorpropamide (Diabinese), tolbutamide (Orinase), flyburide (Diabeta, Flucotrol), flipizine (Micronase), and tolazamide (Tolinase)—act by increasing the production of endogenous insulin. Biguanides such as phenformin (DBI) act by enhancing the action of available insulin. However, phenformin has been associated with life-threatening lactic acidosis and has been removed from the market in the United States.

The management of patients with juvenile-onset diabetes mellitus is different from that of patients with adult-onset diabetes. These patients are usually not obese and do not require limitation of caloric intake. Because their disease is largely the result of insufficient insulin, their management depends on the use of insulin. The goal of therapy is to control the blood glucose level and thereby minimize complications arising from hyperglycemia and prevent the development of ketoacidosis.

Because of the increasing evidence that tight diabetic control can minimize diabetic end-organ damage, patients are now encouraged to monitor their blood glucose frequently in order to carefully titrate the insulin dosing.

The determination of the hemoglobin A1c (Hgb A1c) concentration allows for monitoring of the adequacy of control (Table 14–1). Hemoglobin A1c reflects the proportion of the hemoglobin A that is glycosylated. Normal patients usually have about 5% of their hemoglobin glycosylated, whereas diabetic patients can have as much as 20% of their hemoglobin glycosylated. Optimal diabetic control results in hemoglobin A1c levels of less than 7%.

Numerous preparations of short-, intermediate-, and long-acting insulin are available. Short-acting preparations such as crystalline (regular) insulin, Semilente, and globin insulin have an onset of action in 30 to 60 minutes and a duration of action of 6 to 12 hours, with maximal action usually at 4 to 6 hours. Intermediate-acting preparations such as isophane insulin suspension (NPH) and Lente have an onset of action in 2 to 3 hours, a duration of action of 18 to 24 hours, and a peak effect at 8 to 12 hours. Long-acting preparations such as Protamine Zinc Insulin (PZI) and Ultralente have an onset of action in 3 to 4 hours, a duration of action of 24 to 36 hours, and a peak effect at 14 to 18 hours (Summary Table 14–VI). The most commonly used short-acting insulin is crystalline (regular) insulin.

The cornerstone of insulin therapy is intermediate-acting insulin (NPH), which can often be administered subcutaneously on a daily basis. In some patients, mixtures of short- and intermediate-acting insulins may be used to maximize control. Other patients may require multiple insulin injections for optimal regulation of their blood glucose level.

Hypoglycemia is the most serious complication of therapy. Because the consequences of hypoglycemia can be drastic, the dentist should be aware of the common presenting symptoms and clinical settings leading to hypoglycemia. Hypoglycemia usually occurs as a result of excessive insulin or hypoglycemic agents. Inadequate oral intake may aggravate the situation. The clinical signs and symptoms

Table 14–1. HEMOGLOBIN A1c LEVEL AS INDICATOR OF ADEQUACY OF CONTROL OF DIABETES MELLITUS

Hgb A1c (%)	Level of Control
<7%	Good
7–9%	Fair
>9%	Poor

of hypoglycemia include weakness, nervousness, tremulousness, palpitations, and excessive sweating. The patient's sensorium may progress from confusion and agitation to seizure and coma.

Hypoglycemia should be recognized and promptly treated (Summary Table 14–VIII). The treatment of patients with mild symptoms of hypoglycemia includes the administration of sugar in the form of candy or glucose solutions such as orange juice. Lethargic patients who are unable to take oral fluids are treated with the intravenous administration of concentrated glucose solutions such as 50% dextrose in water ($D_{50}W$). Usually, patients respond within 3 to 5 minutes of the administration of glucose.

Patients on insulin can develop local reactions at the site of injection, allergies to one or more forms of insulin, insulin resistance, and lipodystrophy. In the appropriate patient, pancreatic islet cell transplant can be considered.

DENTAL EVALUATION

Patients Not Known to Have Diabetes Mellitus

It is estimated that for every known diabetic patient, there is one patient with undiagnosed diabetes mellitus. The dentist must therefore be vigilant to detect previously undiagnosed diabetes. The dental history should include questions regarding polyuria, polydipsia, polyphagia, and weight loss. Patients giving a positive history should be referred either to a clinical laboratory for evaluation of the blood glucose level (Chap. 1) or to their physician for further evaluation prior to the initiation of comprehensive dental treatment.

Patients Known to Have Diabetes Mellitus

The dental evaluation of a patient known to have diabetes should determine the form of diabetes (adult-onset or juvenile-onset), the therapy being employed, the adequacy of diabetic control, and the presence of neurologic, vascular, renal, or infectious complications.

The patient should be specifically asked about the duration of disease, the occurrence of hypoglycemia, the history of hospitalizations for ketoacidosis, and any changes in therapeutic regimen. For patients who monitor their blood glucose level at home, the results of recent blood testing should be recorded. The patient's physician may be consulted to clarify the medical status. When available, the most recent fasting blood glucose and hemoglobin A1c levels are also of interest.

Based on the information gathered, patients can be assigned to specific risk categories. These risk categories should suggest some specific guidelines for management.

Patients at Low Risk. Patients with good metabolic control on a stable medical regimen are at low risk. These patients are asymptomatic and have no neurologic, vascular, or infectious complications. Their fasting blood glucose level should be less than 200 mg/dl. Patients with a hemoglobin A1c concentration lower than 7% are deemed to be under excellent control and are at low risk for dental interventions.

Patients at Moderate Risk. These patients have occasional symptoms but are in reasonable metabolic balance. There is no recent history of hypoglycemia or ketoacidosis, and few of the complications of diabetes are present. The fasting blood glucose should be less than 250 mg/dl. Patients with a hemoglobin A1c concentration of 7 to 9% are deemed to be under reasonable glucose control and are at moderate risk for dental interventions.

Patients at High Risk. These patients have multiple complications of the disease and are under poor metabolic control. There is a history of frequent hypoglycemia or ketoacidosis, and there is often a constant need to adjust insulin dosages. The fasting blood glucose may fluctuate wildly, often exceeding 250 mg/dl. Patients with a hemoglobin A1c concentration greater than 9% are deemed to be under poor long-term glucose control and are at high risk for dental interventions.

DENTAL MANAGEMENT OF OUTPATIENTS

Dental management is different for the diabetic having limited dental therapy as an outpatient and the hospitalized diabetic patient requiring more extensive treatment.

General Guidelines

The primary goal should be to avoid untoward metabolic imbalances during the period of dental therapy. Patients should be carefully instructed about their diet and their medications during the course of therapy so as to minimize problems related to either hyperglycemia or hypoglycemia. The dentist should attempt to minimize stress and the risk of infection.

Diet. Unless specifically instructed, an anxious patient may miss a meal prior to a dental appointment. This can increase the risk of hypoglycemia. The patient should be scheduled for a midmorning appointment and instructed to eat a normal breakfast. This minimizes the likelihood of hypoglycemia during the dental procedure, when the blood glucose level should be relatively high. Attention should also be paid to the length of dental sessions. If a session runs into normal meal time, arrangements should be made to allow interruptions for appropriate snacks (e.g., orange juice). Finally, some patients may have limited ability to chew after certain dental procedures. These patients should be prescribed soft foods or liquids (e.g., powdered instant breakfast drinks, milk shakes, soups, or scrambled eggs) to maintain their caloric intake.

Oral Hypoglycemic Agents. Patients should be instructed to take their normal dosage of oral hypoglycemic agents for all outpatient dental procedures.

Insulin Therapy. Modification of insulin therapy must be considered for patients with diabetes who have their meal timing altered or are about to undergo stressful dental procedures. When necessary (see the following specific guidelines) the patient may be instructed to take half of the normal morning dose of insulin and to have a normal breakfast. The patient can often be given the other half of the insulin dose when a normal diet is resumed after the dental procedure.

Minimization of Stress. The dentist should try to minimize stress to the diabetic patient. Whenever feasible, lengthy procedures should be spread over several shorter appointments. Adjunctive sedation techniques should be considered, when appropriate.

Minimizing the Risk of Infection. Diabetics are at increased risk of developing dental and other infections, a risk that can be minimized by preventive and therapeutic maneuvers. The patient with diabetes should have aggressive preventive dental services including frequent recall examinations, oral hygiene instruction, prophylaxis, and treatment of periodontal dis-

ease. The patient should also be considered for antibiotic prophylaxis following surgical procedures, endodontic therapy, and subgingival scaling in the presence of suppurative periodontitis. Antibiotics are important in the treatment of all acute infections. Nonabsorbable suture materials should be used in patients with diabetes, because these patients heal slowly.

Medical Consultation. The physician should be consulted on specific management issues to ascertain the severity of the patient's disease and the degree of control over it. *The physician should also be involved in decisions about insulin coverage during dental treatment.*

Specific Guidelines

Patients at Low Risk. These patients may be treated with normal protocol for all restorative dental procedures (types I to III). Careful attention should be paid to diet control, minimization of stress, and risks of infection in all surgical procedures (types IV to VI). Adjunctive sedation techniques should be considered for all surgery. Usually, no adjustment in insulin therapy is necessary.

Patients at Moderate Risk. General guidelines regarding diet control, minimization of stress, and risk of infection are increasingly important for patients at moderate risk. These patients can undergo restorative dentistry (types I to III procedures) using normal protocol, but the use of adjunctive sedation techniques should be considered. Moderate and advanced dental surgery (types IV to VI) should be performed only after consultation with the patient's physician. Adjunctive sedation techniques should be used, and hospitalization should be considered for advanced surgical procedures (type VI). Insulin dosage adjustments in consultation with the patient's physician should be considered for simple dental surgery (type IV procedures) and is recommended for moderate and advanced dental surgery (types V and VI procedures).

Patients at High Risk. These patients can undergo oral examination after appropriate measures are taken to minimize stress. All other procedures should be deferred until the medical status is stabilized.

An important exception is the patient whose diabetic control is compromised by active dental infection. In this case, the simplest procedure to bring infection under control should be performed. Often, insulin requirements decrease and better diabetic control can be achieved.

DENTAL MANAGEMENT OF HOSPITALIZED PATIENTS

Hospitalization should be considered for patients with extensive surgical needs and in patients at moderate to high risk. The guidelines for minimizing metabolic imbalances, stress, and risks of infection are the same as those delineated for the outpatient. However, the procedures involved often interfere with the patient's dietary intake, in which case adjustments in the medical regimen are necessary.

Management of Patients Taking Oral Hypoglycemic Agents

Oral hypoglycemic therapy should be continued whenever feasible, and patients should be managed on their normal diets. Occasionally, therapy with oral hypoglycemic agents may have to be interrupted for patients requiring general anesthesia. These patients are usually not allowed to have any oral intake on the morning of surgery and may not be able to have oral intake for some period of time after the procedure. Therefore, precautions must be taken to minimize the likelihood of hypoglycemia. An intravenous infusion of D5W (5% dextrose in water) at the rate of 100 ml/hour should be started on the morning of surgery and continued until the patient can resume adequate oral intake.

Most patients undergoing dental surgical procedures can resume oral intake by the evening after the procedure. In rare instances, the patient may not be able to resume oral intake for more than a day, and oral hypoglycemic intake may have to be interrupted. During these periods, the patient's urine and blood glucose levels should be closely monitored, and a sliding scale should be used to prevent hyperglycemia (see next section). The patient's physician should be involved in the determination of appropriate insulin coverage.

Management of Patients on Insulin Therapy

Whenever feasible, patients should be continued on their normal diets. The hospitalized patient may have a slightly lower insulin requirement because of decreased activity. Med-

ical consultation and close monitoring of the patient's urine and blood glucose levels are essential for adjustments of the insulin dosage.

When the patient's oral intake may be compromised by surgery and anesthesia, the following procedures should be followed to minimize the likelihood of hypoglycemia and yet ensure reasonable blood glucose control. On the morning of surgery, a fasting blood glucose should be drawn, and an intravenous infusion of 5% dextrose at the rate of 100 ml/hour should be started and continued until the patient can resume adequate oral intake. The patient should be given half the normal morning insulin dose subcutaneously. The urinary and blood glucose levels should be monitored closely while the patient's oral intake is compromised, and the metabolic status should be regulated by the use of a sliding scale. The sliding scale has to be individualized in close consultation with the patient's physician, because insulin requirements may vary greatly from patient to patient. In general, the sliding scale is designed to regulate the blood glucose level when the patient's normal routine is interrupted. The sliding scale is usually based on the blood glucose level:

>250 mg/dl	8 U regular
200–250 mg/dl	6 U
<200 mg/dl	No coverage

Blood glucose determinations and coverage should be performed at 8 AM and 3 PM while the patient is receiving the glucose infusion. Additional blood glucose determinations (e.g., 11 PM) may be necessary if control is inadequate.

Once the patient resumes oral intake, the glucose infusion can be stopped and the sliding scale coverage can be terminated. The patient can be placed back on the original regimen of insulin. It should be stressed that the postoperative insulin requirement may be slightly different from the preoperative requirement because of stress and changes in diet and activity, and close monitoring of the patient's metabolic status is essential. Management should be carefully tailored to the patient's individual needs, and close consultation with the patient's physician is essential for the optimal delivery of care.

ORAL FINDINGS IN DIABETES

Periodontal disease is the most consistent finding in patients with poorly controlled diabetes mellitus. Approximately 75% of these patients have periodontal disease with increased alveolar bone resorption and inflammatory gingival changes. Diabetics whose disease is under good control are also found to have a higher incidence and greater severity of periodontal disease.

Diabetics may demonstrate xerostomia and recurrent abscesses. Enamel hypoplasia and hypocalcification can result in an increased frequency of caries. The oral flora is often altered by colonization with *Candida albicans*, hemolytic streptococci, and staphylococci.

Abnormal eruption patterns may be noted in children with diabetes. Advanced eruption may be seen before the age of 10, whereas delayed eruption occurs after the age of 10.

■ Examples of Dental Evaluation and Management

EVALUATION

Patient 1. A 50-year-old man who was diagnosed as having diabetes mellitus 2 years ago presents for dental treatment. He has been managed on diet alone and has been asymptomatic. He does not test his urine. His dental needs include a full range of operative procedures, simple extractions, periodontal surgery, and the removal of four impacted third molars. On examination, his blood pressure is 110/70 and his pulse rate is 64 beats per minute (bpm).

Consultation with his physician reveals that the patient had an elevated blood glucose level with glycosuria at the time of his diagnosis but has had blood glucose readings between 150 and 200 mg/dl on the current dietary therapy. He was last examined 2 months ago, when his fasting blood glucose level was 115 mg/dl and his hemoglobin A1c was 7%.

Patient 2. A 30-year-old woman with a 16-year history of type I diabetes mellitus presents for dental treatment. She is on 22 units of isophane insulin suspension (NPH) each morning and has had blood glucose testings showing 200 to 250 mg/dl in random testings. She has not been hospitalized recently. Her dental needs are similar to those of Patient 1. On examination, her blood pressure is 100/80 and her pulse is 64 bpm.

Consultation with her physician reveals that the patient has been clinically stable for the past 2 years. She was last examined 2 months ago, when her blood glucose level was 215 mg/dl and her hemoglobin A1c was 8.7%.

Patient 3. A 31-year-old man who was diagnosed to have type I diabetes at age 9 presents

for dental treatment. He has had multiple admissions because of ketoacidosis and is currently on 14 units of CZI and 12 units of NPH each morning. He tests his blood glucose intermittently and usually has readings in excess of 250 mg/dl. He has severe retinopathy and early renal disease. His dental needs are similar to those of Patients 1 and 2. On examination, he has a blood pressure of 140/80 and a pulse of 80 bpm.

Consultation with his physician reveals that the patient has very brittle diabetes with blood glucose level usually between 200 and 300 mg/dl. He was last examined 2 months ago, when his fasting blood sugar was 268 mg/dl and his hemoglobin A1c level was 12%.

MANAGEMENT

Patient 1. This patient is in the low-risk category. He has good metabolic control with fasting blood glucose readings of less than 200 mg/dl and a hemoglobin A1c level of less than 7%, no history of ketoacidosis, and no evidence of complications of diabetes. Routine operative procedures (types I to III) can be performed using a normal protocol. For surgical procedures (types IV to VI), certain general guidelines should be followed: stress should be minimized, the patient should be instructed about diet, and care should be taken to reduce the risk of infection. Sedation techniques including N_2O-O_2 inhalation and oral diazepam (Valium) should be used when appropriate (Chap. 51). When infection is a concern, antibiotics can be given prophylactically after the dental procedure.

Patient 2. This patient is an insulin-dependent diabetic under reasonable metabolic control. She has glycosuria, her fasting blood glucose level is more than 200 mg/dl, and her hemoglobin A1c level is between 7 and 9%. Although she has no history of ketoacidosis or hypoglycemia and no evidence of diabetic complications, her metabolic status places her in the moderate risk category. This patient can undergo any dental procedure provided certain details are noted.

For the majority of the simple operative, simple surgical, and moderately advanced surgical procedures (types II to V), the patient is expected to be able to resume oral intake shortly after the procedure. She should be instructed to take her normal dose of insulin and have a normal breakfast on the morning of the procedure. Dental sessions should be scheduled in the midmorning and kept short. Care must be taken to minimize stress during the procedure, and adjunctive sedation techniques should be employed. The patient should be instructed to maintain good oral intake after the procedure. If she cannot take solid food, she should be given a liquid diet.

For advanced surgical procedures (type VI), it is likely that oral intake may be compromised after the procedure. After consultation with the patient's physician, she should be instructed to take half the normal dose of insulin on the morning of the procedure and to resume her oral intake later in the afternoon. Lengthy procedures should be divided into several short sessions. With this patient, it would be prudent to remove one or two of the impacted third molars at each session, rather than all four molars at the same time. Similarly, the periodontal surgery should be carried out over several short sessions. When oral intake is expected to be compromised for more than several hours, a short hospitalization may be necessary.

Patient 3. This patient is a brittle diabetic with poor metabolic control. He has had multiple hospital admissions, his fasting blood glucose level is often more than 250 mg/dl, and his hemoglobin A1c level is greater than 9%. He has multiple complications of diabetes. After a comprehensive dental examination, medical consultation should be obtained from his physician prior to further dental therapy. If it is apparent that the clinical status cannot be optimized further, dental intervention should initially be palliative and directed at the eradication of oral infection that may be contributing to the poor metabolic control. The patient should be electively admitted to the hospital, and the metabolic status should be closely monitored. Adjunctive sedation techniques or general anesthesia may be necessary. On the morning of surgery, the patient should be given half the normal dose of insulin, and an intravenous infusion of dextrose in water should be started at the rate of 100 ml/hour and continued until the patient can resume adequate oral intake. All teeth with active periapical disease or advanced periodontal destruction should be extracted. If the third molar bony impactions are not acutely infected, it would be advisable to defer their removal. In the operating room, the teeth should be thoroughly scaled and the roots planed. Where appropriate, soft tissue curettage should also be performed.

After the operation, blood glucose levels should be closely monitored. Insulin administration can be gauged according to a sliding scale based on blood glucose concentrations.

Follow-up outpatient care includes strict oral hygiene measures, frequent recall examinations, and prophylaxis. Carious lesions should be treated aggressively. For this brittle diabetic, dental prosthetics should be of the most simple design until his metabolic status is more stable, at which point more comprehensive dental therapy can be planned.

SUMMARY TABLE **14–I**

Diabetes Mellitus: General Information

DEFINITION
Diabetes mellitus is absolute or relative insulin insufficiency, low insulin output from the pancreas, or unresponsiveness of peripheral tissues to existing insulin.

INCIDENCE
It affects 3 to 4% of all adults.

RISK FACTORS
Hereditary: relatives of diabetics have 2½ times the risk of developing the disease

SYMPTOMS
Polydipsia

Polyuria

Polyphagia

Weight loss

SIGNS
Glycosuria

Complications of Diabetes

METABOLIC

Glucose intolerance

Abnormal protein metabolism

Abnormal fatty acid metabolism with ketoacidosis:
    Gastrointestinal symptoms with nausea and vomiting
    Cardiovascular instability
    Dehydration
    Changes in mental status
    Coma
    Death

INCREASED INCIDENCE OF LARGE AND SMALL VESSEL DISEASE

Coronary artery disease

Peripheral vascular disease

Diabetic retinopathy

Diabetic nephropathy (renal disease)

NEUROLOGIC COMPLICATIONS

Peripheral neuropathy with prominent sensory losses

Autonomic neuropathy:
    Postural hypotension
    Sexual impotence

Changes in gastrointestinal motility

INCREASED RISK OF INFECTION

Increased risk of skin, urinary tract, and oral infections

14–III

Medical Evaluation of the Patient with Diabetes Mellitus

LABORATORY EVALUATION

Fasting blood glucose level consistently elevated above 120 mg/dl

Glucose intolerance, as demonstrated by the glucose tolerance test

Glycosuria

Hemoglobin A1c level greater than 7 to 9%

CLINICAL COURSE

May be asymptomatic, with only chemical evidence of glucose intolerance

In other patients may be progressive, with metabolic, vascular, neurologic, and infectious complications

AGE OF ONSET

Adult onset (90% of patients): Type II
  Insidious onset, usually after age 40
  Often in obese patients
  Complications such as ketoacidosis are rare
  Disease often results from resistance of peripheral tissues to action of insulin

Juvenile onset (10% of patients): Type I
  Onset often before age 25
  More prone to ketoacidosis
  Patients are often underweight
  Disease often the result of decreased endogenous secretion of insulin
  Often associated with progressive complications

14–IV

Medical Management of the Patient with Diabetes Mellitus

GOALS

Establish optimal metabolic control.

Prevent ketoacidosis.

Prevent hypoglycemia.

ADULT-ONSET DIABETES

Attempt to normalize the patient's weight.

Monitor the blood glucose level and monitor the hemoglobin A1c level

In patients with persistent glycosuria, use oral hypoglycemic agents (Summary Table 14–V) or insulin (Summary Table 14–VI).

JUVENILE-ONSET DIABETES

Patients are often insulin-dependent.

Oral Hypoglycemics Commonly Used in the Treatment of Patients with Diabetes Mellitus

SULFONYLUREAS

Acetohexamide (Dymelor)

Chlorpropamide (Diabinese)

Tolbutamide (Orinase)

Tolazamide (Tolinase)

Glyburide (Glucotrol, Diabeta)

Glipizide (Micronase)

There is some concern over the association between the use of these hypoglycemic agents and cardiovascular deaths.

BIGUANIDES

Phenformin (DBI) has been associated with severe lactic acidosis.

Insulin Preparation and Effects After Subcutaneous Injection

TYPE OF INSULIN	SUSPENSION	EFFECTS BEGIN (hr)	MAXIMAL ACTION (hr)	DURATION OF EFFECT (hr)
Short-Acting				
Regular (crystalline)	Solution	$1/4$	4–6	6–8
Semilente	Amorphous	$1/2$	4–6	12–16
Intermediate-Acting				
NPH	Crystalline	3	8–12	18–24
Lente	Amorphous 30%, crystalline 70%	3	8–12	18–28
Long-Acting				
PZI	Amorphous	3–4	14–20	24–36
Ultralente	Crystalline	3–4	16–18	30–36

Modified from Manual of Medical Therapeutics, 23rd ed. Freitag, J. J., and Miller, L. W. Copyright 1980. Published by Little, Brown & Co.

14–VII

Complications of Therapy for Diabetes Mellitus

ORAL HYPOGLYCEMIC AGENTS
Hypoglycemia

Increased cardiovascular deaths associated with use of sulfonylureas

Life-threatening lactic acidosis with phenformin

INSULIN THERAPY
Hypoglycemia

Allergy to insulin

Resistance to insulin

Local reactions at injection sites

14–VIII

Hypoglycemia

DEFINITION
Hypoglycemia is a low blood glucose level as a result of excessive oral hypoglycemic agents, insulin, or inadequate dietary intake.

SIGNS AND SYMPTOMS
Weakness, nervousness, tremulousness, palpitation, and excessive sweating

Lethargy, agitation, and confusion, progressing to seizure and coma

TREATMENT
Administration of oral glucose: orange juice or soft drinks

Administration of intravenous glucose: $D_{50}W$ given as bolus

Dental Evaluation of the Patient with Diabetes Mellitus

PATIENTS NOT KNOWN TO HAVE DIABETES MELLITUS

Patients with signs and symptoms suggesting the possible diagnosis of diabetes should have a blood glucose determination.

Patients with a positive family history of diabetes should have a blood glucose determination.

Patients documented to have an elevated blood glucose level should be referred for medical evaluation.

PATIENTS KNOWN TO HAVE DIABETES MELLITUS

Time of onset of diabetes

Type of therapy required:
  Control of diet
  Oral hypoglycemic agents
  Insulin therapy

Adequacy of control:
  Fasting blood sugar
  Hemoglobin A1c level
  History of hypoglycemia
  History of ketoacidosis

Complications of diabetes:
  Vascular
  Neurologic
  Renal
  Infectious

Risk Categories for the Patient with Diabetes Mellitus

PATIENTS AT LOW RISK

Good metabolic control on stable medical regimen

No history of ketoacidosis or hypoglycemia

No complications of diabetes

Fasting blood glucose level less than 200 mg/dl

Hemoglobin A1c level of less than 7%

PATIENTS AT MODERATE RISK

Reasonable metabolic control on stable regimen

No recent history of ketoacidosis or hypoglycemia

Few complications of diabetes

Fasting blood glucose less than 250 mg/dl

Hemoglobin A1c level of 7 to 9%

PATIENTS AT HIGH RISK

Poor metabolic control

Frequent symptoms

Frequent problems with ketoacidosis and hypoglycemia

Multiple complications of diabetes

Fasting blood glucose level greater than 250 mg/dl

Hemoglobin A1c level of greater than 9%

SUMMARY TABLE **14–XI**

Management of the Patient with Diabetes Mellitus

MINIMIZE STRESS
Short midmorning appointments

Adjunctive sedation techniques, when appropriate

DIETARY INSTRUCTIONS
Instruct patient to continue normal dietary intake before the operation.

If a lengthy dental appointment is planned, especially if the session extends into normal meal or snack time, interrupt the appointment with an appropriate snack, such as orange juice.

Patients expected to have difficulties with solid food after dental procedures should be given a diet of soft solids or liquids.

MINIMIZE THE RISK OF INFECTION
Recommend frequent recall examinations and prophylaxis.

Treat periodontal disease aggressively.

Consider postoperative antibiotic prophylaxis for surgical procedures.

Treat acute infections aggressively.

Consider adjunctive antibiotics for suppurative periodontitis.

SUMMARY TABLE **14–XII**

Insulin Therapy for the Dental Patient

OUTPATIENT
1. Midmorning dental appointment should be scheduled.
2. A normal breakfast should be eaten.
3. *Insulin doses should be tailored to the procedures proposed:*
   a. Patients expected to be able to resume normal oral intake immediately after the procedure can take their normal dose of insulin.
   b. Patients expected to have some delay in the resumption of normal oral intake following the procedure should take half their normal morning insulin dose, following physician consultation.
4. Resume normal diet following procedure.

INPATIENT
1. Schedule early morning surgery.
2. No oral intake after midnight.
3. A fasting blood glucose level should be determined on the morning of surgery.
4. Begin intravenous infusion of D_5W at 100 ml/hr on the morning of surgery.
5. Administer half the normal dose of insulin.
6. Maintain the intravenous fluid infusion until oral intake is resumed.
7. Use a sliding scale based on blood glucose determinations to optimize blood glucose control.
8. Blood glucose determinations should be made at 3 PM and 11 PM.
9. Resume oral intake as soon as possible.
10. The patient should be on a normal insulin regimen 1 to 2 days after surgery and can usually be discharged and followed as an outpatient.

Dental Management of the Patient with Diabetes Mellitus

RISK CATEGORY	PROCEDURES	PROTOCOL
Low risk	I–III	Normal protocol with attention to the general guidelines applicable to all diabetic patients
	IV–VI	Consider adjunctive sedation techniques; half the normal insulin dose only if oral intake is expected to be compromised after consultation with physician
Moderate risk	I–III	Normal protocol; consider adjunctive sedation techniques
	IV	Possible adjustment of insulin dose after consultation with physician
	V–VI	Possible adjustment of insulin dose after consultation with physician; consider hospitalization
High risk	I	Normal protocol
	II–VI	Deferred until metabolic status is stabilized; palliative rather than extensive restorative interventions; aggressive control of oral infections

CHAPTER 15

Adrenal Gland Disorders and Corticosteroid Therapy

The adrenal glands are small, multifunctional endocrine organs located above the kidneys. Each gland is divided into an inner zone called the adrenal medulla and an outer zone called the adrenal cortex (Fig. 15–1). The adrenal medulla produces the catecholamines epinephrine and norepinephrine, which play an integral role in the maintenance of blood pressure, the control of myocardial contractility and excitability, and the regulation of body metabolism. The adrenal cortex produces three different classes of hormones: (1) the glucocorticoids, which help regulate carbohydrate, protein, and fat metabolism and are important in the suppression of inflammation; (2) the mineralocorticoids (principally aldosterone), which help maintain sodium and potassium balance; and (3) the sex hormones, which play a secondary role in sexual maturation.

Many factors intricately regulate the secretion of the hormones. Glucocorticoid production is controlled by adrenocorticotropic hormone (ACTH), which is produced by the anterior pituitary gland. ACTH production is controlled by corticotropin-releasing factor (CRF) produced by the hypothalamus. Circulating cortisol, in turn, feeds back and regulates hypothalamic and pituitary function. Thus, the hypothalamus, the anterior pituitary

gland, and the adrenal glands interact continuously to regulate glucocorticoid production carefully (Fig. 15–2). Mineralocorticoid secretion is also regulated by multiple factors—partly by the renin-angiotensin hormone system, partly by serum potassium concentration, and to a much lesser extent by ACTH.

MEDICAL EVALUATION OF PATIENTS WITH ADRENAL GLAND DISORDERS

Abnormalities in the secretion of the adrenal hormones can be a result of diseases affecting the adrenal gland or diseases affecting factors that regulate adrenal function.

Hyperfunction of the Adrenal Medulla. Tumors called pheochromocytomas, affecting the adrenal medulla, can lead to hypersecretion of epinephrine and norepinephrine (Fig. 15–3). Patients affected by this tumor experience episodic hypertension, headaches, sweating, palpitations, and flushing. The diagnosis can be confirmed by determination of serum concentrations of epinephrine and norepinephrine (catecholamines) or by the detection of elevated levels of metabolites of catecholamines such as vanillylmandelic acid (VMA) or metanephrines in the urine.

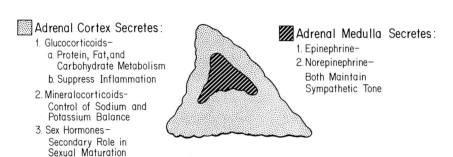

Adrenal Cortex Secretes:
1. Glucocorticoids–
   a. Protein, Fat, and Carbohydrate Metabolism
   b. Suppress Inflammation
2. Mineralocorticoids–
   Control of Sodium and Potassium Balance
3. Sex Hormones–
   Secondary Role in Sexual Maturation

Adrenal Medulla Secretes:
1. Epinephrine–
2. Norepinephrine–
   Both Maintain Sympathetic Tone

Figure 15–1. Normal adrenal function. Each gland is divided into an inner zone (the adrenal medulla) and an outer zone (the adrenal cortex). Each zone functions independently.

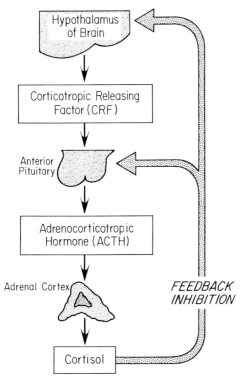

Figure 15–2. Feedback regulation of adrenal function.

Hyperfunction of the Adrenal Cortex. Glucocorticoids, mineralocorticoids, and sex hormones can all be produced in excessive amounts in pathologic states (Fig. 15–4).

Hypersecretion of glucocorticoid hormones can result from diseases that affect the hypothalamus, the anterior pituitary gland, or the adrenal gland itself. Hypersecretion caused by dysfunction of the hypothalamus accounts for about half of cases of cortisol hypersecretion. Excessive ACTH production from tumors of the anterior pituitary gland or from ectopic sources, such as oat cell carcinoma of lung, accounts for another 25% of cases of excessive glucocorticoid production. Benign and malignant tumors of the adrenal glands account for the remaining 25%.

Patients with glucocorticoid hypersecretion have Cushing's syndrome, which results in characteristic changes in body habitus including "moon facies," truncal obesity, muscle wasting, and hirsutism. They are often hypertensive because of tendencies in fluid retention. Long-term glucocorticoid excess can also result in decreased collagen production, easy bruisability, poor wound healing, and osteoporosis. Patients with Cushing's syndrome are often at increased risk for infection. Laboratory studies may reveal increased blood glu-

cose levels because of interference with carbohydrate metabolism, and examination of the peripheral blood smear may demonstrate slight decreases in eosinophil and lymphocyte counts.

The medical evaluation of the patient suspected of having Cushing's syndrome includes measurement of plasma ACTH, plasma cortisol, urinary 17-hydroxycorticosteroids, and 17-ketosteroids. Patients suspected of having adrenal tumors often undergo evaluation of the adrenal area with the aid of ultrasonography, computed tomography (CT), magnetic resonance imaging (MRI), and arteriography to determine the size and location of the tumor. Similarly, patients with suspected anterior pituitary tumors usually undergo tomography of the sella, cranial CT, and cranial MRI.

Hypersecretion of mineralocorticoids can be the result of a tumor or bilateral hyperplasia of the adrenals. Patients with hypersecretion of mineralocorticoids have low serum potassium concentrations, fluid retention, mild hypertension, and possibly symptoms of muscle weakness and transient paresthesias. Radiologic evaluation may include the use of ultrasonography, CT, MRI, and arteriography.

Hypersecretion of the sex hormones can also result from tumors or enzymatic defects. Excessive sex hormone production can produce masculinization in females and in prepubertal boys.

Hypofunction of the Adrenal Glands. Chronic loss of adrenal function is called Addison's disease. The most common cause of this disease is the autoimmune destruction of the adrenal gland, which accounts for well over half of all cases of adrenal hypofunction. Tubercular, fungal, and (rarely) viral diseases can also destroy the adrenal glands and result in chronic adrenal insufficiency. Acute adrenal insufficiency can occur as a result of bilateral adrenalectomy or overwhelming gram-negative sepsis causing bilateral adrenal hemorrhage (Waterhouse-Friderichsen syndrome). Occa-

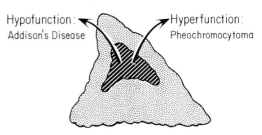

Figure 15–3. Diseases of the adrenal medulla.

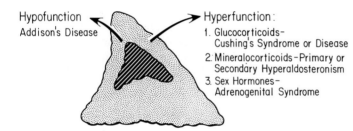

Hypofunction — Addison's Disease

Hyperfunction:
1. Glucocorticoids—Cushing's Syndrome or Disease
2. Mineralocorticoids—Primary or Secondary Hyperaldosteronism
3. Sex Hormones—Adrenogenital Syndrome

Figure 15–4. Diseases of the adrenal cortex.

sionally, hyposecretion is a result of pituitary insufficiency (Figs. 15–3 and 15–4).

Patients with decreased adrenal gland hormone production experience weakness, weight loss, orthostatic hypotension, nausea, and vomiting. Patients with severe adrenal insufficiency cannot increase steroid production in response to stress and in extreme situations may have cardiovascular collapse. On examination, the patients may be hyperpigmented. Intraorally, this is most noticeable on the buccal and labial mucosae, although other areas of the mouth such as the gingiva may be involved (Chap. 38). The hyperpigmentation is the result of hypersecretion of ACTH, which can stimulate melanocytes to produce pigment. Blood studies indicate hyperkalemia and hypoglycemia. Examination of the peripheral smear may reveal increased eosinophil counts. The diagnosis can be made on the basis of serum cortisol determinations. An ACTH stimulation test can also be performed to examine the response of the adrenal gland to an exogenously administered dose of ACTH. An inadequate response suggests adrenal gland hypofunction.

Corticosteroid Therapy. Corticosteroids are potent anti-inflammatory agents frequently used to treat a number of systemic diseases, including rheumatoid arthritis, temporal arteritis, systemic lupus erythematosus and other collagen vascular disorders, nephrotic syndrome, inflammatory bowel disease, asthma, hemolytic anemia, thrombocytopenia, and a variety of dermatologic disorders. These patients do not have primary disease of their adrenal glands. However, the exogenous steroids suppress the functional capabilities of the adrenal glands, which may then be unable to mount an appropriate adrenal response at times of stress, possibly resulting in serious sequelae, including cardiovascular collapse. Prolonged high doses of exogenously administered steroids can cause iatrogenic Cushing's syndrome. Patients on chemotherapy for some malignancies may also have steroids as a part of their chemotherapeutic regimen, and pa-

tients with renal transplants may receive steroids to suppress rejection.

MEDICAL MANAGEMENT OF PATIENTS WITH ADRENAL GLAND DISORDERS

Hyperfunction of Adrenal Medulla. Pheochromocytoma is usually managed by surgical excision. On rare occasions, when metastatic pheochromocytoma is noted at the time of examination, patients may be managed medically with alpha-blocking drugs such as phentolamine or phenoxybenzamine for control of hypertension.

Hyperfunction of the Adrenal Cortex. Adrenal adenoma and adrenal carcinoma are usually treated by surgical excision. Bilateral adrenal hyperplasia may require bilateral adrenalectomy. Patients with an adenoma causing hyperaldosteronism are usually treated surgically, whereas patients with bilateral hyperplasia and aldosterone hypersecretion may sometimes be managed medically. Patients with adrenogenital syndrome may be managed either medically or surgically. The surgical approach requires bilateral adrenalectomy.

Hypofunction of Adrenal Glands. Patients with Addison's disease are managed by steroid supplements. Some steroid preparations in common use are listed in Summary Table 15–III. Prednisone is perhaps the most frequently used because of the ease of administration and the low mineralocorticoid effect. Steroid dosages ought to be as low as possible to avoid side effects. The usual daily maintenance dose of prednisone is 10 to 15 mg. In some patients, mineralocorticoid deficiency may require supplementation with fluorocortisone (Florinef). It is important to remember that patients on chronic replacement therapy for adrenal insufficiency cannot increase endogenous steroid production in times of stress and therefore become relatively adrenally insufficient unless steroid supplements are administered.

Patients on Corticosteroid Therapy. The medical indications for steroid therapy have been outlined. Generally, patients should receive the minimal dose necessary to produce the desired effect. Whenever possible, they should be given steroid therapy on alternate days, because this regimen is least likely to suppress the hypothalamic-pituitary-adrenal axis. If alternate-day therapy is not successful, daily therapy is used. Usually, the entire dose is given in the morning, because this also minimizes the impact on the hypothalamic-pituitary-adrenal axis.

DENTAL EVALUATION OF PATIENTS WITH ADRENAL GLAND DISORDERS

If a patient with a known adrenal disorder requires dental treatment, the physician should be consulted. The nature of the disease and the patient's therapy should be carefully reviewed.

A patient with an adrenal adenoma usually has had the tumor surgically removed and still has normal adrenal function with the one remaining adrenal gland. This patient is not at any increased risk.

Patients with bilateral adrenal hyperplasia may have had bilateral adrenalectomy, in which case they require chronic steroid replacement. The type and dosage of steroids taken should be reviewed. Patients with adrenal insufficiency also require chronic steroid therapy.

DENTAL EVALUATION OF PATIENTS ON STEROID THERAPY

A number of patients presenting to the dental office may either be on steroid therapy or have had steroids in the past. These patients deserve careful evaluation and should be asked about the indications for the steroid therapy, the types and dosages of steroids taken, and the duration of therapy. If the history is ambiguous, the patient's physician should be consulted and the details reviewed. Because hypothalamic-pituitary-adrenal suppression may result from as little as 20 to 30 mg of prednisone given daily for 7 to 10 days and may not completely return to normal for 9 to 12 months, *patients giving a history of daily steroid use for more than a week during the past year may have some degree of adrenal suppression.*

DENTAL MANAGEMENT OF PATIENTS WITH ADRENAL DISORDERS

Hyperfunction of Adrenal Medulla. Patients who have had one adrenal gland removed for a pheochromocytoma should have normal adrenal function because of the one remaining adrenal gland. They can undergo dental treatment using normal protocols. Patients who have had bilateral adrenalectomy for disease affecting both adrenal glands and are on chronic steroid replacement should be treated like patients with hypofunction of the adrenal gland (see later).

Hypofunction of Adrenal Glands. Patients with chronic adrenal insufficiency for any reason, including bilateral adrenalectomy, are normally on chronic steroid replacement therapy. The usual daily replacement dosage is about 10 to 20 mg of prednisone or its equivalent, which is reasonable for maintenance therapy but inadequate during periods of stress. In patients with normal adrenal reserves, the maximal output of cortisol in response to severe stress is estimated to be equivalent to about 60 mg of prednisone.

Although it is sometimes difficult to assess the degree of stress the patient may experience during dental therapy, the problems associated with adrenal insufficiency far outweigh the dangers associated with a short course of increased steroid therapy. It is prudent, therefore, to increase the steroid dosage during periods of possible stress for those patients known to have limited adrenal reserves. The patient's physician should be consulted, the proposed dental procedures and the anticipated stress should be determined, and the patient's medical status and medications should be reviewed. Adjunctive sedation techniques should be used whenever appropriate to minimize stress.

In general, oral examinations (type I procedures) can be carried out without additional steroid coverage.

Nonsurgical procedures and some simple surgical procedures (types II to IV) are associated with mild to moderate degrees of stress, and the steroid dosages should be adjusted. In general, it is reasonable to double the daily steroid dosage on the day of surgery and to return to the maintenance dosage the following day.

Moderate and advanced surgical procedures such as quadrant or full-arch periodontal and oral surgery (types V and VI) are associated with significant stress, and maximal steroid coverage for a short period of time is appropriate. Dosages should be increased to 60 mg of prednisone (or equivalent; see Summary Table 15–III) on the day of the dental procedure and *tapered* rapidly over the ensuing 3 days to the maintenance dosage levels. If the patient is unable to take medications orally after the dental procedure, it is important to continue the therapy using parenteral forms of steroids (300 mg of hydrocortisone given intravenously for maximal steroid coverage). The patient should be returned to the maintenance dosage within 3 to 4 days unless there are secondary problems that require continuing steroid coverage such as infection, severe protracted pain, or compromised oral intake.

Antibiotic Coverage

It is reasonable to prescribe a short course of prophylactic antibiotics if significant soft tissue manipulation is anticipated. Penicillin VK, erythromycin, or tetracycline given in 250-mg oral doses qid can be started on the day of the procedure and continued for 3 days.

Patients on Alternate-Day Steroid Therapy for Nonadrenal Diseases

In general, patients on *alternate-day* steroid therapy have considerably less adrenal suppression than patients on daily steroid therapy. The need for steroid supplementation in this group is questionable. However, because the potential consequences of short-term steroids are minimal, *it is prudent to schedule dental procedures for a day when the patient is taking steroids as opposed to an off-steroid day.* On the day of the procedure, the normal dose should be doubled; a single dose should be given the following day and the normal schedule resumed thereafter. If the patient requires general anesthesia for dental treatment, a more complete assessment of steroid function should be performed and may include, at the physician's discretion, an ACTH stimulation test that directly measures the ability of the adrenal gland to respond to an exogenously administered dose of ACTH. Alternatively, the patient's physician may elect to increase the steroid coverage empirically to maximal doses (60 mg of prednisone daily) after the operation. Again, the doses should be reduced over the next 2

to 3 days to maintenance alternate-day therapy unless there are complications requiring continuation of stress doses of steroids. Patients on alternate-day steroid therapy are immunosuppressed and possibly susceptible to infection, so they may require prophylactic antibiotic coverage.

Patients on Daily Steroid Therapy for Nonadrenal Diseases

Patients on *daily* steroids may be on doses ranging from 5 mg to more than 60 mg of prednisone (or its equivalent) each day. The degree of adrenal suppression depends on the dosage and duration of steroid therapy. With these patients, oral examination can probably be carried out without additional steroids. Nonsurgical procedures (type II and some type III) and simple surgical procedures (type IV), which are associated with mild to moderate amounts of stress, should be performed with steroid supplementation: the maintenance steroid dose should be doubled up to a maximum of 60 mg on the day of the procedure and tapered back to the original dose in 2 days. More advanced surgical procedures (types V and VI) should be carried out under maximal steroid coverage, and the patient should receive 60 mg of prednisone on the day of surgery. If the patient is unable to take oral medications, the steroid coverage should be continued using parenteral preparations such as hydrocortisone. The dosage can be decreased by 50% daily starting the day after the procedure until the maintenance dosage is reached.

Patients Formerly on Steroid Therapy

Occasionally, the dentist may have to manage a patient who is not currently on steroids but has had a history of previous steroid use. It is difficult to assess the adrenal reserve of the patient without conducting a full ACTH stimulation test. Because adrenal suppression can result from as little as 20 to 30 mg of prednisone daily for 7 to 10 days and can persist for 9 to 12 months after the termination of a course of therapy, *patients giving a history of having had more than 20 mg of prednisone daily for more than 1 week during the previous year should receive steroid supplementation.* For procedures associated with mild to moderate degrees of stress (types II to IV), 20 to 40 mg of predni-sone should be administered on the day of the procedure and tapered as previously discussed. For moderate to advanced dental surgery (types V and VI) and for procedures requiring general anesthesia, the patient should receive maximal steroid coverage: 60 mg of predni-sone on the day of surgery rapidly tapered over the next 2 to 3 days.

It should again be stressed that consultation with the patient's physician is crucial to the optimal delivery of care.

ORAL FINDINGS

Patients with Addison's disease frequently develop hyperpigmentation of the skin. Brown or black pigmentation may also be noted in the mouth and is most frequent on the buccal and labial mucosae (Fig. 15–5). There is no particular configuration or distribution to these lesions.

A significant therapeutic effect of steroids is their anti-inflammatory and immunosuppres-sive activity. They are used frequently to treat autoimmune disease and to prevent graft re-jection. As a consequence of induced immu-nosuppression, patients are at risk for infec-tion. Candidiasis may occur with regularity in this group, and viral and bacterial infections are not uncommon. Antibiotic prophylaxis for patients taking steroids is suggested, as noted earlier.

■ Examples of Dental Evaluation and Management

EVALUATION

Patient 1. A 38-year-old woman who has had bilateral adrenalectomy because of Cushing's disease presents for dental treatment. She was diagnosed as having the disease at age 32 and underwent surgery. She has been on steroid re-placement since and is currently on 15 mg of prednisone daily. Her dental needs include a full range of operative procedures (types I to III) and the removal of several teeth (types IV to V). On examination, she appears cushingoid. Her blood pressure is 130/80 and her pulse rate is 64 beats/minute (bpm).

Consultation with her physician reveals that she has been clinically stable since her surgery. She was last examined 3 months ago.

Patient 2. A 42-year-old woman with a long history of rheumatoid arthritis presents for den-

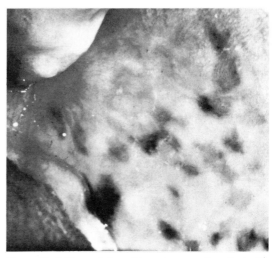

Figure 15–5. Pigmentation of buccal mucosa in patient with Addison's disease.

tal treatment. She noted joint swelling at age 18 and has had progressive joint deformities since. She is currently on two tablets of aspirin every 4 hours for control of symptoms. A review of her past medical regimens reveals that she was on 30 mg of prednisone daily for 4 months and that the steroids have only recently been ta-pered off and stopped. Her dental needs are similar to those of patient 1. On examination, she has a blood pressure of 140/86 and a regu-lar pulse rate of 80 bpm.

Patient 3. A 44-year-old man with a past history of "having had adrenal surgery" presents for dental treatment. The adrenal surgery was per-formed 18 years ago for the removal of a tumor. He has been asymptomatic since and is not on medications. His dental needs are the same as those of the other two patients. On examina-tion, his blood pressure is 130/70 and his pulse rate is 72 bpm.

Consultation with his physician reveals that the patient had a pheochromocytoma removed from his left adrenal gland. He was last exam-ined a year ago and was found to be in good health.

MANAGEMENT

Patient 1. The patient has no endogenous ad-renal reserve and is dependent on exogenous adrenal replacement. She is at high risk and requires steroid supplementation for all dental procedures (types II to VI).

For procedures that would subject the patient to moderate stress, the steroid dose should be doubled to 30 mg of prednisone on the day of the procedure and returned to the original dose of 15 mg on the following day. For moderate and advanced surgical procedures (types V and VI), maximal stress doses of prednisone should be used—60 mg on the day of the procedure, 30 mg on the second day, and 15 mg on the third day. If protracted pain, secondary infection, or compromised oral intake occur, steroid supplements should be continued until the stressful situation has resolved. For all surgical procedures (types IV to VI), prophylactic therapy with an antibiotic such as penicillin is recommended for 3 days.

Patient 2. The patient has a history of recent use of significant doses of steroids (prednisone in doses greater than 20 mg daily for more than 7 to 10 days within the past year). She is therefore at significant risk for adrenal suppression and requires steroid coverage for all dental procedures. For procedures that produce minimal to moderate stress (types II to IV), 20 to 40 mg of prednisone should be given on the day of the procedure. This dosage can be halved on the second day and discontinued on the third day. For moderately advanced and advanced surgical procedures (types V and VI), maximal stress doses of steroids should be given—60 mg of prednisone on the day of the procedure, tapered over the next 2 days. Steroid therapy should be extended if patients develop difficulties such as protracted pain, secondary infection, or compromised oral intake. Antibiotic prophylaxis may be used for moderate and advanced surgical procedures (types V and VI).

Another concern with this patient is the regular ingestion of significant amounts of aspirin. The antiplatelet effect of the drug prolongs bleeding time and may compromise hemostasis. If feasible, aspirin should be discontinued 7 to 10 days prior to the procedure (Chap. 26).

Patient 3. The patient should have intact adrenal function, because only one of his adrenal glands was removed during the surgery for pheochromocytoma. The patient is doing well without medication and should be treated with a normal protocol.

SUMMARY TABLE **15–I**

Adrenal Glands: General Information

FUNCTION

The adrenal cortex produces glucocorticoids, mineralocorticoids, and sex hormones.

The adrenal medulla produces epinephrine and norepinephrine.

CONTROL

Adrenal cortical function is controlled by the adrenocorticotropic hormone (ACTH) from the anterior pituitary, which in turn is controlled by corticotropin-releasing factor (CRF) from the hypothalamus. The balance is maintained by feedback inhibition by circulating cortisol on the pituitary and hypothalamus.

Adrenal medullary function depends on the renin-angiotensin system, serum potassium level, and plasma volume.

SUMMARY TABLE **15–II**

Diseases of the Adrenal Glands

HYPERFUNCTION OF THE ADRENAL CORTEX

Cushing's syndrome: hypersecretion of glucocorticoid as a result of various diseases affecting the hypothalamus (50%), the anterior pituitary (25%), or the adrenal gland itself (25%)

Clinical presentation: "moon facies," truncal obesity, muscle wasting, hirsutism, easy bruisability, poor wound healing, osteoporosis, increased susceptibility to infection, and hyperglycemia

Management: unilateral adrenalectomy, bilateral adrenalectomy, pituitary surgery, or medical management (rarely)

HYPOFUNCTION OF THE ADRENAL CORTEX

Addison's disease: hyposecretion of glucocorticoid as a result of autoimmune destruction of the adrenal cortex (50%), exogenous steroid therapy, or therapeutic bilateral adrenalectomy

Clinical presentation: weakness, weight loss, orthostatic hypotension, nausea, vomiting, hyperpigmentation, hyperkalemia, and hypoglycemia

Management: steroid supplementation

HYPERFUNCTION OF THE ADRENAL MEDULLA

Pheochromocytoma: primary adrenal medullary tumor

Clinical presentation: episodic hypertension, headaches, sweating, palpitation, and flushing

Management: surgical excision or medical management of hypertension only (rarely)

HYPOFUNCTION OF THE ADRENAL MEDULLA

Mineralocorticoid deficiency

Clinical presentation: hyperkalemia

Management: mineralocorticoid replacement

SUMMARY TABLE **15–III**

Principles and Parameters of Therapeutic and Physiologic Levels of Steroids

Typical maintenance dosage of therapeutic steroids: 5–20 mg prednisone/day or equivalent

Continuous steroid therapy dosage: generally ranges from 5–60 mg prednisone/day or equivalent

Alternate-day steroid therapy dosage: generally ranges from 5–60 mg prednisone or equivalent every other day

Maximal normal physiologic steroid production response to severe stress: equivalent to 60 mg prednisone/day

Therapeutic steroids: suppress ability of adrenal glands to increase cortisol production under stress (adrenal suppression)

Maintenance doses of steroids: can be inadequate under stress

SUMMARY TABLE **15–IV**

Clinical Correlates of Steroid Therapy

Adrenal suppression is the physiologic inability of the adrenal glands to produce maximal cortisol levels (equivalent to 60 mg prednisone/day) in the face of maximal stress.

Any patient who has received 20 mg prednisone/day or the equivalent for 7–10 days in the past year or who is receiving typical maintenance dose levels of steroids daily (10–20 mg prednisone/day or the equivalent) is considered to have adrenal suppression.

Patients on long-term, alternate-day steroid therapy have less adrenal suppression.

Adrenal insufficiency can be precipitated by severe stress.

SUMMARY TABLE **15–V**

Steroid Potency and Dosages

DURATION OF ACTION	GLUCOCORTICOID POTENCY	DOSE (mg)	MINERALOCORTICOID ACTIVITY
Short-Acting			
Cortisol (hydrocortisone)	1	20	Yes
Cortisone	0.8	25	Yes
Prednisone	4	5	No
Prednisolone	4	5	No
Methylprednisolone	5	4	No
Intermediate-Acting			
Triamcinolone	5	4	No
Long-Acting			
Betamethasone	25	0.60	No
Dexamethasone	30	0.75	No

SUMMARY TABLE **15–VI**

Dental Evaluation of the Patient with Adrenal Disease and/or Steroid Therapy

1. Confirm original diagnosis of adrenal or nonadrenal disease.
2. Determine past therapy:
   a. Surgery
   b. Steroids (dose, duration, history)
   c. Radiation
3. Determine present adrenal status (adrenal suppression?).
4. Obtain medical consultation.

Dental Management of the Patient with Adrenal Disease or Steroid Therapy for Nonadrenal Disease

1. Assess potential for adrenal suppression.
2. Administer supplemental steroids proportional to the presumed adrenal suppression and the anticipated stress.
3. Taper supplemental steroid doses rapidly over 2–3 days to maintenance levels, unless there is infection, severe protracted pain, or compromised oral intake.
4. Provide steroid supplementation: moderate stress, 20–40 mg prednisone/day or equivalent (types II–IV procedures); maximal stress or general anesthesia, 60 mg prednisone/day or equivalent (types V and VI procedures).
5. Use appropriate sedation techniques (Chap. 51) to minimize stress.
6. Use antibiotic prophylaxis to minimize the risk of infection if significant soft tissue manipulation is anticipated: penicillin VK, erythromycin, or tetracycline 250 mg orally qid for 3 days.

Dental Protocol for Steroid Supplementation

RISK OF ADRENAL SUPPRESSION	PROCEDURES	PROTOCOL
Low Risk		
Patients on alternate-day steroids for nonadrenal disease (5–60 mg prednisone every other day)	II–VI	Procedures should be performed on a day when the patient is taking steroids; day of surgery: double maintenance dose to a maximum of 60 mg prednisone or equivalent; day 2: maintenance dose of steroids; day 3: resume alternate-day schedule
	General anesthesia	Same regimen as low-risk II–VI, beginning with 60 mg or equivalent of prednisone on day of procedure
Significant Risk		
Patient formerly on steroid therapy (20 mg prednisone or more for 7–10 days within past year)	II–IV	Day of surgery: 20–40 mg prednisone or equivalent; day 2: 10–20 mg prednisone or equivalent; day 3: off steroids
	V, VI, or general anesthesia	Day of surgery: 60 mg prednisone or equivalent; day 2: 30 mg prednisone or equivalent; day 3: off steroids
High Risk		
Patient on maintenance dose therapy for adrenal disease (10–20 mg prednisone/day)	II–IV (moderate stress)	Day of procedure: double steroid dose up to a maximum of 60 mg prednisone or equivalent; day 2: maintenance dose
Patient on steroid therapy for nonadrenal disease (5–60 mg prednisone/day)	V, VI, or general anesthesia (severe stress)	Day of procedure: supplement daily dose to 60 mg prednisone/day; taper 50% dose/day over 2–3 days to maintenance dose

CHAPTER 16

Thyroid Disorders

The thyroid gland is an endocrine structure located in the neck superior to the suprasternal notch and inferior to the cricoid cartilage (Fig. 16–1). The major function of this gland is the production of the hormone thyroxine, which is important in the regulation of the metabolic rate of the body and affects carbohydrate, protein, and lipid metabolism. In addition, thyroxine potentiates the action of other hormones, such as catecholamines and growth hormones.

Thyroid hormone secretion is regulated in an intricate fashion. The hypothalamus produces a hormone called thyrotropin-releasing hormone (TRH), which stimulates the production of thyroid-stimulating hormone (TSH) from the anterior pituitary (Fig. 16–2). TSH, in turn, stimulates the production of thyroxine from the thyroid gland. Circulating thyroxine can negatively feed back to the pituitary and the hypothalamus to halt the secretion of TSH. This feedback mechanism permits fine control of the secretion of the thyroid hormone.

Abnormalities in either the anterior pituitary or the thyroid can result in disorders of thyroid hormone production. Thyroid disorders are the second most common class of endocrine disorders and affect approximately 1% of the dental population.

MEDICAL EVALUATION

Hyperthyroidism

Excessive production of thyroxine results in hyperthyroidism. Patients with hyperthyroidism present with symptoms of heat intolerance, nervousness, tremor, excessive sweating, muscular weakness, diarrhea, increased appetite, and weight loss. In the elderly patient, excessive thyroxine may precipitate atrial fibrillation, angina, or congestive heart failure.

On examination, the patient is tremulous and tachycardic. Palpation of the neck may reveal an enlarged thyroid gland. The skin is thin and soft, and the reflexes are often hyperactive.

A number of disease processes can result in hyperthyroidism. In patients under the age of 40, Graves' disease accounts for about 90% of all cases of hyperthyroidism. The disease is thought to be secondary to an autoimmune disorder and is associated with prominent exophthalmos. Middle-aged and elderly patients are more likely to have hyperthyroidism as a result of toxic multinodular goiter. Less commonly, a single toxic nodule can produce excessive thyroid hormone. Transient hyperthyroidism is seen in patients with subacute or chronic thyroiditis. Hyperthyroidism can also result from excessive ingestion of thyroid hormone (factitious hyperthyroidism).

When hyperthyroidism is clinically suspected, thyroid function tests are used to confirm the diagnosis. Patients with hyperthyroidism have high serum concentrations of free thyroxine or triiodothyronine (T_3). Radionuclide thyroid scans are helpful in delineating the nature of the disease.

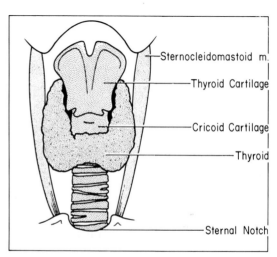

Figure 16–1. Clinical location of the thyroid gland relative to other areas of palpable anatomy.

Sternocleidomastoid m.

Thyroid Cartilage

Cricoid Cartilage

Thyroid

Sternal Notch

156

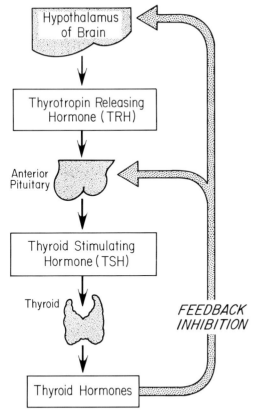

Figure 16–2. Feedback mechanisms that regulate thyroid hormone secretion.

Hypothyroidism

Insufficient production of thyroid hormone results in hypothyroidism. Initially, the patient complains of fatigue, cold intolerance, weakness, and weight gain. Subsequently, hoarseness and impaired mental activity may be noted. In severe cases (myxedema) there is increasing lethargy, culminating in coma.

On examination, the patient has dry, doughy skin, a puffy face, a large tongue, and slow mentation. Bowel sounds are diminished, and the reflexes are abnormal, with slowing of the relaxation phase.

The majority of patients with hypothyroidism have diseases of the thyroid gland, with chronic thyroiditis (Hashimoto's disease), idiopathic thyroid atrophy, previous radioactive iodine therapy, neck irradiation, and thyroidectomy being the leading causes. Pituitary insufficiency can result in secondary hypothyroidism. Rarely, hypothalamic disease is the source of the problem (Summary Tables 16–I and 16–II).

The diagnosis can be confirmed by the determination of free thyroxine and TSH levels.

Patients with primary thyroid disease have low free thyroxine levels and increased TSH levels. The TSH determination is a more sensitive indicator in patients with mild hypothyroidism. Secondary hypothyroidism is identified by a TSH level that is not appropriately elevated in the setting of inadequate thyroid function. TSH may be given to these patients to test pituitary reserve.

Thyroid Tumors

Some patients may have tumors involving the thyroid gland. These are usually detected on routine physical examination as nodules. Benign thyroid tumors are called adenomas. Several different types of malignant tumors— including papillary carcinomas, follicular carcinomas, and medullary carcinomas—can affect the thyroid gland. The tumors can be evaluated by radionuclide scanning and the pathology can be determined by a needle biopsy or by surgical excision.

MEDICAL MANAGEMENT

Hyperthyroidism

Patients with hyperthyroidism can be treated symptomatically with propranolol. Definitive therapy involves the use of antithyroid drugs such as propylthiouracil or methimazole (Tapazole). Side effects of antithyroid drugs include skin rashes, joint pain, and occasionally a decreased white cell count (leukopenia). After the cessation of antithyroid drugs, only 30% of patients remain clinically euthyroid. Patients who cannot be maintained on antithyroid drugs are treated with either radioactive iodine or surgery. Patients are followed closely clinically and with serial determinations of thyroid function tests, because hyperthyroidism resulting from inadequate therapy or hypothyroidism resulting from excessive therapy can occur.

Hypothyroidism

Patients with hypothyroidism are generally treated with a thyroid preparation such as L-thyroxine. The treatment is usually begun with 25 to 50 μg of L-thyroxine and slowly increased to a maximal dose of between 150 and 250 μg. The patients are followed clinically, and serial determinations of free thyroxine and TSH levels are used to monitor adequacy of replacement.

The major side effect of thyroid treatment is hyperthyroidism from excessive replacement (Summary Table 16–III).

Thyroid Tumors

Tumors determined to be benign by needle biopsy can be managed conservatively. Malignant thyroid tumors are usually treated surgically. Postoperatively, the patient is followed for signs of hypothyroidism.

DENTAL EVALUATION

The patient with severe hyperthyroidism is particularly susceptible to catecholamines. Catecholamines used as vasoconstrictors in local anesthetic preparations or gingival retraction cords, when coupled with the stress of a dental procedure, can precipitate thyroid storm. This emergency situation is characterized by marked exacerbation of the symptoms of hyperthyroidism, including very high fever, major central nervous system (CNS) alterations (severe agitation, frank psychosis), vomiting, and diarrhea. Most importantly, there is a high risk of life-threatening arrhythmias and/or congestive heart failure. Short of frank thyroid storm, the use of catecholamines in a patient with severe hyperthyroidism carries a high risk of exacerbating underlying cardiovascular pathology. Even the patient with mild hyperthyroidism may experience tachycardia, tremulousness, and palpitations, as well as run the risk of aggravating pre-existing cardiovascular disease.

The patient with hypothyroidism has pre-existing CNS depression and is acutely sensitive to drugs with CNS depressant side effects. These include the narcotic analgesics commonly prescribed by dentists (Chap. 50) and several of the drugs used in routine dental sedation techniques (Chap. 51). The patient with severe hypothyroidism who is given a CNS depressant drug is at risk of respiratory and cardiovascular depression and/or collapse. The patient with mild hypothyroidism may have an exaggerated response to routine doses of narcotics and sedatives. Because of these possible complications, the dentist must determine relative risk categories for each patient with a thyroid disorder.

Patients at Low Risk. The most common situation for the dentist is the patient with known and treated thyroid disease. Appropriate medical follow-up for patients with thyroid disease includes regularly scheduled physical examinations and laboratory testing. Any patient who is asymptomatic and has had a physical examination and normal thyroid function test results within 6 months is at low risk for complications during dental therapy.

Patients at Moderate Risk. The patient with hypothyroidism treated with thyroid replacement may become hypothyroid again through lapses in medication or subtle metabolic shifts. A similar problem may occur in the patient with hyperthyroidism, especially those treated with propylthiouracil or radioactive iodine. As noted earlier, about 30% of patients who are rendered euthyroid by antithyroid medication remain euthyroid. In addition, a complication of radioactive iodine therapy for hyperthyroidism is the insidious onset of hypothyroidism. Therefore, in the absence of a recent determination of thyroid function tests and physical examination, the risk of recurrent mild hyperthyroidism or hypothyroidism increases. Any patient who is asymptomatic and has not had a medical evaluation within 6 months is at moderate risk for dental therapy complications.

Patients at High Risk. The situation of a patient with undiagnosed thyroid disease presenting to the dentist is rare. However, as noted earlier, both hyperthyroidism and hypothyroidism can occur long after the termination of a course of therapy for thyroid disease. Any patient with a past history of a thyroid disorder should, therefore, be asked about heat or cold intolerance, weight gain or weight loss, changes in appetite or bowel habits, muscular weakness, tremors, and palpitations. Any patient who is symptomatic, regardless of the timing of the most recent medical evaluation, is at high risk for complications of dental treatment.

DENTAL MANAGEMENT

Patients at Low Risk. Patients who are asymptomatic, with a comprehensive medical and laboratory re-evaluation within 6 months of the proposed dental therapy, may undergo all dental surgical and nonsurgical procedures using a normal dental protocol.

Patients at Moderate Risk. Patients who are asymptomatic but who have not had a recent medical and laboratory evaluation must be treated with caution. Although a normal protocol may be used for most procedures, the dentist should avoid the use of vasoconstrictors (e.g., epinephrine in local anesthesia preparations) and minimize the prescription of analgesics and sedatives with CNS depressant side effects. For surgical procedures (types IV to VI) and particularly for moderate to advanced surgery (types V and VI), a medical consultation and/or referral for medical and laboratory re-evaluation prior to dental therapy may be advisable.

Patients at High Risk. Patients who are symptomatic regardless of the timing of their most recent medical evaluation can undergo only dental examination (type I) procedures. All other dental therapy is contraindicated. A medical and laboratory re-evaluation is mandatory before proceeding with dental therapy.

■ Examples of Dental Evaluation and Management

EVALUATION

Patient 1. This patient is a 44-year-old woman with Graves' disease who underwent a thyroidectomy 10 years ago. She has been on 125 μg of L-thyroxine since and has done well. She is asymptomatic. Her last examination was 3 months ago, and thyroid function tests at that time were normal. Her dental needs involve comprehensive periodontal therapy including curettage and full mouth surgery. On examination, her blood pressure is 130/88 and her pulse rate is 64 beats/minute (bpm).

Patient 2. This patient is a 44-year-old woman who was recently diagnosed as having hyperthyroidism. She has been on propylthiouracil for 10 months and is asymptomatic. Her last physical examination was 8 months ago. Her dental needs include comprehensive mandibular periodontal care, mandibular caries control, the extraction of the remaining periodontally involved maxillary teeth, and the placement of a full maxillary denture. On examination, she is anxious and her blood pressure is 140/88. She has a regular pulse rate of 100 bpm.

Patient 3. A 50-year-old woman with no known medical problems presents for dental treatment. She has had symptoms of cold intolerance, slow weight gain, easy fatigability, constipation, and hoarseness. Her family has noticed that she is considerably less active than before. Her dental needs are similar to those of patient 2. On examination, her blood pressure is 110/74 and her pulse rate is 58 bpm. She has dry, doughy skin and a prominent tongue.

MANAGEMENT

Patient 1. This is an asymptomatic patient with a known thyroid disorder and a recent comprehensive medical evaluation. All dental procedures can be completed using a normal protocol.

Patient 2. This is an asymptomatic patient with a known thyroid disorder. She has not had a recent physical examination or thyroid function test. Impressions for the maxillary denture and periodontal prophylaxis can be completed using a normal protocol. Caries control and periodontal scaling and curettage can be done if local anesthesia without a vasoconstrictor is used and no adjunctive sedation techniques are required. If sedation techniques are required for the type II and III procedures, or if the use of vasoconstrictor and postoperative analgesia is anticipated for the periodontal surgery and multiple extractions (types V and VI procedures), a preoperative referral to her physician is in order. Once the physical examination is complete and the thyroid function tests are found to be within normal limits, the balance of dental therapy can be completed using a normal protocol.

Patient 3. This patient reports several symptoms suggestive of hypothyroidism. Routine pulse rate determination reveals a bradycardia, and physical examination supports the possibility of a thyroid disorder. Type I examination procedures may be completed using a normal protocol. However, all other dental therapy is contraindicated at this time. The patient should be referred to her physician to rule out frank thyroid disease. The physician should be advised of your findings and referral before seeing this patient.

Thyroid Disorders: General Information

HYPERTHYROIDISM

Excessive production of thyroxine

Causes

Graves' disease (autoimmune): 90% of patients under age 40

Toxic multinodular goiter, common after age 40

Single toxic nodule (uncommon)

Subacute and chronic thyroiditis—transient hyperthyroidism

Factitious—excessive ingestion of exogenous thyroid hormone

HYPOTHYROIDISM

Insufficient production of thyroid hormone

Causes

Chronic thyroiditis (Hashimoto's disease)

Idiopathic thyroid atrophy

Previous radioactive iodine therapy

Neck irradiation

Thyroidectomy

Secondary hypothyroidism (pituitary deficiency, hypothalamic deficiency)

Effects of Thyroxine

SITE OR TYPE OF EFFECT	EXCESSIVE THYROXINE	INSUFFICIENT THYROXINE
Metabolism	Weight loss with polyphagia; muscle wasting; weakness, fat store depletion; thin skin; heat intolerance	Weight gain, thick skin, cold intolerance
Bone marrow		Anemia
Carbohydrate metabolism	Increased intestinal glucose uptake and hepatic glycogen depletion; transient hyperglycemia and exacerbation of diabetes; possible chronic liver damage	Hypoglycemic syncope
Cardiovascular system	Increased cardiac output, heart rate, pulse pressure; common cause of atrial fibrillation and arrhythmia	Decreased cardiac output, heart rate, pulse pressure
Central nervous system	Rapid mentation; irritability, restlessness	Slow mentation (adults), retardation (infants), poor memory
Gastrointestinal system	Increased motility, diarrhea	Reduced motility, constipation
Other	Potentiation of catecholamines and growth hormones	Amenorrhea; infertility

Medical Management of the Patient with Thyroid Disease

HYPERTHYROIDISM

Propranolol for symptomatic therapy

Antithyroid therapy (propylthiouracil, methimazole)

Radioactive iodine

Surgery

Major Complications

Hypothyroidism

Recurrent hyperthyroidism

HYPOTHYROIDISM

Thyroid replacement therapy

Major Complications

Iatrogenic hyperthyroidism (excessive replacement)

Persistent hypothyroidism (inadequate replacement)

Medical follow-up, medical evaluation, and repeat thyroid function tests every 6 months

Dental Evaluation of the Patient with Thyroid Disease

PATIENTS WITH UNDIAGNOSED THYROID DISORDERS

Patients with symptoms suggestive of disease should be referred for medical evaluation and thyroid function tests.

Hyperthyroidism

Nervousness, irritability, recent weight loss, intolerance to heat, tachycardia

Hypothyroidism

Slow mentation, apathy, recent weight gain, intolerance to cold, bradycardia

PATIENTS WITH KNOWN THYROID DISEASE

Original diagnosis

Past therapy (surgery, medication)

Present medication

Assessment of clinical status (absence of symptoms, normal physical and thyroid function tests within 6 months)

Dental Implications of Thyroid Disease

HYPERTHYROIDISM
Adverse interaction with catecholamines (e.g., epinephrine)

Severe Hyperthyroidism
Life-threatening arrhythmias and congestive heart failure

Exacerbation of underlying cardiovascular pathology

Thyroid storm

Mild Hyperthyroidism
Tachycardia, tremulousness, palpitations

Exacerbation of underlying cardiovascular pathology

HYPOTHYROIDISM
Exaggerated response to central nervous system depressants (narcotic analgesics, sedatives)

Severe Hypothyroidism (Myxedema)
Respiratory depression

Cardiovascular depression

Mild Hypothyroidism
Exaggerated effects of analgesics and sedatives in routine doses

SUMMARY TABLE **16–VI**

Risk Categories for the Patient with Thyroid Disease

PATIENTS AT LOW RISK
Asymptomatic patients
Physical and thyroid function tests within normal limits (within past 6 months)

PATIENTS AT MODERATE RISK
Asymptomatic patients
No recent physical or thyroid function tests

PATIENTS AT HIGH RISK
Patients with symptoms

SUMMARY TABLE **16–VII**

Dental Management of the Patient with Thyroid Disease

RISK CATEGORY	PROCEDURES	PROTOCOL
Low risk	I–VI	Normal protocol
Moderate risk	I–VI (esp. IV–VI)	Minimize use of epinephrine and CNS depressants (e.g., narcotic analgesics, barbiturates, diazepam); consider medical and laboratory re-examination
High risk	I	Normal protocol
	II–VI	Deferred until after medical examination, evaluation, and treatment; thyroid function tests should be normalized prior to procedures

17

Pregnancy

The pregnant patient poses a number of unique management issues for the dentist. Not only is the practitioner responsible for providing safe and effective care for the mother, but the health of the fetus also becomes a concern. In addition, a number of maternal oral changes may be observed as a consequence of the multiple physiologic changes that occur. In view of the dual responsibility that the dentist faces in treating the pregnant patient, a brief review of the physiology of pregnancy and the course of fetal development may be helpful.

PHYSIOLOGIC CONSIDERATIONS

Maternal Changes

The major physiologic changes that occur in the pregnant female are attributable to endocrine, cardiovascular, hematologic, and respiratory alterations. During pregnancy, the placenta becomes an active endocrine organ secreting three major hormones—estrogen, progesterone, and chorionic gonadotropin—all of which function to ensure the viability of the placenta and fetus. Chorionic gonadotropin prevents the normal involution of the corpus luteum at the end of the monthly reproductive cycle. Progesterone, secreted from the corpus luteum and the placenta, affects the uterine endometrium to ensure adequate nutrition for the developing fetus. Progesterone affects the breasts in preparation for lactation and decreases spontaneous contractions of the uterus. Estrogen also prepares the breasts for lactation by increasing glandular tissue. In addition, it enlarges the uterus and external genitalia and relaxes the pelvic ligaments in preparation for delivery.

A 20 to 40% increase in cardiac output is frequently noted in the pregnant female in response to the growing demands of the fetus. A 30% increase in maternal blood volume is

also observed. Generally, maternal cardiovascular changes are most profound at the beginning of the third trimester. Tachycardia and flow murmurs are not uncommon. In some cases, the fetus may put pressure on the inferior vena cava when the mother is supine. This may result in impaired venous return, hypotension, and syncope.

Hematopoiesis of the fetus places large demands for iron on the mother, approximately 55% more than normal requirements. Maternal anemia has been largely reduced by the use of iron supplements during pregnancy.

Changes in maternal respiration may be noted during pregnancy. An increase in the basal metabolic rate increases maternal oxygen demand and the rate of respiration. An increase in the respiratory rate also results when the gravid uterus restricts the movement of the diaphragm and thus reduces the lower lung volume.

Fetal Development

Fetal development is divided into three trimesters of 3 months each. From the standpoint of organ development, the first trimester is the most critical, although most growth occurs during the second and third trimesters (Fig. 17–1). During the first month, the organ systems are organized; by the fourth month, for the most part, organogenesis is grossly completed. However, cellular development of organs occurs throughout the pregnancy and may not be entirely completed until after birth.

MEDICAL EVALUATION AND MANAGEMENT

Normal Pregnancy

The woman who suspects that she is pregnant often calls on her physician or nurse-

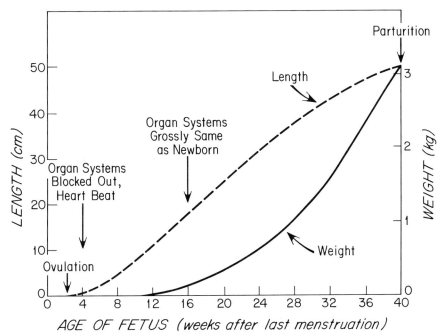

Figure 17–1. Fetal organ development during pregnancy. (Adapted from Guyton, A.: Textbook of Medical Physiology, 8th ed. Philadelphia, W. B. Saunders, 1990.)

practitioner soon after a menstrual period is missed. The patient may complain of nausea or breast tenderness. To confirm the diagnosis of pregnancy, the first urine voided in the morning is collected about 40 days after the last menstrual cycle or 10 days after the first missed period and analyzed for human chorionic gonadotropin (HCG). A positive or negative pregnancy test of this nature does not by itself prove or disprove pregnancy; it must be interpreted in conjunction with the patient's clinical presentation. The measurement of serum beta subunits of HCG is a more sensitive test and should be used when there are ambiguities.

The pregnant female should be followed closely during the entire term. Her weight, blood pressure, blood count, and urinalysis are monitored each trimester to ensure a normal course of pregnancy. Fetal heart sounds can be monitored during the later stages of the pregnancy.

Patients with a family history of genetic disorders and patients over the age of 35 have an increased incidence of fetal abnormalities, and it may be necessary to perform amniocentesis or carry out chorionic villi sampling for genetic counseling. This is usually done during the first trimester or early in the second trimester.

Complications of Pregnancy

Spontaneous Abortion

Spontaneous abortion, or miscarriage, occurs in a significant number of pregnancies. Approximately 15% of pregnancies terminate before the end of the first trimester. The frequency of spontaneous abortion after that period decreases. There is some question as to whether stress may precipitate spontaneous abortion; this issue is unresolved. The relationship between bacteremia and spontaneous abortion is also unclear, as is the relationship between bacteremia and abnormalities in fetal development. However, there is significant evidence that links chronic bacteremia with low infant birth weight. Although this relationship has been studied in a number of chronic infections, such as urinary tract infections, it has not been verified in mothers with chronic oral infections such as periodontitis.

Ectopic Pregnancy

In a small percentage of pregnancies, the fertilization and implantation of the ovum may occur abnormally in a fallopian tube instead of in the uterus. This results in lower abdominal pain and bleeding during the first trimester. Since the bleeding can be massive, it is important to be alerted to this possible complication in any pregnant woman.

Eclampsia

Rarely, patients may present with hypertension and proteinuria during the third trimester. These patients have pre-eclampsia and should be carefully followed. The condition is particularly common in primigravidas who have poor dietary habits. Treatment of pre-eclampsia includes complete bed rest and attempts to control hypertension. Pre-eclampsia may progress to eclampsia, in which patients present with malignant hypertension, seizures, and encephalopathy. In the woman with progressive symptoms of eclampsia, pregnancy may have to be terminated (Summary Table 17–I).

DENTAL EVALUATION AND MANAGEMENT

The issue of dental treatment during pregnancy is not clear-cut. Many obstetricians do not place any restrictions on the dental care of their pregnant patients. Our approach remains conservative, based on the fact that the pregnancy is finite, the sequelae of dental therapy are not always predictable, and the ramifications of problems could be significant. After the first trimester, the patient should be seen for dental prophylaxis. Nondeferrable treatment such as caries control can be performed during the latter part of the second trimester, when the fetus is well developed but not so large as to hinder the mother significantly.

During the second trimester, we do not recommend any elective dental treatment. The pregnancy will be completed in a few months, and to subject the mother and fetus to stress and possible bacteremia during nonemergency dental care is unnecessary.

Prophylaxis should be repeated at the start of the third trimester. By the middle or end of the third trimester the fetus can impinge on the inferior vena cava and cause hypotension in the mother when she is in a supine position. As mentioned earlier, cardiac changes are most noteworthy during the third trimester. Dental procedures during the last months of pregnancy are therefore not recommended.

Two additional concerns regarding the pregnant patient involve the use of radiography and medications. As a general rule, both are to be avoided during pregnancy. The risks are particularly significant during the first trimester. If radiographs must be taken, lead shielding is mandatory. Some texts have stated that there is no contraindication to dental radiography in the pregnant patient when adequate shielding is used. Although the risk to the fetus is minimal, it seems unwise, at best, to take even the slightest risk of injury if it can be avoided.

Our approach is similar with respect to medication. Although there is no evidence to indicate any maternal or fetal problems related to lidocaine, penicillin, or some forms of erythromycin, the elective use of any drug is to be avoided. In the patient requiring care, these agents may be used judiciously. There is a relative contraindication to the use of any aspirin-containing compounds and vasoconstrictors in local anesthetics.

Certain drugs are to be avoided absolutely. Among those frequently in use in dentistry are antianxiety agents such as diazepam and some antibiotics such as tetracycline. Nitrous oxide has been shown to be teratogenic among operating room personnel, and should not be administered to the pregnant patient. Any agent causing respiratory depression is discouraged. The dentist should consult with the patient's physician before prescribing any medication or undertaking treatment. The risk to mother and fetus must be constantly weighed against the therapeutic benefit of treatment. The dentist must be alert to protect pregnant employees from the hazards of stray radiation and gases.

ORAL FINDINGS

The major oral changes attributable to pregnancy are those related to increased vascularity of the gingiva and an exaggerated response to local factors by the periodontal soft tissues. Pregnancy gingivitis is characterized by swelling, redness, and bleeding (Fig. 17–2). It represents an increased response to local factors and is not directly caused by the pregnancy. It can be controlled by eliminating plaque and other local irritating factors. Pregnancy gingivitis progresses with the pregnancy and is most severe during the third trimester. Occasionally, an area of gingiva, most frequently a papillary area, responds more emphatically and produces a localized area of intense capillary and inflammatory proliferation. Such lesions, which are identical to pyogenic granulomas, are known as pregnancy tumors. Professional

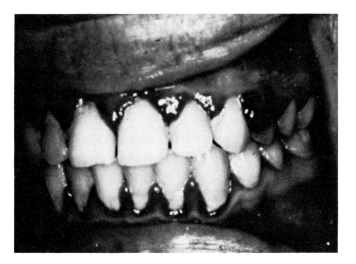

Figure 17–2. Pregnancy gingivitis. Note the severe inflammatory changes of the marginal and papillary gingiva. A developing pyogenic granuloma (pregnancy tumor) is present between the patient's maxillary left canine and first premolar.

prophylaxis, coupled with good patient education and oral hygiene, can minimize the frequency and severity of pregnancy gingivitis. Generally, pregnancy tumors may be left untreated until after delivery. However, if the lesion becomes symptomatic and results in discomfort, dysfunction, or excessive bleeding, it should be excised.

Changes Related to Puberty, Menstruation, or Oral Contraceptives

Hormonal changes resulting from puberty, menstruation, and birth control pills may affect oral tissues. The major changes are associated with an exaggerated gingival inflammatory response to local factors. These are usually well controlled by adequate oral hygiene measures.

■ Examples of Dental Evaluation and Management

EVALUATION

Patient 1. A 22-year-old woman in her second month of pregnancy presents for a routine dental follow-up. She was last seen 6 months ago; this is a scheduled return appointment for dental prophylaxis. She has recently seen her gynecologist and has had a normal pregnancy thus far. Her medical history is unremarkable. Her blood pressure is 110/80, and her pulse rate is 90 beats/minute (bpm).

Patient 2. A 19-year-old woman in her sixth month of pregnancy presents because of severe toothache. She has not had dental care for the past 4 years. She has been followed by her obstetrician and has had a normal pregnancy. Her medical history is otherwise unremarkable. Her blood pressure is 108/80, and her pulse rate is 88 bpm. On examination, she is found to have exquisite tenderness in a left mandibular molar.

Patient 3. A 37-year-old woman in her seventh month of pregnancy presents because of bleeding and pain in her gums. She has had no consistent dental follow-up. Her blood pressure is 180/110, and her pulse rate is 100 bpm. Oral examination reveals extensive periodontitis.

MANAGEMENT

Patient 1. Clearly, any routine radiographic examinations, such as annual bite-wings, are contraindicated in this patient. A review of oral hygiene and patient education with regard to outpatient oral care is appropriate. Examination for caries can be completed, but restoration should be deferred. Dental prophylaxis should be deferred until the beginning of the second trimester and repeated at the beginning of the third trimester. The use of local anesthetics and analgesics should be discussed with the patient's physician. All nonemergency dental care should be deferred.

Patient 2. This patient is in the second trimester of her pregnancy. At this stage, both the mother and fetus are best able to tolerate dental treatment. She presents with an acute process that requires immediate intervention. A diagnostic radiograph may be obtained with the patient and fetus appropriately shielded by a lead apron. The patient's physician should be consulted regarding prospective treatment, anesthesia, and medication. Endodontic therapy or extraction may be performed with local anesthesia. Antibiotics, if needed, should exclude tetracycline; penicillin or erythromycin is generally most appropriate. Definitive restorative treatment or tooth replacement should be deferred until after the pregnancy.

Patient 3. This patient's condition should arouse considerable concern. She is in the third trimester of her pregnancy and has a markedly elevated blood pressure. The possibility of pre-eclampsia should be considered, and the patient should be referred to her physician immediately. The oral changes observed are a result of an exaggerated inflammatory response to local factors. After clearance from the patient's physician, dental appointments directed at prophylaxis, scaling, and oral hygiene instruction are appropriate. Aggressive curettage and possible periodontal flap surgery should be deferred until after the pregnancy.

SUMMARY TABLE **17–1**

Pregnancy

MATERNAL CHANGES

Endocrine: multiple hormonal changes

Cardiovascular: increase of 20 to 40% in cardiac output, tachycardia, and flow murmurs

Hematologic: increase of 30% in maternal blood volume

Respiratory: increased rate of respiration

COMPLICATIONS

Spontaneous abortions: probability of 15% during first trimester; possible relationship to stress of bacteremia

Ectopic pregnancy: fertilization and implantation of the fetus in a fallopian tube, resulting in abdominal pain and heavy bleeding

Eclampsia: pre-eclampsia marked by hypertension and proteinuria; eclampsia characterized by malignant hypertension, seizures, and encephalopathy

Hypertension and syncope: secondary to fetal compression of the inferior vena cava

Anemia: secondary to increased hematologic demands

Cardiovascular disease: exacerbation of underlying disease in response to increased demand

Oral: exacerbation of underlying periodontal disease; increased risk of pyogenic granuloma

Dental Evaluation and Management in Pregnancy

GENERAL GUIDELINES
Take a history of the trimester and note complications and blood pressure.

First Trimester
The fetus is especially susceptible to teratogenic influence and abortion.

Second Trimester
This is the optimal trimester for dental care.

Third Trimester
Syncope and hypertension risk are greatest secondary to fetal position.

Cardiovascular demands are greatest. There is increased risk of anemia, the highest risk of eclampsia, and increased risk of hypertension.

SPECIFIC GUIDELINES
1. Preventive dental prophylaxis should be undertaken at the beginning of the second trimester and the third trimester.
2. All elective dental care should be deferred.
3. Nondeferrable treatment (e.g., caries control) should be completed during the second trimester.
4. Radiographs are contraindicated in all but emergency situations. When taken, lead shielding is mandatory.
5. There should be medical clearance for all drugs, including local anesthetics, analgesics, and antibiotics.
   a. Lidocaine, penicillin, erythromycin, and acetaminophen (Tylenol) are generally approved.
   b. Aspirin and vasoconstrictors in local anesthesia and all drugs causing respiratory depression (e.g., narcotic analgesics) are relatively contraindicated.
   c. Diazepam (Valium), nitrous oxide, and tetracycline are absolutely contraindicated.

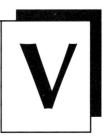

Evaluation and Management of the Patient with Pulmonary Disease

Asthma

Asthma is a condition characterized by episodic reversible narrowing of the airways. The disease affects 2% of the population and accounts for about 5000 deaths each year in the United States. The disease can begin at any age, but about half of patients develop symptoms before the age of 10.

Clinically, the patient presents with episodic shortness of breath and wheezing. The reversible airway obstruction is a result of constriction of the smooth muscles lining the bronchi, edema of the bronchial mucosa, and the formation of tenacious mucus (Fig. 18–1).

A variety of disorders can result in asthma. The most common is an inherited immunologic abnormality that allows inhaled antigens (allergens) to trigger a hypersensitivity response mediated by immunoglobulin E (IgE) and thus produce bronchial narrowing (Fig. 18–2). Asthma may be induced by aspirin ingestion in some individuals, who often have associated nasal polyps and sinusitis. Less common disorders associated with asthma include types of systemic vasculitis such as polyarteritis nodosa and Churg-Strauss syndrome (Summary Table 18–I).

MEDICAL EVALUATION

A detailed history is crucial in the medical evaluation of the patient with asthma. The age at which symptoms of asthma appear is of some prognostic value, because patients developing asthma in childhood often have amelioration of symptoms as adults. This transition may be so marked that many patients with severe asthma as children may have minimal symptoms in later years. Patients developing asthma as adults tend to have less dramatic improvement with time.

The circumstances leading to an episode of asthma should be analyzed to identify possible precipitating factors. Exercise, cold air, emotional stress, respiratory infections, and air pollutants may all be important in precipitating attacks.

The severity of the patient's airway disease can be assessed clinically and by the determination of arterial blood gas levels during an acute episode. Patients with mild airway obstruction (stage I) present with dyspnea, mild expiratory wheezing, and often episodic bouts of coughing. Arterial blood gases show normal oxygenation but a decrease in carbon dioxide (CO_2) content, reflecting hyperventilation. Patients with moderate airway obstruction (stage II) are in more obvious respiratory distress. Arterial blood gases demonstrate mild hypoxemia (low oxygen content) as well as hypocarbia (low carbon dioxide content). With progression of bronchospasm, patients have to use accessory muscles for respiration and may have difficulties with ventilation despite maximal respiratory efforts. Arterial blood gases show progressive hypoxemia, and the carbon dioxide content may be normal (stage III) or high (stage IV) because of progressive respiratory failure. These patients may progress to status asthmaticus, in which severe bronchospasm persists despite aggressive therapy.

The frequency of asthmatic attacks is also important in determining the need for chronic therapy.

MEDICAL MANAGEMENT

The goal in the management of the patient with asthma is to minimize the frequency and severity of episodes of acute bronchospasm. The medications commonly used include beta-adrenergic agonists, inhaled steroids or cromolyn, theophylline, anticholinergic drugs, and oral steroids.

For patients with mild asthma, the first line of therapy is often the use of beta$_2$-adrenergic bronchodilators. There are no indications for the administration of nonselective beta-adrenergic agonists, such as isoproterenol, which are associated with a high incidence of cardio-

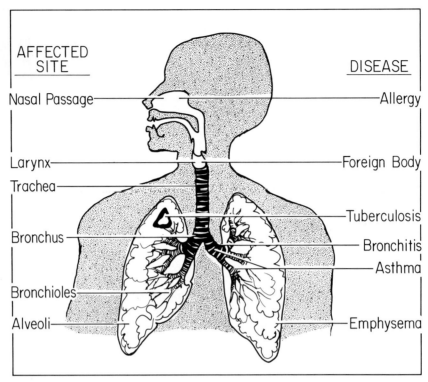

Figure 18–1. Relationship between anatomic sites of the respiratory tree and disease states associated with those sites.

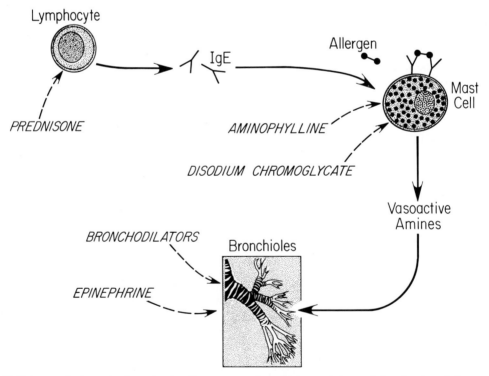

Figure 18–2. Immunologic mechanism whereby allergens cause bronchial constriction and site of action of pharmacologic agents used to prevent the development of those symptoms. Prednisone is directly immunosuppressive; it inhibits lymphocyte activity and thereby reduces levels of IgE. Aminophylline and disodium chromoglycate inhibit the synthesis of vasoactive amines by mast cells once the allergen has complexed with IgE on the cell surface. Bronchodilators and epinephrine work at end-organ sites to reduce or eliminate clinical symptoms.

vascular side effects even when given in an inhaled form. It is now understood that human airway smooth muscles and mast cells have only β_2-adrenergic receptors. Inhaled selective beta$_2$-adrenergic agonists include albuterol (Proventil, Ventolin), terbutaline (Brethaire), metaproterenol (Alupent, Metaprel), isoetharine (Bronkosol, Bronkometer), and bitolterol (Tornalate). Many of these sympathomimetic agents are also available in oral and parenteral forms. Other sympathomimetic agents that are not as beta$_2$-selective include epinephrine (Adrenalin, Primatene, Medihaler-Epi) and isoproterenol (Aerolone, Isuprel). These agents have more cardiovascular side effects, including tachycardia, tremor, and palpitations. Long-term administration of beta-adrenergic agonists does not reduce bronchial hyperresponsiveness, and it is common clinical practice to prescribe long-term treatment with beta-adrenergic agonists (tid or qid). Unwanted side effects are uncommon when selective beta$_2$-adrenergic agonists are given by inhalation. When administered orally or by nebulizer, tremor, tachycardia, and palpitations are the most common side effects.

For patients who are not adequately managed on bronchodilators alone, low-dose inhaled steroids are often helpful. These agents are used because of the increasing understanding that some bronchospastic tendencies are related to inflammatory responses, which can be managed with anti-inflammatory agents. Inhaled beclomethasone (Beclovent, Vanceril), triamcinolone (Azmacort), and flunisolide (Aerobid) are all effective.

Methylxanthines, such as theophylline (Elixophyllin, Quibron, Slo-Bid, Slo-Phyllin, Theo-Dur, Theolair, Uniphyl), oxtriphylline (Choledyl), and aminophylline (Aminophyllin) preparations, are bronchodilators that can be taken orally or parenterally. Theophylline is a less effective bronchodilator than beta-adrenergic agonists, although it has often been used as first-choice therapy for asthma in the United States; it also may have a synergistic effect. Methylxanthines are particularly useful for patients with nocturnal asthma, because many of the preparations are available in a slow-release form. The major problem with theophylline therapy is the relatively high incidence of unwanted effects. The most common side effects are gastrointestinal symptoms (e.g., nausea and vomiting) and cardiac symptoms (including tachycardia and arrhythmias). Cardiac side effects are of particular concern in patients with underlying cardiac disease, because lethal arrhythmias can result.

Cromolyn sodium (Intal) is believed to inhibit the release of mediators from mast cells; it can be used in either an inhalation or an oral form. Cromolyn protects against various indirect bronchoconstrictor stimuli, such as exercise. It is particularly effective in children, because many of these patients have allergic asthma, and is the anti-inflammatory drug of first choice in children because it has few side effects. Its effects in adults are less predictable, but it should be tried in the appropriate patient because there is no way of determining who is likely to respond. Unwanted side effects are rare with cromolyn therapy.

Anticholinergic agents such as ipratropium bromide (Atrovent) inhibit vagal cholinergic tone, resulting in bronchodilation. They are less effective than beta-adrenergic agonists and are usually used in combination with other bronchodilators. They appear to be most useful in patients with predominantly bronchitic symptoms. Side effects are uncommon, because ipratropium bromide is poorly absorbed.

Oral steroids should be used only when other agents have been tried without success. Steroids are remarkably effective in suppressing the inflammation induced by asthma and are associated with more side effects, but they are still needed to control asthma in a minority of patients. Short courses of orally administered steroids are indicated in instances of acute and severe asthmatic exacerbations, particularly if the patient has previously responded to steroids. Treatment with prednisone (30 mg daily) for 1 to 2 weeks is usually effective. There is no need to taper the steroids when a short course is given.

DENTAL EVALUATION

A detailed history is crucial in the evaluation of the patient with asthma. The age of onset of symptoms, the frequency and severity of disease, and the need for hospitalization should all be recorded. Asthma may range from a childhood disease with no symptoms in adulthood to one requiring chronic maintenance therapy and frequent hospitalizations.

The dentist should specifically inquire about events that can result in bronchospasm. Of particular importance is the role of emotional stress in precipitating asthmatic attacks. Patients should also be asked specifically about aspirin intolerance.

The patient's medications are important, because they may influence dental therapy. The types of bronchodilators used should be recorded and their cardiac side effects should be assessed. Of particular interest is the history of corticosteroid usage, because long-term steroid therapy may result in adrenal suppression and adrenal insufficiency during stressful situations (Chap. 15). Because the patient can still have suppressed adrenal function months after the termination of a course of steroids, the dentist should ask specifically about steroid use during the past year. The duration of therapy and dosages should also be recorded. If a patient is not certain about the medications that are being used, the physician should be consulted before any extensive dental treatment.

The physical examination should include a brief assessment of the patient's respiratory status; patients with shortness of breath, audible wheezing, and bouts of coughing should not have elective dental procedures. The pulse should also be taken, and an irregular pulse or sinus tachycardia should alert the dentist to the possibility of excessive medication.

Based on the medical history and the simple physical assessment of respiratory symptoms, patients with asthma can be assigned to various risk categories (Summary Table 18–III).

Patients at Low Risk. Patients with childhood-onset asthma who have had infrequent symptoms as adults and patients with rare bouts of bronchospasm requiring no maintenance therapy are at low risk.

Patients at Moderate Risk. Patients with intermittent episodes of asthma requiring chronic maintenance therapy are at moderate risk. These patients are asymptomatic on medications.

Patients at Significant Risk. Patients who are unstable despite chronic medications are at significant risk. These patients give a history of frequent exacerbations that require adjustments of their medications and occasional hospitalizations for severe bronchospasm. These patients are asymptomatic on chronic maintenance medications at the time of their dental appointments.

Patients at High Risk. Patients presenting with audible wheezing and respiratory symptoms are at high risk regardless of the medical history and drug therapy.

DENTAL MANAGEMENT

The goal of the dental management of the patient with asthma is to avoid precipitating an acute attack.

General Guidelines

Minimization of Stress. Patients with asthma can occasionally have an exacerbation of symptoms under stress, and efforts should be made to identify patients whose bronchospasms are precipitated by emotional stress. Whenever possible, lengthy procedures should be spread over several appointments. Adjunctive sedation techniques should be considered when appropriate (Chap. 51).

Sedation Techniques. Sedation techniques might include the use of N_2O-O_2 inhalation or diazepam (Valium). Antihistamines such as promethazine (Phenergan) or diphenhydramine (Benadryl) should be avoided, because they have a drying effect that can exacerbate the formation of tenacious mucus in an acute attack (Chap. 51).

Use of Epinephrine. Many patients are already on significant dosages of sympathomimetic drugs for bronchodilatation, and care should be taken before epinephrine is used. In patients with concomitant cardiac disease, additional epinephrine can precipitate arrhythmias, angina, or congestive heart failure. Different bronchodilators have different cardiac effects (Summary Table 18–II): isoproterenol, epinephrine, and ephedrine have prominent cardiac stimulatory effects; isoetharine, terbutaline, and metaproterenol have intermediate cardiac stimulatory effects; and salbutamol has minimal cardiac stimulatory effects. The use of epinephrine in local anesthesia or in gingival retraction cord should therefore be adjusted according to the type and amount of bronchodilator the patient is taking.

Use of Aspirin. Some patients have an acute exacerbation of asthma after ingestion of aspirin. They should avoid aspirin-containing drugs (Chap. 50). Alternative aspirin-free drugs that the dentist may prescribe for analgesia are listed in the same chapter.

Use of Antibiotics. The use of the commonly prescribed antibiotics erythromycin and clindamycin concurrently with a methylxanthine preparation (e.g., theophylline) is associated with an increased risk of methylxanthine toxicity. These antibiotics are therefore relatively contraindicated in patients with asthma who are receiving methylxanthine medication as a bronchodilator.

Specific Guidelines

The dentist should consider dental therapy only in asymptomatic patients. Dental therapy should be deferred in patients presenting with symptoms of wheezing or coughing even in the absence of respiratory compromise, because emotional stress in these patients can markedly aggravate the existing bronchospasm. Similarly, dental treatment should be deferred in asthmatic patients presenting with upper respiratory tract infections, because acute exacerbations are more likely in this setting.

In asymptomatic patients, a risk categorization based on the history, the list of medications, and the physical examination can provide some guidelines for dental management.

Patients at Low Risk. These patients have rare attacks and are not on medication. They can be treated with normal operating protocols, with special attention to sedation techniques and minimization of stress.

Patients at Moderate Risk. Asymptomatic patients on chronic maintenance therapy are usually on bronchodilators or steroids.

Patients on bronchodilators may be on isoproterenol, ephedrine, or theophylline, agents with pronounced cardiac stimulatory effects, and caution is advised in the use of epinephrine in these patients. Other patients may be on isoetharine, terbutaline, or metaproterenol, which have milder cardiac stimulatory effects. In general, the pulse should be taken to determine the regularity and the rate. This should provide some clue to the extent of cardiac stimulation caused by medications, because arrhythmias and tachycardias are the major side effects of excessive use of these agents (Chap. 8).

Patients on chronic steroid therapy deserve special attention. The long-term use of steroids can result in adrenal suppression (Chap. 15). Major operative procedures in these patients can precipitate adrenal insufficiency if the steroid dosage is not adjusted appropriately. Adrenal suppression may occur after only 20 to 30 mg of prednisone are given daily for 7 to 10 days, although the duration of adrenal compromise is usually brief. Prolonged steroid therapy may result in adrenal suppression that does not return to normal for 9 to 12 months after the termination of therapy. It is therefore important to determine steroid usage during the year prior to the patient's dental visit. Patients on alternate-day steroids are less likely to develop adrenal suppression. Because it is impossible to specify the exact minimal duration that would suppress endogenous function, it is wise to err on the side of giving

steroid supplements to any patients treated with steroids for more than 7 to 10 days during the preceding year. For procedures anticipated to induce moderate stress (nonsurgical and simple surgical therapy; types I through IV procedures), supplemental doses of prednisone up to a total dose of 20 to 40 mg should be given on the day of the procedure and tapered rapidly to the maintenance dose. For moderate to advanced surgical procedures (types V or VI, or general anesthesia) that are presumed to induce maximum stress, steroids should be supplemented to the equivalent of 60 mg of prednisone on the day of the procedure and tapered rapidly thereafter. Protracted pain, infection, or inability to resume normal dietary intake necessitates extended steroid use. A medical consultation is advised prior to dental therapy (Chap. 15).

It should also be borne in mind that patients on chronic steroid therapy are often immunocompromised and thus more prone to infections. It is therefore reasonable to use a short course of prophylactic antibiotics if significant soft tissue manipulation is anticipated. Penicillin VK or tetracycline given in 250-mg oral doses qid can be started on the day of the procedure and continued for 3 days. Because of the increased risk of toxicity associated with concurrent use of methylxanthines and erythromycin or clindamycin, the latter two drugs are usually contraindicated.

Patients at Significant Risk. These patients give a history of frequent exacerbations despite chronic maintenance therapy. They should have close medical follow-up to ensure optimization of their clinical status prior to extensive dental treatment, and their physicians should be consulted. All dental procedures (types II to VI) should be carried out with attention to the minimization of stress and the use of adjunctive sedation techniques. Hospitalization may be considered for the patient requiring moderate to advanced surgical procedures (types V and VI) to provide adequate monitoring. Patients on steroids should have their dosages supplemented on the day of dental therapy as indicated earlier to minimize the possibility of precipitating adrenal insufficiency.

Patients at High Risk. Patients who are audibly wheezing or coughing or are in the midst of an upper respiratory tract infection should have active dental treatment deferred, because the risk of precipitating an acute attack in these instances is high. Patients with acute episodes of bronchospasm should immediately be referred to their physicians for medical attention.

■ Examples of Dental Evaluation and Management

EVALUATION

Patient 1. A 38-year-old man with a history of childhood asthma presents for dental therapy. He had frequent asthmatic attacks between the ages of 3 and 8 but has rarely been symptomatic since age 20. His last attack was 4 years ago, when he had mild wheezing in the midst of a bout of tracheobronchitis. He is currently on no medications, and his examination reveals no respiratory signs. His dental needs include advanced periodontal therapy, caries control, and extensive fixed prosthetic therapy.

Patient 2. A 24-year-old man with an 8-year history of asthma presents for dental therapy. He has had about four asthmatic attacks each year and has been on chronic bronchodilator therapy. He is currently taking theophylline (Slo-Phyllin), 200 mg orally qid, and metaproterenol (Alupent) aerosol, two puffs qid, and has been asymptomatic for the past 2 months. He has no respiratory difficulties on physical examination, and his resting pulse rate is 88 beats/minute (bpm), with a regular rhythm. His dental needs are the same as those of Patient 1.

Patient 3. This patient is a 33-year-old woman with a 12-year history of asthma with frequent exacerbations. She has been on chronic steroid maintenance therapy for 2 years and is currently on 15 mg of prednisone each morning, Slo-Phyllin 200 mg orally qid, and terbutaline 5 mg orally qid. Her last episode of bronchospasm was about 2 months ago, when she required hospitalization because of severe respiratory compromise. On examination, she has cushingoid facies and truncal obesity. Her blood pressure is 130/84 and her pulse rate is 94 bpm. She has no respiratory symptoms or signs. Her dental needs are the same as those of the previous patients.

Patient 4. A 42-year-old woman with no history of asthma presents for dental evaluation. She had a history of multiple allergies as a child and has been evaluated on several occasions for bouts of severe coughing, but no definite diagnosis has been established. She is not currently on medications. On examination, she is noticeably short of breath and audibly wheezing. She has a pulse rate of 110 bpm and a blood pressure of 150/94. Her dental needs are the same as those of the previous patients.

MANAGEMENT

Patient 1. This patient has childhood-onset asthma and has not had significant symptoms as an adult. He can be treated with normal operating protocols combined with elective sedation techniques and minimization of stress. The procedures can be spread over several short appointments, and care should be taken to avoid antihistamines and aspirin.

Patient 2. This patient is asymptomatic on chronic maintenance therapy and is therefore at moderate risk. He is on bronchodilators, including a theophylline preparation with significant cardiac stimulatory effects (Slo-Phyllin). The normal physical examination is reassuring and there is no evidence of drug toxicity as suggested by the normal pulse rate and rhythm. His dental therapy should be spread over a number of short appointments. Nitrous oxide sedation is appropriate for the simple operative procedures (type II). Oral sedatives such as diazepam (Valium) may be added to N_2O-O_2 inhalation for some complicated operative procedures (type III) and simple to advanced surgical procedures (types IV to VI). Because he is already on sympathomimetic agents, epinephrine should be used cautiously and care should be taken to avoid antihistamines and aspirin. The patient's clinical condition should be evaluated at each appointment to ensure that it has not changed.

Patient 3. This patient is also asymptomatic on chronic maintenance therapy, but she is clinically a bit less stable than Patient 2. The same precautions to minimize stress and to ensure adequate sedation should be followed. She is on significant bronchodilator therapy and the use of epinephrine should be minimized. She is also on chronic steroid therapy, which requires special attention. The fact that she has been on significant dosages of prednisone for 2 years should alert the dentist to the possibility that she is adrenally suppressed and requires an increased steroid dose on the day of the dental procedure. For most procedures involving minimal to moderate stress, doubling her maintenance steroid dose to 30 mg of prednisone orally may be appropriate. For procedures involving significant stress, such as general anesthesia or after moderate or advanced dental surgery (types V and VI), 60 mg of prednisone or an equivalent may be used on the day of the procedure. The steroid dosage should be tapered over the next 2 to 3 days back to her maintenance dose.

The patient is also more susceptible to infection because of the immunocompromises resulting from chronic steroid therapy. She should therefore be treated with prophylactic antibiotics and followed closely if significant soft tissue trauma is anticipated. Penicillin VK 250 mg or tetracycline HCl 250 mg orally qid should be started on the day of dental therapy and continued for 3 days. Erythromycin or clindamycin is relatively contraindicated because of its ad-

verse interaction with methylxanthine preparations (theophylline).

Hospitalization should be considered for moderate and advanced surgical procedures (types V and VI).

Patient 4. Despite the fact that the patient is not known to have asthma, the clinical presentation with shortness of breath and audible wheezing should be adequate grounds for deferral of dental treatment and referral for medical attention. In retrospect, the bouts of severe coughing were probably episodes of bronchospasms as well. Dental therapy can be resumed after optimization of her medical status.

SUMMARY TABLE **18–1**

Asthma: General Information

DEFINITION

Asthma is a condition characterized by episodic reversible narrowing of the airways.

PREVALENCE

2% of the population

Onset before age 10 in 50%

CLINICAL CHARACTERISTICS

Episodic shortness of breath (dyspnea), wheezing, bouts of coughing

Childhood-onset disease often ameliorates with age

Adult-onset disease often more refractory

PATHOPHYSIOLOGY

Constriction of the smooth muscles of the bronchi

Edema of the bronchial mucosa

Formation of tenacious mucus

TYPES

Inherited immunologic abnormality (most common)

Environmental precipitation

Aspirin-induced

Systemic vasculitis with concurrent asthma

POSSIBLE PRECIPITATING FACTORS

Emotional stress

Exercise

Cold air

Respiratory infection

Air pollutants

Aspirin

Medical Management of the Patient with Asthma

GOAL
Minimize frequency and severity of episodes of acute bronchospasm.

MEDICATIONS
Beta$_2$-adrenergic agonists (more selective)
  Albuterol (Proventil, Ventolin)
  Terbutaline (Brethaire)
  Metaproterenol (Alupent, Metaprel)
  Isoetharine (Bronkosol, Bronkometer)
  Bitolterol (Tornalate)

Other sympathomimetic agents (less selective)
  Epinephrine (Adrenalin, Primatene, Medihaler-Epi)
  Isoproterenol (Aerolone, Isuprel)

Inhaled steroid preparations
  Beclomethasone (Beclovent, Vanceril)
  Triamcinolone (Azmacort)
  Flunisolide (Aerobid)

Methylxanthines
  Theophylline
  Oxtriphylline (Elixophyllin, Quibron, Slo-Bid, Slo-Phyllin, Theo-Dur, Uniphyl)
  Aminophylline (Aminophyllin)

Mast cell inhibitor
  Cromolyn sodium (Intal)

Oral steroids

Dental Evaluation of the Patient with Asthma

AGE OF ONSET

FREQUENCY AND SEVERITY OF ATTACKS

PRECIPITATING FACTORS
Emotional stress and aspirin (significant factors)

MEDICATIONS
Bronchodilators and their risk of cardiac side effects (e.g., tachycardia, arrhythmias)

Corticosteroid use (present and within past year), potential adrenal suppression and immunosuppression

PHYSICAL EXAMINATION
Respiratory status (shortness of breath, wheezing, bouts of coughing, upper respiratory tract infection)

Medication side effects

Pulse rate and rhythm (tachycardia or irregular pulse rhythm—suggest toxic drug side effects)

RISK CATEGORY
Patient at low risk: infrequent episodes, no chronic medication

Patient at moderate risk: intermittent episodes requiring chronic maintenance therapy

Patient at significant risk: frequent episodes in spite of chronic maintenance therapy, asymptomatic at the time of the dental appointment

Patient at high risk: symptomatic (e.g., audible wheezing) or physical signs of medication side effects (e.g., tachycardia, irregular pulse)

SUMMARY TABLE **18–IV**

Dental Management of the Patient with Asthma

GENERAL GUIDELINES

Minimization of stress:
  Shorter appointments
  Adjunctive sedation techniques (Chap. 51)
  Antihistamines (e.g., promethazine, diphenhydramine) contraindicated

Minimization of epinephrine use relative to potential cardiac side effects of medications; erythromycin and
  clindamycin relatively contraindicated if patient is taking methylxanthine preparations

Avoidance of aspirin-containing drugs

SPECIFIC GUIDELINES

Patients at low risk:
  Normal protocol for all procedures

Patients at moderate risk:
  Assessment of cardiac side effects of medication, adjustment of epinephrine use, pulse monitoring
  Supplement steroids (see Chap. 15) in patients with adrenal suppression
  For patients on steroid therapy, prophylactic antibiotics when significant soft tissue manipulation is antici-
    pated

Patients at significant risk:
  Medical consultation
  Sedation techniques for all types II–VI procedures recommended
  Consideration of hospitalization for moderate and advanced dental surgery (types V and VI procedures)
  Steroid supplements for patients with adrenal suppression
  For patients on steroids, prophylactic antibiotics when significant soft tissue manipulation is anticipated

Patients at high risk:
  All elective dental procedures contraindicated

Chronic Obstructive Pulmonary Disease

Emphysema and chronic bronchitis, the two most common forms of chronic obstructive pulmonary disease (COPD), are the result of persistent airway obstruction.

The prevalence of COPD is almost 30 cases/1000 population. After cardiovascular disease, COPD is the most common cause of death, accounting for approximately 50,000 deaths annually in the United States. The leading cause of COPD is smoking. Rare individuals may have COPD because of genetic disorders such as α_1-antitrypsin deficiency. COPD primarily affects men over the age of 40 but, as smoking habits change, increasing numbers of women are affected. The social and economic consequences of the disease are considerable, especially because sufferers tend to be incapacitated for several years of their working lives.

Patients with COPD may present clinically with coughing, sputum production, wheezing, and shortness of breath, which are exacerbated by exertion. The presentation depends on the relative contributions of emphysema and chronic bronchitis. The majority of patients have mixed features of both diseases, although one often predominates.

Emphysema is a disease affecting the distal airways, causing destruction of the lung parenchyma and loss of elasticity of the alveolar walls. This results in compromise of air flow during expiration, overinflation of the lungs, and collapse of some airways. A patient with emphysema frequently complains of dyspnea, particularly on exertion. Coughing is a minor part of the clinical picture, and sputum production is usually scanty. As the disease progresses, the patient has tachypnea with minimal exertion, uses accessory respiratory muscles for breathing, and breathes with pursed lips.

Chronic bronchitis is characterized by hypertrophy of and hypersecretion by the mucous glands of the bronchial tree. Mucus plugging compromises airways and produces progressive symptoms. The patient with chronic bronchitis is often a smoker who gives a history of a chronic, productive cough. By definition, the cough must be present for at least 3 months during 2 consecutive years. Initially, symptoms occur during the winter months, but the patient then becomes symptomatic year-round. As the disease progresses, the patient develops dyspnea on exertion, hypoxia, and finally carbon dioxide retention.

The clinical course of COPD is usually progressive, with a steady decline in pulmonary function over the years. Patients with severe disease have markedly increased pulmonary vascular resistance that eventually leads to right-sided heart failure (cor pulmonale). Respiratory failure, often precipitated by pulmonary infection, leads to death (Summary Table 19–I).

MEDICAL EVALUATION

Patients with COPD can present with any combination of symptoms of chronic cough, sputum production, or shortness of breath. Medical evaluation is directed at the identification of the major physiologic deficits, the assessment of the severity of the disease, and the detection of any potentially reversible processes.

The history includes the delineation of the types of symptoms and the degree of limitation of activity. A history of smoking and exposure to pulmonary irritants is often found.

In the physical examination, attention is given to tachypnea, tachycardia, wheezing, use of accessory muscles, cyanosis, an increase in the anterior-posterior diameter of the chest, the degree of hyperresonance on percussion, prolongation of expiration, evidence of consolidation, and right-sided heart failure.

Laboratory evaluation includes a chest x-ray, arterial blood gas determinations, and pulmonary function tests. The chest x-ray is helpful in detecting complications of COPD such as pneumonia, pneumothorax, or right-sided heart failure. Arterial blood gas levels are important for assessment of the severity of disease. Normally, patients should have a Po_2 of about 100 mm Hg, a Pco_2 of about 40 mm Hg, and a pH of 7.40. Patients with mild disease of the airways have normal gas exchange, patients with moderate disease have hypoxemia, and patients with severe disease have carbon dioxide retention in addition to hypoxemia. Pulmonary function tests are important in determining the degree of airway obstruction. The most helpful measurement is the forced expiratory volume at 1 second (FEV_1). The results are compared with predicted values. With increasing airway obstruction, the volume of air expired within the first second is compromised. Patients with a 50% reduction in the ratio are often dyspneic on exertion, and patients with a 75% reduction are often dyspneic at rest. Determination of the FEV_1 before and after the administration of a bronchodilator can provide a quick estimate of the benefit a patient may derive from bronchodilator therapy. Young patients or nonsmokers with COPD should be screened for α_1-antitrypsin deficiency. When acute infection is suspected, sputum examination is important (Summary Table 19–II).

MEDICAL MANAGEMENT

Regardless of the severity of COPD, all patients are urged to stop smoking. The best hope for preventing progression of COPD is to stop the continuous insult to the airways produced by smoking. Patients exposed to other pulmonary irritants are advised to minimize the exposure whenever feasible. This may necessitate a change of job or residence if the relationship between the exposure and the disease is strong.

Patients with tenacious sputum production are encouraged to maintain adequate fluid intake and a humid environment. Expectorants are also used to help mobilize sputum.

Patients with bronchospasm are given a trial of bronchodilators (Chap. 18), especially if they show an improvement in their FEV_1 after receiving bronchodilators during pulmonary function testing. The bronchodilators commonly used include theophylline preparations and beta$_2$-sympathomimetic bronchodilators such as metaproterenol or terbutaline. Corticosteroids may be used in patients with severe bronchospasm refractory to other measures. Corticosteroids can be given systemically or in an inhaled preparation such as beclomethasone. Continuous use of steroids can result in significant morbidity (Chap. 15), so systemic steroids are rapidly tapered as soon as control of bronchospasm is attained.

During periods of acute exacerbation, when the patient suffers from increased coughing and purulent sputum production, antibiotic therapy with ampicillin, tetracycline, or trimethoprim-sulfamethoxazole is often prescribed.

For individual patients with severe hypoxemia, chronic oxygen therapy can be prescribed. Low-flow oxygen therapy can lower pulmonary vascular resistance and minimize symptoms. Oxygen therapy is not attempted until it has been established that the patient does not retain carbon dioxide when given oxygen. Oxygen can be provided by portable units.

Patients with severe COPD and right-sided heart failure (cor pulmonale) may require diuretic therapy. Digitalis preparations are reserved for refractory cases and are used only when objective improvement can be demonstrated (Summary Table 19–III).

DENTAL EVALUATION

Evaluation of the patient with COPD is geared toward assessing the severity of the disease. This can be done by determining the symptoms, current medications, and past hospitalizations. The patient with a history of smoking or signs of respiratory distress such as wheezing should be asked about exertional dyspnea, coughing, wheezing, and sputum production. All patients should be asked about symptoms of acute respiratory infections. The use of medications required to control respiratory symptoms should also be noted.

If a patient has been hospitalized for respiratory difficulties, the physician should be consulted about the patient's current clinical status. *It is particularly important to know whether a patient retains carbon dioxide. Patients who retain carbon dioxide have severe disease and are most prone to respiratory failure when given oxygen and sedatives.*

Based on the evaluation, patients can be grouped into the following risk categories:

Patients at Low Risk
1. Patients with dyspnea only on significant exertion
2. Patients with normal blood gases

Patients at Moderate Risk
1. Patients with dyspnea on exertion

2. Patients on chronic bronchodilator therapy
3. Patients with a recent history of corticosteroid use
4. Patients with hypoxemia but not carbon dioxide retention

Patients at High Risk

1. Symptomatic patients with previously unrecognized COPD
2. Patients with an acute exacerbation (e.g., acute respiratory infection)
3. Patients with significant dyspnea at rest or cor pulmonale
4. Patients with histories of carbon dioxide retention

DENTAL MANAGEMENT

The dental management of the patient with COPD depends on risk category.

Patients at Low Risk. These patients can be managed using a normal protocol for all dental procedures.

Patients at Moderate Risk. The patient should have had a recent medical evaluation and the patient's physician should be consulted. The dentist should be prepared to discuss overall treatment plans, alternatives, and use of local anesthetics, possible sedation techniques, and postoperative analgesics.

Patients on bronchodilator therapy deserve special attention (Chap. 18). Many bronchodilators have cardiac stimulatory effects and, in patients with underlying cardiovascular disease, additional epinephrine may precipitate arrhythmias. It is therefore prudent to use local anesthetics without epinephrine in these patients. Because of the risk of increased methylxanthine toxicity with the concurrent use of erythromycin or clindamycin, these antibiotics are relatively contraindicated for dental infection in patients taking theophylline preparations.

Patients who are currently on steroids and patients who have had significant doses of steroids during the past year deserve special attention. Management of patients on chronic steroid therapy is discussed in detail in Chapter 15.

Patients at High Risk. Patients with symptoms suggesting COPD who have not been medically evaluated should be referred to their physicians prior to dental procedures. Patients with acute exacerbations of symptoms should have all nonemergency procedures deferred until the acute episodes have resolved.

Patients with severe COPD should be managed in close cooperation with their physicians. Stress should be minimized, and short dental sessions should be employed. *The use of any agent that may depress respiratory function— such as sedatives (including nitrous oxide), tranquilizers, and narcotics—must be discussed with the patient's physician. This is particularly true when the patient has a history of carbon dioxide retention.* In most cases non-narcotic analgesics are preferred.

Patients with cor pulmonale are prone to have arrhythmias. The use of local anesthetics with epinephrine should be limited. Moderate and advanced surgical procedures (types V and VI) may best be accomplished in the hospital. Elective complex periodontal-prosthetic treatment plans involving multiple appointments are generally contraindicated.

ORAL FINDINGS

The oral findings associated with COPD are those associated with a chronic smoking habit. Hyperkeratosis and the risk of dysplastic changes in the smoker are discussed in Chapter 40.

■ Examples of Dental Evaluation and Management

EVALUATION

Patient 1. A 56-year-old man with a 40-year history of smoking (about two packs of cigarettes daily) presents for dental treatment. He has had mild dyspnea on exertion for several years, as well as intermittent nonproductive coughing. He is at his baseline state of health at the time of the evaluation. He is not taking any medication. He was last seen by his physician 3 months ago, when he was told that he should stop smoking. Consultation with his physician reveals that he has mild airway obstruction with an FEV_1 70% of predicted value. His dental needs include the treatment of advanced periodontal disease, the removal of four teeth, and the placement of an extensive maxillary periodontal fixed prosthesis.

Patient 2. A 54-year-old man with a 37-year history of smoking has had progressive dyspnea over the past 6 years and is currently dyspneic, even at rest. He has been hospitalized twice in the past 18 months because of acute tracheo-bronchitis complicating his chronic obstructive pulmonary disease. He is currently on amino-phylline 200 mg orally qid. He has not been on steroids during the past 2 years. He has occasional episodes of coughing that produce small amounts of sputum. Consultation with his physician reveals that he has baseline arterial blood gases of PO_2 75 and PCO_2 36, and a pH of 7.38. There is no history of carbon dioxide retention. His medical history is otherwise unremarkable. On examination, he is audibly wheezing but in no acute distress. His blood pressure is 130/86, and his pulse rate is 88 beats/minute (bpm). His dental needs are identical to those of the first patient.

Patient 3. A 54-year-old man with a 38-year smoking history presents for dental treatment. He has had progressive respiratory difficulties and, despite aminophylline and steroid therapy, has had four hospitalizations in the past year. During the last hospitalization, he had significant carbon dioxide retention and required intubation and mechanical ventilation. He is currently on aminophylline 200 mg orally qid and prednisone 20 mg orally daily. Consultation with his physician reveals that he has severe airway obstruction with an FEV_1 40% that of predicted value. On examination, he is tachypneic at rest and audibly wheezing. His blood pressure is 140/80, and his pulse rate is 98 bpm. His dental needs include multiple simple operative procedures, the treatment of generalized periodontitis, and the extraction of the four remaining maxillary molars that are nonrestorable.

MANAGEMENT

Patient 1. This patient is at low risk because he is not hypoxic and is not on bronchodilators or steroids. Dental procedures can be performed using normal protocol. Sedation techniques—including the use of inhalation analgesics (N_2O-O_2), oral sedatives, or intravenous seda-

tives—can be performed in an outpatient setting.

Patient 2. This patient is at moderate risk. He is chronically on medication and is hypoxic at rest (PO_2 of less than 85 mm Hg). Most dental procedures can be done using normal protocols with some minor modifications. Because the patient is on bronchodilator therapy, care should be taken to minimize the use of local anesthetics with epinephrine. As an example, the periodontal surgery should be sextant or quadrant rather than full mouth surgery to limit the amount of local anesthetics and epinephrine. In the setting of oral infection, the use of erythromycin or clindamycin may increase the risk of theophylline toxicity and therefore alternative antibiotics are preferred. Intravenous sedatives and general anesthesia should be used in a hospital setting in view of the hypoxemia.

Patient 3. This patient has severe chronic obstructive pulmonary disease and is at high risk. Medical consultation should be obtained prior to the initiation of dental therapy. The patient is on chronic steroid therapy and is probably adrenally suppressed. The fact that he retains carbon dioxide places him at significant risk of respiratory compromises. With this patient, care should be taken to minimize stress. Short appointments should be used for simple operative procedures (types I to III), prophylaxis, and scaling. The periodontal disease should be managed conservatively with oral hygiene instructions, subgingival débridement, and frequent recall evaluations. Steroid supplementations are necessary for all stressful procedures. The guidelines for steroid supplementation have been discussed in detail in Chapter 15. Moderate to advanced surgical procedures can be performed only in a hospital. Care should also be used in the prescription of analgesics. Sedatives, including N_2O-O_2 inhalation sedation, and narcotics are contraindicated because of the patient's tendency to retain carbon dioxide.

Chronic Obstructive Pulmonary Disease: General Information

DEFINITION
Chronic obstructive pulmonary disease is irreversible airway obstruction and destruction, most often in two forms, emphysema and chronic bronchitis, occurring in a mixed pattern.

PREVALENCE
30 cases/1000 population

IMPORTANCE
Second most common cause of death

CAUSE
Smoking

Genetic disorders such as α_1-antitrypsin deficiency (rare)

PRESENTING SYMPTOMS
Coughing

Sputum production

Wheezing

Shortness of breath

CLINICAL COURSE
Progressive steady decline over years

COMPLICATIONS
Cor pulmonale (right-sided congestive heart failure)

Respiratory failure

Medical Evaluation of the Patient with COPD

HISTORY

Symptoms

Degree of limitation of activity

Smoking history

Exposure to pulmonary irritants

PHYSICAL EXAMINATION

Tachypnea

Tachycardia

Wheezing

Use of accessory muscles

Cyanosis

Prolongation of expiration

Right-sided heart failure (cor pulmonale)

LABORATORY EVALUATION

Chest x-ray

Arterial blood gases (P_{CO_2}, P_{O_2})

Pulmonary function tests (FEV_1, others)

α_1-Antitrypsin deficiency (young patients and nonsmokers only)

SUMMARY TABLE **19–III**

Medical Management of the Patient with COPD

GENERAL GUIDELINES
1. Stop smoking.
2. Avoid pulmonary irritants.
3. Ensure adequate hydration.
4. Humidify the environment.
5. Use expectorants.

BRONCHODILATORS
1. Methylxanthines—aminophylline, theophylline; side effects: nausea, vomiting, tachycardia (low risk), arrhythmias (low risk)
2. Sympathomimetic agents:
   a. Nonspecific beta-adrenergic agents—isoproterenol (Isuprel), ephedrine; side effects: tachycardia (high risk), arrhythmias (high risk)
   b. Beta$_2$-receptor adrenergic agents (selective bronchodilators)—terbutaline (Brethine), isoetharine (Bronkosol), salbutamol, metaproterenol (Alupent); side effects: tremulousness, tachycardia (intermediate risk), arrhythmia (intermediate risk); salbutamol has minimal cardiac side effects

CORTICOSTEROIDS
1. Systemic—prednisone or other steroids; side effects: adrenal suppression, immunosuppression with increased susceptibility to infection, poor wound healing
2. Inhalants—beclomethasone (Vanceril); side effects: oral and nasopharyngeal candidiasis, same side effects as systemic steroids but much lower risk

ANTIBIOTICS
During periods of acute exacerbation

CHRONIC OXYGEN THERAPY

DIURETICS AND DIGITALIS
For cor pulmonale

SUMMARY TABLE **19–IV**

Dental Evaluation of the Patient with COPD

PATIENTS AT LOW RISK

Patients with dyspnea only on significant exertion

Patients with normal blood gases (P_{CO_2}, 40 mm Hg; P_{O_2} 100 mm Hg; pH, 7.40)

PATIENTS AT MODERATE RISK

Patients with dyspnea on exertion

Patients on chronic bronchodilator therapy

Patients who have recently used corticosteroids

Patients with hypoxemia (P_{O_2} less than 85 mm Hg) but not carbon dioxide retention

Erythromycin and clindamycin—relatively contraindicated for patients on methylxanthines

PATIENTS AT HIGH RISK

Patients with previously unrecognized symptoms of COPD

Patients with acute exacerbation (e.g., acute respiratory infection)

Patients with significant dyspnea at rest or cor pulmonale who require chronic oxygen therapy

Patients with a history of CO_2 retention (P_{CO_2} greater than 45 mm Hg)

SUMMARY TABLE **19–V**

Dental Management of the Patient with COPD

PATIENTS AT LOW RISK

Normal protocol for all dental procedures (types I–VI)

PATIENTS AT MODERATE RISK

Recent physical and medical consultation regarding treatment plan and dental drug therapy

Avoid local anesthetics with vasoconstrictors in patients on bronchodilating therapy, especially those with high-risk cardiac effects (see Summary Table 19–III).

Evaluate for adrenal suppression for all patients with histories of steroid therapy within 1 year (Chap. 15).

PATIENTS AT HIGH RISK

Dental therapy (types II–VI) is contraindicated in patients with symptoms suggesting undiagnosed COPD.

All nonemergency dental care should be deferred for patients with acute exacerbations (e.g., acute respiratory infection).

All dental drug therapy must be approved by the patient's physician, especially any agent that may depress respiratory function, such as N_2O-O_2 inhalation sedation, tranquilizers, or narcotics. Non-narcotic analgesics are preferred.

Patients with cor pulmonale are at risk for arrhythmias and the use of vasoconstrictors should be minimized.

Hospitalization should be considered for moderate and advanced dental surgery (types V and VI) procedures.

Tuberculosis

Tuberculosis is clearly making a resurgence in the setting of increased numbers of patients with immunosuppression and with the emergence of new and drug-resistant strains. In addition, atypical mycobacterial diseases, previously rarely human pathogens, are gaining increasing importance.

The tubercle bacillus is transmitted from infected individuals by small aerosolized droplets and is carried into the airways of susceptible persons. Primary pulmonary tuberculosis is usually a mild disease, presenting with fever, chills, cough, and sputum production. In the majority of instances, infected foci in the lung form granulomata, which can heal by scarring and calcification (Fig. 20–1). These lesions can be detected on chest x-rays as scars in the apices of the lungs. In rare instances, the disease can spread contiguously by erosion into the pleural or pericardial spaces, producing pleurisy or pericarditis.

After the primary pulmonary infection, tuberculosis can remain dormant for varying periods. Reactivation can occur later in life, causing pulmonary and systemic disease. Tubercle bacilli in the granulomatous lesions may become disseminated (miliary tuberculosis) and result in involvement of the liver, kidneys, vertebral bodies of the spine (Pott's disease), gastrointestinal tract, or even meninges (tuberculous meningitis). Oral involvement may be the result of infection from pulmonary lesions or the result of seeding from the blood, in the case of disseminated tuberculosis (see later, Oral Findings).

Because oral tuberculosis is highly contagious, it is important for the dentist to be familiar with the disease and its management to minimize the likelihood of inadvertent infection.

MEDICAL EVALUATION

Because patients may have had minimal symptoms during the primary stage of tuber-

culosis and have reactivation of the disease years later, medical evaluation is directed at the detection of both active and dormant disease.

Tuberculosis may be diagnosed in a variety of ways. Most commonly, patients undergo evaluation because of a history of exposure to the disease, a positive skin test for tuberculosis, or a scar detected on chest x-ray. Less commonly, patients may present with symptoms of fever, chills, night sweats, productive cough, and weight loss. The most common presentation is a patient with a positive tuberculin skin test but no active infection; up to 7% of the population in the United States today may fit into this category.

Medical evaluation includes a detailed history of exposure. Tuberculosis in other family members raises a high index of suspicion. Patients may have known tuberculosis that has been treated. The degree of involvement, the form, and the duration of treatment are carefully reviewed to assess adequacy of therapy.

Laboratory tests may detect evidence of prior infection. Tuberculin skin tests, either the Mantoux test using purified protein derivative (PPD) or the tine test, are the most sensitive tests for the diagnosis of infection. A positive skin test does not by itself prove that there is active disease, but it does indicate that infection has occurred. Negative tuberculin skin tests have been documented in some patients with tuberculosis, particularly those with overwhelming disease. A false-positive tuberculin skin test can be seen in patients who have received bacillus Calmette-Guérin (BCG) vaccine as biologic prophylaxis against tuberculosis. A chest x-ray can also suggest prior infection with the finding of apical scars, which progress to frank cavitation.

When there is active pulmonary disease, diagnosis of pulmonary tuberculosis is usually confirmed by examination of the sputum. Sputum specimens are examined either by the Ziehl-Neelsen (acid-fast) stain or the Truant fluorescent stain. Cultures of sputum or first

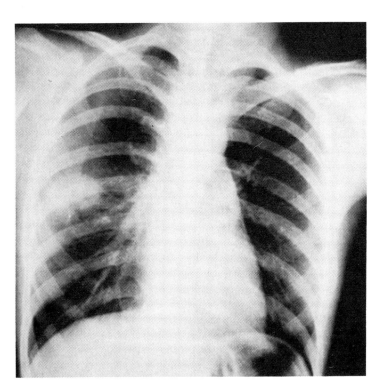

Figure 20–1. Radiograph demonstrating scar formation and calcification of infected pulmonary foci of tuberculosis. (From Rubin, R.H., and Young, L.S.: Clinical Approach to Infection in the Compromised Host. New York, Plenum, 1981.)

morning fasting gastric aspirates are necessary for definitive diagnosis. *Mycobacterium tuberculosis* is a fastidious and slow-growing organism, and often takes weeks before growing in culture media.

Tissue biopsy is often required for the diagnosis of tuberculous pleurisy or extrapulmonary disease, because sputum and gastric aspirates are usually negative for organisms in these situations. Biopsy is the definitive technique for diagnosis of the oral lesions of tuberculosis (Fig. 20–2).

MEDICAL MANAGEMENT

Medical management of tuberculosis is dependent on the clinical setting and the activity of the disease.

Prophylaxis in Uninfected Individuals

In some parts of the world where tuberculosis is common, vaccination with BCG, a live-attenuated strain of *Mycobacterium bovis,* is used for the prevention of primary infection. The vaccine is effective more than 80% of the time. Patients who have received the vaccine demonstrate a positive tuberculin skin test.

Prophylaxis in Patients with Positive Tuberculin Skin Tests But No Active Disease

In the past decade, increasing numbers of cases of active tuberculosis have been reported. This is due in part to the rapid spread of tuberculosis among immunosuppressed patients and in part to the emergence of resistant strains of tuberculosis. Furthermore, an increasing number of atypical mycobacterial in-

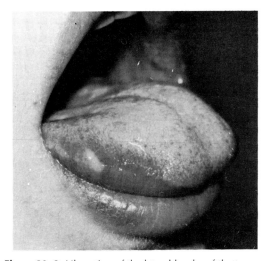

Figure 20–2. Ulceration of the lateral border of the tongue caused by infection with tuberculosis.

fections has been reported, particularly among immunocompromised patients.

Patients with positive tuberculin skin tests can be treated with isoniazid (INH) to prevent active disease. The drug is not without toxicity, however; it can cause hepatocellular damage, particularly in older patients. The risk of reactivation of tuberculosis should be weighed against the risk of drug-induced hepatitis. In general, INH prophylaxis is given to individuals under the age of 35 with a recent conversion of tuberculin skin tests and to patients under age 25 with positive skin tests. The medication is given for a year, with close monitoring of hepatic function. Isoniazid is given to close contacts of patients with active tuberculosis, particularly children or adolescents. Older individuals who have recovered from clinical tuberculosis, have no evidence of active disease, and have never received chemotherapy are often considered for INH therapy. However, the decision to treat asymptomatic older patients needs to be tempered by the increased risk of INH-induced hepatitis in this age group.

Treatment of Patients with Active Tuberculosis

Patients with active disease require combination chemotherapy. Those with mild pulmonary or extrapulmonary disease are usually treated with a two-drug regimen of INH plus ethambutol for 18 to 24 months.

Patients with far advanced cavitary disease or miliary disease are treated with triple-drug therapy such as INH, ethambutol, and streptomycin. Rifampin may be substituted for streptomycin in some instances. Therapy must be continued for 18 to 24 months.

Increasingly, physicians are confronted with strains resistant to multiple drugs. These pose a management challenge and often necessitate use of new and innovative antituberculous drugs. Equally important, atypical mycobacterial infections are causing increasing morbidity. These are often slow-growing organisms that are resistant to conventional therapy and whose eradication may require a combination of drugs such as rifampin, INH, clarithromycin, and ciprofloxacin.

DENTAL EVALUATION

Dental evaluation is directed at the identification of patients with active disease, particularly those with oral involvement.

The medical history should include questions regarding the presence of tuberculous infection in family members as well as other possible exposure to the disease. Prior tuberculin skin test results should be recorded. Patients with known tuberculosis should be asked about the degree of disease involvement, the type and duration of therapy received, and the current status of disease activity. The patient's physician should be consulted for confirmation. Based on detailed history and consultation, patients can be grouped into three risk categories.

Patients at High Risk
1. Patients with known tuberculosis showing symptoms of active disease (fever, chills, night sweats, sputum production, and weight loss)
2. Patients with oral manifestations of tuberculosis (see later, Oral Findings)

Patients at Moderate Risk
1. Patients with positive tuberculin skin tests but no evidence of active disease
2. Patients with chest x-ray findings suggestive of prior tuberculous involvement but no evidence of active disease
3. Patients with inadequately treated tuberculosis but no evidence of active disease

Patients at Low Risk
1. Patients with known tuberculosis who have been adequately treated with no evidence of active disease
2. Patients with history of exposure to tuberculosis but negative skin tests and no evidence of disease involvement.

DENTAL MANAGEMENT

Precautions should be taken to minimize inadvertent infection. Because transmission of infection is largely by aerosolized droplets, masks should be used when treating patients with a history of tuberculosis. Close attention should be paid to sterilization techniques. Gas sterilization should be used for handpieces that cannot be autoclaved.

Specific Guidelines

Patients at High Risk. Patients with evidence of active disease, particularly patients with oral involvement, are highly contagious. Dental procedures should be deferred and patients referred to their physician for further evaluation and management.

If an oral lesion suggesting tuberculosis is

identified during oral examination (see later, Oral Findings), the dental procedure should be terminated and the patient referred for further evaluation and management. If emergency dental care is needed, gowning, double mask and gloves, and strict adherence to aseptic techniques are mandatory. Handpieces that cannot be autoclaved must be gas-sterilized.

Patients at Moderate Risk. These patients have had tuberculous infection and the disease can be reactivated. They have no evidence of active infection, however, and are theoretically noninfectious. Dental procedures can be carried out using appropriate precautions. Masks and gloves should be used. Handpieces that cannot be autoclaved must be gas-sterilized.

Patients at Low Risk. Dental procedures can be carried out using normal protocol.

ORAL FINDINGS

The frequency of the oral manifestations of tuberculosis is somewhat controversial. Whereas most studies indicate a low frequency, Katz found that about 20% of patients with the disease in the lungs had oral involvement at the time of autopsy (Table 20–1). It is generally believed that oral tuberculosis represents infection by organisms brought to the mouth in sputum from pulmonary lesions. Apparently, traumatized mucosal surfaces are predisposed to the development of oral tuberculosis. In the case of miliary tuberculosis, infection may also occur in the mouth as the result of seeding from the blood.

The most common site of oral tuberculosis is the base of the tongue. The gingiva, lip, tonsils, tooth sockets, and soft palate have also been reported to be fairly frequent locations (Table 20–2). The oral lesions of tuberculosis caused by secondary spread from primary lung lesions are ulcerative. The ulcers are usually uneven, with jagged, undermined soft borders. Frequently, they are linear. The lesions are painless, although they may have a purulent center. Lymphadenopathy is a common finding.

Lesions may also occur at the corners of the mouth and present as shallow granulating ulcerations with pebbly surfaces. Such lesions are called cutix orificialis. Granulomatous lesions of tuberculosis have also been reported in the mouth. Involvement of unilateral nodes by organisms produces a firm enlargement called scrofula. Miliary involvement of the skin produces lupus vulgaris.

Tuberculosis-induced oral ulcerations are impossible to differentiate clinically from malignancy. Therefore, biopsy is required for definitive diagnosis with demonstration of organisms in tissues (Fig. 20–3). Smears of saliva may demonstrate organisms when stained with Ziehl-Neelsen stain. Cultures are necessary for confirmation of diagnosis.

■ Examples of Dental Evaluation and Management

EVALUATION

Patient 1. A 45-year-old man presents for dental treatment. His older brother died of tuberculosis at age 15 and he is known to have a positive PPD. He has been treated for a year with isoniazid (INH) and he has no evidence of active disease. His last medical examination was 4 months ago and his chest x-ray at that time was normal. His dental needs include extraction of a fractured maxillary premolar, fabrication of a three-unit bridge, and prophylaxis.

Table 20–1. INCIDENCE OF ORAL TUBERCULOSIS

Author(s)	Year	No. of Cases	Total Tuberculous Patients	Cases with Oral Lesions (%)
Cipes	1926	4	2800	0.14
Rubin	1927	72	5000	1.44
Martin and Koepf	1938	5	3835	0.13
Cameron	1939	1	1892	0.05
Farber et al.	1940	9	9000	0.1
Katz	1941	28*	141*	19.9*
Pratap et al.	1972	7	1241	0.56

From Fujibayashi T, Takahashi Y, Yoneda T, et al.: Tuberculosis of the tongue: A case report with immunologic study. Oral Surg., 47:427, 1979.

*Determined by autopsy.

Table 20–2. INTRAORAL SITES OF TUBERCULOSIS

Author(s)	Year	Tooth Socket	Tongue	Gingiva	Lip	Palate	Buccal Fold	Retromolar Trigone	Buccal Mucosa	Maxilla	Mandible
Primary oral tuberculosis											
Boyes et al.	1956	3	—	3	—	—	1	—	—	—	—
Browne	1959	—	—	1	—	—	—	—	—	—	—
Gardner and Hanft	1961	—	—	—	—	—	1	—	—	—	—
O'Neil	1963	—	—	1	—	—	—	—	—	—	—
Secondary oral tuberculosis											
Collins and Cook	1940	—	—	1	—	—	—	—	—	—	—
Brodsky	1942	—	3	2	3	1	—	—	1	—	—
Wolfer et al.	1948	—	1	—	—	—	—	—	—	—	—
Shengold and Sheingold	1951	9	4	—	4	1	1	—	—	—	1
Bruce	1954	—	—	1	—	—	—	—	—	—	—
Thilander and Wennstrom	1956	1	—	—	—	—	—	—	—	—	—
Radden and Reade	1961	—	—	—	—	—	—	1	—	—	—
Lagerlof et al.	1964	—	1	—	—	1	—	—	—	—	—
Brennan and Urabec	1970	—	—	—	—	—	—	1	—	—	—
Pratap et al.	1972	—	1	—	1	2	—	—	1	2	—
Harris et al.	1973	—	—	—	—	1	—	—	—	—	—
Ramula et al.	1973	1	—	—	—	—	—	—	—	—	—
Bhatt and Dholakia	1974	1	—	—	—	—	—	—	—	—	—
DeLathouwer et al.	1975	—	1	—	—	—	—	—	—	—	—
Sachs and Eisenbud	1977	—	—	—	—	—	—	—	—	—	1
Total		15	11	9	8	6	3	2	2	2	2

From Fujibayashi T, Takahashi Y, Yoneda T, et al.: Tuberculosis of the tongue: A case report with immunologic study. Oral Surg., 47:427, 1979.

On examination, his blood pressure is 103/80 and his pulse is 72 beats/minute (bpm) and regular.

Patient 2. A 33-year-old woman presents for dental therapy. She has no known exposure to tuberculosis, but a recent tuberculin skin test was positive. She is asymptomatic and her evaluation has included a normal chest x-ray and negative sputum culture. She has not received antituberculous chemotherapy. Her most recent physical examination 2 months ago was normal. Consultation with her physician revealed that there is no evidence of active disease. INH prophylaxis has not been started because of a history of viral hepatitis 6 months ago. Her liver function tests are normal and tests for hepatitis surface antigen are negative. Her dental needs

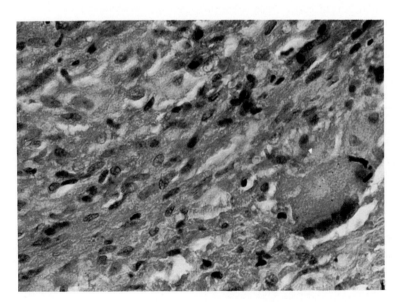

Figure 20–3. Histologic section of a biopsy specimen from a patient with tuberculosis. Note the presence of giant cells and acid-fast organisms in the tissue.

include prophylaxis, localized curettage, and multiple amalgams.

Her blood pressure is 110/70 and her pulse is 94 bpm and regular.

Patient 3. A 45-year-old Portuguese man presents for dental treatment. He had tuberculosis as a child and was treated with "daily injections" for several months. He has had a "lingering cold" for 4 months with fever, chills, and night sweats and has lost 8 lb (3.6 kg) during that period. His dental needs include multiple extractions, fabrication of a mandibular partial denture, and relining of the existing full maxillary denture.

On examination, his blood pressure is 110/80 and his pulse is 90 bpm and regular. He is pale and appears chronically ill.

MANAGEMENT

Patient 1. This patient has a positive PPD but has been adequately treated for a year with INH. He has no evidence of active disease and is at low risk for being infectious. He can be managed with normal dental protocol.

Patient 2. This patient has had a recent positive PPD. She has not been treated because of concern over possible hepatotoxicity from INH following a bout of hepatitis (Chap. 23). Although she has no evidence of active disease, she is at moderate risk of being infectious. Mask and gloves should be used. Instruments should be sterilized at the end of each procedure. Handpieces that cannot be autoclaved should be gas-sterilized.

Patient 3. This patient is probably contagious and is in the high-risk category. His respiratory symptoms, fever, chills, sweats, and weight loss are suggestive of reactivation of his earlier disease. Elective dental treatment is contraindicated and the patient should be referred for further evaluation and management.

SUMMARY TABLE **20–1**

Tuberculosis: General Information

PRIMARY INFECTION

Mycobacterium tuberculosis generally causes a mild pulmonary disease including fever, chills, cough, and sputum production. Infected foci form granulomata, which heal by scarring calcification.

It is usually evident on a chest radiograph.

30,000 new cases occur annually in the United States.

COMPLICATIONS

Contiguous spread by erosion causing
   Pleurisy
   Pericarditis

Miliary tuberculosis: dissemination of the tubercle bacilli in blood from granulomatous lesions to the
   Liver
   Kidneys
   Vertebral bodies of the spine (Pott's disease)
   Gastrointestinal tract
   Meninges
   Oral lesions—highly contagious

Reactivation of primary disease following periods of dormancy

DIAGNOSIS

Definitive diagnosis requires positive culture of organisms; biopsy required for diagnosis of extrapulmonary disease.

Medical Evaluation of the Patient with Tuberculosis

PURPOSE
Medical evaluation aimed at detection of both *active* and *dormant* forms

RISK FACTORS
Family history

Signs of disease

Positive findings on chest radiograph

LABORATORY TESTING
Tuberculin skin test:
   Positive: indicates either active infection *or* that infection has occurred
   Negative: indicates no past or present infection

SPUTUM SPECIMEN
Staining: acid-fast (Ziehl-Neelsen) or Truant fluorescent

Culture (slow growth, 2+ weeks)

TISSUE BIOPSY

TUBERCULOUS PLEURISY

EXTRAPULMONARY DISEASE

Medical Management of the Patient with Tuberculosis

PREVENTION
Vaccination with bacillus Calmette-Guérin (BCG), a live attenuated strain of *Mycobacterium bovis*
   Used in high-risk areas
   Vaccinated patients have positive skin tests (PPD)

PROPHYLAXIS
Prophylaxis is appropriate in patients:
   With positive skin tests
   With no evidence of active disease
   Under age 35 with recent conversion of tuberculin skin test
   Under age 25 with positive skin test

Therapy: isoniazid (INH) for 1 year

Risks: drug-induced hepatocellular damage; patients receiving INH should have liver function tests monitored periodically

TREATMENT OF ACTIVE DISEASE
Mild pulmonary or extrapulmonary disease: two-drug regimen of INH plus ethambutol for 18–24 months

Advanced pulmonary or miliary disease: three-drug regimen of INH, ethambutol, and streptomycin or rifampin for 18–24 months

Dental Evaluation of the Patient with Tuberculosis

HISTORY
Past infection

Organs involved

Exposure to active infection

Skin testing

Therapy and type

Physician consultation

RISK CATEGORIES
High risk (highly infectious):
    Patients with known tuberculosis and symptoms of active disease (fever, chills, night sweats, sputum
        production, weight loss)
    Patients with oral manifestations of tuberculosis (see Oral Findings)

Moderate risk:
    Patients with positive tuberculin skin tests but no evidence of active disease
    Patients with chest x-ray findings suggestive of prior tuberculosis involvement but no evidence of active
        disease
    Patients with inadequately treated tuberculosis but no evidence of active disease

Low risk:
    Patients with known tuberculosis who have been adequately treated with no evidence of active disease
    Patients with a history of exposure to tuberculosis but negative skin tests and no evidence of disease

Dental Management of the Patient with Tuberculosis

PATIENTS AT HIGH RISK (HIGHLY CONTAGIOUS)
Elective dental care is contraindicated

Emergency dental care:
    Hospitalization recommended
    Strict asepsis regimen:
        Gown
        Double mask
        Double gloves
    Careful attention to instrument sterilization
    Handpieces that cannot be autoclaved *must* undergo gas sterilization (usually available in the hospital)

PATIENTS AT MODERATE RISK (THEORETICALLY NONINFECTIOUS)
Mask and gloves

Strict attention to instrument sterilization procedures

Gas sterilization for handpieces that cannot be autoclaved

PATIENTS AT LOW RISK
Normal dental protocol

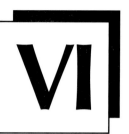

Evaluation and Management of the Patient with Gastrointestinal Disease

Peptic Ulcer Disease

Peptic ulcer disease is a common disorder resulting from damage to the epithelial lining of the stomach or the duodenum. The prevalence of the disease is estimated at 5 to 10% of the population of the United States, with a peak incidence among men between 45 and 65 years of age and among women over 55. About 6% of the dentist's patient population has peptic ulcer disease.

MEDICAL EVALUATION

Patients with peptic ulcer disease can present with pain and gastrointestinal bleeding, obstruction, or perforation. Some patients may have no symptoms and are found to have peptic ulcer disease only when upper gastrointestinal studies are done for other reasons.

Patients with duodenal ulcers outnumber those with gastric ulcers by 4:1 (Fig. 21–1). Patients with duodenal ulcers classically have episodic epigastric pain that is usually absent in the early morning and often starts 2 to 3 hours after a meal. It may occasionally awaken the patient at night. The pain is relieved by eating.

Patients with gastric ulcers often present with epigastric pain radiating to the back. In contrast to the symptoms of duodenal ulcers, the pain is aggravated by eating. In addition, some patients have gastrointestinal bleeding and may vomit blood (hematemesis) or pass black tarry stools (melena). Occasionally, patients may have significant scarring from peptic ulcer disease and present with protracted vomiting secondary to obstruction of the gastric outlet. Rarely, patients with peptic ulcer disease have erosion through the wall of the stomach or intestine and present with acute illness with symptoms of peritonitis secondary to perforation.

The medical evaluation for peptic ulcer includes a detailed history of the location, radiation, and time of occurrence of abdominal pain. A past history of upper gastrointestinal bleeding, gastric outlet obstruction, and gastrointestinal surgery should be documented. Because certain foods and drugs are known to aggravate peptic ulcer disease, patients are asked about the use of tobacco, caffeine, aspirin-containing drugs, corticosteroids, and nonsteroidal anti-inflammatory drugs (NSAIDs), such as indomethacin (Indocin), phenylbutazone, ibuprofen (Motrin), and naproxen.

Clinical examination may reveal epigastric

Figure 21–1. Most common distribution of gastric and duodenal ulcers.

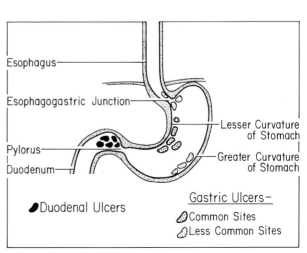

Esophagus

Esophagogastric Junction

Lesser Curvature of Stomach

Pylorus

Greater Curvature of Stomach

Duodenum

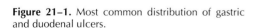
Duodenal Ulcers

Gastric Ulcers–
Common Sites
Less Common Sites

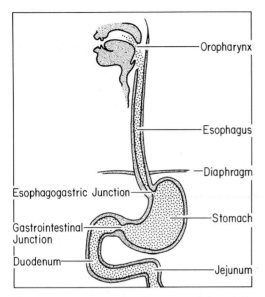

Figure 21–2. Anatomic sites demonstrated through the use of barium examination of the upper gastrointestinal tract.

tenderness, and guaiac testing of the stool may disclose evidence of gastrointestinal bleeding.

If a diagnosis of peptic ulcer disease is suspected, the patient may undergo barium examination of the upper gastrointestinal tract (Fig. 21–2) or endoscopy. The upper gastrointestinal series involves the use of a radiopaque suspension of barium sulfate to outline areas of ulceration or scarring. In some patients, the ulceration may be too superficial to be detected by the upper gastrointestinal series. The diagnosis may then depend on endoscopy, which involves the passage of a flexible fiberoptic scope through the pharynx and esophagus into the stomach and duodenum (Fig. 21–

3). Although more invasive than the upper gastrointestinal series, the examination provides direct visualization of areas of concern and is particularly useful in identifying sites of upper gastrointestinal bleeding.

MEDICAL MANAGEMENT

Because peptic ulcer disease is the result of acid erosion of the gastrointestinal mucosa, medical management is designed either to neutralize the acid produced or to minimize the acid production.

Agents known to damage the lining of the gastrointestinal tract—including aspirin, alcohol, tobacco, corticosteroids, and NSAIDs, such as indomethacin, ibuprofen, phenylbutazone, and naproxen—should be avoided. Emotional stress should be minimized. In addition to these conservative measures, the therapeutic options for peptic ulcer disease include the following.

Diet. Contrary to common belief, alterations of diet do not promote ulcer healing. Milk, bland diets, small frequent meals, and avoidance of spicy or acidic foods do not reduce acid production. Tobacco and caffeine, on the other hand, do increase acid production. Patients usually notice that certain foods may aggravate symptoms, and these should be avoided. Otherwise, dietary restrictions are not necessary.

Antacids. Antacids are the mainstay of therapy. Summary Table 21–II lists commonly used preparations. Antacids are usually given 1 and 3 hours after a meal and before bedtime for maximal effect.

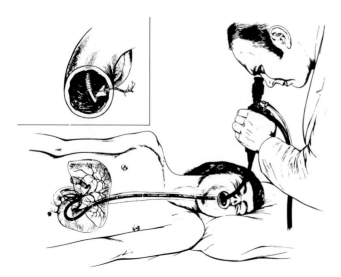

Figure 21–3. Fiberoptic scope used for endoscopy. The scope is passed through the pharynx and esophagus into the stomach and duodenum. (From Stewart, E. T.: Atlas of Cholangiopancreatography. St. Louis, C.V. Mosby, 1977, p. 6.)

Anticholinergics. Anticholinergics such as propantheline (Pro-Banthine) and poldine (Nacton) are sometimes prescribed for patients with peptic ulcer disease. They are useful in reducing acid production at night.

Sucralfate. Sucralfate (Carafate) is a new class of agent designed to coat the stomach and promote healing. The usual dose is 300 to 1000 mg qid, and the medication should be taken on an empty stomach. The drug is designed to be used as a short-term treatment for peptic ulcer disease. It can cause constipation, nausea, and indigestion. Sucralfate can bind to other drugs and decrease the bioavailability of a number of them, including tetracycline, phenytoin, digoxin, and H_2-receptor antagonists.

H_2-Receptor Antagonists. These are important additions to the medical management of peptic ulcer disease. Cimetidine (Tagamet), ranitidine (Zantac), and famotidine (Pepcid) are histamine H_2-receptor antagonists that block the production of acid by the parietal cells of the stomach. These medications have been demonstrated to be effective in reducing acid production and ulcer recurrence.

Patients responding to therapy have resolution of symptoms and evidence of healing on upper gastrointestinal series and endoscopy. Patients with active bleeding can be treated endoscopically by heat or laser cauterization. Patients with intractable symptoms, recurrent upper gastrointestinal bleeding, or gastric outlet obstruction may require surgical intervention.

DENTAL EVALUATION

The dentist often sees patients with a history of peptic ulcer disease. The diagnoses might have been made on clinical grounds alone or in conjunction with radiographic or endoscopic evaluation. These patients should be specifically asked about the occurrence and frequency of symptoms and their medications. Any history of complications of peptic ulcer disease, such as bleeding or gastric outlet obstruction or perforation, should be noted. Previous surgery for peptic ulcer disease should also be reviewed.

DENTAL MANAGEMENT

The dental management of the patient with peptic ulcer disease should avoid aggravation of symptoms. Because stress can increase acid production and worsen peptic ulcer symptoms, it should be minimized. Lengthy procedures should be spread over several shorter appointments, and adjunctive sedation techniques should be used, when appropriate.

The major concern in dental management of the patient with peptic ulcer disease relates to the complications of the drugs used in treatment. Some antacid preparations such as Di-Gel, Gelusil, Maalox, and Mylanta contain aluminum hydroxide (see Summary Table 21–II). These antacids prohibit the effective adsorption of tetracycline, so that effective levels may not be obtained. Alternative antibiotics are therefore preferable. Cimetidine has been rarely associated with thrombocytopenia, and it may be prudent to determine the platelet count prior to moderate (type V) or advanced (type VI) surgical procedures in patients on cimetidine therapy.

Aspirin and NSAIDs should be avoided because of irritation to the mucosal lining of the gastrointestinal tract (Summary Table 21–IV). Summary Table 22–II lists analgesics containing aspirin. Some commonly prescribed analgesics that do not contain aspirin are listed in Chapter 49.

ORAL FINDINGS

Xerostomia is a complication of the chronic use of anticholinergic drugs such as propantheline or poldine. It is associated with a significantly increased risk of caries and periodontal disease (Chaps. 40 and 43).

■ Examples of Dental Evaluation and Management

EVALUATION

Patient 1. A 38-year-old man with a history of "stomach ulcers" presents for dental treatment. He has had midabdominal pain that was aggravated by meals and has had a gastrointestinal series that "showed ulcers." He is currently on Mylanta as needed and has been asymptomatic. He is allergic to penicillin. His major complaint is discomfort in the lower left quadrant of his mouth. Oral examination reveals a periodontal abscess of the lower left first molar. Purulent drainage is evident from the mesial gingival margin. There are shotty lymph nodes in the left anterior cervical chain.

Patient 2. A 28-year-old woman with "ulcer disease" presents for dental therapy. She has had frequent episodes of pain that were relieved by taking food. She continues to have intermittent symptoms, although she takes cimetidine, 300 mg qid. She has not had problems with significant bleeding. She was last examined 6 months ago. Her dental needs include the extraction of two impacted mandibular third molars. On examination, her blood pressure is 140/84, and she has a regular pulse at 90 beats/minute.

MANAGEMENT

Patient 1. This patient presents with an abscess that may be treated conventionally. Local débridement and curettage to maximize drainage should be performed. Because of the presence of the lymphadenopathy, antibiotic coverage is recommended. The drug of choice, penicillin, is contraindicated because of drug allergy. Although tetracycline is often prescribed for periodontal abscesses, the patient's use of antacids precludes its use. Mylanta is an aluminum-containing antacid that binds tetracycline and diminishes its systemic absorption. Erythromycin should be prescribed for this patient.

Patient 2. This patient is on long-term cimetidine. A detailed history should be taken to determine bleeding tendencies. The removal of impacted third molars is a moderately advanced surgical procedure, and the dentist may want to order a platelet count prior to the procedure. Cimetidine therapy is rarely associated with thrombocytopenia. In the postoperative phase, analgesics containing aspirin as well as NSAIDs should be avoided to minimize irritation of the gastrointestinal tract.

SUMMARY TABLE **21–I**

Peptic Ulcer Disease: General Information

DEFINITION
Peptic ulcer disease is the result of damage to the epithelial lining of the stomach (gastric ulcer) or the duodenum (duodenal ulcer).

PREVALENCE
5–10% of the population is affected, most commonly men 45–65 years old and women over 55; the ratio of duodenal to gastric ulcers is 4:1.

CLINICAL CHARACTERISTICS
Episodic epigastric pain is relieved by food (duodenal) or aggravated by food (gastric); occasionally gastrointestinal bleeding, obstruction, or perforation are seen.

Some ulcers are asymptomatic.

PATHOPHYSIOLOGY
Acid erosion of the gastrointestinal mucosa

PRECIPITATING FACTORS
Aspirin
Alcohol
NSAIDs (e.g., indomethacin, ibuprofen, naproxen)
Tobacco
Caffeine
Corticosteroids
Emotional stress

DIAGNOSTIC TESTS
Upper GI series
Endoscopy

Medical Management of the Patient with Peptic Ulcer Disease

AVOID PRECIPITATING FACTORS
Aspirin
Alcohol
NSAIDs (e.g., indomethacin, ibuprofen, naproxen)
Corticosteroids
Tobacco
Caffeine
Stress
Foods that precipitate symptoms

ANTACIDS
Amphojel
Di-Gel
Gelusil
Maalox
Mylanta
Riopan
Sucralfate (Carafate)

ANTICHOLINERGIC AGENTS
Propantheline (Pro-Banthine)
Poldine (Nacton)

H$_2$-RECEPTOR ANTAGONISTS
Cimetidine (Tagamet)
Ranitidine (Zantac)
Famotidine (Pepcid)

ENDOSCOPY WITH CAUTERIZATION

SURGERY

Dental Evaluation of the Patient with Peptic Ulcer Disease

1. Assess frequency and severity of symptoms.
2. Determine history of complications:
   Bleeding
   Obstruction
   Perforation
3. History of surgery
4. History of medications:
   Antacids
   Anticholinergics
   H_2-receptor antagonists

Dental Management of the Patient with Peptic Ulcer Disease

Minimize stress:
   Shorter appointments
   Consider adjunctive sedation techniques

Selective use of analgesics: avoidance of all aspirin-containing compounds

Avoidance of tetracycline in patients taking aluminum-containing antacids

Cimetidine may rarely be associated with thrombocytopenia; consider ordering platelet count before moderate to advanced dental surgery (types V and VI).

Anticholinergics—associated with xerostomia, which is associated with increased risk of caries and periodontal disease; frequent recall prophylaxis and examination recommended

Inflammatory Bowel Diseases

Ulcerative colitis and regional enteritis (Crohn's disease) are the two most common forms of inflammatory disease involving the bowel. The diseases tend to affect patients between 20 and 45 years of age and have a combined prevalence of 1 in 10,000. Both diseases are of interest to the dentist because of their associated oral findings and the dental management problems raised by treatment with corticosteroids.

MEDICAL EVALUATION

Patients with inflammatory bowel disease (IBD) usually present with abdominal pain, fever, and diarrhea. The disease typically begins in young adulthood. Whites are affected more often than blacks, and the prevalence is highest among Jews. Patients suspected of having IBD usually undergo barium enema studies (Fig. 22–1) and sigmoidoscopies or colonoscopies with biopsies. These studies can differentiate between ulcerative colitis and Crohn's disease.

Ulcerative colitis is an idiopathic inflammatory disease causing diffuse ulceration of the colon. Patients may present with symptoms ranging from episodic diarrhea to severe abdominal pain, bloody diarrhea, fever, and prostration. Complications of the disease include bleeding and bowel perforation. Patients with ulcerative colitis develop carcinoma of the colon about 10 times more often than the general population, and the risk increases with the duration of disease.

Crohn's disease is a chronic granulomatous inflammation extending through all layers of the bowel wall. The disease may involve the colon alone (granulomatous colitis, 25% of cases), the terminal ileum alone (ileitis, 25% of cases), or both (ileocolitis, 50% of cases). The cardinal symptoms are diarrhea and lower abdominal pain. Some patients may have symptoms of anorexia, fever, or weight loss. Complications of the disease include fissures

and fistulae involving the abdomen or perineal areas. The risk of carcinoma of the colon is slightly increased over that of the general population.

Both ulcerative colitis and Crohn's disease may have extracolonic manifestations, including oral ulcers (see later, Oral Findings), skin lesions such as erythema multiforme, arthritis, hepatitis, uveitis, and iritis.

Some patients presenting with chronic recurrent abdominal pain, diarrhea, and constipation may have irritable bowel syndrome. The condition has also been referred to as mucous colitis, spastic colon, or irritable colon syndrome. It is defined as a functional disturbance of the bowel precipitated by stress; an extensive gastrointestinal workup does not reveal an organic lesion. The condition tends to occur in young patients and is reportedly the most common gastrointestinal complaint presenting to physicians. It is important to differentiate a functional bowel disorder from IBD.

MEDICAL MANAGEMENT

The medical management of ulcerative colitis includes the use of antidiarrheal agents such as diphenoxylate hydrochloride (Lomotil), sulfasalazine (Azulfidine), metronidazole (Flagyl), and systemic and topical steroids. Patients with ulcerative colitis of more than 7 to 10 years' duration should be followed closely for the development of colonic carcinoma. Patients with severe disease may have to undergo colectomy, which is usually curative.

Patients with Crohn's disease are managed in a similar fashion with antidiarrheal agents, sulfasalazine, and steroids. They are much more prone to the development of fistulae, abscesses, and intestinal obstructions that require surgery. Unlike ulcerative colitis, regional enteritis often recurs despite surgery.

Patients requiring steroid therapy are often adrenally suppressed and require adjustments of their steroid dosages during periods of stress (Chap. 15).

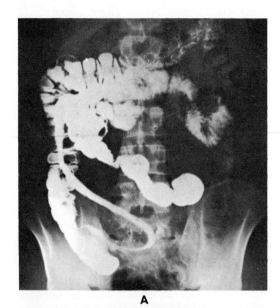

A

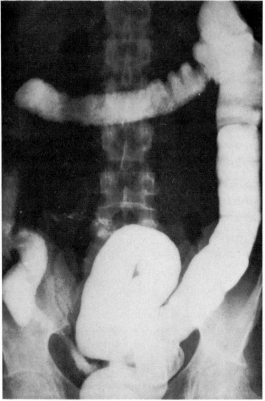

B

Figure 22–1. *A,* Regional enteritis with involvement of the terminal ileum. *B,* Crohn's disease demonstrated with barium enema. Note involvement of the terminal ileum and right side of the colon. (From Beeson, P. B., McDermott, W., and Wyngaarden, J. B. [eds.]. Cecil Textbook of Medicine, 15th ed. Philadelphia, W.B. Saunders, 1979.)

Patients with irritable bowel syndrome are managed with reassurance and symptomatic therapy.

DENTAL EVALUATION

The dentist may be presented with a patient who gives a history of "colitis." It is important to be able to differentiate irritable bowel syndrome from IBD. The patient should be asked about the exact diagnosis, the extent and severity of involvement, the frequency of symptoms, and the medications prescribed. It is particularly important to inquire about steroid use during the previous year and to note the duration and dosages of steroids used. If the nature of the bowel disease is unclear, the patient's physician should be consulted.

Patients who are diagnosed as having irritable bowel syndrome can be treated according to normal dental protocol.

Patients with uncontrolled or poorly controlled IBD are more likely to develop destructive forms of periodontal disease. Preventive care and frequent recall may be prudent in this group. Patients with well-controlled IBD are not at increased risk.

Patients with quiescent IBD can undergo dental treatment using normal protocol, but attention should be paid to minimizing stress.

Patients on steroid therapy deserve special attention. Long-term use of steroids can result in adrenal suppression. Major operative procedures in these patients can precipitate adrenal insufficiency if the steroid dosages are not adjusted appropriately. The details of steroid dosage adjustment for the various types of dental procedures are described in Chapter 15.

Patients formerly on steroid therapy may also have adrenal suppression. For example, 20 mg of prednisone daily for 7 to 10 days can cause adrenal suppression that may not return to normal for 9 to 12 months. It is therefore prudent to consider steroid supplements for patients who were treated with steroids for more than 7 to 10 days during the previous year. The replacement protocol is detailed in Chapter 15.

ORAL FINDINGS

Crohn's Disease and Regional Enteritis

Oral manifestations of Crohn's disease include cobblestone architecture of the mucosa, aphthous-like ulcerations, nonspecific swelling of the mucosa and lips, and lymphadenopathy. The frequency of such lesions has been reported to range from 6 to 20%. The presence of oral lesions may precede small bowel disease.

Symptomatology associated with the oral lesions of Crohn's disease is variable and may fluctuate with the course of the disease. Frequently, patients complain of pain associated with ulcerative lesions. These are best treated symptomatically with palliative rinses or ointments (Chap. 35). Topical steroids may also be helpful.

Rapid alveolar bone loss has been reported in a patient with active Crohn's disease (Fig. 22–2). The patient had more classic oral findings, but there was also significant loss of alveolar bone over a 2-year period. Abnormalities in neutrophil function and the presence of immune complexes have been reported in patients with the disease and may be related to periodontal destruction.

Ulcerative Colitis

The oral changes that occur in ulcerative colitis are nonspecific and fairly uncommon. Aphthous stomatitis of the major and minor variety has been reported in patients with active ulcerative colitis with a frequency of 4 to 20%. There is nothing unique about these lesions either clinically or histologically, and it has been suggested that their appearance with ulcerative colitis is merely coincidental. How-

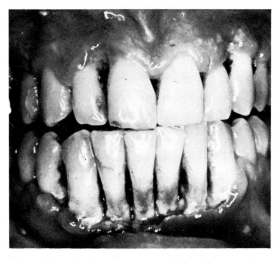

Figure 22–2. Oral manifestations of Crohn's disease. Note the cobblestone appearance and ulceration of the gingiva, as well as evidence of severe alveolar bone loss.

ever, there appears to be some correlation between the clinical course of the bowel disease and the presence of oral ulceration. Other nonspecific forms of ulceration associated with skin lesions have been reported in patients with ulcerative colitis. Pyoderma gangrenosum and hemorrhagic ulcerations have been noted on rare occasions.

Shklar and McCarthy have reported finding vegetating proliferative lesions of the labial mucosa, gingivae, and palates of patients with ulcerative colitis. The condition tends to involve a limited portion of the mucosa. This rare, nonspecific finding has been termed "pyostomatitis vegetans" and is characterized by deep fissure vegetating or proliferative lesions that undergo ulceration and then suppuration.

■ Examples of Dental Evaluation and Management

EVALUATION

Patient 1. A 22-year-old woman with a history of "colitis" presents for dental therapy. The patient has had intermittent bouts of crampy abdominal pain and diarrhea associated with stress. There is no history of rectal bleeding. She is not currently on medication and was last examined by her physician 8 months ago. Her dental needs include the extraction of four severely malposed maxillary incisors and the placement of a six-unit bridge. On examination, her blood pressure is 110/70 and her pulse rate is 64 beats/minute (bpm).

Consultation with her physician reveals that she had a normal gastrointestinal evaluation, including an upper gastrointestinal series and a barium enema study. She is thought to have irritable bowel syndrome.

Patient 2. A 19-year-old man with a 5-year history of ulcerative colitis presents for dental treatment. He was diagnosed as having the disease after an episode of rectal bleeding associated with fever and abdominal pain. He is currently asymptomatic on sulfasalazine (Azulfidine), 1 g qid. His dental needs include routine operative (type II) procedures and the extraction of impacted mandibular third molars (type V procedures). On examination, his blood pressure is 110/70 and his pulse rate is 88 bpm. Consultation with his physician reveals that the diagnosis was based on classic changes seen on barium enema study. The patient has been asymptomatic and was last examined 3 months ago.

Patient 3. A 28-year-old woman with a 6-year history of "colitis" presents for dental treatment. She has had multiple hospitalizations for flares of the disease and has had three abdominal surgical procedures to remove abscesses. She is currently asymptomatic on 20 mg of prednisone each morning. She was last examined by her physician 2 weeks ago. Her dental needs are similar to those of Patient 2. On examination, her blood pressure is 100/82 and her pulse rate is 88 bpm.

Consultation with her physician reveals that she has classic changes of Crohn's disease on her upper gastrointestinal series. She did not respond to Azulfidine and has required steroid therapy intermittently for the past 3 years. She was last hospitalized a month ago for surgical drainage of an intra-abdominal abscess.

MANAGEMENT

Patient 1. This patient does not have IBD. She has the most common form of colitis, a nonspecific stress-related disorder commonly called irritable bowel syndrome. Her dental management can be carried out using normal protocol with attention to the minimization of stress. Adjunctive sedation techniques should be considered for the advanced restorative and simple surgical dental procedures (types III and IV).

Patient 2. This patient has well-controlled ulcerative colitis. He has not required steroid therapy in the past year and is asymptomatic on conventional doses of Azulfidine. Dental therapy can be carried out using normal protocols with attention to the minimization of stress. Adjunctive sedation techniques should be considered for the extraction of the impacted third molars.

Patient 3. This patient has significant problems with multiple flares of IBD. From the standpoint of her dental management, it is particularly important to recognize that she is adrenally suppressed by the large doses of steroids she has required for her bowel disease. Steroid supplements are therefore mandatory for all procedures except for the dental examination (Chap. 15). For operative procedures (types II and III), the maintenance dose of prednisone should be doubled to 40 mg on the day of the procedure and returned to the maintenance level on the following day. For difficult surgical extractions (type V procedure), the prednisone dose should be increased to 60 mg for the day of the procedure and tapered over the next 2 days. Postsurgical antibiotic prophylaxis with penicillin for 3 to 5 days should also be considered.

IBD: General Information

PREVALENCE
1 in 10,000 patients
Young adults (more common among whites and Jews)

TYPES
Ulcerative colitis, primarily involving the colon
Crohn's disease, involving the terminal ileum and colon

SYMPTOMS
Abdominal pain, fever, and diarrhea

DIAGNOSIS
Clinical manifestations—rule out irritable bowel syndrome (functional bowel disease)
Radiographic evaluation, including barium enema and upper gastrointestinal series
Sigmoidoscopy or colonoscopy with biopsy

COMPLICATIONS
Bleeding, bowel perforation, fistula, and colonic carcinoma

EXTRACOLONIC MANIFESTATIONS
Aphthous ulceration (10% of cases)
Skin lesions (erythema multiforme)
Arthritis
Hepatitis
Uveitis and iritis

Medical Management of the Patient with IBD

DISTINGUISH BETWEEN REGIONAL ENTERITIS AND ULCERATIVE COLITIS

ANTI-INFLAMMATORY AGENTS
Sulfasalazine (Azulfidine)
Metronidazole (Flagyl)

CORTICOSTEROIDS
Topical by enema
Systemic steroids

SURGERY
Colectomy often curative for ulcerative colitis
Surgery not curative for patients with regional enteritis with high recurrence rates

SUMMARY TABLE **22–III**

Dental Evaluation of the Patient with IBD

Establish the diagnosis of the type of inflammatory bowel disease.
Determine the severity of disease and the degree of control.
Determine medications used, with special attention to steroid therapy in the past year.
Determine the history of surgical therapy.

SUMMARY TABLE **22–IV**

Dental Management of the Patient with IBD

Minimize stress by shorter appointments and adjunctive sedation techniques (when appropriate).
Prescribe steroid supplements for patients suspected of having adrenal suppression (Chap. 15).
Implement aggressive preventive periodontal protocol for the patient with poorly controlled IBD.

Hepatitis

Viral hepatitis is a contagious disease that affects approximately 500,000 people in the United States each year. The majority of patients have symptoms of an acute mild viral illness, but about 5% proceed to develop chronic hepatitis. Equally important, a number of patients become chronic carriers of hepatitis antigen and are potentially infectious. An understanding of the various types of viral hepatitis and the common modes of transmission is important in the prevention of infection. The dentist is particularly at risk because of exposure to the oral secretions and blood of potentially infectious patients.

TYPES OF HEPATITIS

At least three different types of viruses have been found to cause hepatitis: type A, type B, and type C viruses. At the present time, routine screening is available only for hepatitis B viral antigens and antibodies.

Hepatitis A. Outbreaks of viral hepatitis are usually associated with hepatitis A virus. The virus is shed in the feces and usually transmitted by the fecal-oral route. Children and adolescents are more susceptible to infection than adults. The virus has an incubation period of 30 days (range, 15 to 45 days). Patients usually develop a flu-like illness in the prodromal phase, followed by jaundice, nausea, and vomiting in the clinically ictal phase. Liver function tests show evidence of elevation of transaminases (SGOT and SGPT; Chap. 1) during both the prodromal and ictal phases. The disease is usually mild and resolves spontaneously over the course of several weeks. Infection produces antibodies to the virus and confers lifelong immunity.

Hepatitis A infection appears to be a common occurrence. One survey indicated that more than 80% of patients over the age of 60 have antibodies against hepatitis A virus. There are no chronic carrier states, and fatalities are exceedingly rare.

Hepatitis B. Hepatitis B is a far more serious disease than hepatitis A. The patient with a history of prior hepatitis B infection should be carefully evaluated by the dentist.

Hepatitis B is predominantly transmitted by a parenteral route, although some evidence has suggested that other modes of transmission are possible. Patients with acute hepatitis B infections have been found to have viral particles in saliva, semen, vaginal secretions, and breast milk. These findings explain the high incidence of infection among offspring of infected mothers and among spouses of infected patients. Patients with multiple sexual partners (e.g., some male homosexuals) also have a high incidence of hepatitis B secondary to nonpercutaneous modes of transmission.

Hepatitis B is the only type of hepatitis virus for which there is a screening test. It is now possible to detect antigens on the surface coating of the virus (hepatitis B surface antigen, HBsAg) and on the core material of the virus (hepatitis B core antigen, HBcAg). It is also possible to detect circulating antibodies to hepatitis B virus, which denote prior infection. The e antigen (HBeAg) has been shown to be a predictor of infectivity, and exposure to blood from a chronic carrier who is positive for HBeAg is associated with a high risk of infection.

The clinical course of hepatitis B infection includes a period of incubation, during which the infecting virus replicates, a prodromal phase, when nonspecific symptoms occur, and an ictal phase, when the patient appears jaundiced. The incubation period is about 12 weeks (range, 6 to 24 weeks). About 2 weeks prior to the onset of symptoms, the surface antigen of hepatitis B virus (HBsAg) is detectable in the serum, and enzymes associated with hepatocellular damage (according to liver function tests for SGOT, SGPT, and LDH) begin to increase, denoting inflammatory involvement of the liver (Fig. 23–1). The patient then has a prodromal period with malaise, anorexia, and fatigue before developing jaun-

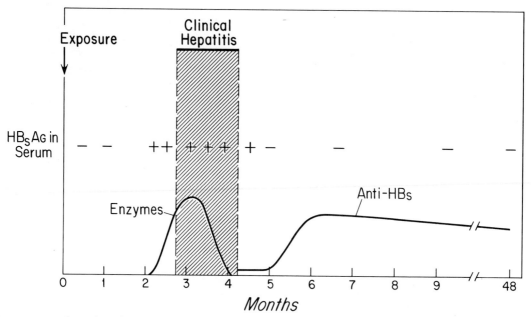

Figure 23-1. Relationship of the presence of hepatitis B surface antigen (HBsAG) in serum, liver enzyme levels, and antihepatitis B antibody after exposure to and recovery from acute viral hepatitis B.

dice, nausea, and vomiting. Symptoms usually last 4 to 6 weeks. About 10% of patients become chronic carriers of the surface antigen and are infectious long after the acute illness.

Dentists exposed to the blood of patients who are antigen-positive are at increased risk of contracting hepatitis B. Prior to the practice of universal precautions, the general dental practitioner was 3 times more likely to contract the disease than the population at large, and the oral surgeon had 10 times the risk. It is therefore essential to practice universal precautions.

Hepatitis C. Hepatitis C is thought to be transmitted parenterally and usually results from a blood transfusion. With the development of screening tests for HBsAg, hepatitis B has decreased significantly as a cause of post-transfusion hepatitis, and hepatitis C largely taken its place. More than 90% of transfusion-related hepatitis is secondary to hepatitis C virus. An assay has been developed to detect antibodies against hepatitis C. Patients developing hepatitis C usually have had a large blood transfusion in excess of 5 units of blood.

The incubation period is 6 weeks (range, 3 to 15 weeks), and the illness is usually mild. Only about 30% of patients develop jaundice; the remaining patients have asymptomatic elevations of serum transaminases. The illness is characterized by periodic increases of transaminases. Up to 40% of patients have persist-

ent abnormalities in liver function tests, and many progress to chronic active hepatitis with the finding of bridging necrosis on liver biopsy. Patients with severe infection can progress to develop cirrhosis and liver failure. Hepatitis C is infective, and patients should be treated with caution.

Delta Agent. A particularly virulent form of hepatitis has been identified among intravenous drug abusers. These patients had the co-existence of hepatitis B and delta agent, an RNA retrovirus, that causes infection only in the presence of hepatitis B.

MEDICAL EVALUATION

Patients may come to a medical evaluation for hepatitis either because of clinical symptoms or because of abnormal liver function tests.

Before jaundice develops, patients usually go through a prodromal period when they may have such nonspecific symptoms as anorexia, malaise, easy fatigability and, in a few patients, skin rashes and urticaria. During the ictal phase, patients develop jaundice and are often symptomatic with fever, nausea, vomiting, dark urine, and light, clay-colored stools. Physical examination may reveal scleral icterus and jaundice, and examination of the right upper quadrant of the abdomen may demonstrate hepatic enlargement and tenderness.

Laboratory examination includes liver function tests (Chap. 1) and tests to determine the presence of hepatitis B antigen and antibodies. Hepatic protein synthesis is determined by tests for prothrombin time and serum albumin concentration. When the diagnosis of viral hepatitis is not clear-cut, special studies may be performed. These can include a liver-spleen scan, which uses radionuclides to depict the anatomy of the liver and the spleen or a cholecystogram, which uses a contrast medium to depict the anatomy of the gallbladder and bile duct (Fig. 23–2).

On the basis of the history of exposure, the incubation period, the clinical manifestations, and the results of the HBsAg determination, it is possible to determine the type of hepatitis infection and to make appropriate treatment recommendations. Patients presenting to their physicians with histories of hepatitis usually have determinations of liver function and HBsAg to detect chronic disease and chronic carrier states.

MEDICAL MANAGEMENT

Acute Hepatitis. Viral hepatitis is usually a self-limiting and benign disease that can be managed on an outpatient basis. Hospitalization is generally reserved for severely ill patients with protracted vomiting or evidence of hepatic failure. The latter usually involves fulminant hepatitis, in which the normal synthetic and metabolic functions of the liver are severely compromised.

Management of the patient with acute hepatitis depends on the clinical status. For pa-

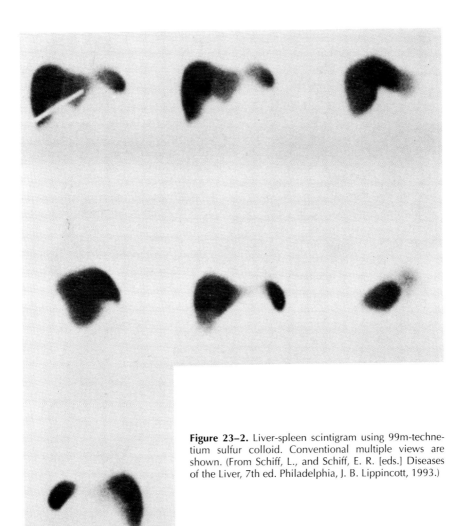

Figure 23–2. Liver-spleen scintigram using 99m-technetium sulfur colloid. Conventional multiple views are shown. (From Schiff, L., and Schiff, E. R. [eds.] Diseases of the Liver, 7th ed. Philadelphia, J. B. Lippincott, 1993.)

tients with mild symptoms, the management is largely conservative, with the aim of maintaining adequate hydration and caloric intake. Strict bed rest, dietary manipulation, and steroids have been shown to be effective. In patients with fulminant hepatitis, steroids, exchange transfusion, and glucose-insulin-glucagon infusions have been tried, all with limited success.

In the majority of patients with viral hepatitis, complete recovery occurs in about 8 weeks. A small number of patients have persistent abnormalities in liver function tests beyond 3 months, indicating that they have chronic hepatitis.

Chronic Hepatitis. Two forms of chronic hepatitis have been identified: chronic persistent and chronic active hepatitis. The distinction is made histologically by liver biopsy. Patients with chronic persistent hepatitis have an excellent prognosis and require no specific therapy. Patients with chronic active hepatitis, on the other hand, have a worse prognosis and can progress to hepatic insufficiency; in most instances, they are treated with steroids and azathioprine. In selected instances, α-interferon has been tried.

Prophylaxis

A major part of the medical management involves preventing the spread of hepatitis.

Hepatitis A. Patients with hepatitis A are advised to wash their hands thoroughly after using the toilet. Intimate contact should be avoided. Household contacts should be given immune serum globulin within 2 weeks of exposure. The immune serum globulin is isolated from patients who have had prior exposure to hepatitis and therefore have circulating antibodies that confer partial protection against viral hepatitis.

Hepatitis B. Patients should not share toilet facilities and personal items with others. Blood and secretions from patients should be carefully handled. Intimate contact should be avoided. Household members should be given immune serum globulin within 2 weeks of exposure. Persons with parenteral exposure to blood that is HBsAg-positive should be given hepatitis B immune globulin, a preparation containing high titers of anti-HBs. A viral vaccine is also available for persons at high risk of infection. Unlike immune globulins, which only confer short-term passive immunity, vaccination confers lifelong active immunity against hepatitis B.

Hepatitis C. Precautions are the same as those recommended for patients with hepatitis B infection. Immune serum globulin and hepatitis B immune globulin have not been of proven benefit in the prevention of this disease.

DENTAL EVALUATION

Because dentists are exposed to the blood and oral secretions of patients, they are particularly at risk for contracting hepatitis. The dental evaluation should therefore identify all patients who are potentially infectious.

Patients giving a history of malaise, low-grade fever, anorexia, nausea, and vomiting should be referred for evaluation. Patients with a prior history of hepatitis or jaundice should also be carefully evaluated. Patients with scleral icterus or jaundice should have dental procedures deferred and should be referred for further evaluation.

Laboratory evaluation of an asymptomatic patient with a past history of hepatitis or jaundice should include determination of liver function, prothrombin time, and hepatitis antigen. Some of these tests, particularly the liver function tests, may have already been performed by the patient's physician, who should be consulted. Patients with persistent abnormalities in liver function tests or with positive HBsAg should be referred for further evaluation.

Based on the history, examination, and laboratory profile, the relative risk of hepatitis infectivity can be assessed.

Patients at Low Risk

1. Patients with histories compatible with hepatitis A infection who have normal liver function tests and negative hepatitis antigen are at low risk.

2. Patients with histories of hepatitis B infection who have normal liver function tests, negative antigen tests, and positive antibody tests are also not infectious.

Patients at High Risk

1. Patients with positive surface antigen for hepatitis B and hepatitis C are at high risk.

2. Patients with abnormal liver function tests are at high risk.

3. Patients with jaundice and symptoms of viral hepatitis are at high risk.

DENTAL MANAGEMENT

Because all patients have to be managed with universal precautions, details of the evaluation of the patient with potential or known hepatitis become less important than strict adherence to universal precautions.

Operative Precautions. Care should be taken to minimize contact with the patient's blood and secretions. The use of air syringes and ultrasonic scalers should be avoided to prevent aerosolization of potentially infective viral particles.

Sterilization Procedures. Strict adherence to sterilization procedures is mandatory (Summary Table 23–IV). With inadequate sterilization, the dentist and other patients can be infected with hepatitis. All instruments should be autoclaved, and those that cannot be autoclaved should be cold-sterilized for an appropriate period of time. Because handpieces are difficult to sterilize adequately using conventional techniques, back-up handpieces should be used. These can be sterilized using ethylene oxide gas, which is available in hospitals at minimal cost.

Cleaning Procedures. Exposed surfaces in the operative field should be wiped clean with antiseptic solutions.

Inadvertent Needle Puncture. When the skin is inadvertently punctured with instruments or needles, it is important to wash the wound thoroughly. Whenever feasible, the patient's hepatitis surface antigen status should be determined. If parenteral exposure to blood that is HBsAg-positive has occurred, the dentist should receive hepatitis B immune globulin.

■ Examples of Dental Management and Evaluation

EVALUATION

Patient 1. A 32-year-old man presents for dental treatment. His past medical history is remarkable in that he contracted hepatitis while he was in the army. He remembers an epidemic of hepatitis during which half of the soldiers in the barracks became jaundiced. He had a brief period of jaundice, malaise, fatigue, anorexia, and nausea, and then he made an uneventful recovery. He has had subsequent blood tests

that did not reveal any residual problems with his liver. His medical history is otherwise unremarkable. He was last seen by his physician 8 months ago and was given a clean bill of health. Consultation with his physician reveals that liver function tests done a year ago were normal. His physician did not have a record of his hepatitis B surface antigen. On examination, the patient appears to be in good health. His blood pressure is 120/80, and his pulse rate is 86 beats/minute (bpm). He does not appear jaundiced. His dental needs include prophylaxis and scaling for severe gingivitis, simple operative procedures, and the extraction of a lower third molar.

Patient 2. A 28-year-old man presents for dental treatment. He was involved in an automobile accident 5 years ago and required massive blood transfusion for a ruptured spleen. During the hospitalization, he developed hepatitis "related to the blood transfusions" and had mild jaundice for about a week. He was told 6 months ago, during a general physical examination, that his liver function tests had all returned to normal. Consultation with his physician reveals that tests for hepatitis B surface antigen have always been negative. His blood pressure is 130/80, and his pulse rate is 76 bpm. He is not jaundiced. His dental needs are similar to those of the first patient.

Patient 3. A 37-year-old homosexual man enters for dental treatment. He gives a history of having contracted hepatitis 5 years ago. He is currently asymptomatic and has not been to a physician for over 3 years. During his last physical examination, he was told that his blood tests still showed residual effects from his hepatitis. Consultation with his physician reveals that he had a positive test for hepatitis B surface antigen when he was last tested 4 years ago. On examination now, his blood pressure is 140/82, and his pulse rate is 86 bpm. He is not jaundiced. His dental needs are similar to those of the other two patients.

MANAGEMENT

Dental management in all these patients is similar, because universal precautions are employed.

Patient 1. The clinical history is most compatible with an episode of hepatitis A that has completely resolved, but there is inadequate information to rule out hepatitis B. Despite the benign clinical course and the normal liver function tests, it is still important to have information about the status of the patient's hepatitis B surface antigen.

Patient 2. The patient's history is most consistent with hepatitis C. He should have liver function tests to determine the extent of hepatic dysfunction, if any. The prothrombin time should also be determined.

Patient 3. The patient has positive hepatitis B surface antigen and elevated liver function tests and is therefore probably infected. These tests are outdated and need to be repeated. The prothrombin time and platelet counts should be determined to assess the risks of bleeding. Universal precautions should be employed. The patient should be referred to his physician for another examination.

Viral Hepatitis: General Information

DEFINITION
Acute infection of the liver by one of three viruses: type A, type B, or type C; chronic hepatitis develops in 5% of cases

SYMPTOMS
Flu-like illness in the prodromal phase

Jaundice

Nausea and vomiting

Fever

Anorexia

SIGNS
Abnormal liver function tests, including elevation of transaminase (SGOT, SGPT, LDH); surface antigen (HBsAg) screening for type B only

TRANSMISSION
Type A
Fecal-oral; incubation, 30 days

Type B
Predominantly parenteral but other modes are possible (saliva, semen, vaginal secretions, breast milk); incubation, 12 weeks

Type C
Parenteral, usually secondary to large blood transfusions in excess of 5 units; incubation, 6 weeks

SIGNIFICANCE
Type A
Common occurrence, high infectivity, low morbidity, generally benign disease (80% of patients over age 60 have antibodies against hepatitis A virus), no chronic carrier states, and rare chronic hepatitis

Type B
Considerable morbidity and infectivity; 10% of patients become chronic carriers of surface antigen (HBsAg) with persistent potential infectivity

Only form of hepatitis with antigen marker

Some patients develop chronic hepatitis.

Dentists are 3 to 10 times more likely than the general population to develop type B hepatitis.

Type C
90% transfusion-related, no antigenic markers; 40% have persistent liver function test abnormalities

Many develop chronic active hepatitis.

Hepatitis C is infective.

CHRONIC HEPATITIS
Two forms are distinguished histologically by liver biopsy and characterized by chronic abnormal liver function tests:
    Chronic persistent form: excellent prognosis, no specific therapy required
    Chronic active form: worse prognosis, can progress to hepatic insufficiency, steroid and azathioprine therapy
Infectivity—both forms

SUMMARY TABLE **23–II**

Medical Management of the Patient with Viral Hepatitis

Preventive measures against transmission:
  Wash hands thoroughly.
  Do not share toilet or personal items.
  Handle blood and secretions carefully.
  Avoid intimate contact.

Rest and supportive care

For types A and B, immune globulin (passive immunity) for household contacts

For type B, viral vaccine (active immunity) for patients at high risk of infection

SUMMARY TABLE **23–III**

Dental Evaluation of the Patient with Viral Hepatitis

CLINICAL APPROACH
All patients with histories of hepatitis or histories or clinical findings of jaundice or scleral icterus should have laboratory testing.

LABORATORY TESTING
Liver function tests (SGOT, SGPT, LDH)

Hepatitis surface B antigen (HBsAg)

Hepatitis antibody titer

Prothrombin time

PHYSICIAN CONSULTATION
Those with persistent abnormal liver function tests should be referred to a physician for further evaluation.

RISK CATEGORIES
Patients at Low Risk
History of hepatitis A with normal liver function tests and negative hepatitis antigen

History of hepatitis B with normal liver function tests and negative hepatitis antigen

History of hepatitis C with normal liver function tests and negative hepatitis antigen

Patients at High Risk
Positive surface antigen for hepatitis B on routine screening (HBsAg-positive patient is probably infected)

Abnormal liver function tests

Jaundice, scleral icterus, and other symptoms of viral hepatitis

Dental Management of the Patient with Viral Hepatitis

PATIENTS AT LOW RISK
Normal dental protocol with the simple addition of mask and gloves for the dentist and assistant

PATIENTS AT HIGH RISK
1. Appointments scheduled at the end of the day to allow for appropriate precautions and sterilization
2. Careful avoidance of exposure to blood and oral secretions
3. Deferring of elective dental care until clinical infection has resolved
4. Strict sterilization procedures: autoclave, chemclave, or cold sterilize (in order of preference) all instruments, including handpieces; *Note:* many handpieces cannot be autoclaved and must be brought to the hospital for ethylene oxide gas sterilization (use of a back-up handpiece is recommended)
5. Use of double gloves and masks; appropriate gowning precautions
6. Draping of all exposed dental equipment where feasible, and wiping of all other surfaces with antiseptic solutions
7. Minimal use of aerosol instruments (air-water syringe, Cavitron)
8. Use of disposable items (e.g., impression trays) when possible
9. Immune globulin for all personnel subjected to inadvertent needle puncture

24

Cirrhosis

Cirrhosis is the result of severe or protracted injury to the liver causing loss of liver cells and progressive scarring. It is the fourth leading cause of death in young men between the ages of 35 and 54. The major cause of cirrhosis is alcoholic liver disease.

The liver is a vital organ responsible for synthesis and detoxification. With destruction of hepatic cells, the liver has a diminished capability to synthesize plasma proteins such as albumin, clotting factors, and lipoproteins. With hepatic insufficiency, the ability to detoxify substances is also markedly compromised, and drugs and toxins normally metabolized by the liver may accumulate. With hepatic failure, the patient may become encephalopathic because of the inability to detoxify even normal products of metabolism. Furthermore, with scarring, the portal circulation of the liver is blocked, resulting in portal hypertension. This in turn leads to the development of ascites and portosystemic collaterals including esophageal varices, a source of frequent massive hemorrhage.

The patient with cirrhosis presents a special problem to the dentist—inadequate synthesis of clotting factors may result in prolongation of prothrombin time and clinical bleeding. The inability to detoxify drugs may result in drug accumulation, and the use of even minor sedatives must be carefully weighed.

MEDICAL EVALUATION

Medical evaluation of the patient with cirrhosis centers on determination of the cause of liver damage and assessment of the severity of liver disease.

The history is important in determining the cause of cirrhosis. In the majority of instances, chronic alcohol abuse is the cause of cirrhosis (Laennec's cirrhosis). In some patients, cirrhosis is the result of chronic hepatitis (postnecrotic cirrhosis), of either viral or toxic origin. Chronic passive hepatic congestion secondary to severe congestive heart failure can result in cirrhosis. Less commonly, diseases such as hemochromatosis, primary biliary cirrhosis, and Wilson's disease result in cirrhosis.

Cirrhosis may be totally asymptomatic and present as an incidental finding at autopsy, or it may be clinically compromising. Cirrhosis often becomes clinically apparent late in life, manifesting itself as portal hypertension, fluid retention, and encephalopathy. Portal hypertension is the result of blockage of the portal circulation by scarred liver parenchyma. It leads to splenomegaly and the formation of a system of collateral veins, which are fragile and can cause massive bleeding (variceal bleeding). Fluid retention is the result of decreased intravascular albumin concentration, a result of compromised hepatic synthesis. Encephalopathy is the result of the inability of the liver to detoxify nitrogenous metabolites. Excessive protein load from diet or from blood in the gastrointestinal tract can precipitate hepatic encephalopathy.

On examination, usually the liver is firm and shrunken and the spleen is enlarged. The patient may have ascites and peripheral edema. Skin findings include spider angiomas and palmar erythema. Patients may have gynecomastia and testicular atrophy. In some instances, patients may have flexion contractures of the fingers (Dupuytren's contractures).

Laboratory evaluation should include complete blood and platelet counts, and determination of prothrombin time (PT), partial thromboplastin time (PTT), and albumin, bilirubin, serum glutamic-oxaloacetic transaminase (SGOT), serum glutamic pyruvate transaminase (SGPT), and alkaline phosphatase levels. These tests provide important information about the patient: patients with cirrhosis caused by alcoholism may have a macrocytic anemia secondary to dietary deficiency of folate or vitamin B_{12} (Chap. 25); they may have decreased platelet counts as a result of both decreased synthesis and increased destruction secondary to hypersplenism; serum albumin and PT tests provide important information about the synthetic ability of the residual liver cells, and patients with significant synthetic dysfunction have a low albumin level and prolonged PT. Liver function tests provide information about the degree of hepatic inflammation and obstruction.

In instances when the cause of hepatic dysfunction is not clear, noninvasive tests such as liver-spleen scan, abdominal computed tomography (CT), and liver ultrasound can be of use. In situations where the diagnosis is obscure even after careful noninvasive evaluation, a percutaneous liver biopsy can be performed to provide a histologic diagnosis.

The clinical course of cirrhosis depends on the nature, extent, and activity of the underlying hepatocellular disease. Patients with Laennec's cirrhosis who have stopped drinking have a 5-year survival rate of 60%, but, if they continue to drink, the survival rate falls to 40%. For patients with postnecrotic cirrhosis, the 5-year survival rate is 25%. Patients with primary biliary cirrhosis usually die within 5 to 10 years of onset of symptoms. Death in patients with cirrhosis is usually caused by variceal bleeding, infection, encephalopathy, and less commonly, hepatoma.

MEDICAL MANAGEMENT

The first objective is to halt further injury to the liver. Alcohol and other potential toxins to the liver should be stopped. In some patients with chronic active hepatitis, corticosteroids and immunosuppressive medications are effective in preventing progression to cirrhosis.

Ascites and edema may be uncomfortable and cause respiratory compromise. Patients are usually instructed to limit salt and fluid intake strictly. If these measures do not suffice, a diuretic program can be judiciously instituted under careful monitoring. It is crucial to avoid volume depletion in patients with cirrhosis. In the rare patient with disabling and refractory ascites, paracentesis may be indicated. Fluid reaccumulates quickly following paracentesis, often at the expense of intravascular volume. A peritoneovenous shunt (LeVeen) has been used in selected patients with refractory ascites, but infection and coagulopathy have limited its use.

Patients with cirrhosis may have significant hemostatic defects, both because of inability to synthesize clotting factors and because of thrombocytopenia secondary to hypersplenism. These defects can be corrected with re-

placement with fresh-frozen plasma and platelets.

Encephalopathy is seen in patients with severe liver disease and reflects the liver's inability to detoxify nitrogenous wastes. Excess dietary protein and gastrointestinal bleeding are important precipitating factors. Dietary protein is limited to 30 to 40 g per day. In patients with a history of encephalopathy, sedatives and tranquilizers should be avoided. In some patients, neomycin or lactulose may be used to treat encephalopathy. Both drugs can change the bowel flora and minimize ammonia production and absorption.

In selected patients, a portacaval or splenorenal shunt procedure may be considered to decompress the portal system and prevent variceal bleeding. However, the risk of hepatic encephalopathy increases after these procedures, and shunts should be considered only in patients with documented and life-threatening variceal bleeding.

In rare instances, a patient with end-stage liver disease may be a candidate for liver transplantation.

DENTAL EVALUATION

The patient presenting with a history of liver disease or cirrhosis deserves special attention.

The patient should be asked about any history of abnormal bleeding, because clotting factor deficiency and thrombocytopenia may be present in the patient with severe liver disease. The patient should also be asked specifically about a history of encephalopathy. Current dietary restrictions and medications also provide important clues about the severity of liver disease. Patients with ascites and peripheral edema are likely to have fluid and salt restrictions, and occasionally they may be using diuretics. Patients with hepatic encephalopathy are likely to have protein restrictions, and may be taking neomycin or lactulose. In all instances in which there may be a concern for significant liver disease, the patient's physician should be consulted prior to dental therapy.

Laboratory evaluation should be directed primarily at an assessment of the bleeding parameters (Chap. 26). Complete blood count, PT, PTT, platelet count and bleeding time should be obtained. Patients with cirrhosis may have prolongation of PT because of an inability to synthesize clotting factors. Some patients may have hypersplenism and thrombocytopenia.

DENTAL MANAGEMENT

The dentist should work in close collaboration with the patient's physician during the entire course of dental therapy.

Patients with Hemostatic Defects

If hemostatic defects have been identified during dental evaluation, these should be addressed prior to elective dental procedures.

In patients with mild prolongation of prothrombin times (less than 1½ times control value), nonsurgical and simple surgical procedures (types I to IV) can proceed with careful attention to hemostasis. For moderate and advanced surgical procedures (types IV to VI) hospitalization should be considered.

In patients who show marked prolongation of prothrombin times (more than 1½ times control value), elective dental procedures should be deferred. The patient's physician should be consulted and the planned procedures carefully discussed. In most instances, dental procedures not expected to cause significant bleeding (some type I to III procedures) can be done on an outpatient basis with careful attention to hemostasis. Mandibular block anesthesia or procedures likely to incur gingival bleeding (types IV to VI, some type III) should be done only after the prothrombin time has been brought to within a reasonable range (PT less than 1½ times control) by replacement with fresh-frozen plasma. Therefore, in the majority of instances, these procedures should be done in the hospital.

If excessive bleeding occurs after the procedure, local measures such as additional suturing, topical thrombin, and Gelfoam should be used. In the rare instance of massive and life-threatening bleeding despite adequate attempts at local control, the patient should be hospitalized, and fresh-frozen plasma should be given.

Some patients may be found to be thrombocytopenic as a result of hypersplenism. Again, the patient's physician should be consulted before dental therapy. Management should be tailored according to the degree of thrombocytopenia and the type of procedures planned.

Patients with mild thrombocytopenia (platelet count of 50,000 to 100,000/mm³) have mild prolongation of the bleeding time (less than 2 minutes beyond the normal range). Some nonsurgical procedures (types I to III) not expected to cause excessive bleeding can be performed with attention to hemostasis. Mandibular block anesthesia and all simple and advanced surgical procedures (types IV to VI) should be performed after correction of the bleeding time prolongation with platelet transfusion.

Patients with platelet counts lower than 50,000 generally require platelet transfusion prior to most dental procedures. A few nonsurgical procedures (types I to III) can be performed without platelet transfusion, after consultation with the patient's physician. Mandibular nerve block, prophylaxis, subgingival scaling and curettage, and any procedure involving even minor tissue trauma (many type II and III procedures and all type IV to VI procedures) should not be performed without platelet transfusion. Hospitalization is advised in these patients.

Patients with History of Encephalopathy

All patients with a history of hepatic encephalopathy have severe liver disease. They often have difficulties detoxifying drugs, and many of the sedatives, tranquilizers, and analgesics used in the dental office cannot be administered because of possible aggravation of the encephalopathy. In all instances, the patient's physician should be consulted before medication is prescribed.

■ Examples of Dental Evaluation and Management

EVALUATION

Patient 1. A 43-year-old man presents for dental evaluation. He gives a history of having had "some kind of hepatitis" at age 21 and has been told that he has some "liver scarring" by a physician. He has recently been evaluated by his physician and was given "a clean bill of health." Consultation with his physician reveals that his most recent visit was 2 months ago, at which time his CBC, blood smear, and liver function tests were all normal. The physician does not know the type of hepatitis the patient has had, but hepatitis B surface antigen and antibody determination 2 years ago were negative.

On examination, his blood pressure is 130/88 and pulse is 68 beats/minute (bpm) and regular.

His dental needs include full mouth scaling, root planing and curettage, full mouth periodontal surgery, and multiple units of fixed prostheses.

Patient 2. A 38-year-old man with a history of alcohol abuse presents for evaluation. He has been told that he has cirrhosis but has been unable to abstain. He has been hospitalized five times for alcohol detoxification and has had a recent hospitalization for upper gastrointestinal bleeding. Consultation with his physician reveals that endoscopy was performed on the patient on that admission and he was found to have gastritis. There was no evidence of esophageal varices and his bleeding parameters during that hospitalization were normal. His most recent examination was a month ago. His CBC and liver function tests were in normal range, albumin was 3.0 mg/dl (normal, 3.5 to 5 mg/dl), and PT was 14.2/11.5 seconds.

On examination, his blood pressure is 140/80 and pulse is 78 bpm and regular. His dental needs are identical to those of Patient 1.

Patient 3. A 42-year-old man with biopsy-proven Laennec's cirrhosis presents for dental therapy. He has had numerous hospitalizations for complications of his liver disease, including variceal bleeding and hepatic encephalopathy. He is currently restricting protein, salt, and fluid intake and is taking 50 mg hydrochlorothiazide bid and lactulose. Consultation with his physician reveals that the patient has severe liver dysfunction. His most recent examination was a week ago when his albumin was 1.8 mg/dl, PT was 20/11.4 seconds, and platelet count was 72,000/mm^3.

On examination, his blood pressure is 130/88 and pulse is 90 bpm and regular. He has obvious ascites and peripheral edema.

His dental needs are similar to those of Patients 1 and 2. He has advanced periodontal disease, multiple caries, and missing teeth.

MANAGEMENT

Patient 1. The patient has a remote history of hepatitis, probably not hepatitis B. His liver function tests and synthetic functions were all normal during a recent evaluation. The patient can be treated using normal dental protocol. A preoperative assessment of the hemostatic status (PT, PTT, platelet count, and bleeding time) is advisable prior to moderate and advanced surgical procedures (types V and VI).

Patient 2. The patient has significant liver function abnormalities and his synthetic functions are compromised: his albumin is below normal and his prothrombin time is prolonged. Because this patient is at increased risk of bleeding, it is important to pay attention to all factors likely to influence hemostasis. All drugs that can impair platelet function (aspirin and nonsteroidal anti-inflammatory drugs, NSAIDs) should be avoided. Special attention should be paid to local hemostasis.

Because of the hepatic compromises, the patient may have difficulties with detoxification of drugs, and the use of sedatives and analgesics should be carefully monitored.

The patient may be less than ideally compliant and the dental therapeutic plans may have to be revised accordingly.

Patient 3. This patient has severe liver dysfunction. His medical regimen reflects considerable hepatic compromises. He is on dietary protein restriction and is taking lactulose to prevent encephalopathy. He has poor synthetic capabilities with hypoalbuminemia and marked prolongation of prothrombin time. Furthermore, he has significant thrombocytopenia (less than 100,000 cells/mm^3).

All these factors make the patient a candidate for palliative dental care only. He is at high risk for bleeding complications and has difficulties detoxifying sedatives and analgesics. Dental procedures should be performed in the hospital in close consultation with the patient's physician. Definitive scaling and simple caries control may be performed to prevent bleeding and abscess formation in the future. Periodontal surgery and ideal crown and bridge care are probably not advisable. In instances where surgery or significant gingival trauma is necessary, fresh-frozen plasma and platelet transfusion should be used to minimize risks of excessive bleeding.

SUMMARY TABLE **24–1**

Description of Cirrhosis

DEFINITION
Loss of liver cells and progressive scarring as a result of severe or protracted injury

COMPLICATIONS
Diminished capability to synthesize protein, albumin, lipoproteins, and clotting factors

Diminished ability to detoxify toxic substances and normal metabolites

Portal hypertension
  Splenomegaly—platelet sequestration
  Ascites
  Portosystemic collaterals: esophageal varices, risk of hemorrhage

CAUSES
Chronic alcohol abuse (Laennec's cirrhosis); 5-yr survival, 40–60%

Chronic hepatitis (postnecrotic cirrhosis); 5–7-yr survival, 25%, viral or toxic

Chronic passive hepatic congestion secondary to congestive heart failure

Others: hemochromatosis, primary biliary cirrhosis, Wilson's disease

SYMPTOMS
Ascites

Peripheral edema

Splenomegaly

Bleeding

Encephalopathy

Esophageal varices

Medical Evaluation of the Patient with Cirrhosis

HISTORY
Alcohol abuse

Hepatitis

PHYSICAL EXAMINATION
Skin changes
  Spider angiomas
  Palmar erythema

Ascites

Peripheral edema

Splenomegaly

Encephalopathy

LABORATORY EVALUATION: ABNORMAL RESULTS
Evidence of macrocytic anemia (secondary to vitamin B_{12} and folate deficiency)

Albumin

Bilirubin

SGOT

SGPT

Alkaline phosphatase

Prothrombin time

Platelet count

OTHER TESTS FOR EVALUATION OF LIVER ABNORMALITIES
Liver scan

Abdominal CT scan

Liver ultrasound

Percutaneous liver biopsy

Medical Management of the Patient with Cirrhosis

Discontinuing toxins to the liver (e.g., alcohol)

Limiting salt and fluid intake

Judicious use of diuretics

Low-protein diet

Liver transplant in appropriate candidates

Neomycin or lactulose

Corticosteroid in some selected instances (e.g., chronic active hepatitis)

LeVeen shunt in rare instances

Platelets and fresh-frozen plasma as needed

Avoidance of sedatives and tranquilizers

SUMMARY TABLE **24–IV**

Dental Evaluation of the Patient with Cirrhosis

Assess severity of liver compromise by history
 History of abnormal bleeding
 History of encephalopathy (neomycin or lactulose use)
 Dietary restrictions
 Alcohol use or abuse
 Salt restrictions or diuretics
 Physical signs
  Spider angiomas
  Palmar erythema
  Ascites
  Peripheral edema

If there are significant findings from the above list, the following should be considered:
 Medical consultation
 Laboratory evaluation (often from physician)
  Albumin, bilirubin
  SGOT, SGPT, alkaline phosphatase levels
  CBC
 Laboratory evaluation prior to dental surgery or significant gingival trauma
  PT
  PTT
  Platelet count, bleeding time (Chap. 26)

SUMMARY TABLE **24–V**

Dental Management of the Patient with Cirrhosis

Avoid use of all antiplatelet drugs:
 Aspirin compounds
 NSAIDs

Minimize use of all sedatives and tranquilizers (physician clearance mandatory).

Manage defects in hemostatic mechanism (physician consultation mandatory; Chap. 26).

If patient's PT is elevated, but less than 1½ times control value
 Nonsurgical and simple surgical procedures (I–IV)—normal protocol with strict attention to hemostasis
 Moderate and advanced surgery (types V–VI) ±* hospitalization

If patient's PT is greater than 1½ times control value
 All surgery (types IV–VI) requires fresh-frozen plasma correction of PT to under 1½ times control value, probable hospitalization

If patient has mild thrombocytopenia (platelet count 50,000–100,000/mm³)
 Nonelective surgical procedures (I–III), normal protocol with strict attention to hemostasis
 Surgical procedures (IV–VI), platelet transfusion, probable hospitalization required

If patient has severe thrombocytopenia (platelet count <50,000/mm³)
 All mandibular nerve blocks, prophylaxis, sublingual scaling, curettage, and any operative procedures involving even minor gingival trauma (most type II and III procedures), and all surgery (types IV–VI), require platelet transfusion and hospitalization.

Combined PT and platelet deficiencies require hospitalization and platelet and fresh-frozen plasma transfusion.

---

* ±, with or without.

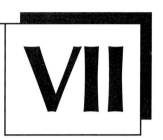
Evaluation and Management of the Patient with Hematologic Disease

25

Anemia

Anemia is a relatively common disorder, with a reported incidence of 17 to 18 cases/1000 population annually. It is defined as a decrease in the number of circulating red blood cells, a decrease in the hemoglobin concentration, and/or a decrease in the hematocrit level. Anemia can result from excessive blood loss or decreased production or increased destruction of red blood cells.

Blood loss is the most common cause of anemia. In young women, excessive blood loss during menstruation is a frequent cause. Blood loss can also result from structural lesions in the gastrointestinal tract, such as peptic ulcers, colonic polyps, or cancers.

Decreased production of red cells most commonly results from dietary deficiencies of iron, folate, or vitamin B_{12}. Other causes include reduced erythropoietin production as a result of renal disease or other chronic diseases, or defects in stem cell proliferation, hemoglobin synthesis, or DNA synthesis. Drugs such as quinidine, alcohol, penicillin, and sulfa compounds may also compromise the ability of the bone marrow to produce adequate red blood cells.

Increased destruction of red cells can result from disorders of the red cell membrane (hereditary spherocytosis), disorders of hemoglobin synthesis (thalassemia, sickle cell anemia), deficiencies of enzymes such as glucose 6-phosphate dehydrogenase (G6PD), or antibody-mediated hemolysis. Increased sequestration and destruction of red cells can also occur in patients with hypersplenism when reticuloendothelial system activity is markedly enhanced.

MEDICAL EVALUATION

Anemia may be symptomatic or may be discovered during a routine examination. A patient with anemia is usually asymptomatic until the hematocrit level falls below 30%. At lower hematocrit levels, the patient may suffer from weakness, fatigability, and dizziness. When the hematocrit level falls still further, dyspnea on exertion may occur. With severe anemia (hematocrit levels of less than 20%), significant orthostatic symptoms appear and patients may have dyspnea even at rest. In patients with cardiac compromises, symptoms of angina pectoris and congestive heart failure may occur.

On examination, pallor of the skin and nail beds may be noted. The patient may have resting tachycardia and orthostatic decreases in blood pressure. Atrophic glossitis and angular cheilitis may be present on oral examination (Fig. 25–1).

The medical evaluation of anemia requires a systematic approach, because there are a great many possible causes, and a vast array of diagnostic tests are available. In most instances, the initial laboratory examination in-

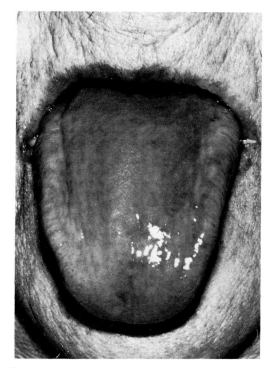

Figure 25–1. Atrophic glossitis and angular cheilitis in a patient with iron deficiency anemia.

cludes a complete blood count (CBC) and determination of mean corpuscular volume (MCV) and mean corpuscular hemoglobin concentration (MCHC). The cells are examined under the microscope, and the morphologic characteristics of the red cells are recorded. Most anemias are treated according to the red cell morphology seen on a peripheral smear. The cells may be small (microcytic), normal-sized (normocytic), or large (macrocytic), and they may contain low (hypochromic) or normal (normochromic) amounts of hemoglobin (Fig. 25–2). The morphologic appearance of the red cells can also help determine the cause of the anemia.

Microcytic Hypochromic Anemia

Iron Deficiency

The most common cause of microcytic anemia is iron deficiency resulting from excessive blood loss, inadequate intake, or poor absorption. Of the various causes, occult blood loss is the most common. In menstruating women, excessive blood loss and inadequate dietary iron replacement are common. In one study, iron deficiency anemia was found in 10 to 20% of the menstruating women studied. In men and nonmenstruating women, blood loss is usually from an occult source in the gastrointestinal tract, such as gastritis or carcinoma, and requires further studies, such as an upper gastrointestinal series and a barium enema, particularly if guaiac-positive stools are documented.

Patients with poor dietary habits and patients with large iron requirements (such as pregnant or menstruating women) may have inadequate iron intake. Malabsorption of iron can occur in patients after partial gastrectomy or excessive antacid use.

Other Causes

Microcytic anemia may also be caused by chronic disease or thalassemia minor. Thalassemia is a genetic disorder that results in abnormal hemoglobin production and occurs

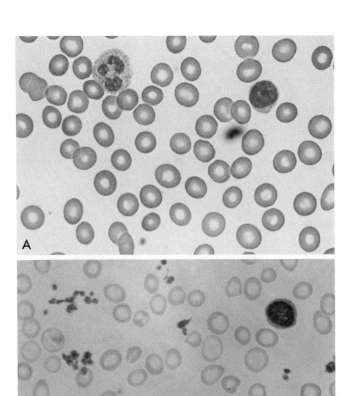

Figure 25–2. *A,* Normal smear of peripheral blood showing red cells, a neutrophil, and a lymphocyte. *B,* Smear of peripheral blood in patient with iron deficiency anemia. Note shape, size, and density of red cells compared with those in the normal smear.

most frequently in patients of Mediterranean heritage. Less commonly, patients with sideroblastic anemia may also have a microcytic smear.

Evaluation of patients with microcytic hypochromic anemia includes the determination of iron levels, iron-binding capacity, and serum ferritin levels. Patients with iron deficiency have low serum ferritin levels, and the iron saturation is usually lower than 15%. The diagnosis can be confirmed by examining the iron stores in a specially stained bone marrow biopsy. Iron deficiency anemia in menstruating women is usually treated with iron replacement. Refractory anemia requires further evaluation. Iron deficiency anemia in nonmenstruating women and in men is evaluated with attention to possible blood loss from the gastrointestinal tract.

When thalassemia is suspected on clinical grounds, a hemoglobin A_2 determination by electrophoresis confirms the diagnosis.

Patients with sideroblastic anemia have high iron saturations, and bone marrow biopsy reveals the presence of ring sideroblasts.

Macrocytic Anemia

Most patients with macrocytic anemia have a deficiency of either vitamin B_{12} or folic acid.

Vitamin B_{12} Deficiency

Severe deficiency of vitamin B_{12} results in pernicious anemia. Vitamin B_{12} is available in most foods; the body reserve of the vitamin lasts about 3 years. B_{12} deficiency therefore usually results, not from dietary insufficiency, but either from deficient gastric production of the intrinsic factor essential for the absorption of vitamin B_{12} or from difficulties with the absorption of the B_{12} intrinsic factor complex. Patients with pernicious anemia can develop neurologic symptoms such as incoordination and difficulties in sensing position and vibration.

Folate Deficiency

Although the body has a 3-month reserve of folate, folate deficiency can occur as a result of dietary inadequacy. Chronic alcohol abuse often leads to macrocytic anemia secondary to poor dietary habits. Patients with malabsorption can also develop folate deficiency. Drugs such as phenytoin (Dilantin) can interfere with folate absorption and produce anemia.

Some patients (pregnant women and patients with hemolysis) may have increased folate requirements and may develop anemia because of an inadequate folate supply.

Other Causes

Macrocytic anemia can also be seen in patients with liver diseases, preleukemic conditions, accelerated red cell production, or hypothyroidism.

Evaluation of the patient with macrocytic anemia includes determination of the serum folate and B_{12} levels. Patients suspected of having B_{12} deficiency should have a Schilling test to differentiate between malabsorption and an intrinsic factor deficiency. A bone marrow aspirate and biopsy are necessary if diseases that result from bone marrow replacement (such as leukemic infiltration or myelofibrosis) are suspected.

Normocytic Normochromic Anemia

Some anemias produce normal peripheral red blood cell smears, such as anemias caused by chronic diseases, some hemolytic anemias, abrupt blood loss anemia, and early iron deficiency anemia. Other causes of normocytic normochromic anemia include anemia secondary to bone marrow infiltration, hypothyroidism, and aplastic anemia.

Evaluation includes a careful history to uncover evidence of chronic diseases. The reticulocyte count is determined, because an elevated count suggests the possibility of hemolysis. Bone marrow biopsy is necessary if bone marrow infiltration or aplastic anemia is suspected.

Hemolytic Anemia

In some instances, anemia may be the result of accelerated destruction of red cells. Patients with hemolytic anemia characteristically have increased bone marrow production of red cells and increased reticulocyte counts. Hemolytic anemia may be the result of either intrinsic abnormalities in the red cells or extrinsic influences upon the red cells resulting in increased destruction.

Intrinsic red cell abnormalities that can result in hemolytic anemias include diseases affecting the red cell membrane (hereditary spherocytosis), the hemoglobin (sickle cell anemia, thalassemia), or enzymes inside the red cells (G6PD deficiency). These congenital red cell disorders cause accelerated red cell destruction by the reticuloendothelial system and, consequently, anemia.

Extrinsic factors can also cause hemolysis. These factors include drugs such as quinidine, penicillin, and methyldopa (Aldomet), as well as viral infections, transfusion reactions, and autoimmune hemolytic anemias.

MEDICAL MANAGEMENT

Once the cause of the anemia has been identified, therapy can be tailored to the patient.

Microcytic Normocytic Anemia

Patients with clinical evidence of excessive blood loss should have appropriate gastrointestinal and gynecologic evaluations. Patients with dietary deficiencies of iron are usually appropriately supplemented. Patients with malabsorption should have the underlying gastrointestinal difficulties corrected. Because patients with thalassemia usually have mild anemia, they require no specific therapy. Sideroblastic anemia may be successfully treated with pyridoxine.

Macrocytic Anemia

Patients with folate or vitamin B_{12} deficiencies usually receive supplementation. Patients with intrinsic factor deficiency generally have an upper gastrointestinal radiographic series performed to rule out achlorhydria and gastric malignancy. Patients with liver disease, preleukemia, or hypothyroidism require no specific therapeutic intervention for the anemia unless symptoms occur.

Normocytic Normochromic Anemia

Patients with abrupt blood loss and anemia require prompt intervention to identify the source of blood loss. Blood replacement is necessary if the loss is significant.

In patients with evidence of hemolysis, the first goal of therapy is to identify the cause. All drugs capable of inducing hemolysis are dis-

continued. Splenectomy may be performed in patients with hypersplenism if the hemolysis is significant. Patients with abnormal red cell membranes or hemoglobinopathy are usually managed with periodic transfusions for symptomatic anemia.

In patients with suspected bone marrow infiltration, a bone marrow biopsy may be necessary to confirm the diagnosis. These patients may require transfusions for symptomatic anemia.

In the appropriate situation, erythropoietin therapy can be considered. This is particularly useful in uremic patients with symptomatic anemia.

DENTAL EVALUATION

The dental evaluation should assess the patient's clinical status and identify the cause of the anemia. Consultation with the patient's physician is important for the appropriate management of these patients.

Patients may have symptoms of weakness, dizziness, dyspnea on mild exertion, or easy fatigability. Although these symptoms are not pathognomonic of anemia, determination of the blood count should be undertaken (Chap. 1), because patients may have anemia uncovered during routine laboratory evaluation.

More commonly, patients give a past history of anemia. The patient should be asked about the exact cause of the anemia, the therapeutic interventions undertaken, and the medications used. An assessment should also be made to determine whether symptoms are present. A recent complete blood count (within 6 months) is important in the overall evaluation of the patient.

Based on the history and the blood count, patients can be placed in various categories.

Patients at Low Risk

1. The patient has a past history of anemia that has since been corrected, is asymptomatic, and has a normal hematocrit level.
2. The patient has an identified cause of mild anemia, but does not require therapy and has a hematocrit level higher than 30%.
3. The patient has an identified cause of mild anemia, is on therapy, is asymptomatic (e.g., a menstruating woman on iron replacement), and has a hematocrit level higher than 30%.
4. The patient has anemia as a result of chronic disease, has a stable hematocrit level above 30%, and is asymptomatic.

Patients at High Risk

1. The patient was not previously known to be anemic but had anemia uncovered during dental evaluation.

2. The patient has a hematocrit level of less than 30%. If patients also have coronary artery disease, they are at particularly high risk.

3. The patient has evidence of ongoing bleeding.

4. The patient has a coagulopathy (Chap. 26) and anemia.

5. The patient requires repeated transfusions to prevent symptoms of anemia.

DENTAL MANAGEMENT

The dental management of individuals with anemia should be tailored to the patient's clinical status (Summary Table 25–VII). The dentist must be aware of the cause and extent of the anemia. If the anemia is the result of an underlying disease, the nature and activity of the disease should be assessed *prior to* dental treatment. The patient's physician should be consulted if the clinical status is not clear-cut. It is particularly important to know that the anemia is not secondary to a coagulopathy, because the management of such a condition often requires special consideration (Chap. 26).

Patients at Low Risk. These patients can be managed according to normal protocol.

Patients at High Risk. Whenever possible, elective dental procedures should be deferred until the clinical status of the patient has been optimized. Thus, for the patient with previously undiagnosed anemia, dental therapy should be postponed until the cause of the anemia is identified and treated. Similarly, dental therapy should be deferred for patients with hematocrit levels of less than 30%. Patients with ongoing bleeding, patients with coagulopathies, and patients requiring multiple transfusions for symptomatic anemia all require clinical stabilization prior to dental treatment.

When clinically stable, these patients should have short dental sessions with minimization of stress. Adjunctive sedation techniques should be considered. Outpatient intravenous sedation and general anesthesia is contraindicated. Hospitalization for careful monitoring should be considered for moderate and advanced (types V and VI) surgical procedures.

ORAL CHANGES

Oral changes are noted in both deficiency and hemolytic anemias but are more consistent in the former.

Deficiency Anemia

Iron Deficiency Anemia

Iron deficiency anemia is a relatively common disorder that may produce dramatic oral changes, especially of the tongue. The most consistent oral finding associated with iron deficiency anemia is atrophy of the lingual papilla (Fig. 25–1). Atrophic changes usually begin at the tip and then spread distally, involving the filiform and fungiform papillae. The surface of the tongue develops a glistening, smooth appearance that may be manifested symptomatically as a burning sensation. Increased susceptibility to trauma may result in ulcerations that persist longer than usual as a consequence of slow wound healing. Although gingival and mucosal pallor are associated with this deficiency, they are difficult to see. Treatment is aimed at correcting the underlying deficiency. Palliation may be achieved using topical rinses such as Xylocaine Viscous, Dyclone, or Benadryl and Kaopectate (50% of each). Angular cheilitis is also noted.

Vitamin B$_{12}$ Deficiency

Deficiencies of vitamin B$_{12}$ produce pernicious anemia. The most consistent finding in this disorder is glossitis, which affects 50 to 60% of patients. As with other deficiency anemias, atrophic glossitis produced by a loss of the filiform, fungiform, and circumvillate papillae results in a smooth, "bald," glistening tongue that is sensitive and red. During periods of atrophy, the tongue is especially sensitive to trauma from rough or fractured restorations or prostheses. The oral changes of pernicious anemia respond well to correction of the deficiency, often within 48 hours. Angular cheilitis is less common than it is in iron deficiency anemia and is not a regular feature of pernicious anemia.

Folic Acid Deficiency

The oral changes associated with folic acid deficiency are similar to those seen in pernicious anemia. Angular cheilitis is a more common finding than in pernicious anemia. In addition, it has been suggested that a significant number of patients with recurrent aphthous stomatitis (approximately 15%) suffer from folic acid deficiency and that this deficiency correlates with the presence of lesions. Elimination of the deficiency state results in ulcer resolution.

Hemolytic Anemia

Oral changes associated with hemolytic anemia may result from the compensatory hyperplastic enlargement of marrow spaces, the deposition of destroyed blood pigments in oral tissue, or anemic changes in the gingiva.

Compensatory hyperplasia of marrow spaces may produce expansion of the maxilla in patients with either thalassemia or sickle cell anemia. This expansion may result in dramatic malocclusions with severe diastema formation. Radiographic evidence of a widened trabecular pattern and increased marrow spaces may be noted.

Deposition of blood pigments into tissue may produce discoloration. Patients with erythroblastosis fetalis display a brown-green discoloration of their deciduous teeth as a result of bile pigment incorporation into the tooth structure during dentinogenesis (Fig. 25–3). A subtle yellowish discoloration of the gingiva may be seen in any patient with a hemolytic anemia.

Patients who develop hemolytic anemia as a consequence of heavy metal poisoning may show deposition of RBC-bound metal along the gingival margin, giving way to a characteristic "lead line" (Fig. 25–4). Such patients demonstrate a deep bluish-black collection of pigmentation along the marginal and papillary gingiva.

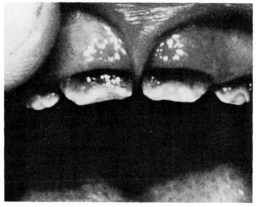

Figure 25–3. Discoloration of the deciduous teeth in a patient with an erythroblastosis fetalis resulting from bile pigment incorporation into the tooth structure during dentinogenesis.

■ Examples of Dental Evaluation and Management

EVALUATION

Patient 1. A 32-year-old woman presents for dental treatment. She is basically healthy but had a history of anemia during her first pregnancy. This was treated with iron supplementation and resolved. She was last seen by her physician a year ago, when her blood count was normal. On examination, her blood pressure is 104/70 and her pulse rate is 76 beats/minute (bpm). Her dental needs include surgical endodontics for an upper first molar.

Patient 2. A 34-year-old woman with thalassemia presents for evaluation. She was diagnosed as having thalassemia at age 18 during an evaluation for anemia. She has been on iron and multivitamin supplementation. She was last seen by her physician 3 months ago, when her

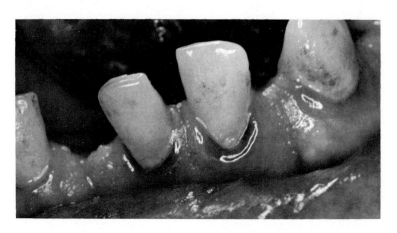

Figure 25–4. Deposition of lead in the marginal gingiva in a patient with heavy metal poisoning showing characteristic "lead line." (Courtesy of Dr. Peter Lockhart.)

hematocrit level was 32%. During the past few weeks, she has suffered from easy fatigability, weakness, and dizziness. On examination, her blood pressure is 110/70 and her pulse rate is 120 bpm. Her skin and nail beds appear to be pale. Her dental needs include caries control with amalgams, scaling and curettage, and four quadrants of periodontal surgery.

Patient 3. A 23-year-old woman with sickle cell anemia enters for dental treatment. The patient has had multiple admissions for sickle cell crises and has required multiple transfusions. She has a chronic hematocrit level of about 25% and has learned to limit her activities accordingly. Consultation with her physician reveals that her most recent hematocrit reading was 27%. On examination, her blood pressure is 110/80 and her pulse rate is 88 bpm. Her dental needs are the same as those of Patient 2.

MANAGEMENT

Patient 1. This patient has a history of anemia, which was corrected with iron supplementation. She has had a recent blood count with normal values. The patient is at low risk and can be managed with normal dental protocols.

Patient 2. This patient has a history of thalassemia and has previously been under reasonable

control, with a recent hematocrit reading of 32%. However, she now presents with symptoms that suggest an exacerbation of her anemia. The elevated pulse rate is also suggestive of significant anemia. All dental care should therefore be deferred, and the patient should be referred to her physician for further evaluation.

Patient 3. This patient has chronic anemia with a hematocrit level of 27%. This places her in the high-risk category, and she should therefore be managed with care. Unfortunately, postponement of dental care is of no value, because this patient is probably as stable as she will ever be. Dental procedures should therefore be carried out with minimization of stress and risk of infection. Preventive dental procedures are particularly important, because oral infection can precipitate a sickle cell crisis. The patient should be aggressively managed with antibiotics for oral infections, including chronic suppurative periodontal disease. The patient's physician should be consulted prior to dental procedures. Examination and simple nonsurgical procedures (types I to III) can be performed on an outpatient basis. All surgical procedures, particularly moderate and advanced procedures (types V and VI), should be performed during an elective hospital admission. Outpatient intravenous sedation and general anesthesia are contraindicated in the high-risk patient.

Anemia: General Information

DEFINITION

Combination of one or more laboratory findings, including
  Decrease in the number of red blood cells
  Decrease in hemoglobin concentration
  Decrease in hematocrit

INCIDENCE

17–18 cases/1000 population/year

CAUSE

Blood loss:
  Menstruation
  Peptic ulcer disease
  Gastrointestinal cancer
Dietary deficiency (iron, folate, or vitamin B_{12})
Drug reactions—quinidine, alcohol, penicillin, sulfa compounds
Decreased production of red cells
Increased destruction of red cells:
  Thalassemia
  Sickle cell anemia
  G6PD deficiency
  Hereditary spherocytosis
  Hypersplenism
  Antibody-mediated hemolysis

SYMPTOMS

Usually asymptomatic until hematocrit falls below 30%

Hematocrit lower than 30%, moderate symptoms—weakness, fatigability, dizziness, dyspnea on exertion

Hematocrit lower than 20%, severe symptoms—dyspnea at rest, orthostatic hypotension, tachycardia

Angina pectoris and congestive heart failure in patients with cardiac compromise

Oral findings—atrophic glossitis, angular cheilitis

DIAGNOSIS

Red cell morphology

MCHC and MCV indices
  Low MCV—microcytic
  High MCHC—macrocytic
  Low MCHC—hypochromic

CATEGORIES

Nonhemolytic anemia
  Microcytic hypochromic anemia
  Macrocytic anemia (megaloblastic)
  Normocytic normochromic anemia

Hemolytic anemia—may have variable MCV and MCHC indices

MEDICAL MANAGEMENT

Recognition of anemia

Diagnosis of underlyihng cause—variable testing

Treatment of underlying cause

Erythropoietin therapy, as appropriate

Transfusion, if necessary

SUMMARY TABLE 25–II

Normal Red Cell Values (Adult)

	MEN	WOMEN	NORMAL VARIATION
Hemoglobin, Hgb (g/dl)	16.0	14.0	± 2 g/dl
Hematocrit, Hct (%)	47.0	42.0	$\pm 10\%$
Red cell count ($\times 10^6$/mm^3)	4.9	4.4	
Mean corpuscular hemoglobin concentration (MCHC)	34.0	34.0	± 2 g/dl
Mean corpuscular volume (MCV)	95.0	95.0	± 5 μ^3

SUMMARY TABLE 25–III

Medical Evaluation of the Patient with Anemia

HISTORY AND PHYSICAL EXAMINATION

LABORATORY PROCEDURES

Hgb and Hct indices (MCV, MCHC)

Peripheral blood smear

Reticulocyte count

Serum iron and iron-binding capacity

Serum vitamin B_{12} and folate

Stools for occult blood

Blood urea nitrogen

Bone marrow studies—iron stain

HEMOLYTIC ANEMIAS (INCREASE IN RETICULOCYTES, LDH, INDIRECT BILIRUBIN)

Sickle cell preparation

G6PD and other enzyme studies

Osmotic fragility

Hemoglobin electrophoresis

Coombs' test

SUMMARY TABLE **25–IV**

Intrinsic Red Cell Disorders (Hemolytic Anemia)

MEMBRANE DISEASES
Hereditary spherocytosis
High-sodium red cells
Spur cell anemia

DISORDERS OF HEMOGLOBIN
Thalassemia
Sickle cell anemia
Unstable hemoglobins

DISORDERS OF ENZYMES
G6PD deficiency
Errors in carbohydrate metabolism (e.g., pyruvate kinase)

SUMMARY TABLE **25–V**

Extrinsic Hemolytic Anemia

INFECTIONS
Infectious mononucleosis
Viral pneumonia

TRANSFUSION REACTIONS

AUTOIMMUNE HEMOLYTIC ANEMIA
Idiopathic
Drug-induced—quinidine, alcohol, pencillin
Secondary to lymphoproliferative disorder
Systemic lupus erythematosus
Trauma

TRAUMATIC HEMOLYTIC ANEMIA
Microangiopathic anemia
Malignant hypertension
Prosthetic valves

Dental Evaluation of the Patient with Anemia

Patients without a history of anemia but with symptoms should have a CBC and MCV and MCH-indices.

Patients with a history of anemia and no recent physical examination should have a CBC and MCV and MCHC indices.

PATIENTS AT LOW RISK

Past history of anemia, asymptomatic, anemia corrected, normal hematocrit

Identified cause of mild anemia, hematocrit higher than 30%, no therapy

Identified cause of mild anemia, hematocrit higher than 30%, current therapy, and asymptomatic

Anemia of chronic disease, hematocrit higher than 30% and stable, asymptomatic

PATIENTS AT HIGH RISK

Patients without previously diagnosed anemia with abnormal CBC and MCV and MCHC indices on screening

All patients with hematocrit lower than 30% with no identified cause

Patients with evidence of ongoing bleeding

Patients with coagulopathy and anemia

Patients requiring repeated transfusions to prevent symptoms of anemia

Dental Management of the Patient with Anemia

PATIENTS AT LOW RISK

Normal dental protocol

PATIENTS AT HIGH RISK

Defer elective dental care until clinical status optimized

Stress reduction protocol
    Shorter appointments
    Consider sedation techniques

Outpatient intravenous sedation and general anesthesia contraindicated

Hospitalization for moderate and advanced surgical procedures

Bleeding Disorders

Hemostasis is a complicated process involving a number of physiologic events. When a blood vessel is damaged, marked vasoconstriction results. Platelets adhere to the damaged surface and aggregate to form a temporary hemostatic plug. Through two separate pathways, involving a cascade of 12 circulating plasma proteins called clotting factors, the conversion of fibrinogen to fibrin is completed. Fibrin tightly binds the aggregated platelets to form a definitive clot. Finally, anticlotting mechanisms in the fibrinolytic pathway are activated to prevent propagation of the clot and to allow clot dissolution and repair of the damaged vessel. Successful hemostasis is therefore dependent on vessel wall integrity, adequate numbers of platelets, proper functioning platelets, adequate levels of clotting factors, and proper functioning of the fibrinolytic pathway (Fig. 26–1).

Patients with bleeding disorders may have one of a number of defects. Management differs depending on the cause. It is therefore important to be familiar with the mechanism of hemostasis, diagnostic tests, and the medical management of patients with bleeding disorders.

MECHANISM OF HEMOSTASIS

When the integrity of a vessel's endothelium is interrupted, underlying collagen fibers are exposed to the circulation. This collagen attracts platelets, and a loose aggregate called the temporary hemostatic plug is formed on the damaged surface. Aggregated platelets release substances that cause local vasoconstriction and facilitate the formation of a definitive clot.

Formation of a definitive clot is dependent on a complex series of biochemical reactions that ultimately leads to the formation of a fibrin clot. These reactions involve conversion of an inactive coagulation plasma protein into an active coagulation factor that activates the

next coagulation factor in the cascade. The final step in this cascade is the conversion of the plasma protein fibrinogen to fibrin. Fibrinogen is a large, soluble protein produced by the liver, and its conversion to fibrin is catalyzed by the enzyme thrombin. The generation of thrombin follows the same general principle as fibrin in that an inactive precursor, prothrombin, is converted to the active enzyme, thrombin. This conversion is mediated by activated Factor X (Xa). Activated Factor X can be generated by one of two pathways:

The intrinsic pathway (Fig. 26–2) is a coagulation cascade initiated by the exposure of Factor XII to endothelial surface agents such as collagen. Each reaction generates an active product that in turn activates the next coagulation factor.

The extrinsic pathway (see Fig. 26–2) involves only one coagulation protein, Factor VII. A tissue factor (tissue thromboplastin) is released with vascular injury. Factor VII complexes with the tissue factor and calcium, and catalyzes the activation of Factor X.

This complicated series of reactions results in the formation of a definitive clot.

LABORATORY EVALUATION OF HEMOSTASIS

Hemostatic defects are caused by abnormalities of platelets or coagulation factors. These defects can be diagnosed with a few simple laboratory tests.

The platelet count provides a quantitative evaluation of platelet function. The normal platelet count should be 100,000 to 400,000 cells/mm^3. A platelet count of less than 100,000 cells/mm^3 is called thrombocytopenia. Mild thrombocytopenia (platelet count in the range of 50,000 to 100,000 cells/mm^3) can result in abnormal bleeding postoperatively. Severe thrombocytopenia (platelet count below 50,000 cells/mm^3) can be associated with major postoperative bleeding.

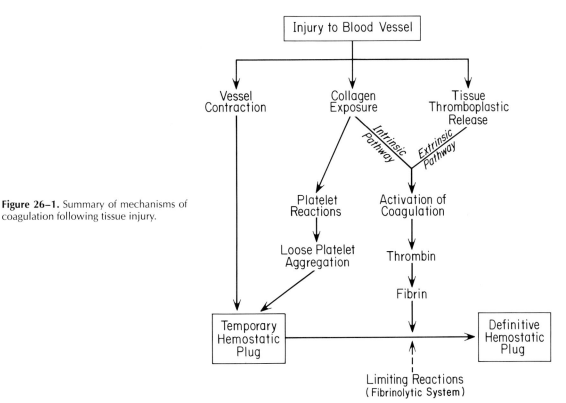

Figure 26–1. Summary of mechanisms of coagulation following tissue injury.

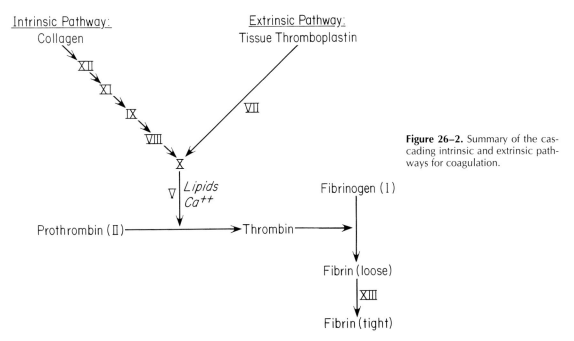

Figure 26–2. Summary of the cascading intrinsic and extrinsic pathways for coagulation.

The bleeding time provides an assessment of the adequacy of platelet count and function. The test measures how long it takes a standardized skin incision to stop bleeding by the formation of a temporary hemostatic plug. The normal range of bleeding time is dependent on the way the test is performed but is usually between 5 and 10 minutes. The bleeding time is prolonged in patients with platelet abnormalities.

The prothrombin time (PT) measures the effectiveness of the extrinsic pathway to mediate fibrin clot formation. It is performed by measuring the time it takes to form a clot when calcium and a tissue factor are added to plasma. A normal PT indicates normal levels of Factor VII and those factors common both to the intrinsic and extrinsic pathways (V, X, prothrombin, and fibrinogen). A normal PT is usually between 11 and 15 seconds. The value is generally compared with a daily control value generated by the laboratory using standardized normal plasma. A prolonged PT can be associated with abnormal postoperative coagulation and bleeding. Prolongation of less than 1½ times the control value is usually not associated with severe bleeding disorders, whereas further prolongation can result in severe bleeding. The PT is most often used by physicians to monitor oral anticoagulant therapy.

The partial thromboplastin time (PTT) measures the effectiveness of the intrinsic pathway in mediating fibrin clot formation. It therefore tests for all factors except Factor VII. The test is performed by measuring the time it takes to form a clot after the addition of kaolin, a surface activating factor, and cephalin, a substitute for platelet factor, to the patient's plasma. A normal PTT is usually 25 to 40 seconds. The values may also be compared with a control value. Prolongation of the PTT by 5 to 10 seconds above the upper limit of normal may be associated with mild bleeding abnormalities. Further prolongation may be associated with significant bleeding. The PTT is most often used by physicians to monitor heparin therapy.

Almost all bleeding disorders can be diagnosed by screening the platelet count, bleeding time, PT, and PTT. In some instances, special tests can be performed to provide additional information about the nature of the hemostatic defect. Several aspects of platelet function can be tested in the laboratory, including platelet adhesiveness and platelet aggregation. Specific factor assays can also be performed in patients with suspected or known factor deficiencies.

DISEASES CAUSING ABNORMALITIES OF HEMOSTASIS

Almost all hemostatic defects are caused by abnormalities of either platelets or coagulation factors. In rare instances, bleeding disorders may be a result of capillary fragility.

Platelet Disorders

Thrombocytopenia

Inadequate platelet numbers can result in clinically significant bleeding. The bleeding usually involves small superficial vessels and produces petechiae in the skin or mucous membranes. Genetic disorders leading to thrombocytopenia are rare; in most instances, thrombocytopenia is acquired. Thrombocytopenia can result from increased platelet destruction, decreased production, or increased splenic sequestration.

Drug-Induced Thrombocytopenia. Drugs can cause thrombocytopenia through marrow toxicity or platelet destruction (Summary Table 26–I).

Cytotoxic drugs, alcohol, and thiazide diuretics are the most common drugs implicated in the suppression of platelet production by the bone marrow. Usually, thrombocytopenia resolves after discontinuation of the drug.

Some drugs can cause thrombocytopenia by increasing peripheral platelet destruction. This is usually mediated by an immunologic mechanism. Quinine, quinidine, and methyldopa (Aldomet) are the most commonly implicated drugs. Other drugs include sulfonamides, heparin, gold, D-penicillamine, and p-aminosalicylic acid.

Immune Thrombocytopenic Purpura (ITP) and Thrombotic Thrombocytopenic Purpura (TTP). Immune thrombocytopenic purpura is a syndrome in which rapid platelet destruction occurs secondary to an immunologic mechanism. The illness may be acute or chronic and may be associated with clinical bleeding. Gingival biopsy is helpful in making a diagnosis in about 30% of cases.

TTP is an uncommon syndrome seen mostly in young women. It is characterized by a clinical pentad of thrombocytopenia, anemia, fever, neurologic signs, and renal failure.

Bone Marrow Failure. Thrombocytopenia can result from failure of the bone marrow to produce platelets. Bone marrow failure can be secondary to drugs, particularly cytotoxic agents. Deficiency of vitamin B_{12} or folate can result in inadequate platelet synthesis. Infiltration of the bone marrow by abnormal cells in patients with leukemia or metastatic cancer can also result in bone marrow failure. Less common causes of bone marrow failure include myelofibrosis and aplastic anemia.

Hypersplenism. Increases in spleen size can lead to sequestration and destruction of platelets. Hypersplenism is most commonly associated with portal hypertension in patients with cirrhosis. Other causes, such as chronic infections, inflammatory diseases, neoplasms, and storage disease, are considerably less common.

Thrombocytopathy

Some patients have adequate numbers of platelets but prolonged bleeding times. In these patients, abnormalities of platelet function must be considered. Platelet dysfunction can be an acquired or a congenital defect.

Inherited Disorders. Several inherited disorders affect platelet function. The most common is von Willebrand's disease, in which there is deficiency in the synthesis of a plasma factor necessary for platelet function as well as a deficiency in the production of Factor VIII. Less common inherited abnormalities of platelet function include Bernard-Soulier syndrome and storage pool diseases.

Acquired Disorders. Acquired abnormalities of platelet function are far more common than inherited disorders.

Drug-Induced Defects. The most common reason for a prolonged bleeding time is the ingestion of drugs that can affect platelet function.

Ingestion of small doses of aspirin (0.3 to 1.5 g) produces impairment of platelet function for 7 to 10 days, a period roughly corresponding to the platelet life span. This finding suggests that aspirin produces an irreversible effect on the platelet.

The effects of other nonsteroidal anti-inflammatory drugs (NSAIDs) (indomethacin, phenylbutazone, meclofenamic acid, ibuprofen, zomepirac sodium, naproxen, fenoprofen, and tolmetin) on platelets appear to be similar to those of aspirin, although they appear to be short-lived (approximately 6 hours).

Concurrent ingestion of alcohol after dosing with acetylsalicylic acid or NSAIDs can markedly increase the latter drugs' impact on bleeding time. A "no alcohol" order is appropriate, for example, when a patient is using NSAIDs as an analgesic following dental surgery.

Drugs that rarely impair platelet function are the tricyclic antidepressants, some anti-histamines and phenothiazines, nitrofurantoin (Furadantin), carbenicillin, dipyridamole, and some cephalosporins.

Clinically, the drug-induced hemostatic effect usually is relatively mild. Some apparently normal subjects display marked sensitivity to the action of aspirin, however, and have marked prolongation of bleeding time. These patients can have significant clinical hemorrhage, particularly during or after surgery. In general, aspirin and other NSAIDs should be avoided when optimum hemostasis is desirable.

Uremia. Patients with renal failure have impaired platelet function that can result in bleeding disorders. The defective platelet function and the hemostatic abnormality largely disappear 24 to 48 hours after peritoneal dialysis or hemodialysis, suggesting the presence of a dialyzable inhibitor in uremic plasma.

Myeloproliferative Disorders. Patients with myeloproliferative disorders such as essential thrombocythemia, polycythemia vera, chronic granulocytic leukemia, and myeloid metaplasia all have impaired platelet function.

Thrombocytopenia Related to Acquired Immune Deficiency Syndrome (AIDS)

Approximately 11% of patients infected with HIV (human immunodeficiency virus) manifest a platelet count of 100,000 cells/mm³ or less. Of interest has been the finding that thrombocytopenia may precede the actual development of symptomatic HIV infection (AIDS). The decrease in platelets observed in these patients is probably related to an effect of the virus on the patient's bone marrow, because other myelosuppressive changes may also be noted.

Based on these findings, the dentist treating patients who are seropositive for HIV, whether or not they are symptomatic, should ascertain the patient's platelet status before performing surgical therapy. As with other patients at risk for bleeding, block anesthesia is to be avoided. Although postoperative bleeding may be a concern following extraction, the use of Gelfoam or similar materials is to be avoided, because they may act as potential sites of infection in the immunocompromised host.

Disorders of Blood Coagulation

Congenital Disorders

A number of congenital clotting factor deficiencies has been described, but three diseases account for more than 90% of all inherited procoagulant deficiencies: hemophilia A, hemophilia B, and von Willebrand's disease.

Hemophilia A. Hemophilia A, or classic hemophilia, is caused by a deficiency of Factor VIII. The disorder is inherited in a sex-linked recessive fashion and is therefore more common in males. The severity of the disease closely parallels the level of circulating Factor VIII. Patients with severe disease have less than 1% Factor VIII; those with moderate disease have 1 to 5% Factor VIII; and those with mild disease have levels of Factor VIII ranging from 6 to 30%.

Patients with hemophilia A, even those with mild disease, have significant bleeding with minor trauma and are at high risk for bleeding after surgical procedures.

Hemophilia B. Hemophilia B, or Christmas disease, is secondary to Factor IX deficiency and is also transmitted as a sex-linked recessive trait. The disease is much less common than hemophilia A but has identical clinical manifestations.

Von Willebrand's Disease. Originally described as a bleeding disorder associated with an autosomal dominant mode of inheritance, von Willebrand's disease is now known to exist in several genetic variants. Patients with the disease have evidence of both abnormal platelet function and deficiency of Factor VIII.

Acquired Disorders

Deficiency of vitamin K–dependent coagulation factors is the most common acquired coagulation disorder. Factors II (prothrombin), VII, IX, and X are made in the liver and require vitamin K for synthesis of their active forms. Among these factors, Factor VII has the shortest half-life (3 to 5 hours), and a prolonged PT is the first laboratory abnormality seen in patients with deficiency of the vitamin K–dependent coagulation factors. The deficiency can result from an inability of the liver to synthesize these factors or from vitamin K deficiency caused by oral anticoagulants, malabsorption, or chronic antibiotic therapy.

Liver Disease. With severe hepatic failure, synthesis of a number of coagulation factors (the vitamin K–dependent Factors II, VII, IX, and X, as well as Factors I and V) may be compromised. Parenteral vitamin K is not helpful, because the defect is not one of vitamin K deficiency but rather of the inability of the liver to perform the necessary synthetic function.

Oral Anticoagulants. Coumarin anticoagulants competitively inhibit vitamin K action. Coumarin is used clinically to prevent thromboembolic events and is useful in patients with deep venous thrombophlebitis, chronic atrial fibrillation, pulmonary emboli, mural thrombi, and cerebrovascular diseases. Anticoagulation therapy is usually monitored by following serial PTs. In most instances, the PT is maintained in a range of 1½ to 2 times the control value.

The effect of these anticoagulants can be reversed with replacement transfusions with fresh-frozen plasma or the administration of vitamin K.

Heparin Therapy. Heparin is an anticoagulant given intravenously. It has a rapid onset of action and is used in hospitalized patients with thromboembolic diseases. Heparin acts by accelerating the inactivation of thrombin. Heparin therapy can be guided by the monitoring of the PTT. In most instances, the PTT is maintained in the 50- to 65-second range, compared to a normal value of 25 to 40 seconds.

Malabsorption. Vitamin K is fat-soluble and requires bile acids for absorption. In patients with intestinal diseases that interfere with bile acid metabolism, vitamin K absorption also is compromised, leading to a deficiency in vitamin K–dependent coagulation factors.

In summary, abnormalities in hemostasis can result from quantitative or qualitative abnormalities of platelets and from deficiencies of coagulation factors. These abnormalities may be inherited or acquired and can lead to significant clinical bleeding in the dental patient if appropriate precautions are not exercised.

MEDICAL EVALUATION

Patients undergo medical evaluation for bleeding disorders under a number of circumstances: a history of abnormal bleeding, either spontaneous or following trauma or surgery; a family history of bleeding disorders; or an abnormal platelet count, PT, PTT, or bleeding time noted during screening evaluation, usually before surgery.

When evaluating a patient for a bleeding disorder, the history is of paramount importance. Excessive menstrual bleeding or abnormal bleeding following trauma or surgery (including dental procedures) provide clues that a bleeding disorder may be present. The type of bleeding may also provide clues about the cause of the disorder. Bleeding resulting from a platelet disorder usually involves superficial small vessels and produces petechiae in the skin and mucous membranes (Fig. 26–3). Coagulation defects are associated with more prominent bleeding in deep tissues; bleeding into a joint with minor trauma, for instance, is characteristic of coagulation abnormalities.

The family history is important in revealing inherited disorders such as clotting factor deficiencies and von Willebrand's disease. Patients giving a positive family history for bleeding disorders require additional evaluation.

When a bleeding disorder is suspected, the medical status of the patient is reviewed. Patients with liver disease may have difficulties with synthesis of coagulation factors. Patients with a number of gastrointestinal problems may have malabsorption and vitamin K deficiency. Patients with dietary deficiencies may have vitamin B_{12} or folate deficiency and decreased production of platelets because of compromised marrow function. It is particularly important to identify patients with alcohol abuse problems and cirrhosis. These patients are particularly at risk for bleeding

disorders: they may have liver dysfunction limiting the synthesis of coagulation factors; they may have dietary deficiency of vitamin K, vitamin B_{12}, and folate; and they may have increased destruction of platelets because of hypersplenism.

In a number of other cases, a medical illness may compromise hemostasis. Patients with disseminated malignancies may have bone marrow failure because of tumor infiltration. Patients with uremia or myeloproliferative diseases may have abnormal platelet function.

Medications taken by the patient should be carefully reviewed. Some drugs, such as oral anticoagulants, have obvious effects on hemostasis. Others, such as aspirin, are less predictable in their effects. Some individuals are sensitive to aspirin and have abnormal bleeding after aspirin ingestion. This abnormality persists for the entire life span of the affected platelets (7 to 10 days).

Other medications that may affect hemostasis include cytotoxic drugs, NSAIDs, and others noted earlier (Summary Table 26–I).

After a detailed history, laboratory evaluation should include platelet count, PT, PTT, and bleeding time. These screening tests can detect almost all significant hemostatic defects.

Patients with a decreased platelet count (less than 100,000/mm³) should be evaluated for diseases that can decrease platelet production or increase platelet destruction.

Patients with a prolonged PT have abnormalities in the extrinsic pathway. In most instances, this defect is secondary to deficiency of clotting factors, either inherited or acquired.

Patients with a prolonged PTT have abnormalities in the intrinsic pathway. Again, the

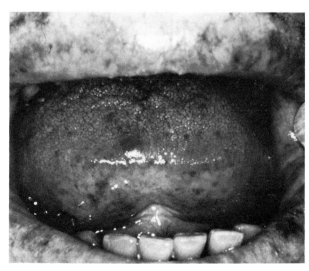

Figure 26–3. Petechiae on both the dorsal and ventral surfaces of the tongue with thrombocytopenia.

defect is usually secondary to a clotting factor deficiency. In rare instances, patients with systemic lupus erythematosus may have circulating anticoagulants that can prolong the PTT without affecting the PT. Interestingly, these patients usually do not have clinically significant bleeding disorders.

In patients with prolonged bleeding time, special studies can help delineate the nature of the platelet defect. In patients with coagulopathy, specific factor assays can be done, both to identify the factor deficiency and to determine the degree of the deficiency.

With a careful history and laboratory evaluation, it is possible to determine the nature of the bleeding disorder and permit medical management.

MEDICAL MANAGEMENT

The medical management of the patient with a bleeding disorder is dependent on the nature of the hemostatic defect.

Platelet Disorders

Thrombocytopenia

All medications that can cause thrombocytopenia should be discontinued. Some of the common offenders are noted in Summary Table 26–I.

In the thrombocytopenic patient, it is also important to avoid drugs that can compromise the function of the remaining platelets. Aspirin and aspirin-containing drugs are the major offenders. Because more than 200 medications contain aspirin, the patient should consult the physician before taking any medication, however innocuous it may appear. Commonly prescribed drugs that contain aspirin can be found in Chapter 50.

Thrombocytopenic patients having significant clinical bleeding and when undergoing surgical procedures need platelet replacement. This is accomplished by the use of platelet packs. Each unit usually raises the patient's platelet count by about 10,000/mm³. In patients undergoing elective surgery, the platelets should be given about 20 minutes prior to the procedure. Washed platelets or whole blood are alternative means of platelet replacement. Whole blood is a poor substitute, however, because platelet survival is poor in whole blood stored for more than a few hours. Platelets are available through blood banks and usually are dispensed on the order of a physician.

Thrombocytopathy

In rare instances, thrombocytopathy is the result of an inherited disorder. The most common of these disorders is von Willebrand's disease. These patients also have a deficiency of Factor VIII and are managed with the use of cryoprecipitates.

In the majority of cases, thrombocytopathy is the result of drugs or systemic illnesses. Drugs capable of impairing platelet function should be discontinued. The bleeding time test should be repeated a week later; elective surgical procedures can proceed if the bleeding time has returned to normal.

In patients with uremia, dialysis should improve platelet dysfunction. Platelet dysfunction can be corrected with desmopressin acetate (DDAVP), estrogen, or cryoprecipitate. DDAVP has been found to be effective in the reversal of bleeding dysfunction in some patients with prolonged bleeding time. DDAVP is administered in doses of 0.4 μg/kg body weight and should be administered 2 to 4 hours before the procedure. The bleeding time determination should be repeated prior to the procedure to monitor improvement. In some patients with prolonged bleeding time, a short course of estrogen therapy may reverse the bleeding diathesis. Estrogen has to be administered for 7 to 10 days to be effective. Determination of the bleeding time has to be repeated prior to the procedure to monitor improvement. Cryoprecipitates are less commonly used now because of concerns that arise from the use of any blood products.

Coagulopathy

The cause of the coagulopathy should be carefully assessed.

Patients with vitamin K deficiency, because of compromised gastrointestinal absorption or dietary deficiency, can have vitamin K replaced parenterally. Vitamin K can be given either intramuscularly or intravenously. The usual dose is 10 mg daily for 3 days.

Patients on warfarin (Coumadin) therapy have inhibition of hepatic synthesis of vitamin K–dependent coagulation factors. This can be reversed in a variety of ways. Withdrawal of the drug leads to slow reversal of the coagulopathy over a period of 7 to 10 days. Administration of parenteral vitamin K leads to reversal of the abnormality over 6 to 12 hours. Rapid reversal of the coagulopathy can also be achieved by clotting factor replacement using fresh-frozen plasma. In view of concerns over the use of any blood products, fresh-frozen plasma should be used judiciously.

Patients with clotting factor deficiency can have parenteral replacement of the clotting factors. Fresh-frozen plasma is most commonly used. It contains all the procoagulants and can be used in the therapy of patients with clotting factor deficiency.

Concentrated Factor VIII with fibrinogen is available as a cryoprecipitate. This is most commonly used in the management of patients with hemophilia A and von Willebrand's disease. Less frequently, it is used in patients with uremia. The available units of Factor VIII in cryoprecipitate are 10 times that found in fresh-frozen plasma. Currently, lyophilized or other purified preparations of Factor VIII are available in the management of patients with hemophilia A.

Prothrombin complex concentrates (Proplex) are lyophilized concentrates of Factors II, VII, IX, and X. Their use is limited because of concerns over hepatitis B and thromboembolism.

Other therapeutic options that are less commonly employed include the use of E-amino-caproic acid (EACA). This agent blocks the lysis of formed clots by blocking the activation of fibrinolytic system. It can be given either intravenously or orally and is sometimes used in the management of patients with hemophilia.

DENTAL EVALUATION

All dental patients should be routinely screened for possible bleeding disorders. The medical questionnaire should include inquiries regarding easy bruisability, bleeding, or clotting problems. Excessive menstrual bleeding, frequent nosebleeds, or unusual bleeding following trauma or surgery provide clues for possible bleeding disorders. Specific questions regarding excessive bleeding following tooth extraction or periodontal surgery should be asked. Family history of bleeding disorders should be noted.

Patient medications should be reviewed. Specific questions regarding aspirin ingestion and anticoagulant therapy should be asked. Patients often fail to report aspirin as a medication. Furthermore, because there are more

than 200 aspirin-containing compounds commercially available, patients may not be aware that they are taking aspirin. Provisions should be made in the dental questionnaire to allow for entry of all over-the-counter drugs the patient uses to detect aspirin-containing medications.

During the dental examination, the dentist should be alert to the physical findings suggestive of a bleeding disorder. Ecchymoses, petechiae, and unusual bleeding are grounds for further screening for possible bleeding disorders.

Finally, prior to moderate and advanced dental surgery, patients should be routinely screened for possible bleeding diathesis. If there are suspicious historical or clinical findings, laboratory screening tests are recommended. The tests should include platelet count, PT, PTT, and bleeding time. These tests can be done in the outpatient departments of hospitals or in commercial laboratories. They screen for almost all clinically significant bleeding diatheses.

Based on the history, examination, and laboratory tests, patients can be grouped into three categories.

Patients at Low Risk
1. Patients with no history of bleeding disorders, normal examination, and normal bleeding parameters
2. Patients with nonspecific history of excessive bleeding but with normal bleeding parameters (normal platelet count, PT, PTT, and bleeding time rule out clinically significant bleeding disorders)

Patients at Moderate Risk
1. Patients on chronic oral anticoagulant therapy and a PT in the therapeutic range (1½ to 2 times the control value)
2. Patients on chronic aspirin therapy

Patients at High Risk
1. Patients with known bleeding disorders: thrombocytopenia, thrombocytopathy, and clotting factor defects
2. Patients without known bleeding disorders who were found to have abnormal platelet counts, PT, PTT, or bleeding time

DENTAL MANAGEMENT

When the dentist is dealing with a patient having a bleeding disorder, the patient's physician should be consulted and the management of dental therapy discussed in detail. The severity of the bleeding defect plays an important part in the management of the patient. A patient with mild thrombocytopenia is treated differently than a patient with a platelet count of less than 10,000/mm³. A patient with 40% Factor VIII activity is managed differently than a patient with less than 3% activity.

The nature of the defect also influences therapeutic decisions. A patient with thrombocytopenia secondary to a recent course of chemotherapy is expected to have bone marrow recovery over a period of weeks. A patient with thrombocytopenia as a result of hypersplenism, on the other hand, is less likely to have improvement in the platelet count with time. It is therefore reasonable to defer elective dental therapy in the former patient until the bone marrow recovers. It is more appropriate to manage the latter patient with platelet transfusion immediately before dental procedures.

Finally, surgical plans should be designed to allow optimal hemostasis. Attention should be paid to bone fragment removal, buccal or lingual plate reapposition following extraction, soft tissue management, tight suturing of mucoperiosteal flaps, and judicious use of local pressure and clotting aids (Gelfoam, local anesthetics with vasoconstrictor, and topical thrombin).

In all patients with bleeding disorders, aspirin and aspirin-containing medications and NSAIDs should be avoided.

Specific Guidelines

Dental management should also be tailored to the cause of the bleeding disorder and the patient's risk category.

Patients at Low Risk. Patients at low risk are at no increased risk of bleeding and can be managed by normal protocol.

Patients at Moderate Risk. These patients are on therapy that can affect hemostasis, and modifications of the therapeutic regimen are necessary before elective dental therapy.

Patients on Anticoagulant Therapy. Patients on oral anticoagulants usually have significant thromboembolic problems, and unless there are severe bleeding complications, the anticoagulation medication should not be totally and abruptly reversed. The dentist is therefore balancing the risks of a bleeding complication with those of the underlying thromboembolic diseases when managing these patients. The patient's physician should be consulted prior to the initiation of dental therapy, and modifications in the anticoagulation therapy can be tailored according to the needs of the patient.

In general, a partial reversal of the anticoagulation problem is necessary. The goal is to bring the PT to below 1½ that of control value over a period of days.

For nonsurgical and simple surgical procedures (types I to IV) and some moderate surgical procedures (type V), the anticoagulation therapy can be regulated on an outpatient basis. Patients on chronic oral anticoagulant therapy usually have had a recent prothrombin time determination. If the prothrombin time is in the therapeutic range (1½ to 2 times control), the oral anticoagulant should be stopped 2 days before the procedure and an immediate PT determined on the morning of surgery. If the PT is indeed less than 1½ times the control value, dental intervention can proceed with careful attention to hemostasis. Oral anticoagulants can be resumed that evening or the following morning.

For many moderate and all advanced surgical procedures (types V and VI), hospitalization should be considered. The same protocol should be followed: oral anticoagulants should be discontinued 2 days prior to admission; PT should be determined on the morning of surgery, and surgery should proceed only if the PT is less than 1½ times control value. Oral anticoagulants can be resumed the day after surgery.

If excessive bleeding occurs after any procedure, local measures such as additional suturing, topical thrombin, and Gelfoam should be used. In the rare instance in which massive and life-threatening bleeding occurs despite adequate attempt at local control, the patient should be hospitalized and fresh-frozen plasma given to reverse the anticoagulation immediately. It must be stressed that this should be undertaken only in extreme circumstances, because complete reversal of anticoagulation would subject the patient to the risk of the underlying thromboembolic disease that necessitated the anticoagulation therapy in the first place. Reversal of anticoagulation should not be done without close medical supervision.

Patients on Chronic Aspirin Therapy. Patients may be on chronic aspirin therapy for a variety of indications; aspirin may be used as an analgesic for headache, toothache, and other minor pain or may be used in patients with arthritis, transient ischemic attacks and, in some patients, to prevent myocardial infarction.

Patients on chronic aspirin therapy should have a template bleeding time test performed prior to elective dental therapy. Aspirin ingestion increases the bleeding time minimally in most patients and the hemostatic effect is usually relatively mild. However, some patients may have marked sensitivity to aspirin and have prolongation of the bleeding time to beyond the normal range. If the prolongation is minimal (less than 2 minutes beyond the normal range), some atraumatic dental procedures unlikely to cause excessive bleeding (types I to III procedures) can be undertaken after consultation with the patient's physician. Mandibular nerve block, scaling, and operative procedures that may induce significant gingival bleeding (some type II and III procedures) and all dental surgery (types IV to VI procedures) should be deferred. Aspirin and aspirin-containing drugs should be stopped for a week and the bleeding time should be redetermined. A repeat bleeding time test within normal limits provides clearance to proceed with dental therapy. Aspirin should not be resumed until adequate soft tissue healing is accomplished and the risk of postoperative bleeding is minimized. This usually requires a "no aspirin" order for from a few days to a week postoperatively. Substitutes for aspirin may be necessary; sodium salicylate or other mild analgesics can be used. NSAIDs should be avoided, however, because they have similar effects on platelet function.

If the bleeding time remains prolonged 7 to 10 days after the termination of all drugs affecting platelet functions, an inherited defect in platelet function should be considered and the patient referred to the physician for further evaluation.

NSAIDs (e.g., Motrin) can also have an impact on platelet adherence similar to that of aspirin. The altered platelet function is more transitory and may have disappeared within 6 hours of taking the medication. Appropriate management of these drugs may involve discontinuing the drug for 1 day prior to the planned procedure, obtaining a repeat bleeding time the day of the procedure, and proceeding accordingly.

It is important to note that alcohol ingestion after acetylsalicylic acid or NSAID dosing will markedly increase the impact of the latter drugs on bleeding time.

Patients at High Risk. Patients with markedly abnormal bleeding parameters are at high risk during dental procedures. In these patients it is important to identify the nature of the bleeding disorder, because management must be tailored according to the cause of the hemostatic defect. Dental management of these patients requires close coordination of care with the patient's physician, and hospitalization is often advisable.

Patients with Thrombocytopenia. Thrombocytopenia can occur as a result of inadequate production, sequestration, or enhanced destruction of platelets. The medical evaluation and management have been detailed in previous sections.

Occasionally, a thrombocytopenic patient may present to the dentist first because of problems with gingival bleeding. If thrombocytopenia is documented, the patient should be referred for medical evaluation before elective dental intervention.

In general, dental procedures should be deferred if the thrombocytopenia is expected to reverse within a reasonable period. This applies to patients with drug-induced thrombocytopenia, dietary deficiency, and transient bone marrow suppression secondary to chemotherapy.

In some instances, the platelet count is not expected to recover. Patients with bone marrow failure secondary to tumor infiltration and patients with hypersplenism are examples. These patients require platelet transfusions prior to most dental procedures.

Platelet transfusion should be given about 20 minutes before the planned procedure. Each unit of platelets is expected to raise the platelet count by 10,000/mm³, and in most instances, patients are given 10 units of platelets prior to the procedure.

For patients with platelet counts in the 50,000 to 100,000 range, nonsurgical procedures not expected to cause excessive bleeding can be done with strict attention to hemostasis. Mandibular nerve block, scaling, and operative procedures that induce significant gingival bleeding and all dental surgery should be performed after platelet transfusion.

It is important to remember that drugs with antiplatelet action should not be used in patients with thrombocytopenia.

Patients with Thrombocytopathy. The dental management of patients with drug-induced thrombocytopathy has been discussed earlier.

Patients with uremia may have significant bleeding time prolongation. In all patients with significant uremia (blood urea nitrogen [BUN] greater than 50 mg/dl), bleeding times should be determined. In the instance when bleeding time is prolonged, the patient's physician should be consulted to tailor the therapy. Dialysis can correct the platelet function abnormality. In patients who are not on dialysis, DDAVP, estrogen therapy and, in special situations, cryoprecipitates may be useful.

Some patients may have inherited disorders in platelet function. The majority of these patients have von Willebrand's disease and are managed with cryoprecipitates, which correct both the Factor VIII deficiency and the platelet function abnormality. The rare patient with other forms of inherited disorders causing thrombocytopathy can be managed with platelet transfusion.

Patients with Inherited Coagulopathy. The patient with an inherited deficiency in clotting factors presents a difficult management problem. Hemophilia A (Factor VIII deficiency), hemophilia B (Factor IX deficiency), and von Willebrand's disease (Factor VIII deficiency with an associated thrombocytopathy) account for more than 90% of patients with inherited disorders of coagulation. In these patients, the severity of the disease is dependent on the plasma activity of the clotting factors. Patients with less than 50% plasma clotting factor activity have some postoperative bleeding. Severe bleeding occurs in patients with less than 20% plasma clotting factor activity.

Most dental procedures should be done in the hospital in patients with significant inherited disorders of coagulation. The dentist should work closely with the patient's physician or hematologist to optimize management.

Patients with hemophilia A require preoperative Factor VIII replacement, usually in the form of cryoprecipitates (concentrated Factor VIII) or a lypholized form of concentrated Factor VIII. Because the half-life of Factor VIII is 12 hours, the patient should receive replacement therapy every 12 hours until bleeding is no longer a clinical concern.

Aminocaproic acid may be used postoperatively to prevent clot lysis at the discretion of the patient's hematologist. Patients with hemophilia B require preoperative Factor IX replacement. The half-life of Factor IX is 24 hours, and daily infusions should be continued until bleeding is no longer a concern.

Patients with von Willebrand's disease present a special problem. The correction of Factor VIII deficiency is sometimes inadequate for control of bleeding because of the associated platelet function abnormalities in these patients. Unlike other thrombocytopathies that respond to platelet transfusions, the thrombocytopathy of von Willebrand's disease is responsive to serum factors found in cryoprecipitates. Cryoprecipitates must be given more frequently than in patients with hemophilia A, and usually 3 to 6 units of cryoprecipitates are given every 6 to 12 hours for bleeding control. The lypholized form of concentrated Factor VIII, on the other hand, does not contain the serum factor and should not be used.

It is also important to remember that many patients with inherited disorders of coagulation have received multiple transfusions and are therefore at high risk for hepatitis infections. Hepatitis B surface antigen and hepatitis B antibody should be determined in these patients (Chap. 23).

Drugs that can affect platelet function such as aspirin or NSAIDs are strictly contraindicated in these patients.

Patients with Acquired Coagulopathy. The management of patients on anticoagulation therapy has been discussed. Other patients with acquired disorders of coagulopathy have either vitamin K deficiency or liver disease. In all instances, close medical supervision is essential.

Patients with vitamin K deficiency can be managed with parenteral vitamin K. Usually, 10 mg of vitamin K given daily for 3 days is sufficient therapy. The PT should be monitored to ensure correction of the coagulopathy.

Patients with severe liver disease are not able to synthesize certain clotting factors (Factors I, II, V, VII, IX, and X). These patients should be managed with fresh-frozen plasma. Replacement therapy should be given about 2 hours before the planned procedure, and the PT should be determined to ensure correction of the coagulopathy.

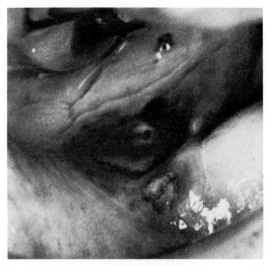

Figure 26–4. Hematoma formation and ecchymosis of the buccal mucosa in a patient with a platelet abnormality.

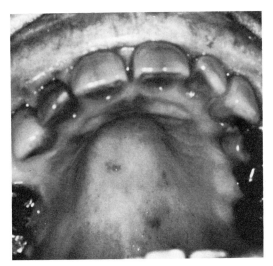

Figure 26–5. Palatal petechiae in a thrombocytopenic patient.

Drugs that can impair platelet function such as aspirin and NSAIDs are contraindicated.

ORAL FINDINGS

The oral findings associated with coagulopathies are discussed in detail under hematologic malignancies (Chap. 27) and cancer chemotherapy (Chap. 42).

Ecchymosis and petechiae are the most common oral findings in patients with bleeding disorders (Figs. 26–4 and 26–5). Their location is most often a mucosal surface. In severe bleeding disorders, spontaneous gingival bleeding may be a presenting symptom to the dentist.

■ Examples of Dental Evaluation and Management

EVALUATION

Patient 1. A 22-year-old woman presents for dental care. The patient gives a history of easy bruisability and heavy menstrual bleeding. Following the extraction of an upper right second bicuspid several years ago, the patient had heavy bleeding and had to return to the dentist "for more sutures." There is no known family history of bleeding disorders. She uses two or three aspirins two or three times each month. Her dental needs include routine operative dentistry, the placement of an upper right quadrant three-unit bridge to replace the missing bi-

cuspid, and extraction of two mandibular third molar impactions.

On examination, her blood pressure is 120/86 and her pulse is 64 beats/minute (bpm) and regular. There are no petechiae or ecchymoses on general inspection.

Patient 2. A 45-year-old woman presents for dental therapy. She has a history of rheumatoid arthritis and has been on chronic aspirin therapy. She is currently taking four aspirins tid. There is no history of use of corticosteroids, gold salts, or penicillamine. Her dental needs are identical to those of Patient 1.

On examination, her blood pressure is 140/86 and her pulse is 75 bpm and regular.

Patient 3. A 54-year-old man presents for dental therapy. The patient had a bout of deep venous thrombophlebitis involving his right leg 4 months ago and is currently taking 7.5 mg of warfarin (Coumadin) each day. He has had blood checks monthly and has not had recent changes in his drug dose. His dental needs include routine operative dentistry in both arches, scaling and root planing for moderate periodontitis, and the removal of six maxillary molars.

His blood pressure is 130/80 and his pulse is 90 bpm and regular.

Patient 4. A 28-year-old man with known hemophilia A presents complaining of bleeding gums. Consultation with his physician reveals that he has a Factor VIII level that is 25% normal. He has had easy bruisability and has required blood and cryoprecipitate transfusions since an automobile accident at age 18.

Clinical examination reveals a generalized advanced gingivitis with heavy plaque and calculus accumulation. In addition, he needs routine operative dentistry in three quadrants.

Physical examination reveals a blood pressure of 130/80 and a regular pulse of 76 bpm.

MANAGEMENT

Patient 1. This patient gives a nonspecific history that is suggestive of a possible bleeding disorder. Prior to the removal of the mandibular impactions, PT, PTT, platelet count, and bleeding time should be determined. If these laboratory values are normal, the patient is at low risk for bleeding, and dental treatment can proceed using normal protocol. Abnormal values for any or all of these tests suggest an undiagnosed bleeding disorder. In these instances, all elective dental procedures should be deferred and the patient referred for further medical evaluation.

Patient 2. This patient is on chronic aspirin therapy and is therefore at moderate risk for bleeding complications during surgical procedures. In many instances, the patient's physician may be able to use alternate forms of analgesics during the perioperative period. Elective dental surgery can then be carried out 7 to 10 days after the patient has stopped aspirin. The bleeding time should be in the normal range prior to any surgical procedure.

For nonsurgical procedures that are not associated with excessive gingival trauma, it is possible to proceed without discontinuation of aspirin therapy provided that the bleeding time is in a reasonable range. In general, if the bleeding time is less than 12 minutes, simple operative procedures not requiring mandibular nerve block may be performed with special attention to local hemostasis. However, if the bleeding time is greater than 12 minutes, even simple operative procedures should be deferred.

Patient 3. This patient is on chronic warfarin (Coumadin) therapy and is at moderate risk for bleeding complications during dental therapy. The patient's physician should be consulted to optimize management. For simple operative dentistry not requiring mandibular nerve block, warfarin may be continued, provided that the PT is in a reasonable range (PT less than twice control value). For surgical procedures associated with gingival trauma, warfarin should be discontinued 2 days prior to the procedure and a PT should be determined prior to surgery. If the PT is less than 1½ times the control value, dental care can proceed. The drug can be resumed the evening after scaling and simple operative procedures. Following multiple extractions, it should be withheld until the day following surgery.

Patient 4. This patient has a significant deficiency in his clotting factor and is at high risk for bleeding complications. The patient should be admitted to the hospital for dental management. The patient's physician should be consulted for perioperative management. Because the patient has a significant deficiency in Factor VIII, cryoprecipitate should be given prior to dental care. Because the half-life of Factor VIII is 12 hours, cryoprecipitate should be repeated at this interval if there is residual bleeding. E-aminocaproic acid may be used postoperatively to prevent clot lysis. The dentist should plan on completing four quadrants of definitive scaling and curettage and all operative procedures under local anesthesia. The lengthy procedure may necessitate adjunctive sedation techniques.

Postoperatively, the analgesics used should not interfere with platelet function, and drugs containing aspirin or NSAIDs are contraindicated.

Thrombocytopenia (Quantitative Platelet Deficiency)

DRUG-INDUCED

Central platelet destruction (marrow toxicity)
   Alcohol
   Thiazide diuretics

Peripheral platelet destruction (immune-mediated)
   Quinidine
   Methyldopa (Aldomet)
   Other (gold salts, sulfonamides, D-penicillamine)

BONE MARROW FAILURE

Drug-induced (see above)

Vitamin deficiency
   Vitamin B$_{12}$
   Folate

Bone marrow infiltration
   Leukemia
   Metastatic cancer

Other (aplastic anemia, myelofibrosis)

HYPERSPLENISM (PLATELET SEQUESTRATION)

Cirrhosis and portal hypertension (most common)

Other (chronic infection, inflammatory diseases, neoplasms, and storage diseases)

IMMUNE THROMBOCYTOPENIC PURPURA (ITP)

THROMBOTIC THROMBOCYTOPENIC PURPURA (TTP)

SUMMARY TABLE **26–II**

Thrombocytopathy (Qualitative Platelet Deficiency)

ACQUIRED: DRUG-INDUCED

Aspirin ingestion (7–10 days irreversible effect with single dose, minor impact common, major impact rare)

Nonsteroidal anti-inflammatory drugs (short-lived, single-dose impact, 6 hr)
  Ibuprofen (Motrin, Advil)
  Naproxen (Naprosyn)
  Fenoprofen (Halfon)
  Indomethacin (Indocin)
  Tolmetin (Tolectin)
  Sulindac (Clinoril)
  Piroxicam (Feldene)
  Ketoprofen (Orudis)

Other (tricyclic antidepressants, phenothiazine, antihistamines, carbenicillin, Furadantin, dipyridamole, some cephalosporins)

ACQUIRED: OTHER

Renal failure (uremia) (BUN >50; creatinine >4)

Myeloproliferative disorders (essential thrombocytopenia, polycythemia vera, chronic granulocytic leukemia, and myeloid metaplasia)

CONGENITAL

Von Willebrand's disease (deficient plasma factor synthesis necessary for platelet function as well as a deficiency in Factor VIII production)

Other (storage pool diseases, Bernard-Soulier syndrome)

SUMMARY TABLE **26–III**

Clotting Factor Deficiencies

CONGENITAL

Hemophilia A (Factor VIII deficiency)
  Sex-linked recessive

Hemophilia B (Factor IX deficiency)
  Sex-linked recessive

} 90%

Von Willebrand's disease (Factor VIII deficiency with platelet function deficiency)
  Several genetic variants

Other factor deficiency

ACQUIRED

Vitamin K–dependent deficiency (Factors II [prothrombin], VII, IX, X)
  Drug-induced (from warfarin)
  Malabsorption disorders
  Liver disease (also affects Factors I [fibrinogen], V)
  Chronic antibiotic therapy

Heparin therapy (accelerates inactivation of thrombin)

Medical Evaluation and Management of the Patient with a Bleeding Disorder

MEDICAL EVALUATION
History
Known history of bleeding disorders
  Easy bruisability
  Frequent nose bleeds
  Heavy menstrual bleeding
  Abnormal history of bleeding following trauma or surgery (dental and other)
  Family history of bleeding disorders

MEDICAL STATUS
Drugs known to cause bleeding disorders

Alcohol abuse

PHYSICAL EXAMINATION
± * petechiae and ecchymosis

LABORATORY ANALYSIS
Basic Screening Tests
Prothrombin time

Partial thromboplastin time

Platelet count

Bleeding time

Other Tests
Fibrinogen levels

Platelet adhesion and aggregation tests

Specific factor assays

Other

MEDICAL MANAGEMENT
Dependent on the nature of the hemostatic defect and its cause (see text)

* ±, with or without.

SUMMARY TABLE **26–V**

Commonly Used Therapeutic Agents in Bleeding Disorders

PLATELET REPLACEMENT

Platelet packs: raise platelet count approximately 10,000/mm^3 per unit given; less effective with multiple transfusions as immunity develops

Uses

Thrombocytopenia: platelet packs given in sufficient units to minimally increase platelet count to greater than 100,000/mm^3; when platelet replacement needed, often given as a 10-unit dose

Thrombocytopathy: if platelet count greater than 100,000/mm^3 and an abnormal BT; often an infusion of 2–4 units of platelet packs is sufficient to correct qualitative platelet defect and allow balance of present platelets to function normally

Other

Washed platelets and *whole blood*—can be used but are less efficient means of platelet replacement; platelet survival in stored whole blood is a few hours, at most

FACTOR REPLACEMENT

1. *Cryoprecipitate:* primarily concentrated Factor VIII (10×/unit versus fresh-frozen plasma) and fibrinogen; primary use—treatment of patients with hemophilia A and von Willebrand's disease; also effective in correcting qualitative platelet disorders found in von Willebrand's disease; half-life of Factor VIII, 12 hr—repeat transfusions at this interval often needed; more frequent infusion required to maintain correction of von Willebrand's qualitative platelet deficiency; cryoprecipitate also used to treat the thrombocytopathy associated with uremia when dialysis correction is not employed
2. *Fresh-frozen plasma:* contains all the procoagulants and is used primarily in the treatment of hemophilia B and all other factor deficiencies, available Factor VIII/unit is 10% that of cryoprecipitate and is therefore not first-choice modality for patients with hemophilia A; fresh-frozen plasma treatment of choice in factor deficiency secondary to liver disease; less commonly, fresh-frozen plasma can be used for rapid reversal of warfarin-induced vitamin K–dependent factor deficiency (II, VII IX, X); half-life of Factor IX is 24 hr—for treatment of hemophilia B, repeat transfusions at this interval are often needed
3. *Prothrombin complex concentrate* (Proplex): lyophilized concentrates of Factors II, VII, IX, X, lyophilized concentrates of Factor VIII also available; use of preparation is limited because of associated complications—thromboembolism, hepatitis B, possibly acquired immune deficiency syndrome (AIDS)

OTHER THERAPEUTIC AGENTS

1. *E-Aminocaproic acid* (EACA; AMICAR): can be given as an IV bolus or orally; blocks lysis of formed clots by blocking activation of the fibrinolytic system; most often used as adjunct to therapy for hemophilia A
2. *Vitamin K:* parenteral vitamin K reverses effect of oral anticoagulants (Coumadin) in 6–12 hr; because associated with difficulty in reinstituting Coumadin therapy, has little use in management of dental patient; 6–12-hr reversal time can be contrasted with 7–10-day reversal with simple withdrawal of Coumadin and rapid reversal with fresh-frozen plasma
3. *Protamine sulfate:* although heparin activity dissipates 4 hr after IV therapy, profamine sulfate rapidly neutralizes heparin
4. *Vasopressin* (DDAVP): found to be effective in reversal of bleeding dysfunction in some patients with prolonged bleeding time; DDAVP in doses of 0.4 mg/kg body weight, should be administered 2 to 4 hr before procedure; bleeding time should be determined prior to procedure to monitor improvement. DDAVP may also be used in mild forms of Factor VIII deficiency.
5. *Estrogen:* in some patients with prolonged bleeding time, short course of estrogen therapy may reverse the bleeding diathesis; estrogen has to be administered for 7- to 10-day period to be effective; bleeding time has to be determined prior to procedure to monitor improvement

Note: All these agents are given by the physician most often in the hospital setting. Their requirement by the dental patient implies mandatory physician consultation.

Basic Laboratory Screening Tests and Normal Values

PLATELET COUNT
Quantitative evaluation of platelet function
  Normal count: 100,000–400,000/mm^3
  Mild thrombocytopenia: 50,000–100,000/mm^3
  Severe thrombocytopenia: <50,000/mm^3

BLEEDING TIME
Assesses adequacy of platelet count (quantitative) and function (qualitative)
  1. In setting of a normal platelet count, bleeding time screens for presence of a thrombocytopathy (qualitative platelet disorder)
  2. Involves assessment of time to stop bleeding following a standardized skin incision
  3. Normal value: 5–10 min

PROTHROMBIN TIME (PT)
Measures ability to form a fibrin clot by extrinsic pathway
  1. Most often used to monitor efficacy of oral anticoagulants (warfarin)
  2. Therapeutic Coumadin maintains PT at 1$^1/_2$–2 times control value range
  3. Patient's PT always reported with daily laboratory control value
  4. Value less than 1$^1/_2$ times control value associated with mild excess bleeding
  5. Value greater than 1$^1/_2$ times control value associated with significant bleeding
  6. Normal value: 11–15 sec

PARTIAL THROMBOPLASTIN TIME (PTT)
Measures ability to form fibrin clot by intrinsic pathway

Prolongation of PTT 5–10 sec above upper limit of normal assoicated with mild bleeding abnormalities

Prolongation of the PTT greater than 10 sec above upper limit of normal associated with significant bleeding abnormalities

Abnormal in the setting of the most common congenital factor deficiencies (VII, IX)

Often used by physician to monitor intravenous anticoagulant (heparin) therapy

Therapeutic heparin maintains PTT in 50–65 sec range

Normal value: 25–40 sec

SPECIFIC FACTOR ASSAYS
Rarely ordered by dentist

Reported as percentage of normal activity
  Severe deficiency: <1% activity
  Moderate deficiency: 1–5% activity
  Mild deficiency: 6–30% activity
  All these above deficiencies are associated with significant bleeding in the clinical setting.

SUMMARY TABLE **26–VII**

Dental Evaluation of the Patient with a Bleeding Disorder

HISTORY
Known history of bleeding disorders

Easy bruisability

Frequent nose bleeds

Heavy menstrual bleeding

Abnormal history of bleeding following trauma or surgery (dental and other)

Family history of bleeding disorders

MEDICAL STATUS
Drugs known to cause bleeding disorders

Alcohol abuse

PHYSICAL EXAMINATION
±* possible petechiae and ecchymoses

LABORATORY ANALYSIS
Prothrombin time (PT)

Partial thromboplastin time (PTT)

Bleeding time

Platelet count

*±, with or without.

SUMMARY TABLE **26–VIII**

Risk Categories for the Patient with a Bleeding Disorder

PATIENTS AT LOW RISK
Patients with no history of bleeding disorders, normal examinations, no medications associated with bleeding disorders, and ±* normal bleeding parameters (tests should be done if patient is taking medications associated with bleeding disorders)

Patients with nonspecific history of excessive bleeding with normal bleeding parameters (PT, PTT, platelet count, bleeding time normal limits)

PATIENTS AT MODERATE RISK
Patients on chronic oral anticoagulant therapy (Coumadin)

Patients on chronic aspirin therapy

PATIENTS AT HIGH RISK
Patients with known bleeding disorders
   Thrombocytopenia
   Thrombocytopathy
   Clotting factor defects

Patients without known bleeding disorders found to have abnormal platelet count, bleeding time, PT, or PTT

*±, with or without.

Dental Management of the Patient with a Bleeding Disorder

RISK CATEGORY	PROCEDURES	PROTOCOL
Low risk	All procedures	Normal protocol
Moderate risk (Coumadin therapy)	I–IV (V)	1. Strict contraindication of aspirin and NSAIDs 2. Strict local hemostatic measures 3. Physician consultation 4. Coumadin management: discontinue drug 2 days prior to procedures; PT day of procedure; If PT <11/2 times control, complete procedure; resume Coumadin day of procedure
	(V) VI	Same as above except resume Coumadin day after procedure 5. Consider hospitalization
Moderate risk (aspirin therapy) if BT is within normal limits (≤10 min) if BT, 10–12 min	I (examination)	Normal protocol
	II–VI	Bleeding time (BT) prior to elective dental treatment
	I–VI	Normal protocol
	I–III	Normal protocol
	IV–VI, or any procedure using block anesthesia or in which patient is at risk for significant gingival trauma	Manage aspirin intake (see below)
BT >12 min	II–VI	Manage aspirin intake 1. Discontinue aspirin for 7–10 days 2. Substitute alternative drug as needed in consultation with physician 3. Repeat bleeding time 4. If bleeding time is normal, continue with procedure 5. Persistent abnormal bleeding time requires further evaluation—refer to physician and/or hematologist 6. Aspirin and NSAIDs contraindicated postoperatively 7. Resume normal aspirin ingestion 7–10 days postoperatively or sooner for nonsurgical procedures
High risk		1. Management varies depending on specific defect 2. Physician consultation mandatory 3. May require hospitalization for use of therapeutic agents (Summary Table 26–V) 4. Complex elective dental care relatively contraindicated

Hematologic Malignancies

LEUKEMIA

The leukemias are a number of diseases characterized by neoplastic changes of the blood-forming elements of the body. The clinical course, cells affected, treatment, and survival vary depending on the form of leukemia. Leukemias are classified by their clinical course into acute and chronic forms and by histologic criteria of bone marrow. Left untreated, leukemic cells proceed from bone marrow to blood and then invade organs and prohibit normal function. The prognosis for untreated leukemia is terrible, with few patients with acute forms of the disease surviving longer than 1 year.

Leukemias are divided histologically into lymphoblastic and nonlymphoblastic forms. The most common form of nonlymphoblastic leukemia, myelogenous leukemia, affects the granulocytic cell line. Each form of leukemia must be treated as an individual disease. For example, acute lymphoblastic leukemia (ALL) is the most common leukemia in children, whereas chronic lymphoblastic leukemia (CLL) is rarely seen before age 20. With the exception of CLL, in which male predominance occurs, there are only slight sex differences in frequency.

A number of possible causes have been associated with leukemia. Almost all have to do with potential modification of cellular genetic material. Chemicals and drugs have been associated with the development of some forms of the disease. Benzene is the compound most frequently associated with its occurrence. Agent Orange, a defoliant used during the Vietnam War, has been implicated as a causative agent.

Following the use of atomic bombs on Hiroshima and Nagasaki in 1945, a large number of exposed individuals developed leukemia at varying times, thereby implicating ionizing radiation as a causative factor of the disease. The role of diagnostic radiation remains unresolved.

Hereditary factors appear to be important in certain forms of the disease. A number of observations support this conclusion. There is a high incidence of leukemia among identical twins when one is affected by the disease. Certain disorders of known genetic cause, such as Down's syndrome, are associated with a high frequency of leukemia.

A number of animal models suggest a role for RNA viruses in the development of leukemia. Experimental and epidemiologic studies in humans are at best equivocal, however, and a viral role in human disease has still not been definitively established.

Medical Evaluation

The presenting signs and symptoms of leukemia are often relatively insidious considering the severity of the disease (Fig. 27–1). Patients may complain of fatigue, malaise, and fever—a symptom complex similar to that of a low-grade viral infection. Unlike a viral syndrome, however, the symptoms do not abate and may progress.

Most symptoms and signs related to leukemia stem from the fact that the bone marrow is overwhelmed with malignant cells, which then spill out into the circulation. Thus, although the absolute white blood count (WBC) of a patient with leukemia may be high, functionally the patient may be neutropenic, because the abnormal cells have crowded out normal cells (Table 27–1). Subsequently, infection caused by a lack of functional neutrophils and bleeding as a consequence of thrombocytopenia are frequent presenting signs. Additionally, tissue infiltrates of leukemic cells into lymph nodes, spleen, or gingiva may occur.

Patients suspected of having leukemia are screened by examining the number of periph-

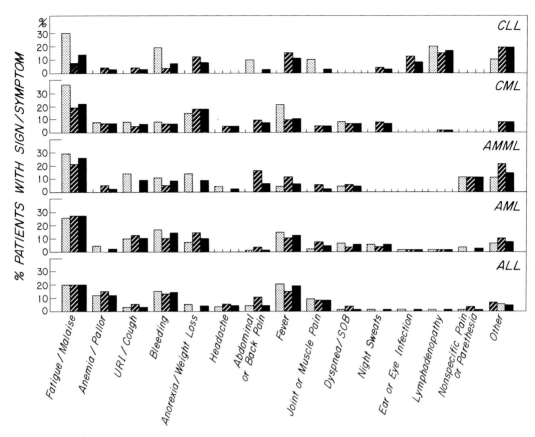

Figure 27–1. Distribution of presenting systemic symptoms in patients with (▨) and without (▦) oral findings compared with the distribution of systemic symptoms in the overall population (■) studied by specific classification of leukemia (CLL, chronic lymphoblastic leukemia; CML, chronic myelogenous leukemia; AMML, acute myelomonocytic leukemia; AML, acute myelogenous leukemia; ALL, acute lymphoblastic leukemia; URI, upper respiratory infection; SOB, shortness of breath). (From Stafford, R.F., Sonis, S., and Lockhart, P.: Oral pathoses as diagnostic indicators in leukemia. Oral Surg., 50:127, 1980.)

eral white blood cells and platelets. Quantitative changes of the WBC are considered characteristic of a leukemic state and result from the presence of increased numbers of malignant cells in peripheral blood. The extent of leukocytosis varies widely, however. Characteristically, it is highest in patients with acute leu-kemia as compared with chronic leukemia. Examination of the blood usually demonstrates many immature or blast forms (Fig. 27–2). Patients with leukemia may also be anemic, as noted by decreased red blood cell production and lowered hemoglobin and hematocrit levels. Similarly, platelet maturation is reduced,

Table 27–1. WBC AND DIFFERENTIAL COUNTS IN LEUKEMIA

Parameter	Normal (%)	Acute Leukemia	CLL	CML
Neutrophils	50–60	10	5–10	20–40
Bands	2–8	0	2–5	10–20
Monocytes	5–8	0	5–8	5–10
Lymphocytes	30–40	5–10	80–80	0–10
Eosinophils	2–5	0	0–2	5–8
Basophils	1–2	0	0–1	2–5
Young forms	0	5–10	0	30–40
Blasts	0	50–80	0	2–5
WBC per mm³	4000–10,000	10,000–100,000	50,000–100,000	100,000–500,000

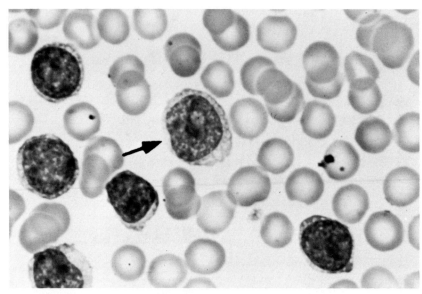

Figure 27–2. Peripheral blood smear demonstrating the presence of immature or blast forms *(arrow)* of a patient with leukemia. (Courtesy of Dr. David Rosenthal.)

and the patient is thus likely to be thrombocytopenic. Definitive diagnosis is dependent on histologic examination of the bone marrow.

Medical Management

All forms of leukemia are treated with chemotherapy. Although the specific agents and regimens vary, much success has been achieved using multimodal therapy. For example, patients with acute myelogenous leukemia (AML) may be treated initially with daunorubicin, cytosine arabinoside, adriamycin, and other agents. Therapy is usually divided into two phases, an induction phase and a maintenance phase. The induction phase is aimed at eliminating or reducing the leukemic population of cells. This is performed immediately after diagnosis. When no leukemic cells are noted in the bone marrow, the patient is said to be in remission. If no further treatment were to be performed, it is likely that the leukemia would again reappear or that the patient would relapse. To prevent this, chemotherapy is given at regular intervals over a 2-year period (maintenance phase). In the case of some forms of leukemia (ALL) in which malignant cells enter the cerebrospinal fluid, radiation therapy may be used to supplement chemotherapy. Chronic leukemia does not generally require as aggressive therapy as acute leukemia.

The prognosis for leukemia varies with the form of the disease and has generally been improving steadily. Acute leukemias (ALL and AML) used to have a universally fatal prognosis. Now, however, the survival rate of children with ALL is over 90% with some treatment protocols. Although the prognosis for AML is not as good, it has shown improvement. The prognosis for the chronic forms of the disease is better; CLL has a better prognosis than chronic myelogenous leukemia (CML).

Dental Evaluation

Undiagnosed Leukemia

Oral pathoses tend to be frequent signs or symptoms in patients with undiagnosed leukemia. Of patients with acute lymphocytic leukemia, approximately 89% have oral problems associated with the onset of their disease. Of these, 22% cite these problems as the reason for seeking medical evaluation for their undiagnosed disease. Almost two-thirds of patients with other forms of acute leukemia demonstrate oral changes during the early, undiagnosed stages of their disease. One-third of these patients seeks medical evaluation because of their oral involvement. Clearly, in patients with acute leukemia, the recognition of oral changes plays a major role in diagnosis of the malignancy.

Oral manifestations of acute leukemia are generally associated with the functionally myelosuppressed state of the patient. The overwhelming presence of malignant cells in the bone marrow results in an actual neutropenia and thrombocytopenia. Hence, patients frequently seek dental care because of gingival oozing, petechiae, hematoma or ecchymosis formation in the case of platelet depletion, or recurrent or unrelenting bacterial infection manifested by profound lymphadenopathy, oral ulceration, pharyngitis, or gingival infection. Patients with high numbers of circulating blast forms may demonstrate gingival hyperplasia resulting from infiltration (Fig. 27–3).

Patients presenting with any of these symptoms or signs must be carefully evaluated to rule out the presence of hematologic malignancy. The clinical approach to a patient who presents with some or all of the symptoms associated with leukemia should include a history, examination, laboratory evaluation and, if required, medical consultation.

Patients should be questioned as to their general health, past episodes of symptoms, systemic signs of myelosuppression (ecchymoses elsewhere, unusually heavy blood flow during menstruation, skin abscess formation, unrelenting pharyngitis, fever, malaise, weight loss), and the course of their oral complaint. Acute leukemia frequently demonstrates a fairly explosive onset; patients having no past oral bleeding may note the sudden onset of spontaneous gingival oozing. Clinical evaluation should include a thorough soft tissue, periodontal, and dental examination, including radiographs. The dentist must question whether the oral findings can be explained on the basis of local factors (bleeding because of plaque or calculus) or whether the oral findings are in disproportion to local factors. If there is any possibility of systemic involvement, the patient should be sent for laboratory evaluation. In screening for leukemia, a complete blood count (CBC), including a differential

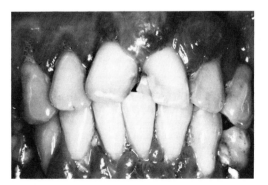

Figure 27–3. Gingival hyperplasia resulting from infiltration of the tissue with circulating leukemic cells (blast forms).

white blood cell count and a platelet count, is recommended. Blood values may vary; however, in the patient with leukemia, the WBC is generally elevated, the differential count demonstrates the presence of atypical cells and a reduction in neutrophils, and the platelet count is reduced. Patients also frequently demonstrate signs of anemia.

Patients in whom the laboratory results are abnormal should be immediately referred to a hematologist for further evaluation.

Diagnosed Leukemia

Frequently, dentists are asked to assess patients with leukemia with respect to the presence of, or potential for, oral infection or other oral problems. Often, this consultation occurs immediately following diagnosis and just prior to the initiation of chemotherapy. As noted elsewhere (Chap. 42), patients with leukemia are in the highest risk category to develop oral problems associated with cancer chemotherapy. Because patients with leukemia are unable to deal with any form of infection effectively, evaluation of the mouth, a frequent portal of entry for microorganisms, is essential. Clearly, the control or elimination of existing or potential sources of infection is critical.

Oral evaluation of the patient with diagnosed leukemia should include soft tissue examination, periodontal evaluation, dental examination, and full mouth radiographs that include the periapical and third molar areas. If the patient has been receiving regular dental care, the dentist providing that care should be consulted.

Evaluation of Patients Prior to Dental Treatment

There are two major considerations in providing dental treatment to the patient with leukemia—preventing infection and preventing hemorrhage. Clearly, before *any* dental treatment is considered, the patient's physician must be consulted and the patient's hematologic status evaluated. In addition, it is important to time treatment appropriately relative to leukemia therapy. Based on these factors, patients may be placed into various risk categories.

Patients at High Risk. Patients at high risk are those with active leukemia. These patients demonstrate a high number of leukemic cells in their bone marrow or peripheral blood. They are thrombocytopenic and neutropenic.

Also in the high-risk category are patients in the midst of antileukemia therapy who are myelosuppressed as a result of treatment (Chap. 42).

Patients at Moderate Risk. Patients at moderate risk have successfully completed the induction phase of therapy and are undergoing maintenance treatment. They do not demonstrate marrow or peripheral blood evidence of malignancy. However, they do demonstrate myelosuppression in association with chemotherapy.

Patients at Low Risk. Patients at low risk have successfully completed therapy and demonstrate no evidence of malignancy or myelosuppression. These patients generally do not receive medication.

Dental Management

Prevention

Because patients with leukemia are especially at risk to develop oral infection, any sources of potential infection or irritation should be eliminated following the guidelines discussed here. Sharp restorations, fractured teeth, removable prostheses, and orthodontic bands and brackets should be replaced, smoothed, or removed. Partially erupted third molars that present the potential for the development of pericoronitis should be extracted. Teeth with caries should be restored if there is no danger of pulpal involvement. Teeth with pulpal involvement should be either definitively treated endodontically or extracted. Any tooth with a questionable prognosis should be extracted. Periodontally involved teeth should be eliminated. Scaling and root planing, oral hygiene instruction, and fluoride rinses (Chap. 42) are all important in minimizing periodontal changes or infection.

Specific Treatment Recommendations

Patients at High Risk. Patients in this category are extremely susceptible to infection and oral hemorrhage. At the initial presentation, many patients with leukemia are in a state in which their marrow and peripheral blood are overwhelmed with leukemic cells, producing a condition termed "blast crisis." Blast crisis is a medical emergency that requires immediate and aggressive medical care. Patients require hospitalization and the institution of chemotherapy. At this time, patients are functionally myelosuppressed.

Dental treatment in this group is limited to emergency care and should generally be restricted to medical management of dental problems. Patients with evidence of oral infection should be treated with intravenous, broad-spectrum antibiotics directed against both gram-positive and gram-negative oral flora. In the patient with periodontal disease, the contribution of anaerobic organisms must be considered. Treatment of these patients represents a complex management problem that requires interaction between dentist and physician.

Patients at Moderate Risk. Patients at moderate risk are those with no evidence of malignancy but who become myelosuppressed as a consequence of maintenance chemotherapy. Generally, myelosuppression is most evident 14 days after the administration of medication. Thus, dental treatment should be avoided at this time.

During periods prior to or 21 days after courses of chemotherapy, dental treatment may be performed. Before any treatment, the patient's physician should be consulted and white blood cell and platelet counts obtained. Elective treatment should be deferred if the WBC is under 3,500 cells/mm^3 or the platelet count is less than 100,000 cells/mm^3. Diagnostic (type I) procedures may be performed using normal protocol. Because of functional white cell modification, antibiotic prophylaxis is recommended for types II, III, and IV procedures. These may be performed in the dental office.

Because of the consequences of potential infection, hospitalization is recommended for types V and VI procedures so that adequate monitoring and intravenous antibiotics may be used. The dentist should consult with the patient's physician concerning the patient's overall ability to tolerate extensive dental treatment and about the prognosis.

Patients at Low Risk. Patients at low risk have been cured of their malignancy. These individuals can be treated using normal treatment protocols.

■ Examples of Dental Evaluation and Management

EVALUATION

Patient 1. You are asked to evaluate a painful swollen operculum overlying the mandibular right third molar of a hospitalized 24-year-old woman with recently diagnosed acute myelogenous leukemia for which she is receiving her first chemotherapy. Her bone marrow demonstrates many myeloblasts.

Patient 2. A 40-year-old woman presents for evaluation of a 1-week history of gingival bleeding. She complains of having a 3-day history of cough, sore throat, and a feeling of being "run down." She is one of your most conscientious patients and has excellent oral hygiene.

Patient 3. A 30-year-old man with acute myelogenous leukemia presents for treatment of a fractured palatal cusp of a maxillary premolar. The patient has had leukemia for the past 9 months and currently goes to the hospital for additional chemotherapy.

Patient 4. A 21-year-old college student presents for the evaluation of treatment of severe gingival recession involving the mandibular incisors. Past medical history is significant for acute lymphocytic leukemia, for which the patient stopped treatment 9 years earlier.

MANAGEMENT

Patient 1. This patient is in the high-risk category because she has recently diagnosed leukemia with malignant cells in her bone marrow. Her myelosuppression is likely to be compounded by the recent administration of chemotherapy. She is also at risk of developing both local and systemic infections from her pericornitis. The objective of treatment in this case is to eliminate infection through the use of intravenous broad-spectrum antibiotics. Local irrigation and reduction of the crown of the opposing third molar would be helpful. When the patient recovers from the chemotherapy (WBC > 1000 cells/mm^3 with at least 50% neutrophils and platelets > 100,000 cells/mm^3), the third molar should be extracted with antibiotic coverage.

Patient 2. This patient presents with symptoms characteristic of undiagnosed leukemia. Her history of malaise and recurrent or prolonged infection should alert the dentist to possible white blood cell dysfunction. A history of spontaneous bleeding in a patient with good oral hygiene is bothersome in that it suggests thrombocytopenia or platelet dysfunction. This patient should be thoroughly examined and sent for a WBC, platelet count, and bleeding time. A consultation with the patient's physician is appropriate.

Patient 3. This patient is in the moderate risk category because he has no evidence of active leukemia, but is still receiving periodic courses of chemotherapy to prevent recurrence of the disease. During these periods, he is likely to develop myelosuppression, which places him at risk for bleeding after dental procedures and infection. The dentist should consult with the patient's physician so that dental treatment can be timed when the patient's hematologic status is optimal. Generally, procedures should be timed following, rather than preceding, the expected nadir.

Patient 4. This patient has no disease and is no longer receiving therapy. He can be treated using a normal protocol.

LYMPHOMAS

Lymphomas are malignancies of lymphoreticular origin that most frequently involve lymph nodes. Although sharing some similarities, lymphomas represent a wide variety of clinical and histologic characteristics and are therefore subclassified. Their cause is unknown. Lymphomas are of major significance to the dentist for three major reasons. First, a significant number of lymphomas initially manifest themselves in the head and neck region, which means the dentist can play an important role in detection of the disease. Second, the oral consequences of therapy for these forms of malignancy are profound and the dentist can prevent and treat many of these problems. Third, the development of head and neck structures may be altered by therapy in children with the disease.

Hodgkin's Disease

Hodgkin's disease is a relatively common form of lymphoma that affects approximately 7/100,000 population annually in the United States. As with other lymphomas, the cause of Hodgkin's disease is unresolved. Hodgkin's disease largely affects individuals between ages 15 and 34 years and those over the age of 50 years.

Clinically, younger patients usually present with a complaint of increasing unilateral painless swelling of the neck. On examination, a well-defined rubbery mass may be noted, often associated with localized lymphadenopathy. If the disease is widespread, patients may complain of symptoms associated with impaired respiratory function because of the involvement of mediastinal nodes. This may include discomfort and shortness of breath. Progressive generalized itching may also be noted, a symptom most often seen in younger women. Older patients tend to develop systemic signs of the disease including night sweats, fever, and loss of weight. These tend to involve men more frequently than women.

A number of studies have indicated that patients with progressive Hodgkin's disease demonstrate suppression of their cell-mediated immune response. This finding may, at least in part, explain the increased susceptibility of patients with Hodgkin's disease to bacterial, fungal, and viral infections. Successful treatment of the disease results in the restoration of normal immune function.

Medical Evaluation

Medical evaluation of the patient suspected of having Hodgkin's disease includes complete history and physical examination and biopsy of suspected lymph nodes. Radiographic evaluation to determine involvement of the chest (chest x-ray and CT) and lymph node involvement (lymphography), in addition to routine laboratory tests, may be performed. The routine use of lymphography has decreased because of the availability of CT scanning. Magnetic resonance imaging (MRI) may also be used to determine the extent of disease. Use of direct visualization of the abdominal cavity through laparotomy has decreased. It is generally used in cases in which only radiation therapy is considered. The objective of these studies is to determine the spread of disease. This categorizing process is known as staging and is of significance in planning therapy and predicting survival. One form of staging is delineated in Table 27–2.

Medical Management

Hodgkin's disease is no longer universally fatal. Almost all patients with the disease exhibit a response to therapy, with a significant proportion being cured.

The role of surgery in Hodgkin's disease is essentially limited to diagnosis and staging (see earlier). Radiotherapy and chemotherapy alone or in combination form the basis for treatment (Table 27–3). Radiotherapy is aimed at eliminating involved nodal tissue. Using specific portals of radiation, the supra-

Table 27–2. MODIFIED ANN ARBOR STAGING CLASSIFICATION FOR HODGKIN'S DISEASE

Stage	
I	Involvement of single lymph node region (I) or of a single extralymphatic organ or site (I_E)
II	Involvement of two or more lymph node regions on same side of diaphragm (II) or localized involvement of an extralymphatic organ or site and of one or more lymph node regions on the same side of the diaphragm (II_E)
III	Involvement of lymph node regions on both sides of diaphragm (III), which may also be accompanied by involvement of the spleen (III_S) or by localized involvement of an extralymphatic organ or site (III_E) or both (III_{SE})
III_1	Involvement limited to the lymphatic structures in the upper abdomen, that is, spleen, or splenic, celiac, or hepatic portal nodes, or any combination of these
III_2	Involvement of lower abdominal nodes, that is, para-aortic iliac, inguinal, or mesenteric nodes, with or without involvement of the splenic, celiac, or hepatic portal nodes
IV	Diffuse or disseminated involvement of one or more extralymphatic organs or tissues, with or without associated lymph node involvement

E = extralymphatic site; S = splenic involvement

Note: The presence of fever, night sweats, and/or unexplained loss of 10% or more of body weight in the 6 months preceding diagnosis is denoted by the suffix letter B. The letter A indicates the absence of these symptoms. Each patient is assigned a clinical stage (CS) on the basis of the initial biopsy, physical examination, and laboratory and radiologic results and a pathologic stage (PS) on the basis of subsequent biopsy results, whether normal or abnormal.

From Wyngaarden, J. B., Smith, L. H., and Bennett, J. C: Cecil Textbook of Medicine, 19th ed. Philadelphia, W. B. Saunders, 1992.

diaphragmatic areas, which include the neck, can be treated with a mantle field and the area below the diaphragm with an "inverted Y" field.

The use of multiagent chemotherapy forms the basis for the treatment of Hodgkin's disease. A number of drug combinations are used, including MOPP (nitrogen mustard, vincristine, procarbazine, prednisone) and ABVD (doxorubicin, bleomycin, vinblastine, dacarbazine). These drugs are given at different times during a 28-day cycle. Patients are typically treated over a period of 6 months.

The success of therapy varies with the extent of the disease (stage) at the time of diagnosis. The more extensive the disease, the poorer the patient's prognosis. Whereas the estimated 5-year survival is 90% for patients with localized disease and no systemic symptoms, it drops markedly in patients with advanced disease. This finding indicates the importance of early diagnosis as an element affecting survival.

Table 27–3. TREATMENT OF HODGKIN'S DISEASE

Ann Arbor Pathologic Stage	Recommended Therapy	Estimated 5-Year Disease-Free Survival (%)
IA, I$_E$A, IIA, II$_E$A*†	Mantle and para-aortic radiotherapy	80–90
IB, I$_E$B, IIB, II$_E$B*	Mantle and para-aortic or total lymphoid radiotherapy	70–75
III$_1$A, III$_S$A*‡	Mantle and para-aortic radiotherapy ± chemotherapy or chemotherapy alone	60–85
III$_2$A	Combination chemotherapy (i.e., MOPP/ABVD or MOPP/ABV hybrid) ± total lymphoid radiotherapy	70–85
IIIB, III$_S$B, III$_E$B	Combination chemotherapy (i.e., MOPP/ABVD or MOPP/ABV hybrid) ± total lymphoid radiotherapy	60–80
IVA, IVB	Combination chemotherapy (i.e., MOPP/ABVD or MOPP/ABV hybrid)	55–70

*Patients with large mediastinal masses (>0.33 of the transverse diameter of the chest) are controlled by irradiation alone in approximately 40 to 50% of cases and should receive combined-modality therapy (chemotherapy followed by irradiation) as primary management, with 5-year disease-free survival of 80 to 85%.

†Patients with subdiaphragmatic stage IA should receive inverted-Y radiotherapy, while patients with subdiaphragmatic stage IIA or II$_S$A with minimal splenic involvement are treated with either total lymphoid radiotherapy or chemotherapy plus inverted-Y radiotherapy.

‡Patients with extensive involvement of the spleen (>four nodules) are controlled by irradiation alone in approximately 40 per cent of cases and should receive combined-modality therapy (chemotherapy and irradiation) or chemotherapy alone as primary management.

From Wyngaarden, J., Smith, L. H., and Bennett, J. C.: Cecil Textbook of Medicine, 19th ed. Philadelphia, W. B. Saunders, 1992.

Dental Evaluation

The dentist may be the first practitioner to detect the presence of Hodgkin's disease during head and neck examination. The presence of an enlarging lymph node warrants investigation.

Approach to Lymphadenopathy. A wide variety of diseases may cause head and neck lymph node enlargement (Fig. 27–4). The patient with such a finding may present a problem to the dentist in terms of determining how extensive a workup and follow-through are required. "Swollen glands" are a frequent patient complaint and may represent residual lymphadenopathy for a mild sore throat or cold or the initial presentation for malignancy such as leukemia or Hodgkin's disease. Thus, a planned approach to lymphadenopathy is important.

The major question that should be addressed by the dentist is the determination of whether the lymphadenopathy is the result of an inflammatory or noninflammatory process. The dentist should try to answer, through examination and history, the following questions:

1. Is the lymphadenopathy painful?
2. How long has the patient been aware of "swollen glands?"
3. Have the nodes changed in size?
4. Does the patient have a sore throat or cold?
5. Did the patient have any recent contact with cats?
6. Are the nodes movable?
7. Are the nodes unilateral?
8. What is the texture of the nodes?
9. Is there evidence of intraoral or facial infection?
10. Is there evidence of oral lesions?

Generally, lymphadenopathy resulting from an inflammatory process tends to be tender to palpation, whereas increased nodal size caused by granulomatous disease or neoplasia is asymptomatic. The acute onset of lymphadenopathy associated with a sore throat, a cold, aphthae, odontogenic infection, or other infectious process or inflammatory oral lesion is usual; although the nodes may persist for a while, they usually regress. This may not be true with young children, who almost always demonstrate the presence of pea-sized lymph nodes in the neck on examination.

In contrast, the patient who complains of progressive enlargement of lymph nodes may have a more serious problem. The symmetry of lymphadenopathy may be important. Most systemic processes, such as cold, flu, or pharyngeal infection, produce bilateral lymphade-

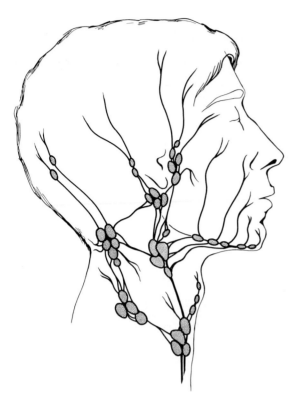

Figure 27–4. Anatomic distribution of the regional lymph nodes of the head and neck.

nopathy, whereas local infections or neoplastic lesions usually cause unilateral lymphadenopathy. However, it is important to note that bilateral lymphadenopathy *does not* necessarily exclude the presence of malignancy (see discussion of staging in Chapter 40). Contact with cats may result in cat-scratch fever or benign lymphoreticulosis, which may present with unilateral head and neck lymph node enlargement. Firm, nonmovable nodes are to be viewed with suspicion for neoplasia.

If, after history and examination, the dentist suspects that the lymphadenopathy is the result of a local process, that process should be treated appropriately (i.e., incision and drainage, pulpectomy, and antibiotics). The patient's lymphadenopathy should be reassessed at a specified interval (2 weeks). If resolution is not progressing, the patient should be referred to a physician for further evaluation. If a local source cannot be found or if the nodes fall into a risk category for noninflammatory disease (increasing painless enlargement), the patient should be referred for biopsy. Clearly, any patient complaining of concomitant symptoms of night sweats, fever, or weight loss in the presence of lymphadenopathy must be assumed to have lymphoma until proven otherwise.

The dentist should also remember that oral cancer or other squamous cell cancers of the head and neck may cause lymphadenopathy. Carcinomas of the nasopharynx and larynx are examples.

Dental Management

There are three major dental management considerations in the patient with known Hodgkin's disease. As mentioned, patients with Hodgkin's disease are functionally immunosuppressed and are at risk for infection. Thus, chronic oral infections may become acute and can seriously threaten the patient. As with other forms of hematologic malignancy, sources of oral infection should be eliminated. Close cooperation between dentist and physician is mandatory in planning dental treatment. Early dental evaluation of the newly diagnosed Hodgkin's disease patient, including radiography, is mandatory.

The second management consideration relates to the effects of radiotherapy on the oral structures. Mantle or supradiaphragmatic radiation involves the neck and the inferior border of the mandible. Thus, as in other forms of head and neck irradiation, one sees xerostomia as a consequence of the radiation to the submandibular and sublingual salivary glands. Although the risk of osteoradionecrosis is minimal, radiation caries, especially in young patients, can be a frequent and troublesome problem. The same preventive protocol as that used for patients receiving radiation for head and neck cancer (Chap. 40) should be followed. This includes frequent prophylaxis, low-sucrose diet, salivary flow stimulation, and routine use of topical fluorides.

Patients with Hodgkin's disease may be treated with chemotherapy. This may cause myelosuppression and place the patient at risk for oral infection or hemorrhage. Management of the patient receiving chemotherapy is discussed in detail in Chapter 42.

■ Examples of Dental Evaluation and Management

EVALUATION

Patient 1. A 23-year-old college student presents for routine evaluation. On examination, the dentist notices a swollen cervical lymph node on the right side of the patient's neck.

Patient 2. This patient has the same findings as Patient 1. On history, however, the dentist finds that this patient has awakened in the morning to find his bedclothes soaked with sweat. Examination reveals a firm, rubbery, nontender unilateral lymph node in the right cervical area. Intraoral examination demonstrates no evidence of pathology.

Patient 3. You are asked to evaluate a 32-year-old woman with recently diagnosed Hodgkin's disease (stage IA).

Patient 4. A 53-year-old business executive presents at your office for dental treatment. She was diagnosed as having Hodgkin's disease 4 months ago (stage IVB).

MANAGEMENT

Patient 1. This patient presents a common problem seen routinely in dental practice—the incidental finding of lymphadenopathy during routine examination. The major differentiation that must be made is whether the enlarged lymph node is the result of an inflammatory or noninflammatory process.

The first step is to obtain a complete history. In this case, you find that the patient has been vaguely aware of the "swollen gland" in his neck over the past 6 months. The patient has been well and feels fine at the time of your examination. The patient hates cats.

Examination demonstrates a unilateral, firm, movable cervical lymph node. The area is somewhat tender on palpation. Intraoral examination demonstrates a partially erupted mandibular right third molar with a red overlying operculum and some slight suppuration on digital pressure. Radiographic examination demonstrates a partially impacted third molar.

In this case, the most likely cause for the enlarged lymph node is inflammation caused by a chronically infected, partially erupted third molar. Extraction of the third molar should resolve the problem.

Patient 2. The approach to this patient is the same as to Patient 1. Based on the patient's history, age, clinical appearance of the lymph node, and lack of intraoral findings, this individual must be suspected of having a noninflammatory process associated with his lymphadenopathy and should be referred for biopsy and further evaluation.

Patient 3. This patient has recently diagnosed Hodgkin's disease. Her staging indicates that the disease is clinically confined to a single supradiaphragmatic lymph node. Her therapy will most likely consist of radiotherapy (Table 27–3). The dentist should consult with the patient's physician. A thorough oral examination should be performed. Any sources of potential infection should be eliminated, if possible. Carious teeth should be restored. The patient should be placed on a preventive protocol for radiation caries (Chap. 40).

Patient 4. This individual is being treated for disseminated Hodgkin's disease (stage IVB). She is most likely being treated with combined chemotherapy and is likely to be myelosuppressed 14 days following the administration of each course of treatment, which will significantly modify dental therapy. Specific dental management for patients in this situation is discussed in Chapter 42.

Non-Hodgkin's Lymphomas

Non-Hodgkin's lymphomas are of significance to the dentist because of their oral presentation and because of the oral complications associated with treatment. They occur about twice as frequently as Hodgkin's lymphomas. Malignant lymphomas are rare in children and increase in frequency with age. The classification of malignant lymphoma has undergone a series of changes. Presently, classification of lymphomas is based on histologic appearance

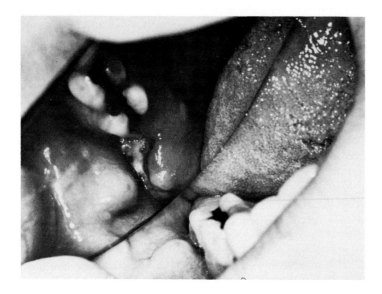

Figure 27–5. Clinical appearance of oral malignant lymphoma. This lesion most often appears as a nonhealing, painless ulceration with a pebbly, uneven surface. Clinically, it is impossible to differentiate from other types of malignancy. Biopsy is required for definitive diagnosis.

into low-, intermediate-, and high-grade forms, which correlate with their clinical behavior. Lymphomas are staged in a fashion similar to Hodgkin's disease.

The cause of malignant lymphomas is not well understood. Viruses have been suggested as causes of the disease. An increased rate of lymphoma in patients who are congenitally immunosuppressed and in patients who receive immunosuppressive therapy has been reported.

Malignant lymphoma may appear in the mouth as a primary tumor or as a secondary manifestation of a tumor elsewhere. The most common clinical appearance of malignant lymphoma in the mouth is a nonhealing painless ulceration (Fig. 27–5). The surface of the ulcer often has a pebbly, uneven surface that

appears to glisten. The borders of the ulcer may not be well defined and may undermine the surrounding mucosa. Malignant lymphoma may affect any aspect of the oral mucosa, although the gingivae, palate, and tonsillar areas are most frequently involved. Lymphadenopathy may also be present. Diagnosis is made by biopsy.

Following histologic diagnosis, patients with lymphoma are staged in a manner similar to those with Hodgkin's disease. The treatment of lymphoma relies on multiagent chemotherapy and radiotherapy. Patients with lymphoma have a high frequency of oral complications associated with chemotherapy (Chap. 42). The prognosis for lymphoma depends largely on the extent of the disease, but has improved significantly.

SUMMARY TABLE **27–1**

Leukemia: General Information

Definition: neoplastic changes of blood-forming elements

Marrow overwhelmed with neoplastic cells (blasts)

Divided into lymphoblastic and nonlymphoblastic forms based on histologic criteria

Each form of leukemia treated as individual disease

Cause unresolved, but thought to be the result of genetic modification

SUMMARY TABLE **27–II**

Medical Evaluation and Management of the Patient with Leukemia

MEDICAL EVALUATION

Presentation often insidious; flu-like symptoms

Laboratory tests demonstrate leukocytosis, neutropenia, thrombocytopenia, and anemia

Bone marrow biopsy needed for definitive diagnosis

MEDICAL MANAGEMENT

Chemotherapy forms basis for treatment
    Drug regimen depends on type of leukemia
    Divided into induction phase and maintenance phase
    Multiple drugs most successful

Radiation therapy may be used as adjunct

Prognosis improving

SUMMARY TABLE **27–III**

Dental Evaluation of the Patient with Leukemia

UNDIAGNOSED LEUKEMIA
1. Oral pathoses frequent presenting sign of disease, especially in acute forms
   a. Oral manifestations of acute leukemia associated with leukemia-induced myelosuppression
      i. Neutropenia: recurrent infection
      ii. Thrombocytopenia: gingival bleeding, hematoma formation
   b. May have gingival infiltrate and/or lymphadenopathy
2. Dental evaluation should include
   a. History
   b. Examination
   c. Laboratory evaluation, including white blood cell count, platelet count, hemoglobin, and hematocrit
   d. Medical referral

DIAGNOSED LEUKEMIA
1. Physician consultation, hematologic status
2. Risk categories (infection and bleeding most significant concerns)
   a. High risk: patients with active leukemia
   b. Moderate risk: patients in remission and receiving chemotherapy
   c. Low risk: patients who have successfully completed therapy with no evidence of malignancy or myelo-suppression

SUMMARY TABLE **27–IV**

Dental Management of the Patient with Leukemia

PREVENTION

Eliminate potential sources of infection or irritation such as sharp restorations, fractured teeth, removable prostheses, or orthodontic bands

Eliminate partially erupted third molars

Eliminate pulpal disease

Scaling, root planing, oral hygiene instruction, use of fluorides

TREATMENT GUIDELINES BY RISK CATEGORY

Patients at high risk
   Control of infection—requires hospitalization and use of broad-spectrum intravenous antibiotics
   Control of bleeding—topical agents, platelets (Chap. 42)

Patients at moderate risk
   Plan dental treatment around chemotherapy or when white blood count $> 3,500$ cells/mm^3 and platelets $>$
     $100,000$ cells/mm^3
   Antibiotic prophylaxis
   Hospitalization for types V and VI procedures
   Physician consultation; dental treatment plan in view of overall patient prognosis

Patients at low risk
   Use normal protocol

SUMMARY TABLE **27–V**

Hodgkin's Disease

FEATURES

Relatively common

Cause unknown

Two age peaks
   Between ages 15 and 34 yr
   Over age 50

CLINICAL PRESENTATION

Young age group: unilateral, painless neck swelling; possible respiratory symptoms and itching

Older age groups: tends to develop systemic signs of disease, including fever, night sweats, and weight loss

Patients with progressive disease are immunosuppressed, with increased frequency of infection

SUMMARY TABLE **27–VI**

Medical Evaluation and Management of the Patient with Hodgkin's Disease

MEDICAL EVALUATION

History and physical examination

Biopsy of neck mass or suspected lymph nodes

Radiographic evaluation to determine extent of pulmonary involvement (chest film, CT) and lymph node involvement

Staging: laparotomy and splenectomy

MEDICAL MANAGEMENT

Surgery limited to diagnosis and staging

Combinations of radiotherapy and chemotherapy routinely used based on stage of disease

Prognosis varies based on stage of disease: 90% 5-yr survival with localized disease versus 20 to 40% survival in patients with advanced disease

SUMMARY TABLE **27–VII**

Dental Evaluation and Management of the Patient with Hodgkin's Disease

MANAGEMENT CONSIDERATIONS

Immunosuppression: increased risk of infection

Radiotherapy: may cause xerostomia and caries

Chemotherapy: complications include stomatitis and increased risk of oral infection and bleeding (Chap. 42)

MANAGEMENT OF RISK OF INFECTION

Physican consultation

Careful and complete oral evaluation

Elimination of potential sources of infection with antibiotic coverage

Avoidance of nonemergent, complicated treatment

Frequent recall

RADIOTHERAPY COMPLICATIONS

Radiation caries prevention protocol (Chap. 40)

Low risk of osteoradionecrosis

ORAL COMPLICATIONS OF CANCER CHEMOTHERAPY (Chap. 42)

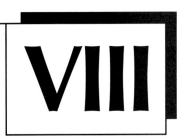

Evaluation and Management of the Patient with Joint Disease

Arthritis

Arthritis is the result of inflammatory or degenerative processes involving joints. Patients with arthritis have pain, deformity, and limited mobility of joints.

Inflammatory arthritis can result from infection (septic arthritis, gonococcal arthritis, and acute hepatitis B arthritis), gout, pseudogout, and a number of immunologically mediated diseases such as rheumatoid arthritis, systemic lupus erythematosus, scleroderma, and spondyloarthropathies.

Noninflammatory arthritis is the result of degenerative changes in the joints. Osteoarthritis is the major cause of noninflammatory arthritis. Less common causes include hemarthrosis and joint infarction.

It is beyond our scope here to discuss the clinical aspects of all the arthritides. The discussion is limited to the more common disorders of rheumatoid arthritis, osteoarthritis, and gout.

MEDICAL EVALUATION

When a patient presents with symptoms involving one or more joints, the medical evaluation is directed at the identification of the cause of the joint symptoms. Of patients with arthritis, 90% have rheumatoid arthritis, osteoarthritis, or gout. The clinical presentation and the associated findings are different in these diseases, as are the therapeutic options.

Rheumatoid Arthritis

Rheumatoid arthritis (RA) is a disease of unknown cause that affects approximately 1% of the population. The disease predominantly affects women and typically has its onset in the third or fourth decade of life. RA has a subacute presentation with the symmetric involvement of multiple joints (polyarticular arthritis). Joints of the hands and wrists are most

commonly affected. Stiffness of these joints in the morning is characteristic. More severe symptoms include pain, swelling, and limitation of joint motion. Joint deformity is seen in the later stages of the disease. Of interest to the dentist is the occasional involvement of the temporomandibular joint in patients with RA.

Examination during an acute episode reveals swelling and tenderness of multiple joints, particularly the small joints of the hands. Patients with long-standing RA may have ulnar deviation of the fingers and subcutaneous nodules (rheumatoid nodules; Fig. 28–1).

Laboratory evaluation reveals a positive rheumatoid factor in about 75% of patients. The erythrocyte sedimentation rate (ESR) is often elevated. Radiographic evaluation may reveal changes that include osteoporosis, reduction in joint space, and bone erosion.

The American College of Rheumatology has established specific criteria for the diagnosis of RA. The criteria stress chronicity of the disease (more than 6 weeks), the symmetric involvement of multiple joints, the presence of subcutaneous nodules, positive rheumatoid factor, and consistent radiographic changes.

Characteristically, RA is a smoldering disease with periodic flares. In rare instances of long-standing disease, patients may have other organ involvement such as rheumatoid lung or secondary amyloidosis.

Osteoarthritis (Degenerative Joint Disease)

Osteoarthritis is the most common form of arthritis. The disease is the result of a breakdown of joint cartilage and secondary mechanical disruption of the joint. The disease may result from trauma but is most often associated with aging.

The weight-bearing joints such as the hips, knees, and spine are most frequently involved.

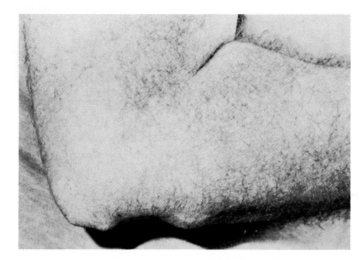

Figure 28–1. Subcutaneous nodules about the elbow in a patient with rheumatoid arthritis. (From Katz, W. A: Rheumatic Diseases. Diagnosis and Management. Philadelphia, J. B. Lippincott, 1977.)

Joints of the hands may also be involved. Typically, the disease has an insidious onset and slow progression. Stiffness, pain, and limitation of range of motion are the predominant signs and symptoms.

On examination, bony enlargement and deformity of the involved joints are apparent. Deformities in the joints of the hands include enlargement of the terminal interphalangeal joints (Heberden's nodes) and, less commonly, the proximal interphalangeal joints (Bouchard's nodes) (Fig. 28–2).

Laboratory evaluation reveals a normal blood count, negative rheumatoid factor, negative antinuclear antibodies (ANA), and normal ESR. Radiologic evaluation may reveal deformities including the formation of osteophytes, reduced joint space, and cysts.

Gout

Gout is an acute inflammatory arthritis usually involving a single joint (monoarticular arthritis). The disease is the result of deposition of uric acid crystals into the joint fluid, which incites a brisk inflammatory response. The condition predominantly affects men above the age of 40. The onset of the attack is abrupt, with peaking of symptoms within 24 hours. The great toe is the classic site of involvement, but the ankles, wrists, olecranon bursae, and knees are other common sites.

On examination, the affected joint is usually warm, red, and tender, with markedly compromised range of motion. The serum uric acid level may be normal or elevated during an attack. The diagnosis can be made by aspirating and examining the joint fluid. The pres-

ence of uric acid crystals in the joint fluid is pathognomonic.

MEDICAL MANAGEMENT

Medical management is in large part dependent on the type of arthritis.

Rheumatoid Arthritis

The goals of therapy are to relieve stiffness and pain, to preserve range of motion, and to minimize joint deformity. Conservative measures such as rest, splinting of involved joints, and exercise are usually prescribed in conjunction with anti-inflammatory drugs.

Rest is usually beneficial for mild disease, but prolonged disuse may lead to the loss of muscle strength or flexion contractures. Splinting is important in selectively resting inflamed joints to prevent contractures. Exercise helps maintain full range of motion and prevent muscular atrophy. These conservative measures are important adjuncts to drug therapy designed to minimize pain and inflammation.

The joint symptoms in RA are secondary to inflammation. Drugs are therefore selected for their anti-inflammatory action.

Aspirin is still the drug of choice in the management of joint symptoms of RA. It is usually started in doses of about three tablets daily. The doses are increased progressively until clinical responses are seen. The dose of aspirin can be increased to the point of tinnitus, which is an early sign of salicylate toxicity. The major adverse effect of aspirin is gastrointes-

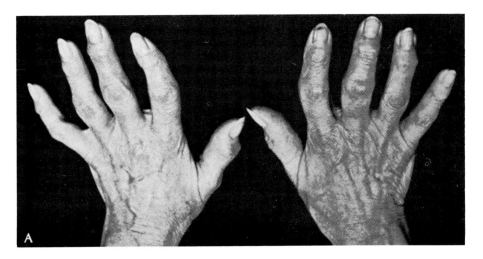

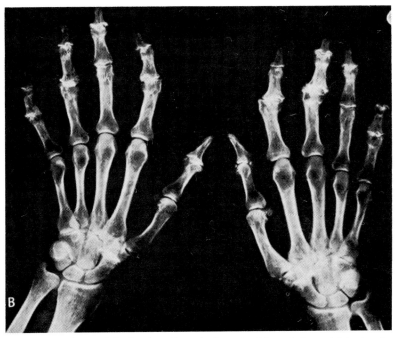

Figure 28–2. *A,* Primary osteoarthritis of the hands with marked proximal interphalangeal joint involvement (Heberden's nodes). *B,* Roentgenographic appearance of same hands. (From McCarty, D. J: Arthritis and Allied Conditions, 9th ed. Philadelphia, Lea & Febiger, 1979.)

tinal irritation and bleeding. Aspirin also has an antiplatelet action and can prolong bleeding time for as long as 7 to 10 days after the termination of the drug. The serum level of salicylate should be determined periodically to maintain a therapeutic level of 15 to 20 mg/100 ml.

Patients who do not respond to appropriate doses of aspirin and patients intolerant of aspirin can be treated with nonsteroidal anti-inflammatory drugs (NSAIDs) such as ibuprofen (Motrin, Advil), naproxen (Naprosyn), fenoprofen (Nalfon), indomethacin (Indo-

cin), tolmetin (Tolectin), sulindac (Clinoril), piroxicam (Feldene), and ketoprofen (Orudis). All these drugs inhibit prostaglandin synthesis and are effective anti-inflammatory agents. Indomethacin (Indocin) also belongs to this family of drugs but is used less frequently in RA because of the gastrointestinal irritation that results from chronic use. The major adverse effect of all the NSAIDs is gastrointestinal upset. Other side effects include headaches, dizziness, and stomatitis. A short-term antiplatelet action can also occur (Chap. 26).

Methotrexate, given weekly, is usually reserved for patients with severe disease unresponsive to aspirin and NSAIDs. The drug is quite effective in the treatment of RA but has significant side effects. The major adverse effects include drug-induced hepatitis and bone marrow suppression with resultant pancytopenia.

Gold salts are generally reserved for patients with severe disease and progressive joint destruction. Gold compounds are effective in RA but have significant adverse effects. Minor adverse effects include skin rashes, buccal mucosal ulceration, and changes in taste. Serious adverse effects include bone marrow suppression and nephropathy. Patients are therefore started on gold therapy slowly, and serial blood counts and urinalyses are monitored.

D-Penicillamine is another agent used for patients with severe erosive joint destruction. Unfortunately, serious adverse effects including severe bone marrow suppression and nephropathy can occur. Other adverse effects include skin rashes and autoimmune syndromes such as myasthenia gravis.

Corticosteroids are also used in the management of patients with debilitating RA. The intra-articular injection of long-acting steroids can reduce inflammation and ameliorate symptoms. Repeated injections, however, may hasten joint degeneration. Systemic steroids have a limited role in treatment because of

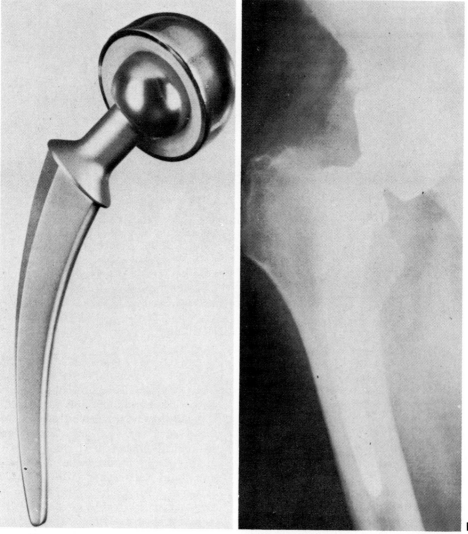

A   B

Figure 28–3. Gillberty bipolar femoral head replacement. *A,* Metallic cup has fixed lining of polyethylene. The head of the femoral component is 32 mm in diameter and snap-fits into the cup. *B,* Roentgenogram of hip with Gillberty components in place. (From Edmonson, A. S., and Crenshaw, A. H. [eds.]: Campbell's Operative Orthopaedics. St. Louis, C.V. Mosby, 1980.)

concern over osteopenia and joint ligament softening. They may be used for short periods of time in instances of severe flares.

Surgery also plays an important role in the management of patients with severe RA. Synovectomy may be needed for joints refractory to conventional therapy. Disabling hip or knee destruction can be managed surgically with arthroplasty or total joint replacement (Fig. 28–3).

Osteoarthritis

Therapy is directed at the reduction of stress placed on the affected joint, the maximization of range of motion, and the relief of pain.

Conservative measures are directed at protection of the involved joints. Patients with osteoarthritis involving the hips and knees are instructed to lose weight. Gentle exercises can be prescribed to preserve range of motion and to maintain muscle tone. Canes and crutches may be used for support. Patients with involvement of the lumbosacral spine are managed with bed rest followed by gentle exercises. Back braces can provide additional support. Patients with cervical arthritis are sometimes given a soft cervical collar for support.

Moist heat, diathermy, and ultrasound treatment may provide symptomatic relief of muscle spasms.

Analgesics are used to control pain. Aspirin, acetaminophen, and NSAIDs such as ibuprofen (Motrin, Advil), naproxen (Naprosyn), fenoprofen (Nalfon), indomethacin (Indocin), tolmetin (Tolectin), sulindac (Clinoril), piroxicam (Feldene), and ketoprofen (Orudis) are commonly used. In general, narcotics are reserved for severe pain.

In some patients, arthroplasty and total joint replacements are indicated.

Gout

During an acute attack, anti-inflammatory agents such as colchicine, indomethacin, phenylbutazone, and NSAIDs are used. Therapy is initiated at the first sign of symptoms, because delay in therapy is usually associated with less dramatic results. The major side effect of these drugs is gastrointestinal toxicity, with nausea, vomiting, and diarrhea.

In patients with frequent attacks of gout, small daily doses of colchicine may be used for a period of 6 to 12 months. Serum uric acid levels are reduced by the use of either allopu-

rinol (Zyloprim), which decreases uric acid production, or probenecid (Benemid) or sulfinpyrazone (Anturane), which increase uric acid excretion. In patients taking the latter agents, it is important to realize that low doses of salicylates block the uricosuric effects of these drugs.

DENTAL EVALUATION

Patients giving a history of arthritis should be asked about the nature, extent, and duration of disease. Medications the patient is currently taking should be recorded, and specific questions should be asked about previous use of corticosteroids, gold salts, and D-penicillamine. Surgery such as arthroplasties or total joint replacements should also be noted.

Many patients with arthritis are on chronically high doses of aspirin or NSAIDs. Aspirin affects platelet function and prolongs bleeding time. This effect persists for the duration of the life of the platelets exposed to the drug (about 7 days). NSAIDs also interfere with platelet adhesiveness. The drug-induced hemostatic effect is relatively mild, but these medications should be avoided when optimum hemostasis is desirable. Some patients display marked sensitivity to the action of these drugs; their bleeding times are very much prolonged, and severe clinical hemorrhage, particularly during or after surgery, can result.

Patients giving a history of use of corticosteroids within the past year deserve special attention, because adrenal suppression can be a concern. The evaluation of patients with a history of steroid use is discussed in detail in Chapter 15.

Patients giving a history of use of gold salts and D-penicillamine should have a complete blood count to assess their bone marrow status, because anemia, leukopenia, and thrombocytopenia all affect dental management.

DENTAL MANAGEMENT

Based on the dental evaluation, specific guidelines can be applied to the dental management of patients with arthritis.

Patients on Aspirin or NSAIDs. Because of the effects of these drugs on platelet function and hemostasis, all patients should have a determination of bleeding time prior to surgical procedures. Patients with prolonged bleeding time should be so advised, their physicians consulted, and surgery delayed until the bleeding time can be normalized. The effects of the drugs may last the entire life of the circulating platelets (7 to 10 days). The patient's physician should be consulted, and alternative forms of therapy for the arthritis may be instituted while aspirin or NSAIDs are discontinued. A detailed discussion of aspirin and nonsteroidal drug management can be found in Chapter 26.

Patients on Methotrexate Therapy. Because methotrexate therapy can be complicated by drug-induced hepatitis and pancytopenia, it is important for the patient to have a recent complete blood count and liver function tests. Patients with anemia, leukopenia, thrombocytopenia, or liver function abnormalities should be referred to their physicians for further eval-

uation, and dental procedures should be deferred.

Patients with a History of Corticosteroid Use. The management of patients who have used corticosteroids for more than 1 week within the past year is discussed in detail in Chapter 15.

Patients with a History of Use of Gold Salts or D-Penicillamine. A patient with a normal blood count can be managed using normal protocols. Patients with anemia, leukopenia, or thrombocytopenia should be referred to their physician for further evaluation, and dental procedures should be deferred.

Oral ulceration associated with gold salt therapy is usually self-limiting (Fig. 28–4). These reactions are noted in about 25% of

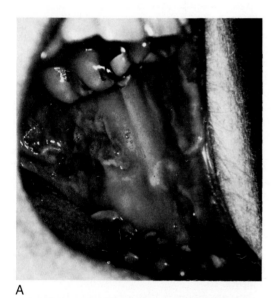

A

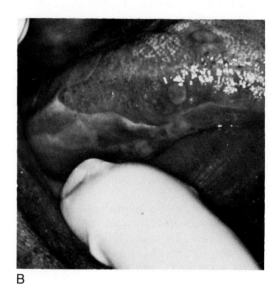

B

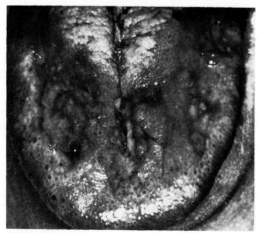

C

Figure 28–4. Mucositis due to gold toxicity. Lesions begin as vesiculobullous lesions *(A)* and then proceed to ulcerate *(B)*. Although lesions usually disappear after gold is discontinued, they may become chronic and lichenoid in appearance *(C)*.

patients receiving gold therapy. Discontinuance of the drug generally results in resolution of lesions within a 14-day period. In the meantime, palliative mouth rinses may be used.

Patients with Gout. Special considerations should be taken into account when prescribing analgesics to patients with a history of recurrent attacks of gout. Low doses of aspirin have an antiuricosuric effect and may, on rare occasions, precipitate an acute episode of gout. It is therefore reasonable for these patients to use drugs that do not contain aspirin.

Patients with Prosthetic Joints. An association has been suggested between dental manipulation and late infection of joint prostheses (not associated with the surgical placement of the prostheses). It has been proposed that bacteremias resulting from dental treatment may seed the prosthesis and produce infection. The evidence to support this conclusion is somewhat circumstantial and may be coincidental. However, until a definitive examination of the subject has been completed, it is prudent to consider patients with prosthetic joints for antibiotic prophylaxis prior to dental treatment. The consequences of infection of the prosthesis far outweigh the risk of antibiotic prophylaxis.

Antibiotic coverage for patients with joint prostheses is also controversial. For many years, patients with prosthetic joints have been managed with the same antibiotic prophylaxis used for the prevention of bacterial endocarditis. However, in a study in which the identity and the drug sensitivity of the causative organisms were determined, *Staphylococcus aureus* was found to be the most common offending organism. Because many of these organisms were penicillin-resistant, it was recommended that a penicillinase-resistant penicillin such as dicloxacillin, erythromycin, or clindamycin be used for prophylaxis. These agents may be taken 1½ hours prior to dental treatment and maintained for 48 hours. Cephalexin (Keflex) therapy is also an alternative.

ORAL FINDINGS

As discussed elsewhere (Chap. 45), the temporomandibular joint may be affected by arthritis. Patients complain of joint tenderness and trismus and may have swelling and erythema over the affected joint. Occasionally, temporomandibular symptoms may induce a patient to seek diagnosis and treatment of joint disease. The evaluation and treatment of arthritis of the temporomandibular joint is the same as for other joints of the body.

Sjögren's Syndrome

Sjögren's syndrome (Chap. 43) is a chronic autoimmune disorder consisting of xerostomia, dry eyes, and connective tissue disease. RA occurs in about 50% of patients with the syndrome. The most striking oral findings associated with Sjögren's syndrome are xerostomia, bilateral parotid gland enlargement, and atrophy of the filiform and fungiform lingual papillae. Angular cheilitis has been noted. The treatment of the oral involvement of Sjögren's syndrome is palliative. Where needed, saliva substitutes may be used. Additionally, because of the high frequency of caries in patients with impaired parotid gland function, the use of fluorides and frequent dental prophylaxis should be considered.

Changes Related to Gold Therapy

Approximately 25% of patients treated with intravenous gold for arthritis develop oral side effects. Stomatitis manifested by mucosal ulcerations is the direct result of treatment. Patients may develop multiple painful ulcerative areas throughout the mouth but most commonly of the movable mucosa. These lesions generally resolve within 2 weeks after gold therapy is discontinued. In the meantime, palliative oral rinses are helpful.

Patients receiving gold therapy may also develop neutropenia. In these cases, secondary oral infection, especially of the gingival margins, may be noted. Patients with pre-existing periodontal disease are at higher risk for this infection than are patients without periodontal disease. Resolution of the myelosuppression results in oral healing. The treatment of oral infection in these cases requires the aggressive use of parenteral antibiotics (Chaps. 42 and 46). The chronic use of gold salts may also produce a faint purplish discoloration of the gingiva.

■ Examples of Dental Evaluation and Management

EVALUATION

Patient 1. A 40-year-old woman with a 6-year history of RA is referred for dental therapy. The patient has had involvement of the small joints of both hands, the wrists, and the left temporomandibular joint. The disease has been quiescent with 12 buffered aspirins a day. She has not been on methotrexate, gold salts, or D-penicillamine, but did have one intra-articular injection of steroids during an acute episode of arthritis involving the left wrist 4 months ago. Her medical history is otherwise unremarkable.

On examination, her blood pressure is 112/68 and her pulse is 88 beats/minute (bpm) and regular. There is no evidence of active joint inflammation on cursory examination. Her bleeding time is 12 minutes (normal range, 2 to 10 minutes). Her dental needs include a prophylaxis, simple amalgam restorations, and the extraction of two maxillary second molars.

Patient 2. A 56-year-old man with a history of "arthritis" is referred for dental treatment. The patient gives a history of increasing pain involving the right knee and right hip over the course of the past 2 years. Nine months ago he had a 4-week course of prednisone (30 mg daily) but did not have significant relief of symptoms. Increasing pain in the knee 6 months ago necessitated a total knee replacement. Although the knee is less symptomatic, he still has considerable pain in his right hip, and a total hip replacement is being considered. He is currently on ibuprofen, 400 mg daily, and occasionally has to use codeine for severe pain.

His blood pressure is 140/88 and his pulse rate is 64 bpm and regular. Examination shows the presence of Heberden's nodes in both hands. Bleeding time is 6 minutes (normal, 2 to 10 minutes). His dental needs are identical to those of the first patient.

Patient 3. A 40-year-old man with a 3-year history of recurrent attacks of gout involving the left great toe and left ankle is referred for dental care. The patient has been managed with indomethacin (Indocin) during the acute attacks and is currently taking allopurinol, 300 mg daily. His last attack was 3 months ago and, according to his physician, his most recent serum uric acid test was normal.

On examination, his blood pressure is 130/88 and his pulse is 64 bpm and regular. His dental needs include a surgical endodontic procedure of the upper right first molar.

MANAGEMENT

Patient 1. This patient is on large doses of aspirin and has an elevated bleeding time. Surgery should be deferred to allow for normalization of the bleeding time. The abnormal bleeding time is presumably secondary to aspirin and should return to normal about 7 days after discontinuation of the drug. A repeat bleeding time test should be performed prior to surgery. The patient's physician should be contacted to arrange for alternate modes of therapy during the time when aspirin is withheld. It should be remembered that NSAIDs are probably not reasonable substitutes, because they also have antiplatelet effects. The physician may recommend non–aspirin-containing analgesics for the short-term period.

The patient has not been on methotrexate, systemic steroids, gold salts, or penicillamine and therefore does not require additional management.

Patient 2. This patient probably has osteoarthritis, as suggested by the involvement of weight-bearing joints and the finding of Heberden's nodes. The patient has been on Motrin chronically, has had a past history of use of systemic steroids, and has a prosthesis in the right knee.

Bleeding time determination is important, because he is on NSAIDs. His bleeding time is in the normal range, and therefore his medical regimen does not require alteration.

Consideration should also be given to the possibility that he may be adrenally suppressed in view of the history of recent steroid use. For prophylaxis and simple operative procedures, the patient should receive 20 to 40 mg of prednisone on the day of the procedure and half that dose on the following day. For moderate and advanced surgical procedures, 60 mg of prednisone should be given on the day of surgery, 30 mg on the following day, and 15 mg on the third day. If protracted pain or infection becomes a problem, steroid coverage for the stressful situation should be continued (Chap. 15).

The prosthesis in the right knee also deserves special attention. Dicloxacillin (125 mg) qid for 2 days beginning 1 hour before the scheduled appointment, with a 250-mg loading dose, can be prescribed for prophylaxis.

Patient 3. This patient has a history of recurrent episodes of gout and is on chronic allopurinol therapy. He is also on an NSAID that may prolong bleeding time. Bleeding time should therefore be determined prior to surgical procedures.

In the choice of analgesics, aspirin should be avoided in view of the possible exacerbation of gout.

Arthritis: General Information

DEFINITION

Arthritis is an inflammatory or degenerative process involving the joints. Rheumatoid arthritis, osteoarthritis, and gout account for 90% of cases.

INFLAMMATORY ARTHRITIS

Infection (septic arthritis, gonococcal arthritis, hepatitis B arthritis)

Pseudogout

Immunologically mediated disease (rheumatoid arthritis, systemic lupus erythematosus, scleroderma, spondyloarthropathies)

NONINFLAMMATORY ARTHRITIS

Osteoarthritis

Hemarthrosis

Joint infarction

INCIDENCE

Rheumatoid arthritis affects approximately 1% of the population; osteoarthritis is at least twice as common; gout is significantly less common

SUMMARY TABLE **28–II**

Arthritis: Common Clinical Presentations

RHEUMATOID ARTHRITIS

Unknown cause

Women predominate

Third and fourth decade of life

Subacute presentation with symmetric involvement of multiple joints (polyarticular arthritis)

Hands and wrists most commonly affected

Morning stiffness characteristic

Laboratory findings
   75% have positive rheumatoid factor
   Erythrocyte sedimentation rate often elevated

Characteristic radiologic changes

OSTEOARTHRITIS (DEGENERATIVE JOINT DISEASE)

Most common form of arthritis; breakdown of joint cartilage with secondary mechanical disruption

Weight-bearing joints (hips, knees, spine) most often affected, hands often affected—Heberden's nodes, Bouchard's nodes

Insidious onset

Laboratory findings
   Negative rheumatoid factor
   Negative antinuclear antibody (ANA)
   Normal erythrocyte sedimentation rate

Characteristic radiologic findings

GOUT

Precipitated by uric acid crystal deposition in joints

Acute onset—a brisk inflammatory response within 24 hr

Usually single joint (monoarticular arthritis)

Large toe most common site; other sites include ankles, wrists, and knees

Laboratory findings
   Serum uric acid level may be elevated
   Diagnosis by aspiration of uric acid crystals in the joint

Medical Management of the Patient with Arthritis

RHEUMATOID ARTHRITIS
1. Rest, splinting of involved joints, controlled exercise
2. Anti-inflammatory drugs
   a. Aspirin (first-choice drug), 3–8 g/day
      Side effects: tinnitus, GI irritation, bleeding, antiplatelet activity
   b. NSAIDs (second-choice drugs)
      i. Ibuprofen (Motrin, Advil)
      ii. Fenoprofen (Nalfon)
      iii. Naproxen (Naprosyn)
      iv. Tolmetin (Tolectin)
      v. Sulindac (Clinoril)
      vi. Piroxicam (Feldene)
      vii. Ketoprofen (Orudis)
      Side effects: GI upset, headache, dizziness, stomatitis
   c. Methotrexate—for severe disease
      Side effects: drug-induced hepatitis; bone marrow suppression
   d. Gold salts—often reserved for severe disease
      Side effects: bone marrow suppression, nephropathy, stomatitis, alterations in taste, skin rashes
   e. D-Penicillamine—reserved for severe disease
      Side effects: bone marrow suppression, nephropathy, skin rashes, autoimmune syndromes (e.g., myasthenia gravis)
   f. Corticosteroids—often reserved for severe disease
      Side effects: repeated intra-articular injections may accelerate joint degeneration
      Systemic steroids (limited role): osteopenia and joint ligament softening, adrenal suppression
3. Surgery
   a. Synovectomy
   b. Arthroplasty
   c. Prosthetic joint replacement

OSTEOARTHRITIS
1. Reduce stress in affected joint, controlled exercise, moist heat, diathermy, ultrasound treatment
2. Analgesics for pain
   a. Aspirin
   b. NSAIDs
   c. Narcotics for severe pain only
3. Surgery
   a. Arthroplasty
   b. Prosthetic joint replacement

GOUT
1. During an attack, anti-inflammatory agents
   a. Colchicine
   b. Indomethacin
   c. Phenylbutazone
   d. Other NSAIDs
2. Chronic therapy
   a. Low-dose colchicine
   b. Medications to lower serum uric acid level
      i. Allopurinol (Zyloprim)
      ii. Probenecid (Benemid)
      iii. Sulfinpyrazone (Anturane)
         (*Note:* Aspirin decreases drug effectiveness.)

Dental Evaluation of the Patient with Arthritis

Determine specific diagnosis

Determine present medications

Specific inquiry regarding
  Corticosteroids
  Methotrexate
  Gold salts
  D-Penicillamine

History of surgical care, especially prosthetic joint replacement

Prostheses at suspected increased risk for bacteremia-induced infection, often *Staphylococcus aureus*

Dental Management of the Patient with Arthritis

1. If surgery planned, bleeding time test to assess qualitative platelet function, mandatory for all patients on ASA or NSAIDs
   If bleeding time elevated and surgery planned, drugs discontinued in consultation with physician; 7 to 10 days later bleeding time test repeated to confirm normal value and surgery can proceed (Chap. 26)
2. Very recent CBC, platelet count mandatory for all patients on methotrexate, D-penicillamine, and gold salts
3. Liver function tests for patients on methotrexate
4. Patients with history of corticosteroid use evaluated for adrenal suppression and need for steroid supplementation (Chap. 15)
5. ASA compounds contraindicated in patients with gout
6. Patients with prosthetic joint replacement may require antibiotic prophylaxis prior to all dental treatment; consultation with orthopedic surgeon often yields suggestion of 2 to 3 days of dicloxacillin, erythromycin, clindamycin, or cephalexin

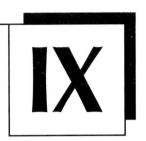

SECTION IX

Evaluation and Management of the Patient with Genitourinary Disease

Chronic Renal Failure, Dialysis, and Transplantation

Patients with chronic renal failure, patients on dialysis, and patients who have had successful renal transplants require special dental management strategies because of their complicated clinical status.

The normal kidney is involved in a number of specialized functions, including maintenance of fluid and electrolyte balance, regulation of acid-base balance, and excretion of nitrogenous waste and drugs. In addition, the kidney is involved in the production or metabolism of a number of hormones including vitamin D, renin, erythropoietin, and prostaglandins. Diseases involving the kidney can therefore cause a variety of metabolic derangements. In the dental management of these patients, the possible existence of problems with hemostasis caused by platelet function abnormalities should also be borne in mind. In addition, some commonly used medications are contraindicated in patients with renal failure.

MEDICAL EVALUATION

Nephrosclerosis secondary to long-standing hypertension, diabetic nephropathy, pyelonephritis, and nephrotoxicity from analgesic abuse are among the more common causes of chronic renal failure. In practice, renal failure is identified by clinical symptoms and laboratory evaluation. The common indicators of renal function are blood urea nitrogen (BUN) and creatinine levels. Normally, BUN level is less than 20 mg/100 ml and creatinine is less than 1.5 mg/100 ml. Values above these levels are abnormal and denote some compromises in renal function. However, patients usually do not have clinical symptoms until the BUN concentration is above 50 mg/100 ml or the creatinine level is above 5 mg/100 ml. Severe renal failure requiring dialysis and transplantation usually occurs at BUN levels above 100 mg/dl and creatinine levels above 10 mg/dl.

Although various diseases can lead to chronic renal failure, the clinical manifestations and functional derangements are remarkably constant. Early in renal failure, the patient presents with anorexia, easy fatigability, lassitude, and weakness. As renal failure worsens, the patient may complain of pruritus, nausea, vomiting, and lethargy. Shortness of breath may occur secondary to cardiomyopathy or fluid overload. The patient may develop hypertension and pericarditis. Late in the course, the patient becomes increasingly lethargic, and seizures and coma can occur terminally.

On examination, patients with chronic renal failure may have hypertension. The skin is usually pale and sallow and areas may be excoriated. There is clinical evidence of fluid retention, with peripheral edema, elevation of jugulovenous pressure, and ascites. Patients may also have congestive heart failure with an enlarged heart and a third heart sound. In patients with severe renal failure, a pericardial friction rub, denoting uremic pericarditis, can be heard. Neurologic examination reveals lethargy and, in patients with severe renal failure, asterixis.

Laboratory evaluation indicates significant metabolic abnormalities. Complete blood count shows anemia as a result of depressed red cell synthesis. Electrolyte determination can show hyperkalemia and acidosis secondary to retention of potassium and acids in renal insufficiency. The serum phosphate level is elevated and the serum calcium level is depressed as a result of phosphate retention and compromised vitamin D synthesis. The BUN and serum creatinine levels are elevated. Bleeding time is also prolonged as a result of inhibition of platelet adhesion by uremic toxins. This prolongation of bleeding time occurs despite normal platelet count, prothrombin time (PT), and partial thromboplastin time (PTT).

The clinical course of chronic renal failure depends on the underlying renal disease. Patients with hypertension and diabetic nephropathy have rapid deterioration, whereas patients with polycystic kidney disease have a slower course. In general, patients with chronic renal failure have progressive deterioration of renal function with rapid worsening during periods of infection or dehydration. With increasing azotemia, patients must be managed with dialysis or transplantation.

MEDICAL MANAGEMENT

The objectives in the management of patients with chronic renal failure are to prevent or minimize the complications of uremia, monitor the disease, and judge when dialysis or transplantation should be considered. Conservative management of renal failure can prolong survival and preserve function.

The kidney is responsible for the removal of nitrogenous wastes. Accumulation of these wastes in renal failure causes some of the uremic symptoms. Reduction of protein intake can prevent worsening of azotemia. Restriction to 0.5 g of protein/kg body weight daily allows sufficient amounts for daily requirements while lessening progression of renal failure.

Judicious fluid and electrolyte management is exceedingly important because patients with chronic renal failure have difficulty adjusting to variations of either excessive intake or rigid restriction of salt and fluids. In patients with a moderate degree of renal failure, salt and water intake must be adequate to match the excess losses that occur as tubular function begins to deteriorate. Restriction of intake at this stage can actually accelerate renal damage by causing decreased extracellular volume and reduced renal perfusion. In later stages, as excretion of sodium and water becomes limited, cautious sodium and fluid restriction becomes necessary.

Acidosis is corrected by the use of sodium bicarbonate. Because patients with renal failure have difficulty with potassium excretion, potassium intake in the diet must be adjusted. Elevated serum phosphate levels are treated with the use of calcium citrate or calcium acetate (PhosLo). Phosphate binders such as aluminum hydroxide (Amphojel, Basaljel, AluCap) are less frequently used because of concerns about long-term aluminum use. Hypocalcemia is treated with vitamin D or its analogues and calcium preparations.

Anemia in the patient with chronic renal failure may be severe enough to cause symptoms. Androgens have been shown to stimulate red cell production and can be used successfully in some patients. Erythropoietin is extremely helpful in the management of patients with anemia resulting from uremia. Unfortunately, the drug has to be administered by injection two to three times a week and is therefore cumbersome to administer.

Patients with chronic renal failure should be cautioned to avoid antiplatelet drugs. Abnormalities in platelet function and prolonged bleeding time can be aggravated by drugs such as aspirin and nonsteroidal anti-inflammatory drugs (NSAIDs).

Doses of drugs that are excreted by the kidney or that are nephrotoxic must be adjusted to avoid toxicity.

When conservative management fails, patients should be considered for dialysis and transplantation. Two major forms of dialysis are available. Hemodialysis involves the use of a machine to remove wastes from the blood (Fig. 29–1). Patients must have either a fistula or a graft established to allow access to the bloodstream. Some patients may have an indwelling catheter placed in either the subclavian or the jugular vein as a temporary access. The presence of these vascular accesses mandates prophylaxis for bacterial endocarditis in all dental procedures. It is important to remember that patients must be given heparin while on the hemodialysis machine, and the effects of heparin last 2 to 3 hours after the dialysis. Patients on chronic hemodialysis are usually dialyzed three times a week for 3 to 5 hours each time.

Another form of dialysis is peritoneal dialysis. In this mode of therapy, a dialysis catheter is placed surgically into the peritoneal cavity. Dialysis fluid is infused into the peritoneal cavity, and the peritoneal membrane is used as the dialyzing membrane for waste removal (Fig. 29–2). The procedure is continuous, with the patient making three to four exchanges each day, 7 days a week (chronic ambulatory peritoneal dialysis). The major drawback in peritoneal dialysis is the possibility of peritonitis, an infection in the peritoneal cavity.

In selected patients, continuous cycling peritoneal dialysis (CCPD) can be used. In this procedure, a machine is used to automate the infusion and drainage of the dialysate. The procedure can be performed at night, allowing the patient increased freedom during the day. This procedure is particularly useful for children.

Patients on dialysis still need to have dietary

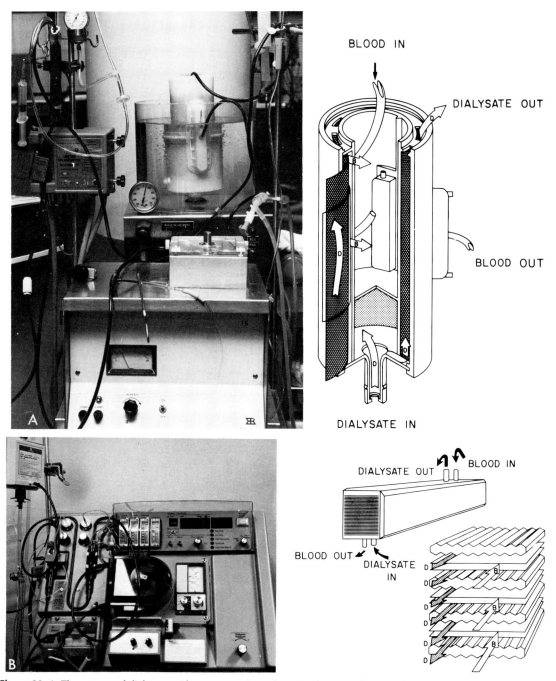

Figure 29–1. Three types of dialyzers with accompanying schematic diagrams showing their functional characteristics. *A,* Coil-type dialyzer. *B,* Flat plate dialyzer.

Illustration continued on following page

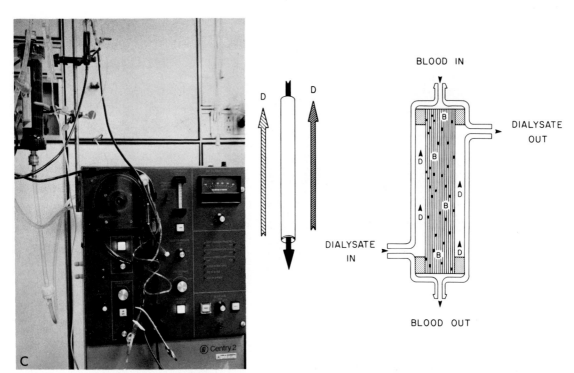

Figure 29–1 *Continued C,* Hollow fiber dialyzer. (*A–C* from Tilney, N. L., and Lazarus, J. M.: Surgical Care of the Patient With Renal Failure. Philadelphia, W. B. Saunders, 1982; diagrams are from Department of Health, Education, and Welfare: Critical Review of Documentation of Artificial Kidney Systems: Hemodialysis. Washington, DC, DHEW, Contract 223-78-5046, 1980, pp. 373–375.)

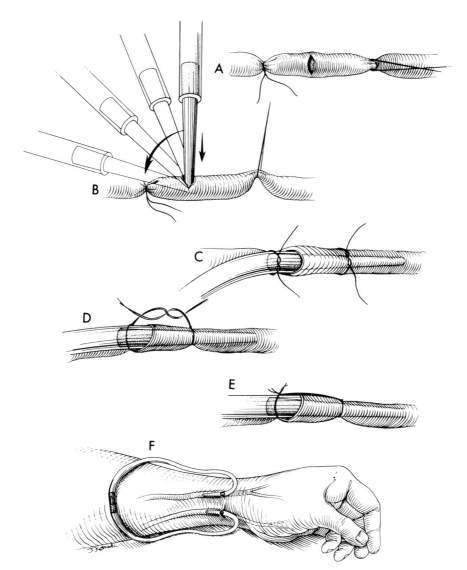

Figure 29–2. Schematic representation of peritoneal dialysis. *A,* The radial artery and a convenient vein are isolated between ligatures, and a small transverse incision is made. Gentle dilatation of this incision is sometimes helpful. *B,* The largest appropriate Teflon cannula is then inserted into the vessel, and its tip is advanced slowly. *C,* The tip and Silastic tubing are then tied in place using both proximal and distal ligatures. *D,* These are then tied together to keep the cannula in place. *E,* The tip should lie comfortably within the vessel without angulation or kinking. *F,* Position of the completed Scribner shunt. (From Tilney, N. L., and Lazarus, J. M.: Surgical Care of the Patient With Renal Failure. Philadelphia, W. B. Saunders, 1982.)

restrictions and medications for metabolic control.

Some patients with end stage renal disease may have to undergo kidney transplantation. These patients receive a kidney from a living related donor or a cadaver. To prevent rejection of the transplanted kidney, patients must be maintained on long-term immunosuppressive therapy. Most are taking azathioprine (Imuran) or cyclophosphamide (Cytoxan), cyclosporine (Sandimmune), and prednisone. Because of these medications, renal transplant patients are particularly prone to infection, including infections in the oral cavity, and they deserve special attention. The management of patients on cytotoxic drugs has been discussed in detail in the chapter on chemotherapy (Chap. 42), and the management of patients on steroid therapy has been discussed in detail in the chapter on the adrenal gland (Chap. 15).

DENTAL EVALUATION

Chronic Renal Failure

Patients with chronic renal failure have special needs that should be considered prior to initiation of dental treatment. They should have had a medical evaluation in the past 3 months. The patient's physician should be consulted to assess the adequacy of metabolic control. Serum electrolyte, BUN, creatinine, calcium, and phosphate levels should be determined. Patients with hyperkalemia, acidosis, and other biochemical abnormalities should have their metabolic status optimized prior to treatment.

Patients should be asked about weakness, easy fatigability, lethargy, pruritus, nausea, and vomiting, and patients with significant azotemic symptoms should be referred to their physicians for evaluation. All medications should be recorded. On examination, the presence of hypertension should be noted. Skin pallor and edema should also be noted.

It is important to recognize that patients with renal failure are often anemic, and a complete blood count should be obtained in order to assess the degree of anemia. These patients may also have a prolonged bleeding time secondary to inhibition of platelet adhesiveness by uremic toxins. If surgery is considered, a bleeding time should be obtained to assess the degree of the defect.

Hemodialysis

The type of vascular access (indwelling catheter, fistula, or graft) should be noted. The times of dialysis should also be noted.

The patient should have had a medical evaluation in the past month, and the metabolic status should be reasonably stable.

Peritoneal Dialysis

The type of peritoneal dialysis used (chronic cycling or chronic ambulatory peritoneal dialysis, CAPD) should be noted. The times of dialysis should also be noted.

Renal Transplantation

Patients who have undergone renal transplantation should be asked about the medications they are receiving and about complications arising from immunosuppression. The patient's physician should be consulted to assess the stability of the clinical status. The physician should be given the details of the proposed dental procedures. Specific questions should include the need for antibiotic prophylaxis and the need for steroid adjustment.

DENTAL MANAGEMENT

Chronic Renal Failure

The management of these patients is in part determined by the associated complications of renal failure. Patients with hypertension should be managed according to the procedures established for hypertensive patients (Chap. 4). Patients with anemia should be managed according to the protocols established for anemic patients (Chap. 25). Those with symptoms and signs of congestive heart failure should be managed accordingly (Chap. 7).

In addition to these management issues, patients with renal failure have metabolic abnormalities that should be optimized prior to the initiation of therapy. Consultation with the patient's physician is therefore important. The physician should be told of the indications for and the nature of the procedures and medications that are likely to be used. Treatment plans should be tailored according to the clinical status of the patient.

Some patients with renal failure have prolonged bleeding times. Studies have demonstrated that transfusion of cryoprecipitates or the use of desmopressin acetate (DDAVP) or estrogen can correct bleeding times in uremic patients and can minimize bleeding tendencies. Consultation with the patient's physician prior to these interventions is mandatory.

In the appropriate patient, oral estrogen therapy may be used. Estrogen therapy has to be continued for 7 to 10 days before its efficacy is realized.

Some patients with chronic renal failure may have a fistula or graft constructed in preparation for hemodialysis. These patients require antibiotics for prophylaxis against intravascular infection (see later).

The dentist should also be aware of drugs that should not be used in patients with renal insufficiency. Of the medications commonly used in dentistry, tetracycline, aspirin, and NSAIDs should be avoided. Tetracycline is an antianabolic antibiotic and can raise BUN levels in patients with renal insufficiency. Because of the compromises of platelet function, it is important to avoid medications with antiplatelet actions such as aspirin-containing analgesics—oxycodone (Percodan), promethazine (Synalgos), or butalbital (Fiorinal)—and NSAIDs, including ibuprofen (Motrin), naprosyn (Naproxcn), zomeperac sodium (Zomax), and indomethacin (Indocin). Similarly, drugs that are potentially nephrotoxic should not be used.

Hemodialysis

In addition to the considerations already noted, patients on hemodialysis present some special management problems.

Patients must be given heparin during hemodialysis, and the heparin effect persists for about 2 to 4 hours after the procedure. Although the residual effect of heparin may be minimal, it is prudent to schedule dental appointments on the day after dialysis to avoid bleeding difficulties.

Patients on hemodialysis have vascular accesses in the form of indwelling catheters, fistulae, or grafts. Although these patients do not usually develop bacterial endocarditis, they are susceptible to intravascular infection and therefore require antibiotic prophylaxis. Patients with good oral hygiene undergoing nonsurgical dental care (types I to III) can usually receive the standard oral regimen (Chap. 11).

Patients with severe local inflammatory disease or patients requiring dental surgical procedures (types IV to VI) might receive the alternate regimen (Chap. 11). One common practice is the use of vancomycin for dental prophylaxis in these patients. Vancomycin is renally excreted and not dialysable. A single dose of vancomycin can thus provide adequate antibiotic prophylaxis. Vancomycin can be given slowly at the time of dialysis and is therefore reasonably convenient. This possibility should be discussed with the patient's physician, and vancomycin can be given with the dialysis session prior to dental treatment. Vancomycin lasts about 4 to 7 days in patients on hemodialysis.

Again, aspirin-containing medications and NSAIDs should be avoided because of their antiplatelet activities.

Peritoneal Dialysis

Heparin is usually not used in peritoneal dialysis, and patients do not have vascular accesses. There is therefore less concern over bleeding or intravascular infection.

Dental procedures should be scheduled at a time when peritoneal dialysis is not in progress.

Renal Transplantation

After careful consultation with the patient's physician, decisions should have been made about the need for and form of antibiotic prophylaxis (Chap. 46) and the need for adjustment of steroid doses (Chap. 15). In the majority of instances, oral amoxicillin or erythromycin is used for prophylaxis. Steroid doses must usually be adjusted if surgical procedures are necessary. Postoperatively, the patient should be followed closely and any infection aggressively managed. In this immunocompromised host, seemingly innocuous oral infection can progress rapidly to cellulitis. Because of the propensity for infection, frequent recalls for dental prophylaxis are desirable.

Concurrent use of erythromycin and cyclosporine is contraindicated. Erythromycin causes increased cyclosporine toxicity, probably by increasing its absorption. Concurrent use of metronizadole and cyclosporine is also contraindicated. Metronizadole reduces the metabolism of cyclosporine, which can result in nephrotoxicity.

ORAL FINDINGS

A number of oral changes have been associated with renal failure and correlate with the severity of the condition. As renal failure develops, patients may complain of bad taste and halitosis, which are probably a result of urea in the saliva. Ammonia may be noted on the breath. Parotid inflammation and enlargement may also be present.

Reduced platelet function may result in mucosal and gingival hemorrhage. An increased frequency of acute necrotizing ulcerative gingivitis and periodontitis have also been reported.

Mucosal ulcerations, termed "uremic stomatitis," can appear anywhere on the mucosa, although the floor of the mouth, ventral surface of the tongue, and anterior mucosal surfaces seem to be most frequently involved (Fig. 29–3). Ulcerations may vary in size, but they are nonspecific and may simply represent a manifestation of a decreased healing capability of the oral mucosa in patients with uremia. Generally, these lesions tend to be painful. It has been hypothesized that they are the result of a reaction of tissue to salivary urea. Ulcerations of this type heal spontaneously with the resolution of the underlying uremia.

Pseudomembrane formation, characterized by a superficial mucosal and/or gingival exudate, has also been reported in patients with chronic renal failure. It has been suggested that such pseudomembrane formation represents superficial fungal infection caused by *Candida* or represents tissue necrosis caused by coagulase-negative staphylococci and streptococci.

Oral lesions in patients with uremia tend to be more severe in patients with poor oral hygiene. Scrupulous oral hygiene seems to reduce the frequency of both pseudomembrane formation and ulcers in this group. Treatment is basically palliative and is aimed at containing the development of oral lesions until the underlying uremia can be effectively managed.

Oral Findings in Transplant Recipients

Cyclosporine is a relatively new immunosuppressive agent used with increasing frequency to prevent rejection in a variety of allogeneic transplant recipients. Although the overall morbidity of cyclosporine is lower than for other antirejection drugs, it is a frequent cause of gingival hyperplasia.

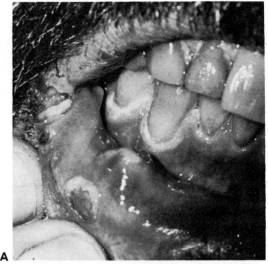

A

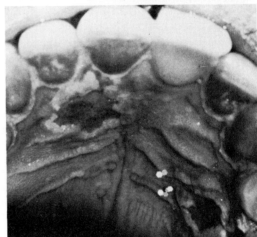

B

Figure 29–3. *A, B,* Uremic stomatitis characterized by ulcerations of the mucosa and hard palate in this patient in renal failure.

Patients on chronic cyclosporine therapy can develop gingival hyperplasia and need to be monitored closely; as many as 70% of individuals taking cyclosporine develop gingival hyperplasia. Young patients taking the drug are more likely to be affected than older patients. Neither the frequency nor the severity of the hyperplasia is related to the serum concentration of cyclosporine. Once a threshold concentration has been surpassed, patients are at risk. It appears that hyperplastic development is most active for the first 3 to 6 months following the initiation of therapy. The hyperplasia plateaus by 1 year. Because poor oral hygiene and the presence of plaque increase the probability of cyclosporine-induced hyperplasia, patients who are to receive the drug should have intensive oral hygiene instruction and aggressive professional follow-up. The use of an antimicrobial mouth rinse such as povi-done-iodine or chlorhexidine may be helpful, although there are no studies to support their use in these cases.

■ Examples of Dental Evaluation and Management

EVALUATION

Patient 1. A 34-year-old man with a history of chronic glomerulonephritis presents for dental treatment. He has had problems with his kidneys for 6 years and is now in "mild renal failure." He was last examined by his physician a month ago and was told that his kidney function had deteriorated further. He has been on hydralazine, 50 mg orally qid, propranolol (Inderal), 80 mg orally bid, and furosemide (Lasix), 80 mg orally bid. He also takes multivitamins, folic acid, and aluminum hydroxide.

Consultation with his physician revealed that he was hypertensive, with a blood pressure of 180/100 on his last examination. Consequently, his diuretics were increased. His hematocrit at last examination was 32%, BUN was 65 mg/dl and creatinine was 6 mg/dl.

He has no symptoms other than easy fatigability.

On examination, his blood pressure is 140/88 and his pulse is 86 beats/minute (bpm) and regular. He has no edema.

His dental needs include routine operative procedures, prophylaxis, scaling, and the extraction of an intermittently symptomatic lower left third molar.

Patient 2. A 22-year-old man who has end stage renal disease on the basis of urethral valves and chronic pyelonephritis presents for dental treatment.

He has had progressive symptoms and was started on hemodialysis 8 months ago. He is currently doing well on dialysis three times a week (Monday, Wednesday, and Friday, from 7 to 11 AM). He was last seen by his physician 3 weeks ago and his chemistries have been at acceptable levels. He is currently on multivitamins, one tablet daily; folic acid, 1 mg daily; and aluminum hydroxide, four tablets qid. He has no symptoms.

His most recent laboratory evaluation (2 weeks ago) revealed a hematocrit of 32%, normal electrolytes, BUN of 76 mg/dl, and creatinine of 7.8 mg/dl. His calcium was 8.6 mg/dl and his phosphate was 5 mg/dl.

His blood pressure is 130/86 and his pulse is 64 bpm and regular.

He needs conservative periodontics (scaling and curettage) and the extraction of an impacted lower left third molar.

Patient 3. A 40-year-old woman with end stage renal disease secondary to diabetes and hypertension presents for dental treatment. She has had diabetes since age 12 and has been insulin-dependent. She has severe diabetic retinopathy and has had a vitrectomy recently. She had progressive renal dysfunction and was started on peritoneal dialysis 7 months ago. She has done reasonably well and is dialyzed with CAPD, four exchanges daily.

She was last examined by her physician 3 weeks ago and was told that she was doing well. Consultation with the physician reveals that her most recent laboratory values were determined 6 weeks ago when her hematocrit was 35%, electrolytes showed mild acidosis, BUN was 45 mg/dl, and creatinine was 11.2 mg/dl. Her calcium and phosphate levels were normal.

Her current medications include aluminum hydroxide, four tablets qid; captopril (Capoten), 25 mg orally bid, ferrous sulfate, 300 mg orally each day; multivitamins, one tablet daily; and folic acid, 1 mg daily. Her insulin requirement has been stable at 34 U NPH (U 100) SC every morning.

On examination, her blood pressure is 110/70 and her pulse is 60 bpm and regular. She has no symptoms.

She needs general operative dental care, scaling and curettage for moderate periodontitis, and extraction of two maxillary second molars.

Patient 4. A 23-year-old man presents for dental therapy. He had end stage renal disease secondary to obstructive uropathy as a child and had a successful renal transplantation 6 years ago, with a kidney donated by his older brother. Consultation with his nephrologist reveals that he has normal renal function on 100 mg of azathioprine (Imuran) and 15 mg of prednisone a day. He has had an uneventful clinical course since his transplant, except for one hospitalization for cryptococcal meningitis 5 years ago. This was successfully treated, and he has had no sequelae.

He needs removal of two impacted lower third molars and replacement of two maxillary central incisors traumatically avulsed during general anesthesia, using a six-unit fixed prosthesis.

The patient's physician believes that antibiotic prophylaxis and steroid dosage adjustment are necessary.

MANAGEMENT

Patient 1. This patient has moderately severe renal insufficiency and should have a bleeding time determination prior to surgical treatment. If the bleeding time is prolonged, the patient's physician should be consulted and the proposed procedures should be explained in detail. If the physician concurs, DDAVP can be given about 2 hours before the procedure to correct the bleeding time and optimize hemostasis.

The patient is also mildly anemic and his blood pressure is in the upper limit of normal. Both factors should be monitored during dental therapy.

Patient 2. This patient has end stage renal disease and is on chronic hemodialysis. It is not unusual for the BUN and creatinine levels to be moderately elevated, even with adequate dialysis. Dialysis is usually effective in correcting the platelet defect seen in uremia and the bleeding time should be normal. Nonetheless, it is important to determine the bleeding time prior to the curettage and removal of the impacted lower left third molar.

Dental procedures should all be scheduled for the day after hemodialysis to minimize the possibility that the heparin used during hemodialysis may have a residual effect.

The patient has a graft for hemodialysis and requires antibiotic prophylaxis before the dental procedures. It would be reasonably easy to administer 1 g of vancomycin intravenously while the patient is on dialysis.

Patient 3. This patient has end stage renal disease and is undergoing peritoneal dialysis. The metabolic parameters are not unusual for such patients; they often have relatively high creatinine levels despite adequate dialysis. There is no need for antibiotic prophylaxis in this instance.

The patient is also a diabetic. Dental procedures should be scheduled for midmorning, and multiple short procedures should be planned. An insulin dose adjustment should be considered for the curettage appointments and is recommended for the planned extractions (Chap. 14). The patient should have 17 units (half her normal dose) of NPH insulin and a full breakfast on the morning of the latter procedure. Care should be taken to minimize stress and prevent infection. If there is concern that oral intake may be compromised after the procedure, the patient requires hospitalization and intravenous therapy. With her dental needs, most of the dental procedures can be performed on an outpatient basis, including the extractions of two maxillary second molars. More involved surgical procedures, had they been necessary, are best done in the hospital.

Although her blood pressure is in the normal range during the initial evaluation, she is on antihypertensive medication (Captopril) and her blood pressure should be closely followed.

Patient 4. Although this patient has been stable clinically after renal transplantation, he is immunosuppressed and has been on long-term steroid therapy.

Prior to the extraction of the third molars, the patient needs antibiotic prophylaxis. The standard regimen is reasonable in this clinical setting. However, because physicians may differ in their preference of antibiotic prophylaxis, consultation is mandatory.

The patient has also been on steroids for 6 years and is adrenally suppressed. Removal of the impacted molars should be performed after increasing his prednisone dose to 60 mg (or its equivalent) on the day of surgery. This can be tapered to 30 mg prednisone on day 2 and to his maintainance dose of 15 mg on day 3. Supplemental steroids should be continued for a longer period if the patient has protracted pain, infection, or compromised oral intake.

The bridge fabrication involves less stress. It is appropriate to give the patient 30 mg prednisone (double the maintainance dosage) on the day of the procedure and his regular maintainance dose on the day following bridge preparation.

The patient should be instructed to return promptly if there is unusual pain, swelling, or local inflammation. Infection should be managed aggressively, with a low threshold level set for admitting the patient for intravenous therapy, if necessary.

Renal Failure: General Information

COMMON CAUSES

Nephrosclerosis secondary to long-standing hypertension

Diabetic nephropathy

Pyelonephritis

Nephrotoxicity from analgesic abuse

LABORATORY MEASUREMENTS OF NORMAL FUNCTION

Bun level, 10–20 mg/dl

Creatinine level, less than 1.5 mg/dl

SYMPTOMS AND SIGNS OF RENAL FAILURE

Anorexia, easy fatigability, lassitude and weakness, pruritus, nausea, vomiting and lethargy

Dyspnea, hypertension, peripheral edema

Symptoms often occur when BUN level is greater than 50 mg/dl and creatinine level is greater than 4 mg/dl

Other laboratory abnormalities:
 Hyperkalemia
 Acidosis
 Hypocalcemia, hyperphosphatemia
 Prolonged bleeding time

Medical Management of the Patient with Renal Failure

CONSERVATIVE THERAPY

Reduction in protein intake

Careful fluid and electrolyte management

Sodium bicarbonate to correct acidosis

Decrease potassium intake in diet

Phosphate binders

Vitamin D or analogues, or calcium preparations, to treat hypocalcemia

Androgens or erythropoeitin to correct anemia

Strict avoidance of antiplatelet drugs
 Aspirin
 NSAIDs

Strict avoidance of antianabolic drugs
 Tetracycline

DIALYSIS

Hemodialysis

Peritoneal dialysis

RENAL TRANSPLANTATION (patients are on life-long immunosuppressive agents following transplantation)

Azathioprine (Imuran)

Cyclophosphamide (Cytoxan)

Cyclosporine (Sandimmune)

Prednisone

SUMMARY TABLE **29–III**

Dental Evaluation of the Patient with Renal Failure

FOR PATIENTS WITH CHRONIC RENAL FAILURE

Medical consultation to ascertain stability

Recent (3-mo) physical examination

Determine cause of renal failure

Determine presence of symptoms–easy fatigability, lethargy, pruritus, nausea, vomiting

Rule out hypertension

Obtain BUN, creatinine, and serum electrolyte values*

Complete blood count to rule out anemia*

Bleeding time

FOR PATIENTS ON HEMODIALYSIS

Determine the type of vascular access (indwelling catheter, fistula or graft)

Determine the time of dialysis

Antibiotic prophylaxis

FOR PATIENTS ON PERITONEAL DIALYSIS

Determine type of peritoneal dialysis (chronic cycling or chronic ambulatory)

FOR PATIENTS AFTER RENAL TRANSPLANTATION

Determine medications

Medical consultation regarding
  Adrenal suppression
  Need for antibiotic prophylaxis

*These values are often available from the physician.

SUMMARY TABLE **29–IV**

Dental Management of the Patient with Renal Failure

Aspirin, NSAIDs (e.g., ibuprofen, indomethacin), and tetracyclines are contraindicated

Determination of bleeding time prior to elective surgery

Medical consultation in patients with abnormal bleeding time for cryopreciptate therapy (Chap. 26)

Management of hypertension, if present (Chap. 4)

Management of anemia, if present (Chap. 25)

Antibiotic prophylaxis for patients undergoing hemodialysis, especially those with indwelling catheters and grafts (vancomycin 1 g over $1/2$ hr given on dialysis)

Avoid procedures on days of hemodialysis (patients may have residual effects from heparin)

Patients with renal transplant may require
  Supplemental steroids (Chap. 15)
  Prophylactic antibiotics

30

Sexually Transmitted Diseases

A number of sexually transmitted diseases (STDs) are highly prevalent in the United States. Oral manifestations of these infections are generally the result of orogenital or oroanal contact. Because these diseases tend to be highly communicable, their recognition is important to prevent the spread of infection to the dentist or to other patients. The identification and treatment of oral manifestations of STDs are becoming increasingly common.

MEDICAL EVALUATION

Gonorrhea, syphilis, and herpes simplex are the most common sexually transmitted diseases in the general population. Infection caused by the human immunodeficiency virus (HIV) is discussed in Chapter 47.

Gonorrhea

Gonococcal infections are seen increasingly and represent the second most common infectious disease in the United States, affecting more than 3 million patients annually. The disease is exclusive to humans and is almost ubiquitously transmitted by sexual contact. The number of reported cases is probably significantly lower than the actual frequency of the disease, because many patients are asymptomatic and a number of cases go unreported.

Gonococcal infections are most frequently seen in patients 15 to 24 years of age, with military personnel, migrant groups, homosexual men, and prostitutes at highest risk. The disease is caused by the gram-negative coccus, *Neisseria gonorrhoeae.* The most common site of infection is the urethra.

In men, following a 2- to 8-day incubation period, a purulent urethritis develops that may be followed by spread to contiguous tissues including the prostate, seminal vesicles, and epididymis. Women also develop a urethritis, but it tends to be more mild. Spread to contig-

uous tissues may also occur in women, and pelvic inflammatory disease may result. Most cases of gonococcal infection in women are asymptomatic, however, as are a significant number of cases in men. Thus, good practice dictates the evaluation and treatment of asymptomatic sexual partners of patients with known infection.

Gonorrhea should be suspected in a man presenting with creamy white urethral discharge. The diagnosis can be made by identification of the organisms using Gram's stain or by culture.

Cultures must be done carefully because of the fragility of the organism. Thayer-Martin medium should be used, because it contains antibiotics that inhibit the growth of organisms that could prevent the growth of the gonococcal organism.

Syphilis

Syphilis is perhaps the most infamous of the STDs, having made its mark throughout history. Unfortunately, it is not a disease of the past. On the contrary, its frequency is increasing. The dentist must be aware of this disease for two major reasons: first, the most common extragenital site for lesions caused by syphilis is the mouth; second, because some stages of the disease are highly contagious, dentists must be able to recognize and deal with the symptoms for their own protection.

Syphilis is caused by the spirochete *Treponema pallidum,* which survives only on moist surfaces. Syphilis can be classified into two major forms, acquired and congenital. Acquired syphilis is transmitted by sexual or other interpersonal contact. Congenital syphilis is transmitted to the newborn by its mother.

The acquired form of syphilis occurs in three longitudinal stages. The initial lesion of syphilis appears about 3 weeks following contact. At the site where the organism enters, a papular lesion develops and quickly becomes a painless, indurated ulceration called a chancre. Frequently, unilateral lymphadenopathy develops. The patient is otherwise asymptomatic. The most common extragenital site of involvement is the mouth, with the lip, tongue, and tonsils affected in decreasing order. The chancre usually lasts for about 1 month, after which it heals spontaneously.

Once the chancre heals, the number of spirochetes increases until the second clinical stage of the disease is reached. This phase is sometimes called the mucous patch phase and occurs between 6 and 8 weeks after initial exposure. Secondary syphilis is a systemic disease. A flu-like syndrome is common, and patients may develop generalized lymphadenopathy. The most characteristic feature is a generalized skin eruption with palm and sole involvement. Mucous patches and split papules often occur on mucous membranes (see later, Oral Findings). Many other organs, including the liver and kidneys, may be involved. Secondary syphilis is highly contagious. As in primary syphilis, the manifestations of secondary syphilis resolve spontaneously, even without therapy, usually within weeks or months.

About one-third of patients with untreated syphilis develop lesions of tertiary syphilis, usually 10 to 40 years after the primary infection. Patients with tertiary syphilis can have cardiovascular and neurologic involvement. Gummas, which are progressively destructive granulomatous lesions, can involve the skin, bone, and other organs.

The diagnosis of syphilis is usually made on the basis of clinical features and serologic testing. *T. pallidum* cannot be cultured in the laboratory. In patients with primary syphilis, darkfield examination may permit the direct visualization of *T. pallidum* from the chancre. This requires special microscopes and experienced observers.

The most widely used serologic tests for syphilis include the VDRL, Hinton, and RPR tests (Chap. 1). These are excellent screening tests but can yield false-positive results. A more specific serologic test is the FTA-ABS test.

Herpes Genitalis

A rapidly increasing form of STD is herpes genitalis, a viral infection caused by the sexual transmission of type 2 herpes simplex virus. After an incubation period of 2 to 10 days, vesicular lesions develop on the genitalia. In the man, penile lesions are seen. In the woman, the lesions may affect the external genitalia, vagina, or cervix. The lesions ulcerate and can be extremely painful. Local lymphadenopathy and fever may accompany the lesions.

In most patients, herpes genitalis is self-limited, but some patients may have a relapsing infection. Herpetic infection during pregnancy is particularly worrisome, because neonatal herpes can be devastating.

Herpes genitalis is usually diagnosed on clinical grounds alone, although viral inclusion bodies can be found using special techniques.

In the medical evaluation of patients with STDs, it is important to remember that these patients may have more than one STD. One should therefore perform serologic testing for syphilis in patients with gonococcal or herpetic infections.

MEDICAL MANAGEMENT

Gonorrhea

The preferred drugs for gonococcal infection are penicillin G, ampicillin or amoxicillin, and tetracycline. Patients with uncomplicated gonorrhea can be adequately treated by any of three drug regimens (Table 30–1).

Syphilis

Syphilis is treated with penicillin. Because the organism multiplies slowly, the goal is to attain relatively low but long-lasting antibiotic levels. The duration of therapy is dependent on the duration of infection (Table 30–2). Penicillin-allergic patients are usually treated with tetracycline or erythromycin.

Herpes Genitalis

In most patients, herpes genitalis is self-limited and the lesions resolve without scarring. In patients with severe pain, topical acyclovir can be used to ameliorate symptoms.

Table 30–1. TREATMENT OF UNCOMPLICATED GONORRHEA

1. Aqueous procaine penicillin G, 4.8 million units injected intramuscularly at two sites with 1.0 g probenecid by mouth, *or*
2. Ampicillin, 3.5 g (or amoxicillin, 3.0 g) single oral dose given with 1.0 g probenecid by mouth, *or*
3. Tetracycline, 0.5 g by mouth qid for 5 days

Table 30–2. TREATMENT OF SYPHILIS

1. Early syphilis (incubating, primary, secondary, early latent stages):
   2.4 million units of benzathine penicillin IM
   600,000 units of procaine penicillin IM daily for 8 days
   For penicillin-allergic patients:
   Tetracycline, 500 mg by mouth qid for 15 days
   Erythromycin, 500 mg by mouth qid for 15 days
2. Syphilis of greater than 1 yr duration (latent or tertiary stages):
   2.4 million units of benzathine penicillin IM weekly for 3 consecutive wk
   600,000 units of procaine penicillin IM daily for 15 days
   For penicillin-allergic patients:
   Tetracycline, 500 mg by mouth qid for 30 days
   Erythromycin, 500 mg by mouth qid for 30 days

DENTAL EVALUATION

The dentist should inquire about past history of STDs and should be familiar with the oral manifestations of these diseases.

Patients may give a history of STD treated in the past. When possible, the dentist should verify the type of disease, its treatment, and its cure.

More commonly, the dentist may see oral lesions suggestive of STDs (see Oral Findings). Prompt recognition minimizes the chances of inadvertent infection.

DENTAL MANAGEMENT

Care should be exercised whenever there is a concern over possible oral involvement with STDs. All forms of STDs are contagious and can contaminate dental instruments, resulting in accidental infection of other patients. Double-glove technique, a mask, and protective glasses should be used. Instruments should be sterilized promptly after use.

Patients who are undergoing treatment for an STD can be infectious. Only emergency treatment should be performed and precautions taken to minimize contamination.

When an oral lesion is suspected to be secondary to an STD, routine dental care should be postponed until the lesion is adequately evaluated.

Diagnosis of the oral manifestations of an STD is based on the demonstration of direct or indirect evidence of bacterial infection, tissue changes, or the production of antibodies to the infecting organisms. Because the organisms that cause syphilis and gonorrhea are relatively fragile, special culture media, other than those commonly found in the dental office, are required for their microbiologic diagnosis. However, the examination of biopsy specimens at times of active infection frequently reveals the presence of these organisms. This is especially true of the chancre. Thus, biopsy of indurated ulcers in patients at risk for STD is often diagnostic. Serologic testing is of value in the diagnosis of syphilis. Almost all hospital and commercial laboratories can easily perform such tests, the VDRL or RPR tests being among those most commonly ordered. It must be remembered, however, that serologic changes may not be noted in the early stages of syphilis. Thus, a repeat serologic examination may be required following the disappearance of the ulcerated lesion. If the dentist is confronted by an area of superficial ulceration in a sexually active patient and gonorrhea is suspected, the patient can be referred to the family physician or a hospital bacteriology laboratory, where culture of the lesion should be performed. Once the diagnosis of an STD has been established, the patient should be referred to the physician for definitive treatment. Routine dental care should be postponed until treatment is completed.

ORAL FINDINGS

Gonorrhea

Oral involvement in gonococcal infections is relatively common, accounting for about 20% of cases in homosexual men and in women who practice fellatio. The oral lesions of gonorrhea tend to be asymptomatic. Clinically, these lesions occur within a week of genital contact and appear similar to those of acute necrotizing ulcerative gingivitis (ANUG), with a necrotic pseudomembrane covering discrete ulcerations (Fig. 30–1). Removal of the surface necrosis often leaves an underlying bleeding surface. Unlike ANUG, areas of the oral mucosa other than the gingivae are frequently involved, including the oropharynx. Diffuse areas of mucosal erythema may be the only manifestation of infection.

Syphilis

Congenital Syphilis

Three characteristic lesions, referred to as the Hutchinsonian triad, have been associated

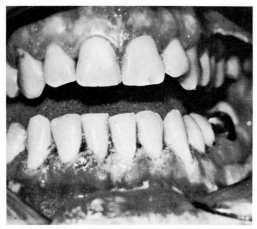

Figure 30–1. Gonococcal stomatitis. Note necrosis of marginal and papillary gingiva and evidence of gingival bleeding.

with congenital syphilis. These consist of interstitial keratitis, eighth nerve involvement, and deformed central incisors, which are screwdriver-shaped and notched. Other manifestations of congenital syphilis include abnormality of first molar anatomy (mulberry molars), saddle nose, atrophic glossitis, and a high palatal arch. Occasionally, diffuse luetic involvement of the skin results in linear lesions around the mouth called postrhagadic scars.

Acquired Syphilis

Primary Syphilis. A chancre may occur in the oral cavity of patients with primary syphilis. The most common intraoral sites for these lesions are the lip, tongue, and tonsils. As with extraoral lesions, the oral chancre appears about 3 weeks after contact. It is characterized clinically as a painless, indurated ulcer (Fig. 30–2). Frequently, submandibular and cervical

lymphadenopathy are noted. The chancre heals spontaneously in approximately 4 weeks.

Secondary Syphilis. The oral mucosa is frequently involved in patients with secondary syphilis. Patients may complain of sore throat and demonstrate diffuse inflammation. Mucous patches may be seen on the tongue, buccal mucosa, tonsil, pharynx, and lips. Clinically, mucous patches appear as raised, grayish-white membranous areas overlying an eroded erythematous base (Fig. 30–3). Generally, the lesions are painless. At times, especially on the palate, the base may not be eroded. The secondary phase of syphilis can affect the corners of the mouth, giving a cheilitis-like appearance. Such lesions are referred to as split papules. Secondary syphilis is the most infectious stage of the disease. Clearly, the dentist must approach patients with suspected lesions cautiously, with attention to protection of any open wounds on the fingers or hands. Serologic tests for the disease are positive at this stage.

Tertiary Syphilis. The oral lesions of tertiary syphilis are relatively common and have been

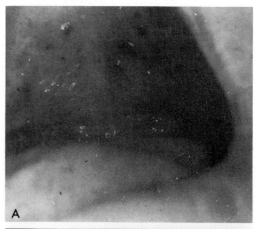

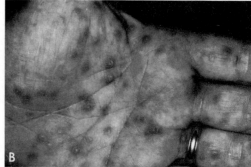

Figure 30–3. Oral manifestations and skin lesions of secondary syphilis. Both lesions are highly infectious. *A*, Mucous patch involving palate. *B*, Papular lesion of the palm.

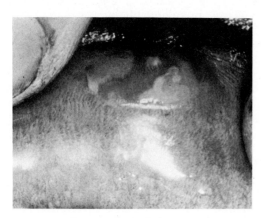

Figure 30–2. Oral chancre.

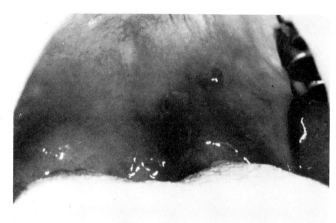

Figure 30–4. Gumma: oral manifestation of tertiary syphilis.

reported to make up over 80% of the oral manifestations of the whole disease. The two most common oral lesions of tertiary syphilis are the gumma and the luetic tongue. The gumma is a destructive ulcerative lesion that is usually necrotic; it begins as a raised ulcerative mass and then degenerates into a large area of tissue destruction. The most common site for gummas is the hard palate, and fully developed lesions may demonstrate destruction of underlying palatal bone with perforation into the nasal cavity (Fig. 30–4). Although dramatic in appearance, the gumma is painless. Its appearance is suggestive of malignancy, and biopsy is required for definitive diagnosis. Spirochetes are not usually found in the lesion.

The atrophic glossitis associated with tertiary syphilis is important as a precursor of leukoplakia and squamous cell carcinoma (Fig. 30–5). Because of its mobility, the tongue is heavily infected during the secondary stage of the disease. A diffuse vasculitis develops and sub-

sequently results in an obliterative endarteritis that produces an impairment of the lingual circulation with resultant atrophy of the filiform and fungiform papillae. At times, shrinkage of the lingual musculature produces a wrinkled appearance. With the loss of surface protection, a significant percentage of patients with luetic glossitis (19 to 30%) develop carcinoma.

Osseous lesions have been described in tertiary syphilis, occurring rarely in the mandible. Luetic osteomyelitis represents gummatous involvement of the bone and is radiographically demonstrated by multiple areas of radiolucency (Fig. 30–6). Meyer and Shklar also described a lesion of the mandible in tertiary syphilis in which there was evidence of resorption and loss of normal bone vitality and strength, so that spontaneous fractures occurred easily. There was no suppuration or mucosal lesions in the cases studied, but all the patients demonstrated other skeletal pa-

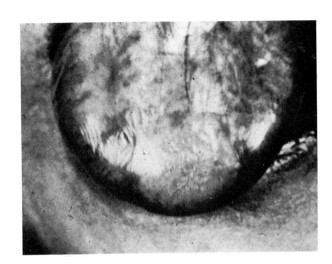

Figure 30–5. Atrophic glossitis associated with tertiary syphilis.

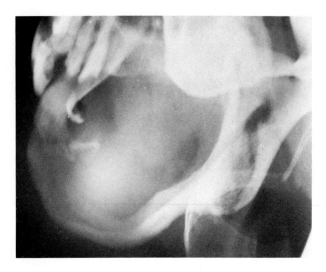

Figure 30–6. Radiograph demonstrating radiolucency as a consequence of luetic osteomyelitis.

thology. They suggested the term "bone syndrome" to refer to these lesions.

Herpes

Originally, herpes simplex type 2 was considered to be anatomically as well as serotypically specific and confined to the genital region. This is no longer the case, however. Oral-genital contact may result in oral infection. Similarly, genital-hand-mouth contact may also produce oral infection.

The oral manifestations of herpes type 2 are essentially the same as type 1. Patients may experience a prodrome of tingling and paresthesia of the lip, which lasts between 24 and 48 hours. This is followed by the appearance of labial vesicles. Generally, these tend to be painful. The discomfort may radiate to surrounding areas. During this period, the virus is communicable and may be passed by direct or indirect contact. The vesicle may rupture and then pass through a drying and crusting stage before healing without scarring. Lubrication in the form of petroleum jelly is helpful. Secondary bacterial infection may occur that, if superficial, can be treated with an appropriate antibiotic ointment, such as bacitracin. The recurrent pattern of oral herpes type 2 has not been studied.

■ Examples of Dental Evaluation and Management

EVALUATION

Patient 1. A 26-year-old woman presents for routine dental care. Examination reveals the presence of an asymptomatic indurated ulcer of the tongue. Submandibular lymph-adenopathy is present. The patient reports that the ulcer has been present for about 3 weeks. She denies smoking. She drinks alcohol socially. She denies ever having prior oral ulceration.

Patient 2. A 32-year-old homosexual man presents for evaluation of an asymptomatic area of ulceration on his palate. Examination demonstrates an area of local superficial necrosis of the palate and attached gingiva that has been present for 2 days. His sexual partner recently noted a discharge.

Patient 3. A 66-year-old retired sailor presents for evaluation of a nontender palatal ulceration. The lesion has been present for an unknown period. Examination demonstrates lingual atrophy, with areas of leukoplakia.

MANAGEMENT

Patient 1. This patient presents with a nonhealing asymptomatic ulcer of more than 2 weeks' duration. Included in the differential diagnosis are malignancy and syphilis. The patient is in a low-risk group for carcinoma. The ulcer should be biopsied and the patient sent to a laboratory for serologic testing. No dental treatment should be performed. The patient should be referred for appropriate treatment.

Patient 2. The history, appearance, and location of this lesion are consistent with those of oral gonorrhea. The patient should be referred to his physician for definitive diagnosis and treatment. Alternatively, the dentist could culture a sample from the lesion if Thayer-Martin medium is available, and make a referral based on the results obtained.

Patient 3. This patient presents with oral ulceration, lingual atrophy, and leukoplakia. Biopsy is indicated for diagnosis of the ulceration and leukoplakia. Included in the differential diagnosis are carcinoma and tertiary syphilis. The palatal lesion is in a characteristic location for gumma. The tongue lesion may represent a luetic change, placing the patient in a high-risk group for carcinoma.

SUMMARY TABLE **30–1**

STDs: General Information

GONORRHEA

Most frequently affects those aged 15 to 24 yr

Caused by *Neisseria gonorrhoeae*

Most common site: urethra

Diagnosis: culture in Thayer-Martin medium

Treatment: penicillin, ampicillin, or tetracycline

SYPHILIS

Caused by spirochete *Treponema pallidum*

Three stages:
    Chancre: 3 wk after contact; indurated ulcer; heals spontaneously after 1 mo; infectious
    Mucous patch phase: 6–8 wk after contact; infectious; resolves spontaneously within weeks or months
    Tertiary syphilis: 10–14 yr after initial contact; cardiovascular and neurologic involvement; gummas can involve skin, oral mucosa, bone, and other organs

Diagnosis: darkfield examination of smears; serologic testing

Treatment: penicillin

HERPES GENITALIS

Caused by herpes simplex virus type 2

Incubation, 2–10 days

Vesicular lesions

May be relapsing

Treatment: topical acyclovir

SUMMARY TABLE **30–II**

Oral Manifestations of STDs

GONORRHEA

Oral involvement common

Oral lesions asymptomatic

Lesions similar to those of acute necrotizing ulcerative gingivitis (ANUG)—surface necrosis with underlying bleeding ulceration; unlike ANUG, may involve mucosal surfaces

SYPHILIS

Primary syphilis—chancre
    Lip and tongue most common intraoral sites
    Indurated ulcer occurs about 3 wk after contact and lasts about 4 wk
    May have lymphadenopathy
    Heals spontaneously
    Infectious

Secondary syphilis—mucous patch
    Most common sites are tongue, buccal mucosa, tonsil, pharynx, and lips
    Raised, painless grayish-white membranes; may cause cheilitis
    Heal in a few weeks to a year
    Infectious

Tertiary syphilis—gumma and luetic glossitis
    Gumma: painless ulceration usually of palate with involvement of underlying bone
    Occurs years after contact
    Atrophic glossitis caused by vasculitis; predisposes to carcinoma

Congenital syphilis
    Tooth abnormalities—incisors and first molars
    Atrophic glossitis
    High palatal arch

SUMMARY TABLE **30–III**

Dental Evaluation and Management of the Patient with an STD

HISTORY

Determine past history of disease and treatment, and verify cure.

CLINICAL MANAGEMENT

Use caution when approaching potentially infectious lesions.

Postpone routine dental care in patient suspected of having active disease.

Biopsy nonhealing ulcerations.

Obtain appropriate microbiologic and serologic examination, where indicated.

Defer routine dental care until patient receives definitive treatment.

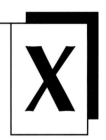
Evaluation and Management of the Patient with Neurologic Disease

Seizure Disorders

Epilepsy is not a disease but rather a symptom complex, the result of diverse neuronal disturbances. Symptoms range from altered consciousness and motor activity to aberrant sensory phenomena and behavior. The incidence of epilepsy in the general population is estimated at 0.5 to 2%.

Seizure disorders are typically classified as generalized or focal (partial). Generalized seizures often involve loss of consciousness, whereas focal seizures do not.

The most common form of seizure is the generalized grand mal (tonic-clonic) seizure. Of patients with seizure disorders, 90% have grand mal seizures at some phase of the disease, and 60% have this form of seizure exclusively. Patients have abrupt loss of consciousness and abnormal motor activities, including tonic and clonic contractions of the muscles of the extremities, usually lasting 2 to 5 minutes. Urinary and fecal incontinence may also be part of the symptom complex. Following the seizure, the patient is usually sleepy and confused and is said to be in the postictal phase.

Petit mal (absence) seizures are the second most common form of seizure. Of all patients with seizures, 25% experience this form at some phase of their disease. Most patients with petit mal seizures also have grand mal seizures, however; only 4% of patients with seizure disorders experience petit mal seizures exclusively. Petit mal seizures are characterized by a 10- to 30-second loss of consciousness, often without loss of motor tone and with little or no abnormal motor activity. Patients typically stop in the middle of activity and stare blankly or blink their eyes rapidly during the attack. They rapidly resume normal activity and usually do not have a postictal phase.

The third most common form of seizure disorder is psychomotor seizures. These seizures are partial seizures, because there is usually no loss of consciousness. During psychomotor seizures, patients often exhibit bizarre behavior, make unintelligible sounds, and cannot com-

municate. These seizures usually last a few minutes, followed by a short period of confusion. As with petit mal seizure, most patients with psychomotor seizures also have grand mal seizures; 6% of patients with seizure disorders have psychomotor seizures exclusively.

Less common seizure disorders include akinetic seizures (drop attacks) seen in children, jacksonian seizures involving focal motor or sensory disturbances, and the myoclonic seizures commonly seen in patients with metabolic derangements or degenerative brain disease.

MEDICAL EVALUATION

The physician usually classifies seizures into two categories, symptomatic or idiopathic.

Patients with symptomatic seizures have identifiable underlying disorders causing the seizures. The disorders include tumors, cerebrovascular diseases, and scars from head trauma. Other causes include high-grade fever in young children (febrile seizures), central nervous system infections (meningitis, encephalitis), excessive alcohol ingestion, and metabolic derangements such as hypoglycemia, hypocalcemia, and uremia.

Patients with idiopathic seizures have no identifiable underlying disorders.

When approaching a patient presenting with seizures, the physician obtains a detailed history from people who have witnessed the seizures to determine the type. Careful general and neurologic examinations are performed to see whether there are focal neurologic abnormalities that suggest an underlying disorder.

Laboratory evaluation of the patient includes metabolic screening with determinations of serum glucose, electrolyte, calcium, BUN, and creatinine levels. The patient may undergo lumbar puncture, particularly if meningitis is suspected. Lumbar puncture is usually deferred if there is concern over increased intracranial pressures. When a central nervous system lesion is suspected, a CT or isotope brain scan can be obtained. The electroencephalogram (EEG) is the single most useful modality for the evaluation and monitoring of patients with seizure disorders. The test provides information about the origin as well as the type of seizures involved.

MEDICAL MANAGEMENT

Whenever possible, the causative factor in patients with symptomatic epilepsy should be eliminated. Correction of metabolic imbalances, treatment of infection, and surgical removal of tumors or abscesses are all approaches that are used.

Drug therapy is used to prevent recurrent seizures. Different types of seizures respond differently to anticonvulsant drugs. Classically, a single drug is used initially, and other drugs may be added subsequently if needed to achieve control of seizure activity.

Except in patients with petit mal seizures, the barbiturate phenobarbital is often tried first. The principal side effect of the drug is drowsiness. If seizures are not well controlled, a second drug, typically phenytoin (Dilantin), may be added. Common adverse reactions to phenytoin include confusion, ataxia, skin rash, and gingival hyperplasia. The combination of phenobarbital and phenytoin is the most commonly used regimen for control of grand mal seizures.

Primidone (Mysoline) is increasing in popularity as a treatment for grand mal seizures. It is the drug of choice for patients with psychomotor seizures. Phenobarbital is a major metabolite of primidone. Ethosuximide (Zarontin) is the most commonly used medication for isolated petit mal seizures. Other anticonvulsants include carbamazepine (Tegretol), diazepam (Valium), and clonazepam (Clonopin).

DENTAL EVALUATION

The dental evaluation of the patient with a seizure disorder should include questions about the type of seizures, the medications used, and the frequency of seizures while taking medication. The dentist should understand the more important complications of anticonvulsant drugs and be familiar with the potential problems that may occur during dental therapy.

Patient Evaluation

Some patients may give a history of having had a single seizure in the distant past with no sequelae. These patients are asymptomatic without medications. Usually, these patients have symptomatic seizures that have resolved with the correction of the underlying disorder.

Of patients with seizure disorders, 90% have grand mal seizures as the sole or primary component of the disorder. Petit mal and psychomotor seizures are less common. Patients should be asked about the type of seizures they have. The patient's physician should be consulted if there are ambiguities about the diagnosis.

The majority of patients with seizure disorders are on phenobarbital, phenytoin, or both. The patient should be asked about current and past medications. The duration of therapy, particularly that of phenytoin therapy, should be recorded.

The frequency of seizures should also be carefully evaluated. Patients on medical therapy should have seizures infrequently. Patients having more than one seizure a month are under poor seizure control, and elective dental therapy should be deferred until control is optimized.

Gingival Hyperplasia with Long-term Phenytoin Therapy

Patients receiving long-term phenytoin therapy deserve special attention, because they may develop gingival hyperplasia (Figs. 31–1 and 31–2). The frequency of this complication is not well established, and reports have given a varying incidence ranging from 25 to 85% of patients on long-term phenytoin therapy.

Gingival hyperplasia is more common among younger patients. Tissue irritation by orthodontic bands, defective restorations, and unrestored broken teeth accelerate gingival hyperplasia. The level of oral hygiene is important, because gingivitis also accelerates the process.

Gingival hyperplasia can be generalized but is most often worse in the anterior teeth and the buccal aspect of teeth.

Dental evaluation of a patient on chronic phenytoin therapy should include a specific determination of the degree and distribution of gingival hyperplasia. Assessment should also be made of the role gingival hyperplasia may be playing in aggravating periodontal disease,

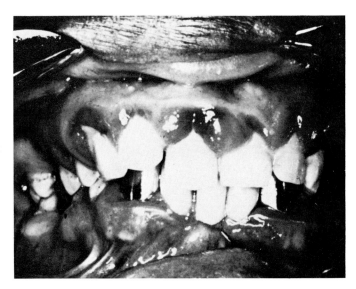

Figure 31–1. Gingival hyperplasia caused by Dilantin. Note the inflammatory component occurring simultaneously.

in compromising esthetics, in preventing adequate mastication, and in the restoration of the dentition.

DENTAL MANAGEMENT

A patient with a past history of symptomatic epilepsy who has had correction of the underlying disorder and is currently asymptomatic on no medication can be treated using a normal protocol.

Elective dental therapy should be deferred for patients with poor control of seizure activity and for patients who are in the midst of a change in their anticonvulsant therapy.

For patients who are stable on an anticonvulsant regimen, dental therapy can proceed with attention to specific guidelines.

Specific Guidelines

Risks of Aspiration

Patients with a seizure disorder are at increased risk of aspiration during a seizure. The dentist should therefore consider the possibility of a seizure during the dental procedure with aspiration of loose intraoral material. A clinical approach that maximizes the ease of rapid removal of all dental instruments and aids must be taken. A rubber dam and a rubber dam clamp with an attached floss lead are preferable to the use of multiple cotton rolls.

In patients with seizure disorders, the choice of restorations may also be influenced by con-

cern over possible aspiration during a seizure. In general, fixed, permanently cemented restorations are preferred over a removable partial denture. Unilateral "Nesbit-type" partial dentures should not be used. When a partial or full denture is necessary, full palatal coverage with metal designs for the major connector are preferred over primarily plastic prostheses.

Attention must also be paid to the preparation of "temporary restorations." Whereas all-acrylic, office-cured temporary bridges may normally suffice, the dentist may choose laboratory-processed metal-reinforced temporary bridges for the patient with a seizure problem.

Use of Drugs

The dentist should be aware of possible interactions between anticonvulsant drugs and commonly prescribed drugs used in dentistry.

Phenobarbital and primidone are medications that can depress the central nervous system. It is therefore reasonable to avoid the use of other drugs that can depress the central nervous system for sedation or analgesia. Whenever feasible, non-narcotic analgesics should be employed.

Phenytoin, phenobarbital, and primidone are potent stimulants for hepatic enzymes responsible for drug degradation. This is important because a number of the drugs commonly prescribed by the dentist are degraded by liver enzymes. Tetracycline and doxycycline (Vibramycin) are two commonly used drugs that have an accelerated degradation. It is therefore important to use alternative antibiotics for

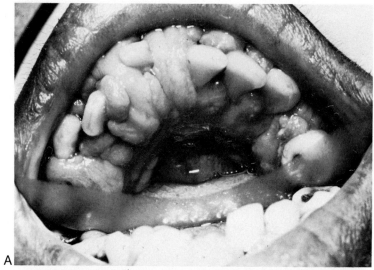

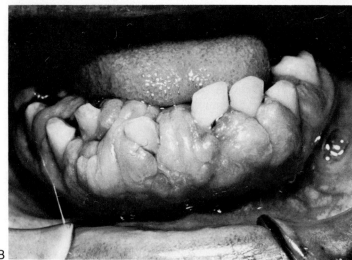

Figure 31–2. *A, B,* Dilantin-induced gingival hyperplasia of long-standing duration. Note the fibrotic appearance of the gingiva, which has almost "buried" the teeth.

patients on chronic phenytoin, phenobarbital, or primidone therapy.

Gingival Hyperplasia

Prevention should be emphasized in patients with gingival hyperplasia. Poor oral hygiene accelerates the development of gingival hyperplasia, and the disease may itself be a deterrent to adequate plaque removal, leading to secondary gingival inflammatory changes.

Patients should be carefully instructed about oral hygiene. The use of a brush, dental floss, rubber tip, Water Pik, or other interproximal aids must be demonstrated. In patients with severe gingival hyperplasia, flossing may be difficult, but the use of the brush and rubber tip should be encouraged.

Dental management should also revolve around the elimination of factors that can irritate the gingivae. Defective restorations should be replaced, carious lesions restored, and orthodontic bands removed.

Gingival inflammation should be eliminated by appropriate subgingival débridement, scaling, and curettage. Prophylaxis and subgingival débridement should be performed every 3 months.

Gingival resection should be considered if severe hyperplasia prevents adequate oral hygiene or compromises mastication. Left unattended, gingival hyperplasia increases the risk of caries and periodontal disease.

It is important to stress to the patient that gingival hyperplasia recurs after surgery. A diligent oral hygiene program, coupled with prophylaxis and débridement every 3 months, is necessary if recurrence is to be minimized.

In all instances, when gingival hyperplasia is detected, the patient's physician should be consulted to see whether alternative anticonvulsant therapy can be used. With the increasing numbers of anticonvulsant drugs currently available, an alternative drug may be effective. Alternative anticonvulsant therapy is particularly important in patients with recurrent gingival hyperplasia following adequate therapy and in patients giving limited dental cooperation.

Management of Seizures in the Dental Office

Despite careful evaluation, a patient may have a seizure in the dental office. Management should be directed at preventing self-inflicted injury.

In some instances, the patient may have an "aura" and may be able to inform the dentist of an impending seizure. The dental procedure should be terminated immediately. The patient should be placed in a supine position on the floor, preferably on a carpeted area away from hard surfaces and objects. A seizure can sometimes occur without prodrome in the dental chair. The patient should be left in the dental chair, which should be placed in the supine position, and instruments removed from the area. The patient can be gently but not forcibly restrained to prevent injury.

If possible, part of a towel or a padded tongue depressor can be placed between the teeth to prevent biting of the tongue and lips. Extraordinary efforts to introduce objects between the teeth should not be made, because tissue injury and bleeding can be caused by improper placement.

During a seizure, airway patency should be established by gently extending the patient's head. Vital signs should be monitored carefully.

Most seizures last 2 to 5 minutes, followed by a postictal phase. During the postictal phase, the patient is still confused and should be closely monitored. Usually, the patient recovers in about an hour. The patient should be discharged from the dental office in the custody of a responsible person. If there is concern about possible complications such as aspiration during the seizure, the patient should be referred to the emergency room for further evaluation.

In rare instances, recurrent episodes of seizures or persistent seizure activity (more than 5 minutes) may occur (status epilepticus). Medical assistance should be obtained immediately and arrangements made for emergency transport to the hospital. Anticonvulsant drugs may be administered in an attempt to terminate the seizure. Because the drugs must be administered intravenously and may cause significant respiratory and cardiovascular depression, only adequately trained personnel comfortable with intravenous therapy should attempt the intervention. The drug of choice for the management of seizures is diazepam (Valium), 5 to 10 mg (1 to 2 ml of a 5 mg/ml solution), given slowly over a period of 1 to 2 minutes. Complications of the drug include respiratory depression, transient hypotension, and bradycardia and, in rare instances, cardiac arrest. Intravenous therapy should therefore be reserved for patients with status epilepticus while emergency transport is being arranged.

■ Examples of Dental Evaluation and Management

EVALUATION

Patient 1. A 26-year-old woman presents for dental therapy. She gives a history of having had a seizure when she was 4 years old during a high fever. She has been asymptomatic since and has not been on medications.

On examination, her blood pressure is 110/80 and her pulse is 88 beats/minute (bpm) and regular. Her dental needs include the restoration of several carious lesions, endodontics, crown placement for two molars, and the extraction of four impacted third molars.

Patient 2. A 33-year-old woman presents for dental treatment. She has had recurrent seizures since age 6 and is currently taking phenobarbital, 60 mg orally tid, and phenytoin (Dilantin), 100 mg orally tid. She has had infrequent seizures on this regimen; the last seizure was 18 months ago. She has had close medical follow-up and had an examination 4 months ago. Consultation with her physician reveals that the patient is thought to have idiopathic seizures under excellent control. She has had sporadic dental care, and her last dental examination was 4 years ago.

She presented to the dental office complaining of "ugly bleeding gums."

On examination, her blood pressure is 120/86 and her pulse is 86 bpm and regular.

Clinical examination reveals moderately severe inflammatory gingivitis superimposed on severe anterior and posterior hyperplasia. There is heavy plaque and calculus accumulation. A full series of radiographs reveals incipient horizontal alveolar bone loss in the molar regions. The patient brushes her teeth daily but does not use other oral hygiene aids.

Patient 3. A 24-year-old college student with an 18-year history of recurrent seizures enters for dental therapy. He is currently on phenytoin (Dilantin), 200 mg orally bid, and phenobarbital 200 mg tid. He has had frequent seizures and his Dilantin dose was raised by his physician 3 days ago. He is allergic to penicillin.

He presents in acute distress with a nonrestorable cariously exposed lower left first molar. His physician is not immediately available for consultation.

On examination, his blood pressure is 130/80 and his pulse is 90 bpm and regular.

MANAGEMENT

Patient 1. This patient has a history of symptomatic seizures. The acute episode occurred along with a high fever as a child and has not recurred since. The patient is not expected to have residual problems and all her dental care can be completed using a normal protocol.

Patient 2. The key to successful management in this patient is education and prevention. The patient should be made to understand the importance of oral hygiene and frequent recall prophylaxis. This patient should undergo comprehensive conservative periodontal therapy and should be given detailed instruction in the use of the toothbrush and rubber tip for plaque removal and gingival massage. Definitive supragingival and subgingival débridement and curettage should be done. As the inflammatory component of the gingivitis resolves, the patient should be instructed to use floss.

Surgical correction of the gingival hyperplasia should be considered only after a proper oral hygiene program has been instituted. The patient's physician should be consulted prior to surgery. Gingivectomy with flap entry surgery for the maxillary molars may be planned as an office procedure. Following surgery, the patient should be placed on a 3-month recall prophylaxis schedule.

If conservative and surgical therapy fail to control gingival hyperplasia, the patient's physician should be consulted with respect to possible alternative to phenytoin therapy.

Patient 3. In an otherwise uncomplicated patient, the appropriate therapy would be the simple extraction of the acutely infected nonrestorable molar. However, this patient has a seizure disorder that is under poor control and has had recent changes in his medical regimen. It would be more appropriate to manage the abscess medically until the medical status of the patient can be clarified. The patient has a history of penicillin allergy and can be managed with erythromycin. Tetracycline should not be used, because it is rapidly degraded in patients on phenobarbital and phenytoin.

The patient also requires analgesia for the abscess. Because phenobarbital is a central nervous system depressant, non-narcotic analgesics are preferred. A nonsteroidal anti-inflammatory drug (NSAID) can be used.

Seizure Disorders

GRAND MAL (TONIC-CLONIC) SEIZURES

Occur in 90% of patients with seizure disorders; 60% have this form of seizure exclusively

Generalized seizure disorder, with loss of consciousness and abnormal motor activities

Seizure usually lasts 2 to 5 min

Urinary and fecal incontinence may be part of symptom complex

"Postictal" phase with confusion and sleepiness may follow

PETIT MAL (ABSENCE) SEIZURES

Second most common seizure disorder; 25% of patients with seizures experience this form of seizure

4% of patients experience petit mal seizures exclusively

Seizure often lasts 10 to 30 sec

Generalized seizure characterized by loss of consciousness without loss of motor tone and with little or no abnormal motor activity

"Postictal" phase usually absent

PSYCHOMOTOR SEIZURES

Third most common form of seizure disorder; 6% of patients have this form exclusively

Partial seizure characterized by no loss of consciousness; patients often exhibit bizarre behavior, making unintelligible sounds with failure to communicate

Duration is several minutes

LESS COMMON SEIZURES

Akinetic seizures (drop attacks), often in children

Jacksonian seizures: focal motor and sensory disturbances

Myoclonic seizures: often in patients with metabolic derangements or degenerative brain disease

Medical Evaluation of the Patient with a Seizure Disorder

APPROACH TO DIAGNOSIS

Primary differential diagnosis: classification into symptomatic or idiopathic category
    Symptomatic seizures have underlying disorders as cause
        Tumors
        Cerebrovascular disease
        Scars from head trauma
        High-grade fever in a young child (febrile seizures)
        CNS infection
        Excessive alcohol ingestion
        Metabolic derangements
            Hypoglycemia
            Hypocalcemia
            Uremia
    Idiopathic seizures have no identifiable underlying disorder

EVALUATION

History and physical examination

Laboratory screen: serum glucose, electrolyte, calcium, BUN, and creatinine levels

Electroencephalopathy (EEG)

± Lumbar puncture

± Computed tomography (CT scan)

±, with or without.

Medical Management of the Patient with a Seizure Disorder

SYMPTOMATIC SEIZURES

Eliminate or control causative factor
    Correct metabolic imbalance
    Treat infection
    Surgically remove tumors or abscesses, when possible

Drug therapy to control recurrent seizures

IDIOPATHIC SEIZURES

Drug therapy to control recurrent seizures

DRUG THERAPY

Sequential addition to initial single drug until combination therapy controls recurrent seizures

Drugs: combination of phenobarbital and phenytoin is most common regimen for grand mal seizures
    Phenobarbital; side effects: drowsiness, CNS depression
    Phenytoin (Dilantin); side effects: confusion, ataxia, skin rashes, gingival hyperplasia
    Primidone (Mysoline)
        Increasing popularity as alternative for grand mal seizure control
        First drug of choice for psychomotor seizure
        Phenobarbital is major metabolite
    Ethosuximide (Zarontin): most commonly used drug for isolated petit mal seizures
    Carbamazepine (Tegretol)
    Diazepam (Valium): recommended "emergency" drug for dental patient in status epilepticus
    Clonazepam (Clonopin)

SUMMARY TABLE **31–IV**

Dental Evaluation of the Patient with a Seizure Disorder

Type of seizure

Medications, including recent changes in regimen

Frequency of seizures—"poor control": seizure more frequently than once a month

Specifics of oral examination for patients on phenytoin therapy
Determine extent of hyperplasia (degree and distribution)
Determine extent of coincident inflammatory disease
Evaluate hyperplasia as contributory factor to periodontitis
Evaluate hyperplasia with regard to compromise in esthetics and masticating function
Determine oral hygiene level
Rule out presence of defective restorations, caries

SUMMARY TABLE **31–V**

Dental Management of the Patient with a Seizure Disorder

Dental therapy contraindicated for patients with poor control (i.e., more than one seizure per month)

Non-narcotic analgesics (i.e., NSAIDs) preferred for patients receiving the CNS depressant drugs phenobarbital and primidone

If narcotic analgesics necessary, reduce dosage for patients concurrently receiving CNS depressant drugs

Tetracyclines relatively contraindicated for patients on phenytoin, phenobarbital, or primidone; degradation of antibiotic accelerated

Management of gingival hyperplasia
Control oral hygiene
Thoroughly débride local factors and control superimposed inflammatory gingival changes
Frequent recall prophylaxis and oral hygiene review schedule
Consider surgical therapy if there is
Major esthetic compromise
Major compromise of masticatory function
Concurrent alveolar bone destruction (i.e., periodontitis)
Inability to control inflammatory tissue changes conservatively because of anatomic predisposition to plaque retention
Consider medical consultation for alternate anticonvulsant therapy (i.e., substitute for phenytoin) if
Adequate conservative therapy and surgery have failed (recurrent hyperplasia)
Conservative therapy, especially proper oral hygiene and close dental follow-up are unrealistic (e.g., institutionalized or retarded patient, uncooperative patient or guardian)

Minimize risk of aspiration (acute seizure during dental appointment)
Rubber dam and clamp with floss lead attached preferable to multiple intraoral cotton rolls
Fixed restorations preferred to removable prosthesis
Unilateral "Nesbit-type" partials strictly contraindicated
Laboratory-processed, metal-reinforced temporary crowns and bridges preferred over all-acrylic office-cured temporary prostheses
Metal major connectors or metal plates for all mandatory removable prostheses

Management of Seizures

Primary goal: prevent self-inflicted injury
1. Place patient in supine position.
2. Gently, but not forcibly, restrain the patient.
3. If possible, place part of a towel or padded tongue depressor between teeth (to prevent biting lips and tongue).
4. Ensure airway patency by extending patient's head.
5. Monitor vital signs.
6. Most seizures last 2 to 5 min, followed by a postictal phase.
7. During postictal phase, the patient may be confused and recovers over a 1-hr period.
8. Discharge patient from the dental office in the custody of a responsible person.
9. With recurrent seizures or persistent seizure activity (more than 5 min)
    Obtain medical assistance.
    Call for immediate transportation to an emergency room.
    Administer 5–10 mg IV diazepam (1 to 2 ml of 5 mg/ml solution) slowly* over 1 to 2 min.

*Significant respiratory and cardiovascular depression may accompany IV diazepam; personnel must be thoroughly familiar with the use of IV medications and complications.

32

Cerebrovascular Disease

Cerebrovascular disease is the third leading cause of death in the United States, ranking behind heart disease and cancer. The clinical entities of major importance to the dentist include transient ischemic attacks (TIAs) and cerebrovascular accidents (CVAs), or stroke. TIAs result in reversible neurologic disability, but the damage of CVA is irreversible. The most significant cause is the formation of thrombi (aggregations of platelets and debris) at the site of ulcerated atherosclerotic plaques in the cardiovascular system. A thrombus may cause damage at the site of origin if it is in the cerebrovascular tree or may do so after embolization from a distant site (most often the heart). Once a thromboembolism occludes a vessel, distal ischemia results. Clinical symptoms relate to this ischemia and, in the case of TIAs, are transient as the thrombus is fragmented or dissolved, thus restoring normal circulation. The impact of the vessel occlusion is rapid because of the brain's constant high demand for oxygen and glucose substrate, with little or no storage of the latter. The TIA may last just a few minutes or up to 24 hours, depending on the extent of vessel occlusion and the body's response to dissolving the thrombus. If the ischemia persists too long, cerebral infarction occurs, causing an irreversible stroke. If the vessel occlusion is complete initially, then the infarct may be the primary event. The most important risk factor is the presence of atherosclerosis (Chap. 3), especially that complicated by untreated hypertension. Diabetes mellitus, smoking, and hypercholesterolemia and hyperlipidemia as risk factors for atherosclerosis are also risk factors for cerebrovascular disease, as are age, the use of oral contraceptives, and heart disease. Emboli from defective heart valves or valvular prostheses, emboli in atrial fibrillation, systemic hypotension from myocardial infarction, or heart block may cause cerebrovascular disease. Indeed, the aggressive treatment of longstanding hypertension may itself be a causative factor, making that disease a dual-edged sword. Finally, in addition to thrombosis and embolism, stroke may be the product of cerebral hemorrhage resulting from an interplay between hypertension and a vascular aneurysm.

MEDICAL EVALUATION

The medical evaluation of transient ischemic attacks is critical. Because one-third of all untreated patients with TIAs suffer a complete stroke, and because more than 30% of all patients having TIAs die within 5 years, a correctible cause must be sought. By definition, a TIA leaves no neurologic deficit. The physician's primary source of information is the past history of the episode. Depending on the visual, sensory, or motor loss patterns, localization to the carotid artery and to the vertebrobasilar artery syndrome may be made. Clinical examination may reveal a diminished or absent carotid pulse or a carotid bruit, all suggestive of carotid stenosis as the primary cause. The critical diagnostic decision for the physician is whether to perform carotid arteriography. Definitive diagnosis and distribution of carotid stenosis may suggest curative surgical therapy (endarterectomy). Unfortunately, the diagnostic arteriography itself carries a significant risk of morbidity or mortality. Other less invasive, lower risk procedures such as radionuclide angiography may suggest or rule out surgical therapy. Emphasis is then placed on medical management of the cerebrovascular disease.

Stroke patients fall into two distinct categories: the patient with ongoing or evolving stroke and the patient with completed stroke. A stroke in evolution is one with a progression or worsening of neurologic symptoms within 24 to 72 hours of the original signs. Aggressive medical therapy may limit the area of infarct and the residual neurologic damage. A completed stroke is one in which the neurologic deficiency has been stable for 24 to 72 hours.

MEDICAL MANAGEMENT

The cornerstone of medical management for cerebrovascular disease is prevention. Underlying conditions that contribute to reversible TIAs are treated aggressively before stroke occurs. This usually involves aggressive therapy for hypertension, but treatment may also include carotid endarterectomy, therapy to correct atrial fibrillation, and prosthetic valve replacement for defective heart valves. No uniform medical regimen exists. However, antiplatelet aggregation drugs and anticoagulants are typically prescribed for 6 to 12 months for most TIAs and often longer for CVA victims. Typically, aspirin (300 mg, bid to qid) or warfarin (Coumadin) therapy is used. Therapeutic warfarin maintains the prothrombin time at two to three times the normal control value and is generally monitored by the physician using repeat bimonthly tests. The physician pays special attention to the blood pressure in both controlling hypertension and preventing hypotension to avoid recurrent disease. Stress reduction, limited physical exertion, and controlled physical rehabilitation are important. The patient with cerebrovascular disease is at particular risk during surgical procedures using general anesthesia, and blood pressure must be strictly controlled.

DENTAL EVALUATION

The primary concerns for the dentist relative to the patient with cerebrovascular disease are fourfold. First, the dentist must realize that the presence of any significant cerebrovascular disease suggests the probability of advanced atherosclerosis. Therefore, the patient is at a higher risk not only for stroke but also for the full range of heart pathology (Chap. 3). Second, the dentist should be aware of possible known causative factors that would affect care in other ways. An example is a patient with a history of TIA secondary to atrial fibrillation and mitral stenosis. Antibiotic prophylaxis to prevent subacute bacterial endocarditis and an appropriate sedation technique may be in order. Third, the relative stability of the cerebrovascular disease is important. *Patients who are within 6 to 12 months of diagnosed TIA or CVA are at higher risk for exacerbation of disease than other patients.* Patients with frequent TIAs or TIAs of increasing frequency are also high-risk patients. Finally, a detailed drug history is in or-

der. Specific questions regarding aspirin and warfarin use are imperative.

For all these reasons a medical consultation is advisable. In addition to specific answers for these questions, the dentist should discuss a stress reduction protocol and choice of analgesics with the physician. Narcotic analgesics, sedative-hypnotics, and several antianxiety drugs have CNS depressant effects that might contribute to an episode of hypotension and an exacerbation of the cerebrovascular disease.

DENTAL MANAGEMENT

Elective dental therapy in high-risk patients with cerebrovascular disease is contraindicated. Patients within 6 to 12 months of an acute event (TIA or CVA) should receive palliative dental care. This might involve the aggressive antibiotic management of an abscessed tooth or the root canal débridement aspect of endodontic therapy rather than extraction. Multiple extractions and comprehensive dental care should be deferred.

When surgical procedures are planned, normal hemostasis must be ensured. Patients on warfarin require cessation of the drug for 2 days to allow the warfarin level to fall below 1.5 times the control value (Chap. 26). Consultation with the physician and possible hospitalization are recommended. For patients on chronic aspirin therapy, a preoperative normal bleeding time must be determined. An abnormal bleeding time requires discontinuing the aspirin for 7 to 10 days and repeating the bleeding time test prior to surgery. Again, a medical consultation is advised (Chap. 26).

The dentist must also carefully select an appropriate sedation technique. Although stress reduction to maintain normal blood pressure, heart rate, and rhythm is important, the selection of techniques must minimize the risk of hypotensive episodes. Therefore, the practitioner might rely on N_2O-O_2 conscious inhalation sedation, possibly supplemented by small doses of oral diazepam (Valium). This low-potential CNS depressant regimen is preferred to the use of oral barbiturates or any of the intravenous sedation techniques. The use of the latter is relatively contraindicated for all but the most skilled operator in the ideal setting for emergency back-up.

Outpatient general anesthesia for patients with cerebrovascular disease is strictly contraindicated because of the labile nature of the blood pressure in this setting, particularly for those patients being treated for concomitant hypertension (Chap. 4).

For similar reasons, the dentist may wish to minimize the use of narcotic analgesics. Non-narcotic alternatives are preferred as long as their potential effects on platelet function have been considered (Chap. 50).

■ Examples of Dental Evaluation and Management

EVALUATION

Patient 1. A 54-year-old man presents with a history of hypertension, heart murmur, and arrhythmia. He is presently on a diuretic, propranolol, and warfarin (Coumadin). Consultation with his physician reveals a 5-year history of well-controlled hypertension, atrial fibrillation, and mitral stenosis. His most recent prothrombin time, done 2 weeks ago, was 25 seconds, with a control of 11 seconds. On physical examination, his resting blood pressure is 138/84 and his pulse is 58 beats/minute (bpm) and irregular.

This patient has hopelessly severe maxillary periodontal disease. The mandibular dentition has moderate periodontal disease, multiple caries, and missing second bicuspids and first molars bilaterally. The mandibular incisors are nearly hopeless.

Patient 2. A 62-year-old woman presents for dental treatment. She was hospitalized 3 months prior to this examination for acute "temporary paralysis on my left side." The patient also reports that "my speech was garbled" at that time. She further states that she has "recovered completely" and is now taking "a blood thinner and a water pill and something else for my blood pressure." Prior to this recent hospitalization, the patient reported "perfect health."

Consultation with the patient's physician reveals a history of a transient ischemic attack occurring 3 months ago that required a 2-week hospitalization. Previously untreated hypertension is now well controlled with a thiazide diuretic and hydralazine therapy. The patient is also currently on warfarin (Coumadin) therapy, which the physician plans to discontinue within the next 6 months.

On physical examination the patient's blood pressure is 138/86 and her pulse is 74 bpm and regular. Her dental needs are identical to those of Patient 1.

Patient 3. A 68-year-old man presents with a history of multiple TIAs preceding a frank stroke (CVA) 1½ years ago. He presents with residual right-sided motor deficiency and is accompanied to the office by his youngest daughter. He is currently on warfarin (Coumadin) therapy as a preventative for recurrent stroke, and digoxin and Lasix for "heart failure." The patient has significant dyspnea on exertion, requiring assistance to negotiate the four steps up to his bedroom.

His blood pressure is 140/88 and his pulse is 78 bpm and regular. The distribution of dental pathoses is similar to that of Patients 1 and 2.

MANAGEMENT

Patient 1. This patient does not have documented cerebrovascular disease. However, the patient's atrial fibrillation in the presence of concurrent mitral stenosis places the patient at risk for embolus-induced TIA or CVA. The appropriate medical management is prevention—hence, the anticoagulant therapy.

The ideal dental treatment plan involves maxillary full-arch extraction (type VI procedure), followed by placement of a full denture. For the mandible, a full range of operative caries excavation (type II), selective extraction of the incisors (type IV), prosthetic fixed temporization (type III), periodontal surgery (type V), and final periodontal fixed prosthesis (type III) would be ideal therapy.

The presence of the mitral stenosis requires subacute bacterial endocarditis (SBE) prophylaxis for all appointments (Chap. 11).

The presence of atrial fibrillation suggests the use of sedation techniques for moderate and advanced dental surgery (Chap. 51).

The PT is greater than 1½ times the control value, and therefore warfarin (Coumadin) management is needed for all procedures causing gingival bleeding or for procedures requiring block local anesthesia (Chap. 26). Aspirin-containing drugs are contraindicated.

In view of the extent of the surgical therapy, the need for sedation, and the warfarin (Coumadin) management, elective hospitalization for maxillary full-arch extraction and mandibular periodontal surgery may be considered.

Patient 2. This patient has a history of a recent TIA (within 3 months), probably precipitated by uncontrolled hypertension and generalized atherosclerotic vascular changes. The hypertension is now well controlled.

The dental treatment plan should include caries control and minimal scaling and oral hygiene instruction (types II and III procedures) only for the next 6 months. This temporary palliative treatment plan requires warfarin (Coumadin) dose adjustment in consultation with the physician for all procedures using mandibular block anesthesia or involving gingival trauma.

After 6 to 12 months have elapsed from the acute TIA and the warfarin (Coumadin) therapy has been discontinued, a more ideal dental treatment plan can be implemented, with greater safety for the patient and an easier protocol for the dentist.

Definitive scaling and curettage can be completed in the dental office. Multiple extractions and periodontal surgery may be accomplished in the outpatient setting or during an elective hospitalization. Sedation techniques and a stress reduction protocol (i.e., shorter appointments) are recommended. A mandibular partial denture prosthetic treatment plan may be considered instead of an extensive fixed periodontal prosthesis, but the latter is not contraindicated.

Patient 3. This patient has had cerebrovascular disease with significant residual physical deficit. He also has congestive heart failure and is significantly debilitated. It is 1½ years since his CVA, and he is on warfarin (Coumadin) therapy for an indefinite period.

A palliative dental treatment plan is recommended. In view of the debilitating systemic disease, a comprehensive ideal treatment plan is relatively contraindicated. Warfarin dose adjustment in consultation with the physician is required for most palliative procedures. Elective hospitalization is strongly recommended for all dental surgery. Only the most simple periodontal and prosthetic treatment measures should be considered.

SUMMARY TABLE **32–1**

Cerebrovascular Disease

CLINICAL ENTITIES

Transient ischemic attack (TIA): reversible neurologic disability for a few minutes to 24 hr

Cerebrovascular accident (CVA): irreversible neurologic damage

CAUSE

Ischemia or infarct secondary to thromboembolic occlusion of a vessel, most often at the site of ulcerated atherosclerotic plaques

RISK FACTORS

Atherosclerosis

Untreated hypertension

Diabetes mellitus

Smoking

Hyperlipidemia (hypercholesterolemia)

Age

Oral contraceptives

Heart disease

CLINICAL IMPORTANCE

Cerebrovascular disease—third leading cause of death in the United States

One-third of all patients with untreated TIAs—suffer complete stroke (CVA)

30% of all patients with TIAs—dead within 5 yr

SUMMARY TABLE **32–II**

Medical Evaluation of the Patient with Cerebrovascular Disease

Neurologic examination
  Localize visual, sensory, and/or motor loss patterns to the carotid artery or vertebrobasilar artery syndrome
Physical examination for diminished carotid pulse or a carotid bruit (suggestive of carotid stenosis)
± Carotid arteriography
Radionuclide angiography

±, with or without.

SUMMARY TABLE **32–III**

Medical Management of the Patient with Cerebrovascular Disease

Prevention: minimize risk factors
  Aggressive therapy for hypertension
  Carotid endarterectomy
  Therapy to correct atrial fibrillation and prosthetic valve replacement

Anticoagulant (Coumadin)-antiplatelet aggregation (aspirin-containing) drugs
  TIA: often 6–12 mo
  CVA: often longer than 6–12 mo

Strict control of blood pressure (hypertension-hypotension increase the potential for recurrent cerebrovascular disease)

Dental Evaluation of the Patient with Cerebrovascular Disease

History of cerebrovascular accident (CVA)

History of transient ischemic attacks (TIAs)

Presence of risk factors
  Hypertension
  Diabetes mellitus
  Smoking
  Hyperlipidemia-hypercholesterolemia
  Age
  Oral contraceptives

Other cardiovascular disease

Hospitalizations

Medications
  Antiplatelet drugs (containing aspirin)
  Anticoagulants (Coumadin)
  Other (antihypertensives, antiarrhythmic drugs)

Blood pressure, pulse (rate and rhythm)

Medical consultation

Dental Management of the Patient with Cerebrovascular Disease

PATIENTS WITHIN 6–12 MONTHS OF TIA OR CVA
Medical consultation mandatory

Elective dental care relatively contraindicated

Advanced outpatient sedation techniques (IV sedation) and general anesthesia strictly contraindicated

Moderate and advanced dental surgery (types V, VI) require hospitalization

Appropriate management of antiplatelet and anticoagulant medication

Minimize use of CNS depressant drugs (i.e., narcotic analgesics, barbiturates)

PATIENTS 6–12 MONTHS OR MORE AFTER TIA OR CVA
Medical consultation recommended

Advanced outpatient sedation techniques (IV sedation) and general anesthesia contraindicated

Consider elective hospitalization for moderate and advanced dental surgery (types V, VI)

Appropriate management of antiplatelet and anticoagulant drugs

Minimize use of CNS depressant drugs (i.e., narcotic analgesics, barbiturates)

Stress reduction protocol (simple and intermediate sedation techniques recommended)

Craniofacial Neurologic Disorders

TASTE DISORDERS

Taste disorders are relatively common problems that, in addition to being annoying to the patient, may lead to nutritional and digestive problems. Three categories of taste disorders have been described: ageusia, or absence of taste; hypogeusia, or diminished taste; and dysgeusia, or distortion of taste.

Taste is mediated by chemoreceptors called taste buds, each an organ of about 50 cells, which are distributed throughout the mouth and oropharynx. Cells within taste buds routinely are replaced over a 10-day cycle. Hence, any disorder or drug that modifies mitoses, such as cancer chemotherapy, alters the patient's ability to taste. The taste buds of the tongue are of major functional significance and are found in fungiform, foliate, and circumvallate papillae. Fungiform papillae are found on the anterior two-thirds of the tongue and are innervated by the facial nerve (cranial nerve [CN] VII). Circumvallate papillae are arranged in a V-shaped configuration on the posterior third of the tongue. Both the circumvallate and foliate papillae are innervated by the glossopharyngeal nerve (CN IX).

The sense of taste results from a combination of stimulation of taste buds and smell. Alterations in either of these result in changes in sensation. The most common causes of taste dysfunction are usually the consequence of local problems such as periodontal disease, poor oral hygiene, dentures, or physical or chemical irritation. Aging, with its resultant decrease in mitotic activity, may also account for changes in taste. Modifications in saliva, although not as frequent, may contribute to a reduced or modified ability to taste. Many drugs affect taste (Table 33–1), some by direct chemical interaction with taste buds, others by modifying saliva or reducing cell renewal.

A variety of systemic diseases (Table 33–2) including diabetes mellitus, cancer, and renal failure have been reported to affect taste to varying degrees. Although not a presenting sign of these diseases, taste alterations can be bothersome and may require alterations in patients' diets. Viral illnesses may temporarily modify taste.

The dentist's approach to patients complaining of taste disorders should be aimed primarily at eliminating or ruling out local factors as a cause of the problem. If this has been done to the dentist's satisfaction and there is no reason to suspect drug-induced changes, the patient should be referred to a physician (usually a neurologist) for additional evaluation.

GLOSSODYNIA

Glossodynia, or burning tongue, is a relatively common complaint (Fig. 33–1). Frequently, the problem is related to some form of local irritation. However, a number of underlying systemic diseases may cause glossodynia. In many instances, the reason for the problem cannot be readily identified.

In taking a history of the patient complaining of glossodynia, the nature of onset, the location (localized versus generalized), the patient's age, and the medical history may provide important diagnostic clues. Patients complaining of pain of abrupt onset or following the placement of a new prosthesis or restoration may be manifesting a form of local irritation. In contrast, patients noting a chronic, progressive onset may have atrophic changes in the tongue resulting from a systemic illness.

On examination, the tongue should first be inspected for signs of local irritation. Most often, this takes the form of areas of ulceration or erythema and erosion. If a lesion can be found and is in proximity to a source of mechanical irritation, treatment is straightforward—elimination of the source of the problem.

Table 33–1. DRUGS AFFECTING TASTE AND SMELL

Classification	Drug
Amebicide, anthelmintic	Metronidazole, niridazole
Anesthetic, local	Benzocaine, procaine hydrochloride (Novocain), and others, cocaine hydrochloride, tetracaine hydrochloride
Anticholesteremic	Clofibrate
Anticoagulant	Phenindione
Antihistamine	Chlorpheniramine maleate
Antimicrobial	Amphotericin B, ampicillin, cefamandole, griseofulvin, ethambutol hydrochloride, lincomycin, sulfasalazine, streptomycin, tetracyclines, tyrothricin
Antiproliferative, including immunosuppressive	Doxorubicin and methotrexate, azathioprine, carmustine, vincristine sulfate
Antirheumatic, analgesic, antipyretic, anti-inflammatory	Allopurinol, colchicine, gold, levamisole, D-penicillamine, phenylbutazone, 5-thiopyridoxine
Antiseptic	Hexetidine
Antithyroid	Carbimazole, methimazole, methylthiouracil, propylthiouracil, Thiouracil
Dental hygiene	Sodium lauryl sulfate (toothpaste)
Diuretic and antihypertensive	Captopril, diazoxide, ethacrynic acid
Hypoglycemic	Glipizide, phenformin and derivatives
Muscle relaxant drugs for treatment of Parkinson's disease	Baclofen, chlormezanone, levodopa
Opiates	Codeine, hydromorphone hydrochloride, morphine
Psychopharmacologic, including antiepileptic	Carbamazepine, lithium carbonate, phenytoin, psilocybin, trifluoperazine
Sympathomimetic	Amphetamines, phenmetrazine theoclate and fenbutrazate hydrochloride (combined)
Vasodilator	Oxyfedrine, bamifylline hydrochloride
Others	Germine monoacetate, idoxyuridine, iron sorbitex, vitamin D, industrial chemicals, including insecticides

From Schiffman, S. S.: Taste and smell in disease. N. Engl. J. Med., 308:1277, 1983.

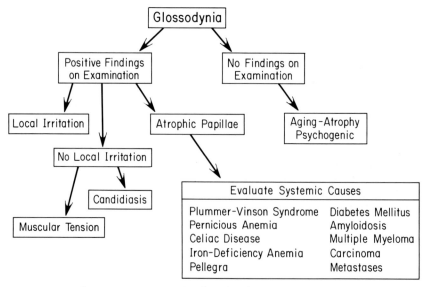

Figure 33–1. Sequence for clinical evaluation of glossodynia.

Table 33–2. DISORDERS AFFECTING TASTE AND SMELL

Disorders	Taste*
Nervous	
Bell's palsy	A/D
Damage to chorda tympani	A/D
Familial dysautonomia	A/D
Head trauma	A/D
Multiple sclerosis	A/D/D
Raeder's paratrigeminal syndrome	Distorted
Nutritional	
Cancer	A/D (sweet); heightened (bitter in some cases)
Chronic renal failure	A/D/D (metallic taste)
Cirrhosis of the liver	A/D
Niacin (vitamin B₃) deficiency	A/D/D
Thermal burn	A/D/D
Zinc deficiency	A/D
Endocrine	
Adrenocortical insufficiency	IDDR
Congenital adrenal hyperplasia	IDDR
Panhypopituitarism	IDDR
Cushing's syndrome	A/D
Cretinism	A/D
Hypothyroidism	A/D/D
Diabetes mellitus	A/D (glucose)
Gonadal dysgenesis (Turner's syndrome)	
Pseudohypoparathyroidism	A/D (bitter, sour)
Local	
Facial hypoplasia	A/D
Sjögren's syndrome	A/D
Radiation therapy	A/D/D
Viral and infectious	
Acute viral hepatitis	
Influenza-like infections	A/D/D
Other	
Cystic fibrosis	Individual variation
Hypertension	A/D (salt)
Laryngectomy	A/D/D

Adapted from information appearing in *The New England Journal of Medicine*. Modified from Schiffman, S. S.: Taste and smell in disease. N. Engl. J. Med., 308:1276, 1983.

*A/D, absent or diminished; A/D/D, absent, diminished, or distorted; IDDR, increased detection, but decreased recognition.

It should be noted that "taste" disorders are often the result of deficiencies in smell rather than taste functioning. Relative losses in smell are sometimes ascribed to losses in taste.

The presence of atrophic papillae may indicate underlying systemic disease, including diabetes mellitus, a number of nutritional deficiencies, and some malignancies. If atrophy is noted, the history is often helpful in delineating the direction of additional workup and studies. Pernicious anemia, iron deficiency anemia, and diabetes mellitus are easily ruled out by laboratory evaluation. If patients also complain of other systemic signs or symptoms, such as weight loss, bone pain, or diarrhea, they should be referred to a physician for further evaluation.

Coating of the tongue may indicate candidiasis, which causes surface necrosis and underlying erythema (Chap. 49). Such infection may produce symptoms of burning or pain. Patients should be questioned about antibiotic therapy, because suppression of the normal oral bacterial flora by such medication may produce fungal infection. Generally, broad-spectrum antibiotics such as tetracycline cause candidiasis more commonly than narrow-spectrum medications. Other causes of candidiasis include generalized immunosuppression caused by medication, disease, or age extremes.

Rarely, glossodynia may accompany congenital abnormalities of the tongue (Chap. 39). Patients with fissured tongue are often sensitive to acidic foods. A similar pattern may be noted by patients with geographic tongue.

In the majority of patients (75%) with glossodynia, no clinically apparent abnormalities can be observed. In this group, atrophic changes resulting from aging or psychogenic causes appear to be the most frequent causes. Patients should be reassured and treated palliatively with local ointments (benzocaine in Orabase) or rinses.

NEUROLOGIC PAIN SYNDROMES

A number of neurologic pain syndromes mimic odontogenic or myofacial pain. Thus, when the dentist evaluates facial pain, a variety of syndromes or conditions may be considered in the differential diagnosis. Among these are idiopathic trigeminal neuralgia, periodic migrainous headaches, migraine headaches, posttraumatic neuropathy, and systemic disease neuropathy.

Trigeminal Neuralgia

Idiopathic trigeminal neuralgia, or tic douloureux, is a localized neuralgia characterized by episodes of extreme sharp or electric pain of short duration. This neuralgia is seen most frequently in patients of middle to old age, although its presence may be symptomatic of multiple sclerosis in younger individuals. Pain is initiated by contact with a specific trigger zone, which is frequently on the face but may be intraoral. For some reason, the neuralgia and trigger zone are more common on the right side than the left. The third (mandibular) branch of the trigeminal nerve is most often affected. Tic douloureux has a slight predilection for females.

The cause of trigeminal neuralgia is unknown. Various mechanisms for the condition have been suggested, including possible circulatory insufficiency and the production of compression of the gasserian ganglion by pulsations of the carotid artery.

The diagnosis of trigeminal neuralgia can usually be made on the basis of the history. Local anesthetic nerve block of the trigger zone prevents the onset of pain for a short period and is therefore a good confirmatory diagnostic technique.

A variety of treatment approaches have been used in patients with trigeminal neuralgia, who often go to great lengths for relief of their excruciating pain. Analgesics are of no help in treating this disease. Carbamazepine (Tegretol), which inhibits the action of polysynaptic reflexes, has been used with reasonable success if taken continually. Although the drug appears safe for most patients, a number of side effects, including dizziness, blurred vision, and myelosuppression, have been reported. Phenytoin (Dilantin) has been used with mixed success.

Surgical or chemical destruction or severance of the affected nerve has enjoyed mixed success. Alcohol injections have historically been used. Absolute alcohol may be injected into the peripheral nerve in small amounts. This technique is relatively safe but may result in edema, necrosis, trismus, or hematoma formation of a few days' duration. Absolute alcohol may also be injected into the foramen ovale, with the placement being guided by radiographic monitoring. Clearly, this technique requires a high level of operator skill. Finally, surgical peripheral neurectomy may be performed.

Migraine and Cluster Headaches

Migraine and cluster headaches are thought to be of vascular origin. Migraine headaches are common, affecting approximately 50% of the American population. Migraine headaches may occur alone or as part of a more widespread syndrome in which patients experience symptoms such as nausea, vomiting, diarrhea, constipation, or photophobia. Migraine headaches are usually first experienced during puberty and are more common in women than men. About half of patients who experience migraines have a familial history of the problem. Women who experience migraines are at risk for stroke, especially if they smoke or use oral contraceptive pills.

Clinically, migraine headaches are often heralded by a prodrome, which may include vertigo, tunnel vision, spots before the eyes, or a feeling of detachment. Headaches are usually unilateral but may spread to involve both sides of the head. The temporal area and upper lateral part of the face are often involved. Pain is characterized by throbbing and aching and may vary significantly in both duration and severity.

Vasodilation has been associated with the onset of migraines. Hence, pressure on the carotid frequently provides symptomatic relief and is a helpful diagnostic sign. Analgesics are not generally effective in managing migraines. In contrast, vasoconstrictors, such as Cafergot tablets, may be beneficial.

Cluster headaches are considered a modification of migraine headaches and are also referred to as periodic migrainous headache. Cluster headaches are more common in men than in women and are usually noted in those in an older age group (thirties to sixties) than classic migraine headache.

Cluster headaches are characterized by an abrupt onset free of any prodromal signs. Usually, the headaches begin in the midfacial region but may progress to involve the forehead. Patients experience intense throbbing, burning, or aching for relatively short periods (5 to 20 minutes). Painful episodes usually are repeated several times a day and then spontaneously disappear. Watery discharge from the nose and eyes usually accompanies the headaches. Alcohol appears to increase the likelihood of cluster headache onset.

Post-traumatic Neuropathy

Occasionally, head injury may cause subsequent neuropathy that results in clinical headache. A number of causes have been associated with this form of headache, including scarring, muscle tenderness, and vascular changes. Rarely, an intracranial cause in the form of hematoma may cause this type of discomfort and is often elicited by deep pressure. Patients complain of burning, numbness, or throbbing. Symptoms may respond to nerve blocks or systemic analgesics.

FACIAL NERVE PARALYSIS

The seventh cranial nerve (the facial nerve, CN VII) controls the muscles of facial expression. Paralysis of the facial nerve is most commonly associated with Bell's palsy. This condition, in which there is unilateral involvement of the facial nerve, is most frequently thought to be polyneuritis that occurs as a sequela to a viral infection (often herpes simplex). Generally, patients demonstrate an acute onset preceded by a viral prodrome. In addition to facial nerve involvement, other cranial nerves may also be involved, especially the trigeminal and glossopharyngeal nerves. Facial nerve paralysis need not be complete; prognosis is often associated with the extent of involvement and whether, over time, there is actual nerve degeneration. In patients with incomplete paralysis, recovery generally occurs in 3 to 6 weeks. In patients in whom there has been partial nerve damage, improvement may be incomplete but is generally noted no later than 12 weeks after the onset of the paralysis. Of patients affected, 80% recover fully.

Bell's palsy is usually treated by neurologists, but otolaryngologists may also become involved. Treatment generally consists of patient reassurance, eye protection, and palliation (pain often accompanies Bell's palsy), which can be achieved with steroids and muscle stimulation. Surgery is sometimes suggested to decompress the facial nerve, but results are not uniformly successful.

Another cause of facial paralysis of special significance to the dentist is the inadvertent injection of local anesthesia into the body of the parotid gland during inferior alveolar nerve block. The body of the parotid contains the facial nerve. Consequently, the introduction of local anesthesia results in the abrupt onset of transient facial paralysis. Treatment of this problem consists of reassurance of the patient and, most importantly, protection of the eye. The latter may be accomplished by the use of dark glasses and artificial tears to prevent drying. Taping the affected eye closed has also been suggested. If the patient experiences any signs of eye irritation, an ophthalmic consultation is indicated. The paralysis should wear off a few hours after injection.

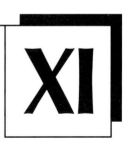
Evaluation and Management of the Patient with Psychiatric Disease

Psychiatric Disease

Approximately 20% of all prescriptions given in the United States are for medications whose primary effect is to alter the mental status of the patient. This figure excludes medications given for other therapeutic goals that have secondary effects on mental status. It is obvious, therefore, that the dentist can encounter a significant number of patients receiving drugs that affect their psychiatric state.

It is far beyond our scope here to discuss at length the variety of mental disorders treated by the psychiatrist or internist. More than in any other specialty in medicine, controversy exists over the definition of disorders and the recommended therapy. Nevertheless, the dentist is asked to treat patients who are receiving a variety of psychoactive drugs, many of which have profound interactions with the drugs common to routine dental protocols. The physician often refers to the use of a particular drug in a pseudoclassification descriptive of the underlying condition. "Antipsychotic" agents are often one of the phenothiazines or haloperidol. "Antidepressants" may refer to one of the monoamine oxidase (MAO) inhibitors (e.g., Nardil), tricyclic antidepressant agents, or the newer selective serotonin reuptake inhibitors (e.g., Prozac). Lithium is often referred to as a "mood-stabilizing" agent used for "affective disorders," such as mania or depression. Finally, the physician may refer to an "antianxiety" or "sedative" medication, such as one of the benzodiazepines or meprobamate. The crossover use of terms with particular drugs is universal and can often seem intimidating to the dentist.

DENTAL EVALUATION

When a patient reports "psychiatric therapy" or the use of a common psychoactive drug (Summary Table 34–I), a physician consultation is always advisable. Prior to this consultation, however, a thorough examination should be completed (type I procedure). An overall ideal treatment plan and potential alternatives consistent with oral health should be developed.

The impact of the patient's medications on the dentist's choice of local anesthetic solutions, sedation techniques, and postoperative analgesics must be reviewed. The effect on caries and periodontal disease susceptibility must also be considered. The dentist must then assess the individual's potential for cooperation. This is a twofold assessment in that the ability to tolerate individual dental appointments as well as to commit to a sequence of interdependent visits must be evaluated.

At this point, preceding any definitive care (types II to VI procedures), the internist or psychiatrist should be consulted.

The physician can first provide an assessment of the patient's status. Can the dentist anticipate a well-controlled patient whose usual demeanor was reflected in the first dentist-patient meeting? Or can the dentist anticipate several acute exacerbations of psychiatric disease over time during an extended dental treatment plan?

The physician may also provide clues as to the manner in which the dentist may secure patient confidence and cooperation.

The dentist should then discuss with the physician the choice of anesthesia, possible sedation techniques, and potential analgesics, because they may interact with the patient's psychoactive medication (see later).

DENTAL MANAGEMENT

Treatment Planning

It is inadvisable to plan complex prosthetic-periodontal treatment for the potentially uncooperative, marginally controlled psychiatric patient. Palliative care only may be the therapy of choice for such patients until better medical control is achieved.

Xerostomia. If the patient is receiving phenothiazines, tricyclic antidepressants, or MAO inhibitors (Summary Table 34–I), aggressive recall is in order. (Recall is especially needed for patients on all tricyclic antidepressants but is not needed as consistently for patients on MAO inhibitors or selected phenothiazines.) These agents, with their atropine-like effect, produce significant xerostomia as a side effect. Therefore, more frequent prophylaxis, caries, and periodontal examinations and adjunctive fluoride therapy may be appropriate for patients at high risk for dental disease. The poorly controlled uncooperative psychiatric patient probably ignores required oral hygiene home care, whereas the cooperative controlled patient needs supportive maintenance for any sophisticated prosthetic treatment undertaken by the dentist.

Dental Drugs

The remainder of the dental management is dictated by the interaction of the particular psychoactive drugs with vasoconstrictors in local anesthesia and central nervous system depressants. There might be a relative or absolute contraindication to the use of these latter agents because of possible synergism with the psychoactive medication.

Use of Vasoconstrictors. If a patient is receiving MAO inhibitor drugs (Summary Table 34–I), the use of vasoconstrictor agents (e.g., epinephrine) in local anesthesia solutions is no longer contraindicated. While human studies are not available, animal models demonstrate no interaction between epinephrine, norepinephrine, levonordefrin, and MAO inhibitors. Indeed, the degradation of these vasoconstrictors is regulated by the enzyme catechol methyltransferase and is not affected by the presence of MAO inhibitors. Only phenylephrine, which is metabolized by monoamine oxidase, is likely to be potentiated severalfold by MAO inhibitors and is therefore strictly contraindicated. Phenylephrine is found in cold and allergy medications and is rarely used as a vasoconstrictor in regional anesthesia.

Other sympathomimetic agents can precipitate a lethal hypertensive crisis in patients on MAO inhibitors. Analogously, it has been reported that the tricyclic antidepressants can potentiate the effects of catecholamines, so local anesthetics with vasoconstrictors should be minimized. Phenothiazines, haloperidol, lithium, and sedative hypnotics have minimal interaction with common dental vasoconstrictors.

Central Nervous System Depressants. All CNS depressants, particularly narcotic analgesics and barbiturates used in some sedation techniques, are strictly contraindicated in patients receiving MAO inhibitors; their interaction carries a significant mortality risk. The phenothiazines also affect these agents and are relatively contraindicated.* Indeed, for all patients taking psychoactive medications, narcotics must be prescribed with caution.

Non-narcotic analgesics are preferred, but if narcotics are indicated, the appropriate dosage of narcotic may be 25 to 50% the normal dose to obtain the same analgesia or sedation. Consultation and clearance with the physician is mandatory. To a lesser but still significant extent, tricyclic antidepressant drugs also potentiate CNS depression, and avoidance or dosage adjustment of CNS depressants is indicated in consultation with the physician. For patients using other psychoactive drugs, caution is recommended in prescribing CNS depressant agents.

Use of Sedation Techniques

If the patient is a cooperative, well-controlled psychiatric patient, more complex periodontal-prosthetic treatment may be planned. However, such patients often require the short-term use of sedation.

Simple to moderate sedation techniques (Chap. 51) often suffice for types I to III (simple to advanced) operative dentistry procedures. The particular agents and dosage planned should be discussed with the physician in view of the potential drug interactions (see earlier). The dentist should also note that there is a higher risk for paradoxic excitation with the use of N_2O-O_2 in psychiatric patients. If advanced sedation techniques (Chap. 51) are planned or if moderate to advanced dental surgical procedures (types V and VI) are required, hospitalization for proper intraoperative and postoperative monitoring may be advisable. Again, dose consultation with the physician is recommended.

---

*Before prescribing any medication, the dentist should be thoroughly familiar with current PDR recommendations.

Common Psychoactive Drugs

CLASS OF DRUG	GENERIC NAME	TRADE NAME(S)
Antianxiety agent Benzodiazepines	Diazepam	Valium
	Alprazolam	Xanax
	Chlordiazepoxide	Librium
	Oxazepam	Serax
	Lorazepam	Ativan
	Hydroxyzine	Atarax
Others	Buspirone	BuSpar
	Meprobamate	Equanil, Miltown
Phenothiazine (for manic-depression and psychoses)	Chlorpromazine	Thorazine
	Thioridazine	Mellaril
	Trifluoperazine	Stelazine
	Fluphenazine	Prolixin
	Promazine	Sparine
Tricyclic antidepressant (for depression)	Amitriptyline HCl	Elavil
	Imipramine HCl	Tofranil
	Nortriptyline HCl	Pamelor
	Protriptyline HCl	Vivactyl
	Maprotiline HCl	Ludiomil
	Doxepin HCl	Sinequan
Serotonin reuptake inhibitor (for depression)	Fluoxetine	Prozac
	Sertraline	Zoloft
Monoamine oxidase inhibitor (for depression)	Isocarboxazid	Marplan
	Phenelzine sulfate	Nardil
	Tranylcypromine sulfate	Parnate
Other psychoactive medications and combination drugs	Haloperidol	Haldol
	Lithium carbonate	Lithium
	Trazodone	Desyrel
	Valproate	Depakene, Depakote
	Perphenazine (phenothiazine) and amitriptyline (tricyclic antidepressant)	Triavil
	Chlordiazepoxide (antianxiety) and amitriptyline	Limbitrol

SUMMARY TABLE **34–II**

Dental Management Considerations: Medications for Psychiatric Disorders

DRUG	INTERACTION WITH VASOCONSTRICTORS IN LOCAL ANESTHESIA	INTERACTION WITH CNS DEPRESSANTS	INDUCES XEROSTOMIA
MAO inhibitor	—	4+ (strictly contraindicated)	1+ (significant)
Tricyclic antidepressant	2+	2+	Severe
Phenothiazine	±*	3+	Significant
Sedative-hypnotic	—	1+	—
Haloperidol	1+	—	—
Lithium	—	—	—

*±, with or without.

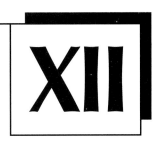

Evaluation and Management of the Patient with Oral Mucosa Disease

CHAPTER

35

Oral Ulcerative Disease

Ulcers are one of the most common types of lesions seen in dental practice. Although some ulcers are symptomatic, a significant number are completely symptom-free. Unfortunately, many of the ulcers that represent serious disease fall into the latter category. Astute observation and thoroughness are the keys to identifying these lesions during routine examination.

The majority of oral ulcers are the consequence of either trauma or aphthous stomatitis. Although these lesions are, for the most part, clinically identical, aphthous stomatitis is recurrent. In both cases, lesions heal spontaneously in 10 to 14 days from the time of onset. A number of important and serious diseases manifest themselves as ulcers of the oral mucosa. Some are infectious, such as syphilis, tuberculosis, and histoplasmosis, and some are malignant, such as squamous cell carcinoma and lymphoma. Frequently, these lesions are asymptomatic, and their presence is not known to the patient. Identification is made by the studious observer. These lesions tend not to heal spontaneously, the chancre of syphilis being the obvious exception. Thus, an important axiom in dealing with oral ulceration is to

perform a *biopsy of any lesion that does not heal spontaneously within 2 weeks following its initial appearance.* In almost all cases, definitive diagnosis can be made by histologic examination.

TRAUMATIC ULCERS

Because of the constant motion of the masticatory mucosa over the teeth and the introduction of hard objects into the oral cavity, traumatic ulcers are frequent. Generally, traumatic ulcers are the consequence of mechanical injury resulting from inadvertent biting of the mucosa (Figs. 35–1 and 35–2), from irritation caused by fractured amalgam restorations or prostheses (Fig. 35–3), or from sharp objects introduced into the mouth. Ulcerations may also occur as a consequence of thermal or chemical burns (Figs. 35–4 and 35–5). Symptomatically, the most outstanding feature of traumatic ulcers is pain. Discomfort usually follows 24 to 48 hours after insult to the tissue. The patient can often identify a specific event or object associated with the trauma although, in the case of faulty restorations, a specific event may be absent. The clinical appearance

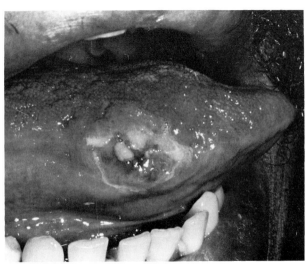

Figure 35–1. Traumatic ulcer of the tongue that resulted from biting when the patient was having a seizure.

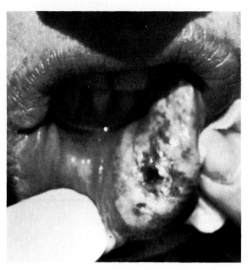

Figure 35–2. Traumatic ulcer of the lip that resulted after the patient chewed his lip following a dental procedure when the lip was anesthetized.

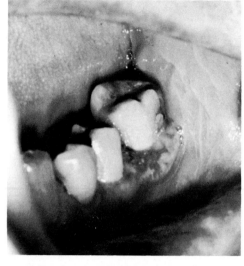

Figure 35–4. Ulceration caused by a chemical burn (aspirin).

of traumatic ulcers is similar to that of aphthous ulcers. The ulcer is usually ovoid and has a yellowish-white necrotic center surrounded by a broad erythematous border. In the case of mechanical trauma, the lesion usually conforms in area and linearity to the source of the trauma. Hence, any ulceration that appears to be linear is usually the result of trauma.

The diagnosis of traumatic ulcer is based on the history or on the identification of a specific source of irritation. Once the source of irritation is eliminated, traumatic ulcers heal in approximately 10 to 14 days. Treatment of trau-

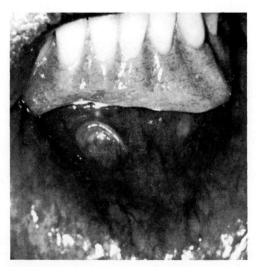

Figure 35–3. Traumatic ulcer secondary to an irritating denture flange. The denture has been adjusted.

matic ulcers is aimed at maintaining cleanliness by frequent rinsing with saline or hydrogen peroxide in water, palliation with anesthetic ointments, and elimination of the source of irritation.

APHTHOUS STOMATITIS

Recurrent aphthous ulcerations, frequently referred to as canker sores, are among the most common lesions of the mouth. Their recurrent pattern and associated discomfort make them extremely bothersome and, at times, debilitating to patients. Aphthous stomatitis may occur as occasional single ulcerations or may be manifested as a never-ending continuum of severe ulcerative lesions.

The prevalence of aphthous stomatitis depends largely on the population studied. Although an overall prevalence of 20% has been reported, individuals in middle and upper middle class economic groups appear to be most frequently affected. An incidence of aphthous stomatitis of 66% was noted among professional students, as compared with only 5% in an indigent population. There appears to be a slight predilection for females. Seasonal peaks have also been noted in winter and spring.

The etiology of aphthous stomatitis has been scrutinized for some time and as yet is not completely resolved. It seems that a specific cause for the condition is identifiable in about 30% of cases. A suspected infectious cause was originally attributed to herpes simplex virus

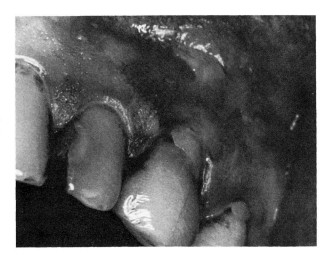

Figure 35–5. Ulceration of gingiva and contiguous mucosa caused by a chemical burn (aspirin and alcohol).

(HSV). However, numerous attempts to isolate HSV from aphthous ulcerations have failed to demonstrate its presence. In addition, no anti-HSV antibodies could be demonstrated in patients with aphthous stomatitis. Furthermore, the relatively high frequency of HSV infection in patients of low economic status is incompatible with the demographic pattern of the disease.

The observation that exacerbations of aphthous stomatitis in women may correlate with the menstrual cycle has led to speculation that there may be a hormonal basis for the disease. However, the nearly equal distribution of aphthous stomatitis in men and women argues against this possibility.

Most likely, multiple factors can initiate aphthous stomatitis. A number of workers have suggested an emotional cause for the disease. The finding of a correlation between stress and severity of the disease, as well as its demographic distribution, supports a psychogenic cause. Animal studies have demonstrated aphthous stomatitis–like lesions following artificially induced stress.

A variety of other conditions have also been identified as causative of true aphthous or aphthous-like lesions. These include deficiencies of vitamin B_{12}, folate, zinc, and iron, cyclic neutropenia, human immunodeficiency virus (HIV) infection, agranulocytosis, Crohn's disease, and food allergies.

The pathophysiologic basis of aphthous stomatitis seems to be clearer. Evidence now suggests an autoimmune mechanism for the tissue destruction noted in aphthous lesions. The histologic appearance of aphthous lesions is one of nonspecific ulceration preceded by a lymphocytic infiltrate. The latter is suggestive of a cell-mediated immune response.

In vitro measurements of cell-mediated immunity (CMI), using lymphocytes from patients with aphthous stomatitis, also support an autoimmune mechanism for the pathophysiology of the disease.

Lymphocyte proliferation (blastogenesis) in response to an antigen correlates with cell-mediated immunity. Lehner allowed peripheral blood lymphocytes from patients with active aphthous stomatitis to react with allogeneic fetal tissue homogenates and measured the amount of lymphocytic proliferation. Lymphocytes from patients with active aphthous lesions were highly reactive in contrast to lymphocytes from patients with no history of aphthous stomatitis or patients in remission.

A role for CMI in aphthous stomatitis is also suggested by the ability of lymphocytes from patients with aphthous stomatitis to mediate the cytolysis of oral mucosal cells. Dolby found that lymphocytes from patients with active aphthous lesions were able to lyse gingival target cells. This work has been confirmed by Rogers and colleagues, who found that, whereas lymphocytes from patients who were free of disease did not effectively lyse oral epithelial target cells, lymphocytes from patients with a known history of aphthous stomatitis could lyse target cells. These studies, coupled with those of Lehner, suggest that an immune mechanism is probably active in the initiation of the destructive phase of aphthous stomatitis.

Clinically, aphthous stomatitis is characterized by the recurrence of oral ulcerations. The ulcer stage is usually preceded by a 2- to 3-day period in which the patient notes a vague feeling of discomfort. The only clinical finding at this time may be an area of erythema. This is soon followed by the appearance of a deep ulcerative lesion. The lesion is usually ovoid,

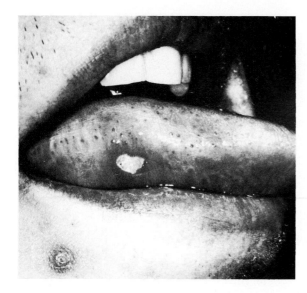

Figure 35–6. Aphthous lesion on tongue. Note the ovoid shape, central necrosis, and erythematous surrounding ring.

has some depth, a yellowish-white necrotic base, and a surrounding zone of erythema in a ring (Figs. 35–6 and 35–7). Rarely do lesions exceed 1 cm in diameter. Most commonly, aphthous lesions are found on the buccal, labial, or alveolar mucosa or on the ventral surface of the tongue. It is uncommon for aphthous stomatitis to involve heavily keratinized areas such as the hard palate or attached gingiva. The major symptom associated with aphthous stomatitis is pain of such severity that eating and speaking patterns may be significantly altered. Because it is relatively common for patients to develop edematous enlargement of the tissue surrounding the ulcer, trauma to the lesion may occur inadvertently. Generally, lesions last a maximum of 7 to 14 days, although they are clinically most painful during the early phases of the disease.

The diagnosis of aphthous stomatitis is based on the clinical appearance and course of the lesion and recurrent history. It is usually difficult to establish a specific stressful incident related to the appearance of lesions, although there may be some correlation with the menstrual cycle. Aphthous lesions must be differentiated from traumatic ulcers, acute herpetic gingivitis, allergy, and erythema multiforme as well as ulcerations caused by systemic disease or conditions described above.

The differentiation between aphthous lesions and trauma is based on the history and the relationship of the lesion to a source of irritation. Essentially, there is no clinical or histologic difference between aphthous and traumatic ulcerations, although any linearity in ulceration suggests a traumatic cause. Acute HSV infection may present as ulcerative le-

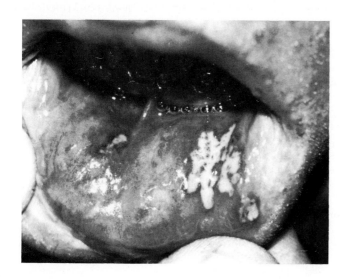

Figure 35–7. Major aphthous stomatitis (Sutton's disease). This is an example of one of many areas of mucosal ulceration occurring simultaneously.

sions after vesicles have ruptured (Chap. 48). This is a concurrent phenomenon, usually involving a number of areas in crop-like fashion. Patients with HSV infection may have experienced constitutional symptoms. These lesions tend to occur in a younger, nonsocioeconomically restricted age group with simultaneous gingival involvement. Allergic lesions tend to be more diffuse than aphthous lesions and although erythematous are usually nonulcerative. Erythema multiforme may present with some ulceration, especially after rupture of bullae. However, these lesions are nonrecurrent and are more diffuse than aphthous lesions. It may be difficult to differentiate ulcerations caused by systemic diseases from aphthous stomatitis. The major difference lies in the lack of recurrence and delayed healing time. Any ulcer that fails to heal in 14 days should undergo biopsy.

Although aphthous ulcers heal spontaneously 10 to 14 days after onset, they are extremely painful. The goal of therapy should be to reduce inflammation, minimize pain and discomfort in affected areas, and speed healing. Currently, no medications meet all three goals. A wide range of treatments have been suggested, including antibiotics, immunomodulators, antimicrobial mouthrinses, and dietary supplements. However, topical steroids remain the mainstay for the treatment of aphthous stomatitis in which a specific etiology has not been identified. These are dispensed either as an ointment (triamcinolone acetonide in Orabase) or as a cream (triamcinolone cream). It has been suggested that the ointment form is not as effective as the cream, because the corticosteroid may be inhibited by the bulk of the ointment. If the cream is used, Orabase ointment can be placed over it to help maintain it in position. In prescribing triamcinolone, it is important to inform the patient to dry the ulcer before application and then to use the drug tid or qid. Some systemic diseases, such as hypertension, preclude the use of corticosteroids (Chap. 4). Corticosteroids may also be administered by injection of small amounts of the drug (0.1 ml) into the lesion. The disadvantages of this form of treatment are its reliance on professional application and the limitation in dosage.

CARCINOMA

Squamous Cell Carcinoma

Carcinoma of the oral cavity is most frequently of the squamous cell type. One of the

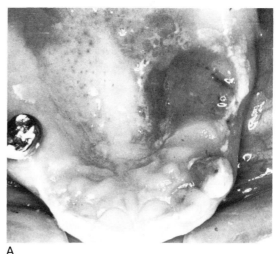

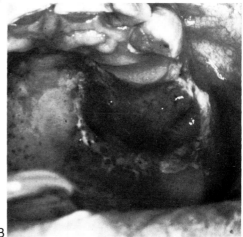

Figure 35–8. *A, B,* Squamous cell carcinoma. Note the combination of ulceration and leukoplakia as well as the expansion of the underlying bone indicative of tumor invasion.

most common presentations of the disease is as a painless, growing, nonhealing ulcer (Fig. 35–8). Ulcers vary in depth. The borders are often firm, and the surface of the ulcer may be smooth or pebbly and somewhat erythematous. Areas of leukoplakia may be associated with the ulcer. The rate of growth is variable and depends largely on the degree of anaplasia of the tumor. The lower lip, tongue, and floor of the mouth are frequent sites of squamous cell carcinoma. Malignant cells spread through the lymphatics, and nodal involvement is common. Secondary infection and hemorrhage may occur as the lesion increases in size. A biopsy is mandatory for definitive diagnosis, although cytologic smears may be of help in screening for the disease, despite the relatively high rate of false-negatives. See

Chapter 40 for a complete discussion of oral carcinoma.

Malignancies Other Than Squamous Cell Carcinoma

Non–squamous cell malignancies of the oral mucosa that present as ulcers are relatively unusual. These lesions do occur, however, and the clinician must be aware of their possible presence. Among these lesions, lymphomas of the non-Hodgkin's variety are the most common. As with squamous cell carcinoma, they present as expanding, painless ulcers (Fig. 35–9), which may occur on any mucosal surface including the gingiva and palate. The borders of these lesions may appear to overlap an erythematous pebbly base. Definitive diagnosis is impossible without a biopsy. Frequently, these lesions may indicate primary disease elsewhere in the body.

Ulcerative lesions may also be the consequence of metastatic spread of malignancies (Fig. 35–10). Although metastases to bone are not unusual, spread to oral soft tissue is not frequent. In most cases, mucosal involvement caused by metastases is a consequence of spread from adjacent bone. Of tumors metastasizing to the mouth, malignancies of the breast, lung, and kidney are the most common.

EROSIVE LICHEN PLANUS

Lichen planus (Chaps. 36 and 37) has three clinical manifestations: a hyperkeratotic form,

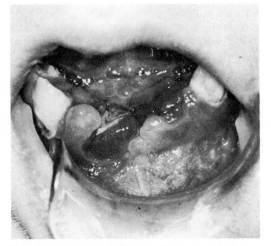

Figure 35–9. Non-Hodgkin's lymphoma presenting as an ulceration of the alveolar mucosa.

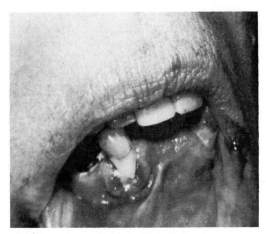

Figure 35–10. Ulceration of gingiva and alveolar mucosa caused by metastases from a primary adenocarcinoma of the breast.

a vesiculobullous form, and an erosive form. The erosive form presents as broad, shallow, painful ulcerative lesions, usually with an erythematous base (Fig. 35–11). The borders of the lesion may be contiguous with papillated areas of the hyperkeratotic form of the disease.

Lichen planus is seen in patients about 40 to 50 years old and is slightly more common in women than men. Frequently related to stress, the disease has an insidious onset and an unpredictable chronic course. In some patients, lesions persist for long periods, whereas in others they spontaneously resolve after a short symptomatic burst. Erosive lichen planus is symptomatic and causes pain and changes in taste; rarely, lesions may become secondarily infected. Lesions tend to be bilateral and may involve any area of oral mucosa, although the cheeks, lips, ventral surface of the tongue, and the attached gingiva are most commonly affected.

The diagnosis of erosive lichen planus is made by histologic examination. Treatment for erosive lichen planus may be palliative with rinses such as Xylocaine Viscous, Benadryl, and Kaopectate or dyclonine HCl. Lichen planus usually responds to steroids. For localized areas, topical steroids such as triamcinolone acetonide or betamethasone valerate 0.1% in paste or ointment form may be helpful. For more diffuse areas, which are resistant to topical treatment, systemic steroids may be required. Controversy exists about whether the immunosuppressive cyclosporine is efficacious in the treatment of severe lichen planus. In these cases, the dentist should enlist the aid of an internist or dermatologist in managing the patient.

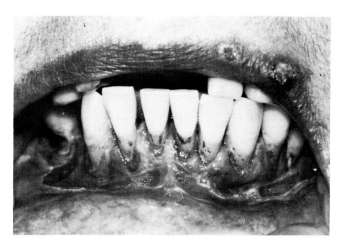

Figure 35–11. Erosive lichen planus. Broad, shallow ulcerative areas are visible. Separation of the epithelium from its connective tissue base can be seen at the margins of the ulcers.

NECROTIZING SIALOMETAPLASIA

Necrotizing sialometaplasia is a benign ulcerative disease affecting the palate that was first described in 1973. Since then, the lesion has been reported in the nasopharynx, retromolar pads, parotid gland, and labial mucosa. Most lesions tend to be unilateral, although approximately 10% present as bilateral ulcerations of the hard palate. The ulcerative appearance of necrotizing sialometaplasia, which affects both soft tissues and the underlying bone, so closely resembles malignancy that aggressive surgical treatment has often been performed. Therefore, histologic criteria are of primary importance in the diagnosis of this entity and consist of squamous metaplasia of ducts and mucous acini, locular necrosis, and evidence of granulation tissues and inflammation.

The cause of necrotizing sialometaplasia remains ambiguous. Among proposed mechanisms by which the lesion develops are infarction, trauma, and arteriosclerotic changes. The lesions have neither an infectious nor an immunologic cause. Characteristically, the clinical appearance is ulcerated with an erythematous border exposing bone, although isolated swelling without ulcerations has been reported (Fig. 35–12). Influential predisposing factors include age, race, sex, geographic location, use of alcohol, and smoking. The mean age of reported cases is 45.5 years. The vast

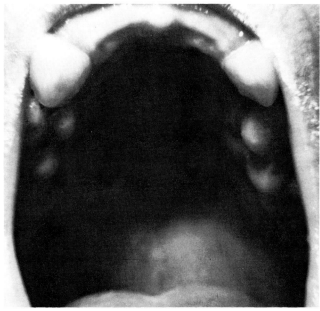

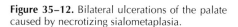
Figure 35–12. Bilateral ulcerations of the palate caused by necrotizing sialometaplasia.

majority of affected individuals are white men and most give a history of regular alcohol consumption and smoking. Over 75% of cases involve palatal tissue. Ongoing systemic illness is not apparent as a predisposing factor. Reported symptoms of pain occur in approximately one-third of cases. Recurrences have not been reported; lesions characteristically resolve in 6 to 10 weeks. The major clinical problem in dealing with sialometaplasia is in differentiating the disease from malignancies. A biopsy is required for definitive diagnosis.

MARROW DISORDERS

Disorders of bone marrow that produce neutropenia frequently result in ulceration of the oral mucosa. Aplastic anemia, hematologic malignancies such as lymphoma and leukemia, cyclic neutropenia, and drug-related leukopenia are among the common causes of such ulceration.

Any area of the mucosa may become ulcerated in the presence of neutropenia. However, the marginal gingiva in a patient with existing periodontal disease is especially susceptible to progressive ulceration (Fig. 35–13). In this group, microscopic sulcular ulceration is no longer kept in check by the patient's defense mechanisms. As a result, necrotizing ulcerative gingivitis occurs, which clinically resembles acute necrotizing ulcerative gingivitis. Patients become febrile and are in pain. They have a bad taste in their mouths and a foul odor to their breaths. Secondary hemorrhage may occur if the patient is also thrombocytopenic. If left untreated, the ulceration may advance to involve the attached gingiva and mucosa (Fig. 35–14).

Mucosal ulcerations occur most frequently in traumatized areas such as the lateral borders of the tongue or buccal mucosa. Lesions appear as penetrating ulcerations and are most often ovoid. The borders may be raised and the base yellowish because of necrosis. Pain is a uniform symptom. Unlike in aphthous lesions, a peripheral band of erythema is usually absent as a consequence of the patient's inability to mount an effective inflammatory response (Fig. 35–15).

Oral ulceration in a patient with known neutropenia may be a life-threatening occurrence, because the ulcer may act as a portal of entry for bacteria. Bacterial invasion in this patient population can proceed to septicemia. Thus, patients with oral ulceration, fever, and neutropenia require hospitalization and parenteral antibiotics (Chap. 42). Patients with persistent ulceration who are suspected of having neutropenia should be appropriately tested to rule out myelosuppressive disease (Chap. 27). A complete blood count and differential white count serve this purpose.

ACUTE NECROTIZING ULCERATIVE GINGIVITIS

Acute necrotizing ulcerative gingivitis (ANUG) is a unique bacterial infection that characteristically affects the marginal and papillary gingiva. The disease has been documented since the time of the early Romans. Outbreaks of ANUG have been consistently reported among the armies of the world, and its presence during World War I led to the name "trench mouth" for the condition. Acute necrotizing ulcerative gingivitis has also been referred to as Vincent's disease, in recognition of one of the individuals who originally documented it. Unlike conventional periodontal

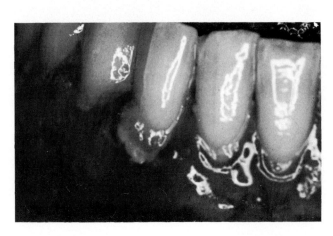

Figure 35–13. Ulceration of marginal gingiva resulting from neutropenia. The presence of gingival inflammation predisposes to the development of ulceration in these patients.

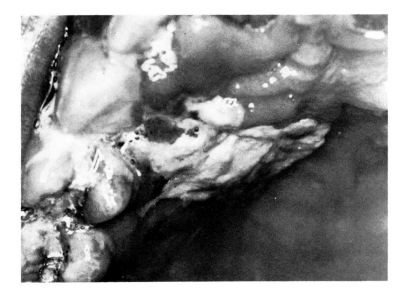

Figure 35–14. Progressive ulceration from the gingiva to the palate in a neutropenic patient.

disease, ANUG is most often observed in young adults in their early twenties. It is the only periodontal infection in which bacterial invasion of the gingival tissue has been observed.

Clinically, ANUG is characterized by the sudden onset of localized or diffuse gingival pain, the former being more common. Patients also note gingival bleeding, bad taste, and fetor oris. About 50% of patients with ANUG experience systemic manifestations of infection, which may include malaise, fever, and lymphadenopathy.

The clinical appearance of ANUG is unique (Fig. 35–16). Gingival examination reveals localized or generalized areas of papillary and marginal necrosis. The disease usually begins interproximally and then spreads laterally.

The necrotic areas form a pseudomembrane overlying an inflammatory base. There is complete loss of the interdental papillae, which appear to be punched-out and crater-like. The tissue is friable and may bleed spontaneously or as a result of the slightest provocation. The patient is usually miserable.

The cause of ANUG has been the subject of a number of studies. The bacterial flora associated with ANUG has been described as a fusospirochetal complex that includes *Fusobacterium fusiforme, Vibrios,* streptococci, diplococci, and filamentous forms. *Treponema vincentii* is the most common spirochete associated with the lesion. Because many of these organisms are normal inhabitants of the oral cavity, smears are of little value in establishing a diagnosis of ANUG. Although once thought to

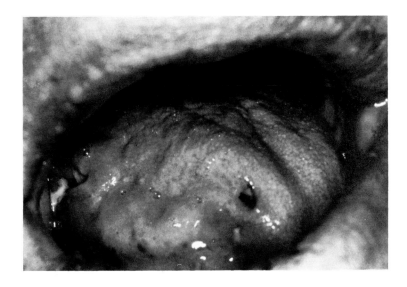

Figure 35–15. Deep ulceration of the tongue in a neutropenic patient. A second ulcer on the lateral border is also visible. Note that although both lesions are deep, the characteristic signs of inflammation are absent.

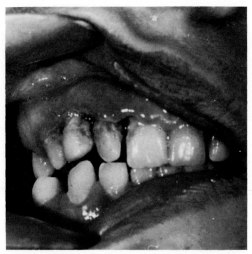

Figure 35–16. Clinical appearance of acute necrotizing ulcerative gingivitis. Note the loss of normal gingival architecture ("punched-out" papillae) and pseudomembrane.

be communicable, the disease cannot be transmitted solely by the transfer of organisms from one individual to another. Rather, it is believed that a localized reduction in tissue resistance, often precipitated by stress, produces an environment in which the fusospirochetes proliferate. The findings of outbreaks of ANUG in military training camps and at universities during examination periods seem to substantiate the relationship between the disease and stress.

The diagnosis of ANUG is made on the basis of the patient's age, history, and clinical appearance. ANUG is most commonly confused with herpetic gingivostomatitis, which usually occurs in a younger age group, is preceded by a viral prodrome, and is characterized by the presence of vesicular lesions on the mucosa in addition to a gingivitis. The clinical appearance of the gingiva reflects a diffuse acute gingivitis (Chap. 48). It should also be noted that a similarity exists between the clinical appearances of ANUG and HIV-related gingivitis (Chap. 47).

The aims of treatment for ANUG are to reduce the presence of local accumulations of bacteria and to eliminate the systemic effects of the infection. Fortunately, the causative organisms of ANUG are generally sensitive to penicillin. Hence, any patient who manifests systemic signs of infection (fever or lymphadenopathy), any patient who is medically compromised such as a diabetic, or any patient with diffuse ANUG should be placed on a regimen of penicillin. We recommend a starting dose of 1 g of potassium phenoxymethyl penicillin followed by a 1-week course of 500 mg qid. In addition, the lesions should be initially gently débrided with cotton pellets soaked with 3% USP hydrogen peroxide. Once systemic symptoms are eliminated, more aggressive local débridement may be done using curettes. Pain medication appropriate to the level of discomfort can be prescribed. The patient should be instructed in oral hygiene and also informed of the tendency for recurrence. Any suggestion of underlying systemic pathology should be investigated.

NOMA (GANGRENOUS STOMATITIS, CANCRUM ORIS)

Noma is an acute, gangrenous process that affects the oral soft tissues. The disease is most commonly seen in children suffering from nutritional deficiencies, dehydration, or some underlying hematologic disorder such as leukemia.

Clinically, the disease is characterized by aggressive destruction of soft tissue, and may progress to erode through skin. Breakdown of adjacent bone may also occur. The disease has been described as starting in the mandibular posterior region as a small area of reddish erosion or ulceration that rapidly progresses. Considered by some to be a virulent form of ANUG, noma possesses common clinical characteristics of bad breath and taste, increased salivation, and pain. Systemic signs of infection are generally present and include fever, malaise, and lymphadenopathy. The presence of a cellulitis usually precedes the appearance of skin breakdown.

The bacteriology of noma is similar to that of ANUG and includes the fusospirochetes *Borrelia vincentii* and *Fusobacterium nucleatum.* Gram-negative organisms have also been reported to play a role in the disease.

Since the advent of antibiotics, the mortality rate from noma has been significantly reduced. Treatment should be directed at controlling any underlying medical condition and at eliminating infection. Penicillin is the preferred antibiotic. In cases in which there is simultaneous malnutrition, dehydration, or anemia, the patient should be hospitalized and receive high-dose penicillin by the intravenous route. Fluid and electrolyte imbalances should be corrected. Localized areas of necrosis should be débrided. When necessary, patients should be given appropriate analgesia to control pain. Scarring may occur.

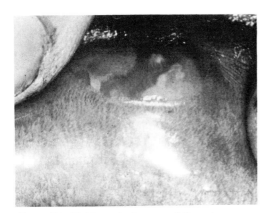

Figure 35-17. Ulcer of primary syphilis—chancre.

SYPHILIS

The oral findings and treatment of acquired syphilis have been discussed in detail elsewhere (Chap. 30) and are reviewed only briefly here. Syphilis has a three-stage clinical presentation, of which the first and third stages present as oral ulcerations.

The primary lesion of acquired syphilis is the chancre, which is most common periorally on the lip or corners of the mouth and occurs approximately 3 weeks after contact with an infected lesion. Clinically, chancres usually present as painless ulcerations. The borders may be raised and the surface of the lesion frequently has a yellowish necrotic base that is heavily populated with organisms and thus is highly infectious (Fig. 35-17). Lymphadenopathy with tenderness is also noted. The chancre heals spontaneously in about a month. Diagnosis of the chancre is confirmed by demonstration of *Treponema pallidum* with darkfield microscopy. Serologic tests for syphilis may not be positive when the chancre is present (Chap. 1). Differential diagnosis includes other infectious ulcers such as tuberculosis, chronic granulomatous disease such as sarcoid, and malignancy. The history and laboratory examination are usually definitive.

The tertiary lesion of acquired syphilis is the gumma. Unlike the other lesions of syphilis, the gumma is not seen in proximity to the initial infection and, in fact, is noted 2 to 10 years later. Only half of patients having primary syphilis eventually manifest signs of tertiary disease. Clinically, the gumma is rare in the mouth but, when present, is seen as a deep penetrating ulcer, often involving the palate or tongue (Fig. 35-18). If tissue overlying bone is involved, osseous necrosis may occur. Unlike the primary and secondary forms of syphilis, the gumma is not infectious.

TUBERCULOSIS

Primary oral infection with tuberculosis is highly unusual. Oral infection is usually the result of secondary infection from a primary pulmonary source. Ulceration of the tongue is the most common oral lesion of tuberculosis. The lesion is infectious and deep, with indurated borders (Fig. 35-19). Frequently, the lesion is painful, unlike the lesion in carcinoma, which it resembles closely. Diagnosis is based on history and biopsy. (For a detailed discussion of tuberculosis, see Chap. 20.)

VIRAL STOMATITIS

The primary oral manifestation of viral infection is vesiculobullous in nature and usually

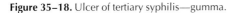

Figure 35-18. Ulcer of tertiary syphilis—gumma.

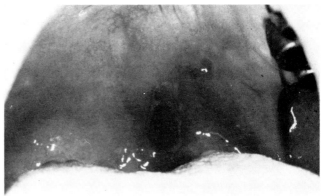

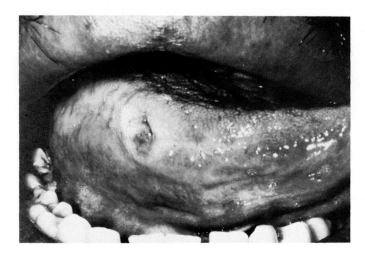

Figure 35–19. Ulcer of tuberculosis. Note the depth of the lesion and the raised, indurated borders.

produces crops of small vesicular lesions. Viral infections and their typical presentation have been discussed elsewhere (Chap. 48). It is not uncommon, however, for virally induced vesicular lesions to rupture before the patient presents for evaluation. In these cases, the disease presents in an ulcerative form.

As mentioned previously, ulcers caused by viral infection are rarely solitary. Rather, they occur as crops of lesions, or at least as a number of ulcerative areas. Clinically, the lesions are similar in appearance to aphthous stomatitis and are frequently confused with this entity (Fig. 35–20). The lesions are painful, with a punched-out ovoid center that is surrounded by an erythematous border. The center of the lesion is frequently necrotic. Unlike aphthous lesions, viral stomatitis, excluding herpes labi-

alis, tends not to be recurrent. These lesions are usually preceded by a viral prodrome of malaise, anorexia, and fever. Smears of the cells at the base of the lesion may reveal viral inclusion bodies of the epithelial cells with ballooning degeneration. Viral lesions tend to occur most frequently on the palate but may occur on the mucosa and gingiva. Distribution of the lesions may be helpful in suggesting a diagnosis. Herpangina is most common on the posterior third of the oral pharynx; herpes zoster is unilateral.

A number of forms of nonspecific viral stomatitis may be encountered. As with other viral infections, croppy unilateral or bilateral ulcerations, preceded by a cold or other viral disease, should suggest a viral cause for oral lesions.

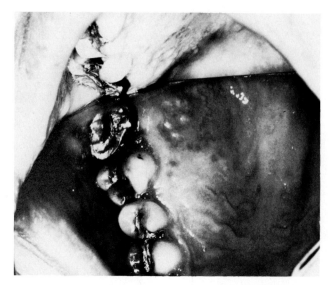

Figure 35–20. Viral stomatitis. Note the distribution of the multiple ulcerations of the palate.

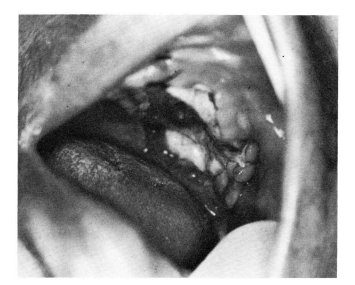

Figure 35–21. Mucormycosis.

Treatment of virally induced ulcers is palliative. The lesions heal without scarring in 10 to 14 days.

HISTOPLASMOSIS

Histoplasmosis is a deep fungal infection that sometimes affects the mouth. The disease is caused by the fungus *Histoplasma capsulatum,* an organism endemic to certain parts of the world. In the United States, the Mississippi River Valley region is the most common location for the disease. Although there are an estimated 500,000 new cases of histoplasmosis in the United States annually, most cases are subclinical or restricted to respiratory tract involvement. Of these cases, 5% are disseminated, however, and it is in these patients that oral involvement has been reported.

The organism is found in spores in the soil. Spores can be spread by birds in endemic areas, thus allowing urbanites to be exposed to the fungus. The spores enter the body through the respiratory tree to the lung. Clinical manifestations of histoplasmosis include cough and dyspnea and frequently weight loss.

Oral manifestations of histoplasmosis are varied and include painful ulcerations, nodules, or vegetative processes. Most patients with oral lesions display more than one oral manifestation. Patients complain of pain, weakness, and the other symptoms discussed above. Fever is an infrequent finding. The appearance of the lesions may also vary; ulcers may be deep or shallow.

Men are more frequently affected by the disease than women. Oral involvement has never been reported in a patient under 20 years of age. Generally, the disease is found in elderly white people.

Oral lesions occur anywhere in the mouth but are most common on the oropharynx, buccal mucosa, tongue, and palate. The clinical appearance of histoplasmosis is generally the same as that of epidermoid carcinoma. Thus, biopsy is mandatory and diagnostic when specimens are stained appropriately (Gomori–methenamine silver). Cultures of smears of lesions may give false-negative results. A skin test for histoplasmin may be an effective diagnostic technique, depending on when the patient was infected.

Treatment of histoplasmosis is reasonably successful with amophotericin B.

PHYCOMYCOSIS (MUCORMYCOSIS NECROSIS)

Mucormycosis is a rare fungal infection most commonly noted in debilitated patients. The infection is caused by organisms of the order Mucorales, especially *Mucor* and *Rhizopus.* Both are common in soil and decaying vegetable matter and can be cultured easily from normal individuals, in whom they are nonpathogenic. The organisms are most easily noted using periodic acid–Schiff (PAS) stain.

Mucormycosis has long been associated with individuals with poorly controlled diabetes mellitus. However, it is now noted with increasing frequency in myelosuppressed patients, notably those with leukemia or patients receiving chemotherapy for other malignancies, and in patients immunocompromised by diseases such as AIDS.

The most common form of the disease is rhinocerebral, in which organisms normally first infect the nasal passages. The infection may then spread to involve the lungs and gastrointestinal tract.

Oral manifestations of mucormycosis are relatively rare but, when present, include a nonhealing, progressive, necrotic ulcer (Fig. 35–21). Underlying bony destruction may occur. Tissue destruction caused by the fungus is the result of vessel thrombosis. The organism has an affinity for blood vessel walls, where proliferation occurs, causing thrombosis and subsequent necrosis. Facial swelling, proptosis, and eye and facial symptoms may be noted in patients with disease extending to the orbit, paranasal sinuses, and cranial cavity.

The diagnosis of mucormycosis is based on the demonstration of infecting organisms in tissue. Biopsy and PAS stain are diagnostic. Cultures are also helpful. Patients with debilitating disease are at risk for developing this infection. Nonhealing ulcers must be dealt with aggressively in this group.

Untreated, mucormycosis proceeds to a fatal conclusion. Treatment of the underlying disease should be undertaken. Amphotericin B is the treatment of choice, given over a long period (months).

Oral Ulcerative Diseases

DIAGNOSIS	RELEVANT HISTORY	APPEARANCE AND SIGNS	LOCATION	PATIENT PROFILE/CAUSE	TESTS	COURSE AND MANAGEMENT
Aphthous stomatitis	Recurrent ulcerations of mucosa	Ulceration of mucosal surface with whitish-yellow necrotic center and erythematous border; painful; sometimes + lymphadenopathy; ovoid; may be multiple	Usually mucosal surface, no gingival involvement, rarely palate	Young adults and up; 30% specific etiology	Rule out systemic component where indicated: CBC Folate level B_{12} level	Heals in 10–14 days; drugs: triamcinolone in Orabase to reduce inflammation; palliation: benzocaine in Orabase, warm salt rinses; remove source of irritation; in severe cases, physician consultation and systemic steroids
Chancre of primary syphilis	History of recent sexual contact	Painless indurated ulcerative area with raised borders and whitish center; lymphadenopathy usually present (unilateral)	Lip or tongue, tonsils	Any sexually active individual; bacterial cause: Treponema pallidum	Darkfield microscopic examination of smear shows organisms; biopsy	Heals spontaneously in about 1 mo; treat with penicillin (Chap. 30)
Tuberculosis	Usually + pulmonary TB	Painless ulceration with purulent center, ragged, undermined edge; yellowish appearance, + nodes	Tongue, tonsils, soft palate	Patient with known or suspected pulmonary TB; bacterial cause: Mycobacterium tuberculosis	Biopsy: smear usually secondary, + PPD (Chap. 20)	TB Rx: streptomycin, INH (Chap. 20)
Carcinoma	Alcohol and cigarette consumption	Painless, indurated ulceration with firm, raised borders; may have leukoplakia associated and may have erythema, bleeding, or erosion, ± nodes; tongue may be fixed	Anywhere; most frequently base of tongue, lip (lower), floor of mouth	Men > 40 yr; women affected more frequently	Biopsy; smear—15% false-negative	Variable, depending on time of diagnosis, size of tumor, degree of spread; treat with surgery, radiation therapy, or chemotherapy (Chap. 40)
Neutropenia	Rapid onset; sick patient—malaise, fever, recurrent infections, bad taste, pain	Destructive broad ulcerations usually affecting attached gingiva and spreading; painful; pseudomembrane; loss of architecture: much necrosis; erythematous borders variable	Usually begin at attached gingiva and spread; may also involve traumatized areas—buccal mucosa or tongue	Variable, can be caused by numerous diseases such as leukemia, aplastic anemia, cyclic neutropenia, drug-induced neutropenia	WBC and differential count shows marked ↑ in PMN	Variable course depending on pathology; treatment: local debridement and palliation, systemic antibiotics; treat underlying disease
Viral stomatitis (usually presents as vesicles, but if they break may be seen as ulcers)	Usually prodrome of 2–3 days of malaise, fatigue, anorexia; oral lesions have rapid onset, go from vesicles to ulcers	Multiple, painful, small shallow ulcerations usually in crops, with whitish centers and erythematous borders; patients feel sick; may have lymphadenopathy, fever, coated tongue, myalgias, gingivitis	Depends on virus	Depends on virus, but may be youngsters to young adults for most except herpes zoster or debilitated patients	Smear of base shows cells with ↑ nuclear:cytoplasmic ratio; viral inclusion bodies; Tzanck preparation; neutralizing antibodies	Self-limiting; palliative treatment (Chap. 48)
Deep fungal infections; histoplasmosis	History of living in region where histoplasmosis is reported—in United States, Mississippi Valley	Ulcers of varying depth; painful; appearance of lesions variable; complaints of sore throat, weight loss, cough, dyspnea, fatigue, weakness, anorexia; fever rare	Oropharynx, buccal mucosa, tongue, palate	Men predominate; oral lesions seen in adults (20 yr); caused by Histoplasma capsulatum	Isolate H. capsulatum from culture; complement fixation; immunodiffusion; histoplasmin skin test; biopsy	Amphotericin B

INH, isoniazid; PMN, polymorphonuclear neutrophils; PPD, purified protein derivative.

CHAPTER

36

White Lesions

White lesions of the oral cavity are common. This category of lesions consists of a wide range of conditions, some of which are mundane and of little consequence and others that, if untreated, are potentially fatal. White lesions can be divided into two broad categories, necrotic lesions and keratotic lesions. The coloration associated with necrotic white lesions is caused by the collection of cells, bacteria, and debris on the tissue surface. Contrastingly, the white coloration in keratotic lesions is the result of excess amounts of surface keratin.

The initial diagnostic step in evaluating white lesions is aimed at differentiating between necrotic and keratotic lesions (Fig. 36–1). Because most necrotic lesions are associated with some form of injury, a thorough history often yields information suggesting a diagnosis. Additionally, necrotic lesions are often painful, whereas keratotic lesions are usually asymptomatic. Clinical differentiation can often be accomplished by scraping lesions with a moistened tongue blade (Chap. 2). Generally, the surface of necrotic lesions can be removed by firm scraping. On the other hand, no amount of scraping can modify keratotic lesions.

Definitive diagnosis of keratotic white lesions is usually made by histologic examination. Because approximately 10% of keratotic white lesions are dysplastic or true carcinomas, biopsy of suspicious white lesions is mandatory. Generally, incisional biopsy is the technique of choice.

NECROTIC WHITE LESIONS

Burns

The mouth may be exposed to a wide variety of physical or chemical agents that can result in burns of the oral mucosa. Usually, such burns are accidental, but they may also occur because of the iatrogenic use of certain drugs or medicaments.

Clinically, burns of the mouth present as areas of white necrotic tissue overlying a connective tissue or mucosal base, depending on the depth of the burn (Fig. 36–2). Almost all cases are painful, although burns may not initially be symptomatic. Depending on the source of injury, lesions may be localized or diffuse. Necrosis resulting from the ingestion of a chemical, for example, tends to involve

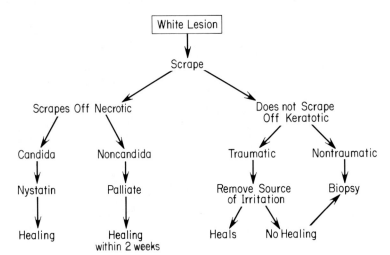

Figure 36–1. Flow diagram of diagnostic sequence for white lesions of the mouth.

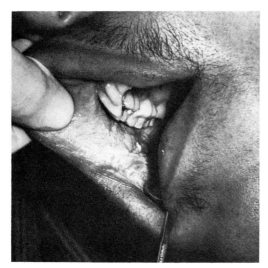

Figure 36–2. Chemical burn of the buccal and labial mucosae.

broad areas of mucosa, whereas physical injury may be more limited. Generally, the epithelial sloughing that accounts for the white necrotic appearance is followed by healing. Epithelialization is usually complete in about 2 weeks from the time of insult.

A number of agents cause burns in the mouth. In children, electrical burns may occur if youngsters are unfortunate enough to chew on live wires. Electrical burns characteristically involve the corners of the mouth and lips and may also involve intraoral mucosa and the tongue. Severe burns may result in scarring and stricture formation, which can lead to reduced oral function. A prosthetic stent may be of help in maintaining the position of tissue and minimizing scar formation.

Chemical burns of the mouth are relatively common and may result from exposure to a variety of agents. Uninformed patients may occasionally place aspirin against the gingiva or mucosa associated with a sensitive tooth (Fig. 36–3). The acetylsalicylic acid produces a contact burn of the oral tissue, evident as a localized area of white necrotic slough, usually in the mucobuccal fold. The lesion is generally painful and may demonstrate bleeding when the necrotic surface is removed.

Patients may use hydrogen peroxide for rinsing. This has become especially popular, combined with baking soda, as a "home remedy" for periodontal disease. Not infrequently, undiluted peroxide results in a generalized superficial necrotic slough of the oral epithelium. Once the rinse is discontinued or replaced by a noncaustic solution such as saline or warm water, healing proceeds rapidly.

Sodium hypochlorite or other such solutions that are routinely used for the irrigation and débridement of root canals are caustic to the skin and mucosa and may cause burns. Routine use of a rubber dam and immediate flushing with water are helpful preventive measures.

Thermal burns of the mouth are not common. Burns caused by food are more often caused by hot, sticky foods, such as cheese, than liquids, which tend to be quickly cleared. A thorough history usually elicits the cause of the lesions, which tend to be localized and occur most frequently on the anterior palate or tip of the tongue. Following a relatively painful course, these lesions heal in about 10 to 14 days. Dental manipulation may result in thermal burns. This occurs most commonly when overheated impression compound comes in contact with the mucosa. Clearly, this may be easily prevented by routine testing of the material before it is inserted into the patient's mouth.

A number of other unnamed agents may cause burning of the oral mucosa. Whenever a diffuse necrotic region is identified, the patient should be questioned regarding intake of chemicals. Similarly, a localized necrotic area may be caused by spot contact with a caustic agent.

Candidiasis

Of the fungal infections that affect the mouth, candidiasis is the most common. Ap-

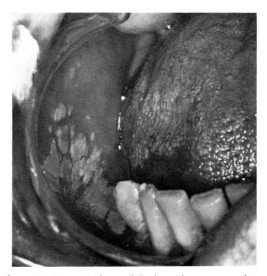

Figure 36–3. Aspirin burn of the buccal mucosa resulting in white necrotic slough.

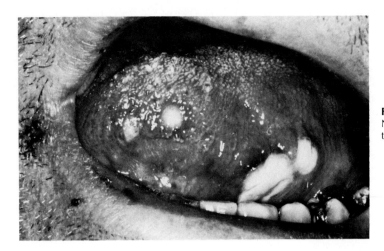

Figure 36–4. Candidiasis of the tongue. Note the clumped areas of white necrotic tissue caused by fungus.

proximately 50% of the population has *Candida albicans* in the normal oral flora. Usually, this organism is of no clinical significance. If changes occur in the oral environment, however, candidal organisms can proliferate and cause infection (Chap. 49).

Candidiasis is most frequent in patients at either age extreme; in newborns the infection is called thrush. It has been reported that fungal proliferation is seen frequently under the palate of maxillary prostheses. Any patient whose marrow status changes because of diseases such as aplastic anemia or drugs is at high risk to develop candidiasis. Similarly, patients receiving immunosuppressive therapy such as steroids or debilitated individuals such

as patients with diabetes may develop fungal infections of this type. Mucocutaneous candidiasis is one of the most frequent signs of symptomatic human immunodeficiency virus (HIV) infection (Chap. 47). Prolonged use of antibiotics, particularly broad-spectrum agents, may produce candidiasis.

Clinically, candidiasis has a wide range of manifestations. Patients may be totally asymptomatic or complain of pain or burning or of having a coated feeling in the mouth. On examination, the clinician may note raised, curdy white areas that often appear to lump in heaps (Fig. 36–4). The tongue may take on a coated, white appearance (Fig. 36–5). The borders of the white areas may be erythematous (Fig. 36–6). The white areas can usually be scraped off with firm pressure using a wooden tongue blade, leaving a raw bleeding surface. A smear of the material reveals the presence of hyphae when observed microscopically.

Candidiasis usually responds well to topical therapy if there is no significant underlying

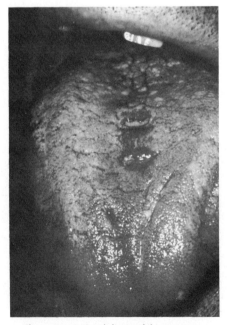

Figure 36–5. Candidiasis of the tongue.

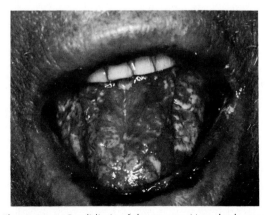

Figure 36–6. Candidiasis of the tongue. Note the hemorrhagic borders.

pathology. Nystatin oral suspension, given at a dose of 200,000 to 400,000 units tid or qid, with instructions to swish and swallow, is effective for most cases of mucosal candidiasis. Alternatively, clotrimazole troches (10 mg), one tablet five times daily for 2 weeks, may be used. Candidiasis beneath dentures can be treated with nystatin ointment applied to the prosthesis. Gentian violet suspension is also an effective topical antifungal agent, but it so discolors tissue that assessment is confounded. Systemic medications for mucosal candidiasis include ketoconazole tablets. Fluconazole, a recently introduced antifungal drug, offers a systemic alternative and has proved effective in the treatment of candidiasis in patients with HIV infection. For patients with systemic fungal involvement or esophageal or pulmonary candidiasis, and who have compromised ability to deal with infection, amphotericin B must be considered. This medication requires intravenous administration and is highly nephrotoxic. Its use should be considered only after consultation with the patient's physician and is confined to hospitalized patients.

KERATOTIC WHITE LESIONS

White keratotic lesions of the oral mucosa are referred to as leukoplakia, which, simply translated, means "white plaque." Unfortunately, the term has been somewhat misused in the past and often is thought to imply malignant changes.

The simplest white lesions that affect the mouth are those caused by an increased production of keratin, most commonly in re-

sponse to chronic irritation. These areas of hyperkeratosis may occur anywhere in the mouth but are most frequent on the buccal mucosa opposite the cusps of the molars and on the lateral borders of the tongue. These lesions are often linear and reflect a "bite line." Most often they are bilateral. Diagnosis is clinical, and no additional therapy is required (Fig. 36–7).

Localized areas of hyperkeratosis are potentially more of a problem. These areas may occur opposite an area of irritation, such as a sharp cusp, fractured restoration, or ragged edge of a prosthesis or clasp. The lesions may be associated with some mucosal inflammation, and most often are asymptomatic. Similar areas may be seen on the palate, especially in smokers. Pipe and cigar smokers usually demonstrate the most dramatic changes, because areas of hyperkeratosis are often interspersed with areas of inflammation of the minor salivary glands. Clinically, this condition presents as a series of speckled, red, raised dots against a white background, and is referred to as nicotinic stomatitis (Fig. 36–8).

The clinical approach to areas of leukoplakia must be made with consideration of the fact that approximately 10% to 15% of these lesions demonstrate histologic evidence of dysplasia or frank malignancy. Obvious sources of irritation should be eliminated, and the patient should be reevaluated in about a week. If the area of leukoplakia is still present, biopsy is mandatory. As already noted, cytologic smears of white keratotic lesions may be useful when mass screenings are performed. However, the high incidence of false-negatives (15%) makes this technique undesirable for

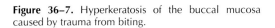

Figure 36–7. Hyperkeratosis of the buccal mucosa caused by trauma from biting.

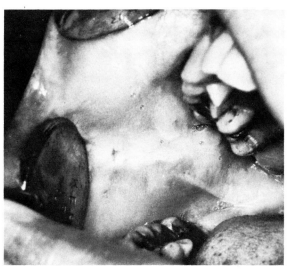

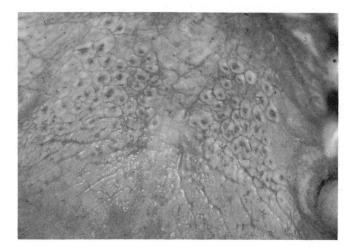

Figure 36–8. Nicotinic stomatitis.

definitive diagnosis. If a lesion is suspicious enough to require a smear, it should undergo biopsy (Fig. 36–9). A complete discussion of carcinoma may be found in Chapter 40.

Lichen Planus

Lichen planus is a relatively common dermatologic condition that often presents with coincidental oral lesions. In addition, a significant number of cases demonstrate oral findings in the absence of skin lesions.

The cutaneous lesions of lichen planus most frequently involve the flexor surfaces of the arms or legs. Most often, the condition is bilateral. Patients present with an itchy rash that manifests itself as individual or contiguous

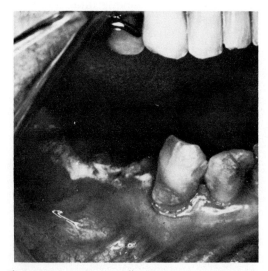

Figure 36–9. Squamous cell carcinoma presenting with a combined clinical appearance of a white lesion adjacent to a nonhealing ulceration.

papules. Thus, the lesion can have a variety of appearances. On close examination, raised, discrete papules may be identified, although the lesions can appear as plaques. In most cases, cutaneous lichen planus appears before or simultaneous with oral lesions. It has been suggested by Shklar and McCarthy that almost all cases of lichen planus progress to involve both the skin and mouth.

The oral lesions of lichen planus may take on a variety of forms, including hyperkeratosis, erosion, or bullae. The latter are discussed elsewhere (Chap. 37).

The hyperkeratotic form of lichen planus is the most common oral manifestation. The lesions are essentially asymptomatic. Most commonly, the buccal mucosa (80%) or tongue (65%) is affected, although 20% of cases involve the lip. The oral hyperkeratotic lesions of lichen planus present as a unique reticulated pattern of a striated network of contiguous, raised, white papules (Fig. 36–10). The lesions, also called Wickham's striae, lace along the mucosa, frequently terminating in areas of erythema. Most often, lesions are bilateral.

Lichen planus is most often a disease of middle-aged adults, although a broad range of ages may be affected. A female predilection of approximately 2:1 has been suggested. Concern has been raised that lichen planus may predispose to or develop into squamous cell carcinoma. The evidence for such a hypothesis appears to be somewhat speculative, and firm data are currently lacking. In view of these studies, however, careful follow-up of patients with lichen planus is probably prudent.

The cause of lichen planus is not resolved. The histologic finding of a lymphocytic infiltrate associated with the subepithelial connective tissue has been interpreted by some to

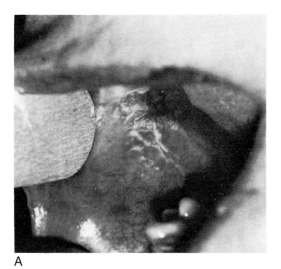

A

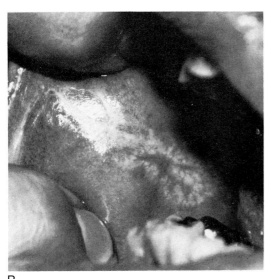

B

Figure 36-10. *A, B,* Lichen planus of the buccal mucosa demonstrating lace-like striations.

suggest a role for autoimmunity in the development of the disease. Alternatively, lichen planus may be the consequence of a cell-mediated immune response directed against induced mucosal antigens. Stress has been discussed at length as a potential causative factor. Many times, in fact, an identifiable source of stress can be ascertained by simply questioning the patient. Examples include family sickness or death or changes in marital status. Generally, if such a cause can be identified, its resolution is followed by elimination of the disease.

A number of drugs produce reactions of the oral mucosa considered to be lichenoid in nature. Drugs associated with lichen planus include chlorpropamide, tolazamide, hydroxyurea, gold, alphamethyldopa, propranolol,

carbamazepine, and phenytoin. Generally, this form of lichen planus tends to be of the vesiculobullous variety, although hyperkeratotic areas may be noted.

Clinically, lichen planus may start as a number of small papular areas that expand to the characteristic striated pattern. Because the hyperkeratotic form of the disease is asymptomatic, the lesions may not be noted by the patient until they have progressed and are clearly visible. Alternatively, the disease may not be noted until routine dental examination. Diagnosis of lichen planus can often be made clinically. This is especially true of patients in whom characteristic bilateral lesions are present. If there is any doubt as to the nature of the lesion, it should undergo biopsy.

Lichen planus runs a benign and often chronic course. Lesions may go through periods of exacerbation and remission. Patients should be reassured regarding the benign nature and clinical insignificance of the disease but re-examined periodically.

White Sponge Nevus

White sponge nevus is a genetically inherited keratotic condition that affects the mouth and other mucosal surfaces. Unlike the majority of other white oral lesions, it is first noted in youngsters.

Clinically, patients present with areas of bilateral, raised spongy hyperkeratosis most frequently involving the buccal mucosa and tongue (Fig. 36-11). White sponge nevus is asymptomatic and of no clinical consequence. Diagnosis is clinically based on the age of the patient, family history, and appearance of the lesion. No treatment is required.

LUPUS ERYTHEMATOSUS

Lupus erythematosus (LE) is a relatively common autoimmune disorder. There are two dissimilar forms of the disease: a chronic discoid form (CDLE) and a systemic form (SLE). The two forms are so unlike that it has been suggested that they may be two different diseases. Whereas SLE is almost uniformly a disease of young adult women, CDLE is seen in both sexes and at a slightly older age level.

Although it is well established that an autoimmune reaction underlies the development of LE, the exact cause is not totally resolved. Genetic and environmental factors have been identified. Among the latter, certain chemi-

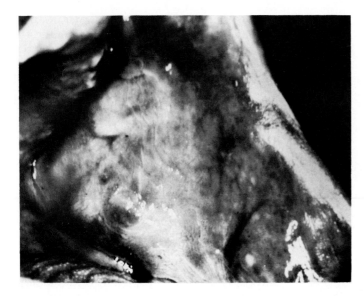

Figure 36–11. White sponge nevus.

cals, hair dyes, drugs, foods, and infectious agents have been mentioned. It appears that an increase in the number of antibody-producing cells results in the generation of antibodies that react with self-antigens. Increases in the number of activated T helper cells have also been reported. Loss of immune tolerance appears to be a key factor in the development of LE (Steinberg et al., 1991).

CDLE is a chronic disease having a mild, relatively asymptomatic onset. As previously noted, the disease is noted in individuals of both sexes; there is a slight female predilection. Clinically, patients with CDLE most often demonstrate an erythematous cutaneous rash, which is most commonly seen in areas exposed

to the sun. Classically, the rash involves the cheeks and bridge of the nose to give a "butterfly pattern." On close examination, scales may be noted. The skin lesions are usually well defined.

It is unusual for patients with CDLE to manifest oral changes of the disease in the absence of skin lesions. However, the opposite situation may be true. Approximately 50% of patients with CDLE demonstrate oral findings of the disease. The oral lesions of CDLE consist of a nonspecific mixture of hyperkeratosis, ulceration, and erythema. A radial arrangement of capillaries at the periphery of the lesion has been described by Shklar and McCarthy. Because of the nonspecific nature of the oral

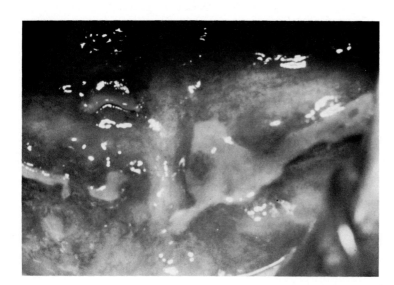

Figure 36–12. Systemic lupus erythematosus. Note the area of white necrotic slough with borders of erythema.

lesions, definitive diagnosis of CDLE based on their presence is almost impossible. Biopsy and appropriate immunofluorescent tests are required for definitive diagnosis.

CDLE demonstrates a chronic, uneven course that goes through periods of exacerbation and remission. The disease may spontaneously disappear as the patient ages. Treatment of CDLE has been successfully achieved using antimalarial drugs. Intralesional injections of steroids have been helpful in resolving some chronic oral lesions. Topical steroids may also be of value.

SLE causes more severe symptoms and consequences than does the chronic form. It is also more rare. Seen almost always in young women, onset of the disease is heralded by a variety of signs and symptoms, including malaise, joint pain, fever, rash, weight loss, kidney and central nervous system involvement, and pulmonary and cardiac problems. Myelosuppressive changes manifested by anemia, leukopenia, and thrombocytopenia may occur during flares of the disease. Antinuclear antibodies are found in 90% of patients and play an important role in the diagnosis of the disease.

The oral changes associated with SLE are nonspecific. Patients present with erosive and vesiculobullous lesions, which may be surrounded by areas of erythema. Heaped-up areas of necrotic slough may be seen coincidentally or eventually become present (Fig. 36–12). Oral lesions of SLE do not occur in the absence of other signs or symptoms of the disease and may simply represent manifestations of myelosuppression.

Diagnosis of SLE is usually complete before the dentist sees the patient and is based on the demonstration of antinuclear antibodies. SLE varies in severity and runs an uneven course. Although there is no cure for the disease, a number of therapeutic measures are available to control the disease. These range from supportive measures and conservative therapy, such as bed rest, aspirin, and antimalarial drugs, to splenectomy and aggressive use of corticosteroids. Recent studies with immunotherapy using α_2-interferon have been encouraging.

White Lesions

DIAGNOSIS	RELEVANT HISTORY	APPEARANCE AND SIGNS	LOCATION	CAUSE	DIAGNOSTIC PROCEDURES	COURSE AND TREATMENT
Burns	Exposure of mucosa to caustic agent, electricity	Necrotic white area, painful, scrapes off	Tongue, mucosa, corners of mouth	Physical injury	Clinical observation	Self-resolving in 10–14 days, palliation
Candidiasis	Broad-spectrum antibiotics; underlying systemic disease; immunosuppression	White, raised curdy areas, erythematous borders, scrapes off; esophageal involvement causes dysphagia	Palate, tongue, buccal mucosa	*Candida albicans*	Clinical microscopic demonstration of hyphae	May be self-resolving after underlying condition eliminated; mycostatin, ketoconazole, clotrimazole, gentian violet, amphotericin B
Leukoplakia Hyperkeratosis	Irritation of mucosa from restoration, smoking, chewing, etc.	Nonscrapable white plaque	Anywhere	Chronic physical trauma	Remove irritating source; if does not resolve in 7–14 days, biopsy	May be chronic; may undergo malignant change
Carcinoma	Smoking, alcohol, snuff dipping, chronic irritation, syphilis	Nonscrapable white plaque	Anywhere	Unknown: tobacco use, alcohol, irritation	Biopsy	Depends on location and extent of involvement

Disease	Clinical Signs / History	Appearance	Location	Etiology	Diagnosis	Behavior
Lichen planus	Stressful event	Lacy, papillated, white striae	Gingiva, tongue, mucosa	Stress, autoimmune	Clinical, biopsy	Chronic, may spontaneously disappear
White sponge nevus	Present since childhood	Spongy, raised white areas, bilateral	Buccal mucosa	Genetic	Clinical	Chronic, no treatment
Lupus erythematosus — Chronic discoid form	Both sexes; mild onset; older age of onset than SLE; skin lesions—butterfly-patterned rash of face	Hyperkeratosis, ulceration, erythema	Mucosa, tongue	Autoimmune, viral	Biopsy	Antimalarial drugs; steroids; chronic, uneven course; α-interferon
Systemic form	Young adult women, symptomatic onset; fever, malaise, weight loss, renal, CNS involvement, myelosuppression	Nonspecific erosive and vesiculobullous lesions; may be caused by myelosuppression	Anywhere	Autoimmune, viral	Biopsy	No curative treatment, uneven course, severe at times

Vesiculobullous Diseases and Autoimmunity

Like the skin, the oral mucosa manifests a variety of vesiculobullous diseases. These vary in frequency, severity, and systemic consequence. All these diseases have some characteristics in common. Vesicles are small, fluid-filled, raised areas of mucosa that are usually ovoid, not exceeding 0.5 cm in diameter. They may appear singularly or in clusters (Fig. 37–1). Depending on when they are seen by the clinician, the actual vesicle may be ruptured, leaving a raw open erosive surface. Bullae are similar to vesicles but larger in size and scope. They may be singular or may coalesce to form extensive areas of involvement. When ruptured, they leave ragged edges, which can be lifted away from the underlying tissue (Fig. 37–2). In this condition, they are extremely painful.

Five major vesiculobullous diseases or conditions affect the mouth: pemphigus vulgaris, mucous membrane pemphigoid, bullous lichen planus, erythema multiforme, and certain drug eruptions. The specific cause of the conditions mentioned is, in many cases, poorly

understood. However, autoimmune reactions are thought to be of importance in the pathogenesis of most vesiculobullous diseases. Additionally, the demonstration of autoantibodies plays a role in the diagnosis and longitudinal assessment of some of these diseases.

Autoimmune diseases may be considered to be systemic when tissue involvement is widespread and many organ systems are involved, or organ-specific when one organ or tissue is affected primarily. Lupus erythematosus is an example of a systemic autoimmune disease. Usually, the oral vesiculobullous diseases represent organ-specific examples of autoimmune diseases in which the oral mucosa and skin are the target tissues.

The concept of autoimmune disease is based on the premise that the patient's immune system loses the ability to distinguish "self" from "nonself." The mechanism for this action is thought to be the consequence of the expression of new or modified antigens by some of the patient's cells, resulting in the sensitization of immune cells and a subsequent

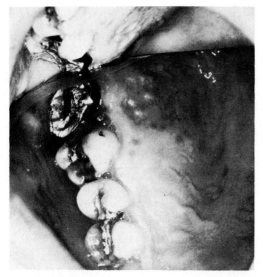

Figure 37–1. Cluster of vesicles on the palate caused by viral stomatitis. Ruptured vesicles are present and have formed ulcers.

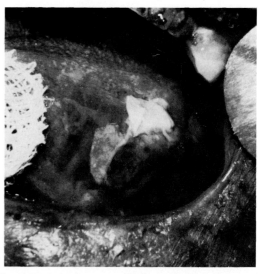

Figure 37–2. Large, ruptured bulla on the lateral aspect of the tongue. The roof of the bulla is easily visualized.

cellular or humoral immune response. The cause for modified or new antigen formation varies. Enzymatic degradation of cell surfaces, viral infection, drug action, or the presence of cross-reacting antigens (cellular antigens that resemble "foreign antigens") may culminate in the initiation of autoimmune disease.

Diagnosis of vesiculobullous disease is usually based on history, clinical examination, and biopsy. Patients suspected of having such a malady should be specifically questioned regarding the type of onset of their lesions (acute or chronic), the length of time the lesions have been present, whether they are cyclical or constant, and whether other areas of the body such as the skin, eyes, or genitalia are involved. In addition, the geographic origin of the patient and history of drug intake should be established. The clinical appearance of the lesion may offer clues to diagnosis. In many cases, however, biopsy is required for definitive diagnosis. Incisional biopsies that include a portion of noninvolved tissue are most effective. Cytologic smears may be useful in the diagnosis of pemphigus vulgaris.

PEMPHIGUS VULGARIS

Pemphigus vulgaris is a serious chronic vesiculobullous disease of mucosa and skin. The disease is seen almost totally in adults over the age of 60 years. Pemphigus is noted most often among individuals of Mediterranean or Middle Eastern background. There appears to be a strong genetic predisposition for the disease. An autoimmune mechanism is suggested by the finding of antibodies in the lesions of skin and mucosa localized in the intercellular spaces between epithelial cells. The presence of antidesmosomal antibodies results in the dissolution of intercellular cementing substance (Fig. 37–3) and the destruction of desmosomes that normally bind squamous epithelial cells together. This process results in intraepithelial separation of the stratum germinativum from the underlying stratum spinosum, with subsequent acantholysis and loss of epithelial integrity. Further corroboration of an immune cause comes from the fact that pemphigus responds well to treatment with corticosteroids as well as antimetabolites; both of these agents are potent immunosuppressors.

Pemphigus vulgaris usually starts with localized vesiculobullous lesions in the oral cavity and skin. The mouth is involved in 70% of cases and is the only site of presentation in 50% of patients with the condition. Early detection and appropriate therapy at early stages often prevents extensive and widespread involvement of the skin. Thus, the need for

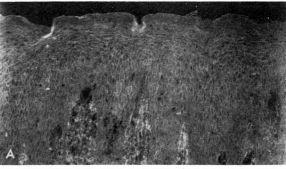
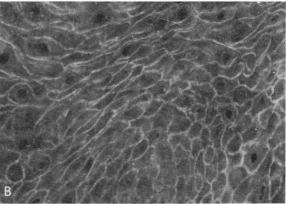

Figure 37–3. Demonstration of intercellular antidesmosomal antibodies by immunofluorescence. The light areas around the cells indicate the presence of antibodies. *A,* Low-power magnification. *B,* High-power magnification.

more aggressive therapy, which is often accompanied by undesirable side effects, may be avoided.

The skin lesions of pemphigus vulgaris are initially vesiculobullous eruptions that subsequently ulcerate and are then prone to secondary infection and poor healing. Untreated, the lesions progress and coalesce to produce large areas of epithelial denudation and infection. Patients become dehydrated and septic, with an almost universal fatal outcome.

Oral lesions are present in almost all cases of pemphigus vulgaris and often precede skin involvement. Prognosis of the disease is always improved if treatment can be instituted prior to the onset of skin lesions. Any area of the mouth may be involved, including mucosal surfaces and gingivae. Pemphigus vulgaris may be manifested as a desquamative gingivitis. In severe cases, almost the entire oral mucosa may be affected, with vesiculobullous lesions in various stages of development, regression, and healing (Figs. 37–4 and 37–5). Even in relatively successful therapy of severe widespread pemphigus, the oral lesions are the last to heal, and minor oral involvement may persist with periodic exacerbation and regression of lesions. Development of oral lesions can be stimulated by traumatic influences, such as abrasion of mucosa by hard fragments of food. Bulla production can be initiated by the clinician simply by rubbing the mucosa with the thumb (positive Nikolsky sign).

Biopsy specimens from oral lesions of pemphigus present a characteristic pattern of acantholysis and are invariably diagnostic for the disease. Cytodiagnostic techniques may be helpful as corroborating evidence for the diagnosis of pemphigus. Smears of oral lesions

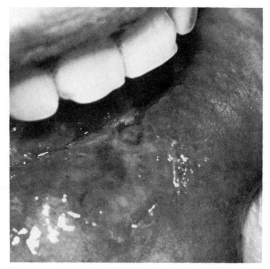

Figure 37–4. Large, broken bulla of the labial mucosa caused by pemphigus vulgaris.

demonstrate large numbers of acantholytic cells with large, hyperchromatic nuclei (Fig. 37–6). Fluorescent antibody techniques may be used to corroborate the histologic and cytologic diagnosis of an early case of pemphigus in which lesions are confined to oral mucosa. Because pemphigus represents a diagnosis with serious implications, all useful tests should be employed in arriving at a definitive diagnosis. However, fluorescent antibody techniques, particularly the indirect technique, may be negative when the involvement is early and confined to the oral mucous membrane. Immunofluorescent techniques are helpful in longitudinal monitoring of antibody titers during treatment.

Although there is no cure for pemphigus

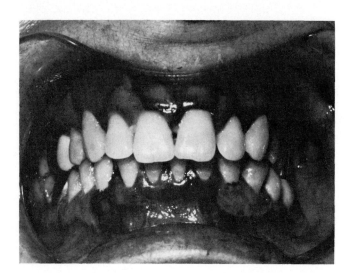

Figure 37–5. Extensive vesiculobullous involvement of gingiva and adjacent mucosa caused by pemphigus vulgaris.

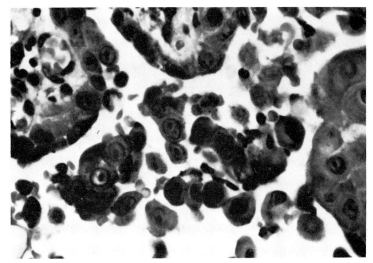

Figure 37–6. Cytologic smear of lesion of pemphigus vulgaris. Note the separation of the cells and hyperchromatic nuclei.

vulgaris, the disease can usually be successfully controlled with immunosuppressive drugs such as azathioprine (Imuran) or prednisone. Because these medications may produce significant side effects, it is recommended that patients with pemphigus be primarily managed by a dermatologist. Patients treated with these agents may develop secondary candidal infections. Local oral symptoms can be controlled with palliative rinses or ointments such as lidocaine (Xylocaine Viscous), dyclonine hydrochloride (Dyclone), and benzocaine in Orabase.

MUCOUS MEMBRANE PEMPHIGOID

Mucous membrane pemphigoid is a relatively rare vesiculobullous disease that affects the oral cavity. The disease is thought to be of autoimmune origin, in which antibodies directed against the basement membrane cause separation of the epithelium from the underlying connective tissue and the formation of subepithelial bullae. These antibodies are readily demonstrable by immunofluorescent techniques. Unlike pemphigus vulgaris or bullous pemphigoid, the oral cavity is almost always involved in mucous membrane pemphigoid, with reported frequencies ranging between 90 and 100%.

Mucous membrane pemphigoid appears to have a predilection for women; 19 of 30 patients with the disease reported by Lever were women. Similarly, of 85 patients with mucous membrane pemphigoid studied by Shklar and McCarthy, 73 were women. While mucous

membrane pemphigoid is seen over a broad age range, it is generally a disease of older patients, with a mean age of onset of 60 years. Although reported in young adults, the disease is extremely rare in children.

The oral cavity is the most consistently affected area of the body, although other mucous membranes may be involved. Lesions are initially vesiculobullous but usually become erosive. The gingiva is almost always affected and manifests a desquamative gingivitis. Keratinized gingivae are affected almost exclusively, appearing red and eroded, with areas of necrotic white slough. Bullae may form (Fig. 37–7). Although edentulous areas are not often affected, lesions may be seen and are aggravated by removable prostheses. They are extremely sensitive. It is rare to observe intact bullae, because these usually rupture prior to presentation. Secondary surface infection of areas of necrosis is not uncommon and appears clinically as ulcers with yellowish centers surrounded by regions of erythema. These lesions generally heal in about 2 weeks, but healing may be delayed. As in pemphigus vulgaris, it is not uncommon for the patient to have lesions at different stages. Thus, an individual may present with forming vesicles (2 to 3 days), erosive lesions, erythema, and ulceration. The disease tends to be chronic, and lesions may persist for years.

The major goal in the diagnosis of mucous membrane pemphigoid is to differentiate it from pemphigus vulgaris, because the former has a much more benign course. Biopsy is critical for diagnosis and reveals nonspecific subepithelial vesiculation, with the separation of epithelium sharply at the basement mem-

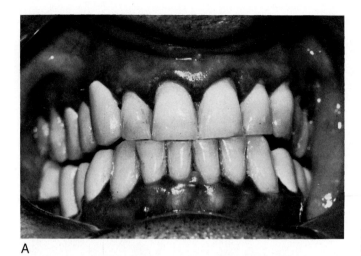

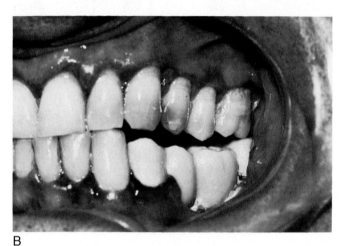

Figure 37–7. *A, B,* Mucous membrane pemphigoid. Note the involvement of the marginal and papillary gingiva with the development of vesiculobullous areas.

brane. Cytologic smears are not useful in the definitive diagnosis of mucous membrane pemphigoid. Immunofluorescence is helpful in differentiating the disease from lichen planus, bullous pemphigoid, and pemphigus vulgaris (Fig. 37–8).

The second most common anatomic site for mucous membrane pemphigoid is the conjunctiva. Conjunctivitis sometimes precedes, but usually occurs simultaneously with, oral lesions. The conjunctiva appears red and swollen, and if the lesions persist, adhesions called symblepharon develop in the eyelid to eyeball area (Fig. 37–9). Because corneal damage may occur as a sequela, ophthalmologic consultation should be routine in any patient with mucous membrane pemphigoid in whom conjunctival involvement is suspected or who has symptoms (burning or pain).

As yet, there is no specific therapy for mucous membrane pemphigoid. Treatment should be directed at palliation, preventing serious complications, and reducing local irrita-

tion, because this aggravates the condition. Periodontal disease should be eliminated. Fixed rather than removable prostheses should be used whenever possible. Palliative mouthwashes can be recommended, but commercial rinses containing alcohol or other irritating compounds should be eliminated. Topical steroids in ointment or paste form can be applied for local control of inflammation and reduction in discomfort. Their usefulness in controlling the disease is variable. Local intralesional injections of steroids may also be helpful. Benzocaine in Orabase, lidocaine (Xylocaine Viscous), diphenhydramine hydrochloride (Benadryl) and Kaopectate, or dyclonine hydrochloride (Dyclone) may be used to soothe sore tissues.

In patients who are extremely symptomatic, systemic corticosteroids may be used to control the disease. Shklar and McCarthy have reported that relatively small doses of systemic steroids are effective and recommend prednisone in initial daily dosages of 20 to 25 mg,

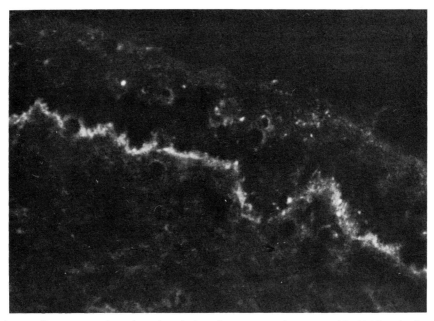

Figure 37–8. Immunofluorescence of specimen from lesion of mucous membrane pemphigoid. Note the linear distribution of antibody between the epithelium and underlying connective tissue.

followed by gradual tapering. Alternate-day administration of steroids may minimize their side effects. Systemic steroids should be used prudently, because they may produce a variety of side effects (Chap. 15). The dentist should work with the patient's physician in any case in which systemic steroid therapy is contemplated. Less invasive local therapy should always be tried first.

Mucous membrane pemphigoid often runs a chronic, protracted course. Patients should be reassured but also realistically apprised of the drawn-out nature of this disease.

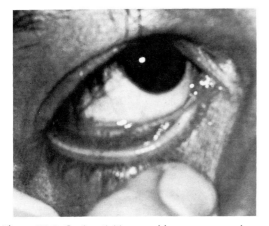

Figure 37–9. Conjunctivitis caused by mucous membrane pemphigoid. Following the mouth, the conjunctiva is the most common site for mucous membrane pemphigoid.

Bullous Pemphigoid

Bullous pemphigoid is an autoimmune disease in which antibodies are demonstrated in the area of the epithelial basement membrane. Consequently, subepithelial vesiculobullous lesions arise, in which separation is noted between the epithelium and the underlying connective tissue.

Unlike mucous membrane pemphigoid, bullous pemphigoid is predominantly a disease of skin; oral involvement is noted in only 20% of patients with the disease. Bullous pemphigoid tends to affect elderly individuals and is most common in those over 60 years old. Oral involvement in bullous pemphigoid generally is noted after cutaneous lesions are present.

The most consistent oral finding in bullous pemphigoid is a diffuse, painful, desquamative gingivitis. The lesions appear on attached gingivae and demonstrate areas of redness and bleeding. Lesions at different stages of development are often seen simultaneously. Vesiculobullous lesions rupture to form ulcerative and eroded areas. The margins of the lesions may actually be noted to peel away. Other areas of the oral mucosa may also be involved. Definitive diagnosis is made by histologic examination. Immunofluorescent tests are also helpful.

Skin lesions of bullous pemphigoid ultimately are vesiculobullous in nature, although

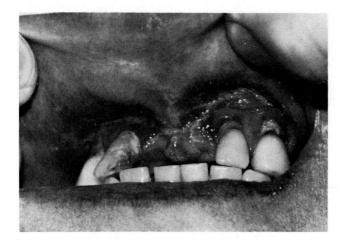

Figure 37–10. Bullous lichen planus. The bullae of the alveolar mucosa and mucobuccal fold have ruptured, leaving an open, raw surface.

the disease begins as a nonspecific rash. Frequently, ruptured vesicles crust over. The limbs are most commonly involved.

The cutaneous lesions of bullous pemphigoid are usually responsive to steroids. Oral lesions may be more persistent and may remain despite the elimination of lesions in other areas. Local palliation of gingival involvement includes débridement, good oral hygiene, and bland mouth rinses. The disease tends to run a chronic course.

LICHEN PLANUS

One of the clinical manifestations of lichen planus is as an erosive or bullous form. Usually, this lesion appears in concert with the hyperkeratotic form of the disease (Chap. 36). The cause of lichen planus is unresolved. Stress, drug reactions, and immune dysfunction have been implicated. Frequently, a specific stressful event can be identified in the history. Lichen planus may occur in transient episodes, or it may become chronic. The disease may disappear following the resolution of a stressful situation, such as the death of an ill relative or the resolution of a divorce. Because of the presence of a lymphocytic infiltrate in histologic sections from patients with lichen planus, an autoimmune component has been suggested in the pathogenesis.

Clinically, patients with bullous lichen planus are usually uncomfortable and complain of burning, pain, and sensitivity to spices. Examination may demonstrate the presence of bullae of varying sizes. Rarely are bullae intact, however. Rather, one observes large, open, raw, eroded areas frequently bordered by lichenoid areas of leukoplakia (Figs. 37–10 and 37–11). The borders of these lesions are usu-

ally uneven, and the bases may be erythematous. Areas of hyperkeratotic striae are often evident in other parts of the mouth. Most frequently, bullous or erosive lichen planus involves the buccal mucosa, ventral surface of the tongue, or attached gingivae. In most instances, lesions are distributed bilaterally and often symmetrically. The flexor surfaces of the arms may concurrently demonstrate the skin lesions of lichen planus.

The diagnosis of bullous lichen planus can usually be based on the appearance of the lesions. However, because lichen planus may resemble other conditions, biopsy is strongly recommended.

There is no cure for bullous lichen planus. Patients who are uncomfortable may receive symptomatic relief through the use of pallia-

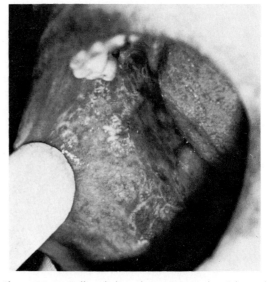

Figure 37–11. Bullous lichen planus. Ruptured vesicles and bullae are present, as are lichenoid areas at the periphery.

tive mouth rinses or ointments. Topical steroid ointments or creams (triamcinolone acetonide) have been reported to be effective in some patients. For patients who are constantly uncomfortable, a short course of systemic steroids may be prescribed in cooperation with the physician. Patients should be advised to avoid spicy foods. Any source of oral irritation should be eliminated.

The issue of whether patients with lichen planus are predisposed to oral squamous cell carcinoma has been raised. The conclusions of a number of studies are conflicting. However, it seems prudent for the clinician to follow patients with lichen planus closely.

ERYTHEMA MULTIFORME

Erythema multiforme is an acute mucocutaneous disease that has extreme clinical variability. Although erythema multiforme is usually grouped with the vesiculobullous diseases, it may also present as ulcerative, erythematous, or erosive lesions.

The cause of erythema multiforme is not well understood, and a variety of causes have been suggested. One popular theory suggested that erythema multiforme represents a sequela of infection with herpes simplex virus. Support for this hypothesis comes from the observation that erythema multiforme is frequently noted 1 to 3 weeks after infection with the virus. In addition, it has been noted that erythema multiforme is relatively common after inoculation with herpes simplex virus vaccine.

Erythema multiforme has also been reported following bacterial and fungal infections. Mycoplasma are the bacteria most often implicated. Many drugs have also been implicated in a causative role for this condition, including quinidine, gold salts, digitalis, phenylbutazone, heavy metals, antibiotics, and oral contraceptives (Table 37–1).

It seems likely, based on the explosive onset of the disease and the suggestion of a multiagent cause, that some form of humoral autoimmune reaction is responsible for the development of the disease. Any of the agents mentioned in discussions of the cause of erythema multiforme can produce modifications in cell surface antigens or the production of cross-reacting antibodies, which could result in tissue destruction.

Unlike other forms of oral vesiculobullous diseases, erythema multiforme is noted most frequently in young adults. Children may also be affected. Whereas mucous membrane pem-

Table 37–1. DRUGS ASSOCIATED WITH ERYTHEMA MULTIFORME

Analgesics	Antidiabetic drugs
Aspirin	Chlorpropamide
Barbiturates	Tolbutamide
Codeine	
Ibuprofen	Antineoplastic drugs
Fenoprofen	Alkylating agents
Sulindac	Methotrexate
Antibiotics	Antihypertensives
Chloramphenicol	Diltiazem
Ciprofloxacin	Hydralazine
Clindamycin	Minoxidil
Dapsone	Verapamil
Penicillin	
Sulfonamide	Antirheumatics
Tetracycline	Gold salts
	Phenylbutazone
Anticonvulsants	
Carbamazepine	Psychopharmacologic
Phenytoin	agents
	Glutethimide
Antituberculosis drugs	Lithium
Isoniazid	Meprobamate
Rifampin	Methaqualone

Adapted from Stampien, T. M., and Schwartz, R. A.: Erythema multiformae. Am Fam Physician, 46:1171–1176, 1992. Published by the American Academy of Family Physicians.

phigoid and pemphigus vulgaris tend to occur more frequently in women, there is a male sex predilection for erythema multiforme.

Clinically, erythema multiforme has an acute onset. A detailed history often reveals mention of one of the causative agents previously discussed. The disease may affect the skin or mucosa; both types of tissue may be simultaneously involved. Skin lesions of erythema multiforme present a unique picture, consisting of a central region of vesiculation surrounded by a circumferential band of erythema. The vesiculation may rupture, leaving a crusting central area of necrosis. Because of the concentric ring appearance, the lesions are commonly referred to as "target lesions" (Figs. 37–12 and 37–13). Skin lesions are usually symmetrically distributed and most often present on the hands and feet.

The oral lesions of erythema multiforme are more variable in appearance than the skin lesions. Almost all are painful. Any area of the mouth may be involved; whereas some authors have claimed that most lesions tend to be toward the anterior portion of the mouth including the lips, others have stated that the tongue, palate, gingivae, and buccal mucosa are most often involved. The severity of the lesions also varies; some areas may demonstrate only subtle areas of mucosal erythema (Figs. 37–14 and 37–15). In contrast, large hemorrhagic vesiculobullous lesions may extend from the mouth

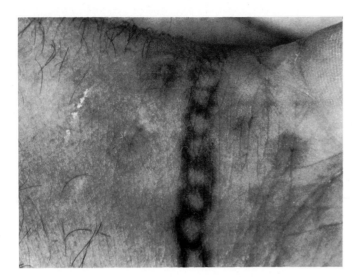

Figure 37–12. Multiple target lesions of erythema multiforme on patient's wrist. The chain-like area is a tattoo.

Figure 37–13. Close-up of target lesion of erythema multiforme.

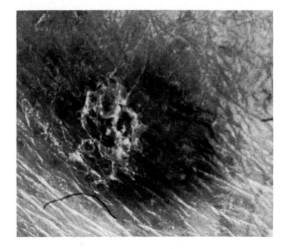

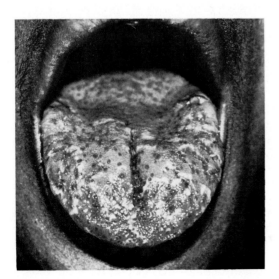

Figure 37–14. Erythema multiforme involving the tongue secondary to drug therapy.

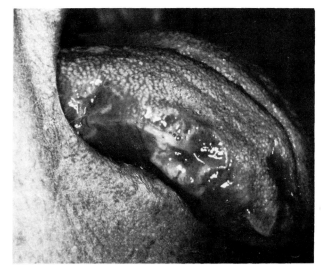

Figure 37–15. Bullae of the tongue caused by erythema multiforme.

beyond the mucocutaneous junction to involve the lips (Figs. 37–16, 37–17, and 37–18). Lesions tend to be symmetric. The onset of erythema multiforme tends to be sudden, but once lesions are established, the disease may become chronic with periods of remission and exacerbation.

Treatment of erythema multiforme is somewhat controversial, especially with regard to the use of systemic steroids. It seems that mild or moderate cases of the condition are self-limiting. In these instances, usually only palliation and treatment of secondary infection are necessary. Patients heal spontaneously in about 2 weeks. More severe or persistent cases may necessitate steroid therapy. In these situa-

tions, a short, intensive, tapering course of prednisone appears to be effective. When oral lesions can be correlated with drug intake, the offending agent should be discontinued. Supportive care may be required, especially in youngsters with severe oral lesions in whom fluid and food intake is compromised. Such patients may require hospitalization so that intravenous fluids and nutrition may be supplied. Systemic analgesics may also be used if needed.

Management of patients with erythema multiforme may represent a complex problem. Cooperation among the dentist and other health professionals is essential in caring for these patients.

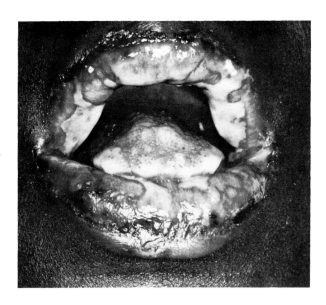

Figure 37–16. Erythema multiforme with extensive lip involvement secondary to herpes simplex infection. Note the extensive vesiculobullous lesions of the labial mucosa.

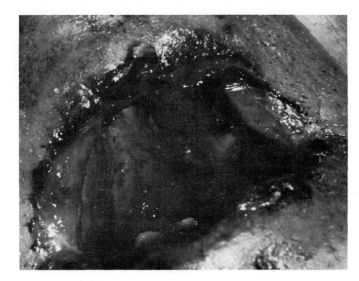

Figure 37–17. Erythema multiforme with extensive palatal involvement and hemorrhagic lesions of the lips.

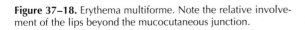
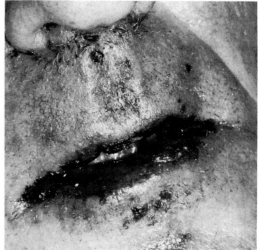

Figure 37–18. Erythema multiforme. Note the relative involvement of the lips beyond the mucocutaneous junction.

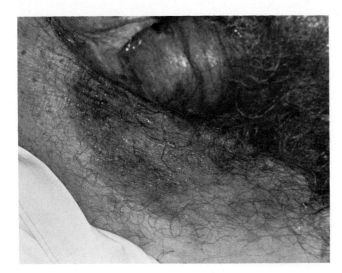

Figure 37–19. Erythema multiforme involving the skin of the groin and penis.

Stevens-Johnson Syndrome

In 1922, Stevens and Johnson described an entity in children that they termed an "eruptive fever associated with stomatitis and ophthalmia." The condition they described had a number of features that made it unique and differentiated it from more common forms of erythema multiforme. Since that time, severe cases of hemorrhagic erythema multiforme in which patients have a specific set of concurrent findings, including either fibromembranous or papulovesicular conjunctival involvement, skin and mouth lesions, fever, and leukopenia, are referred to as Stevens-Johnson syndrome. Other mucous membranes may also be affected, especially the external genitalia (Fig. 37–19). Ocular lesions may be especially severe and, if untreated, can lead to blindness.

Vesiculobullous Diseases

DIAGNOSIS	RELEVANT HISTORY	APPEARANCE AND SIGNS	LOCATION	PATIENT PROFILE/CAUSE	TESTS	COURSE AND TREATMENT
Pemphigus vulgaris	Bulla formation or erosion; may have skin involvement; oral lesions usually painful	Large bullae, sometimes not intact, leaving broad open ulceration; Nikolsky's sign positive	Mucosal surfaces, occasionally attached gingiva, 40% of cases have oral lesions preceding cutaneous lesions, almost all cases have oral involvement	Most commonly seen in adult Jews and other Mediterranean groups; autoimmune cause; age at onset >50	Cytology—Tzanck preparation; biopsy—acantholysis, immunofluorescence	Progressive course with increasing involvement; treated with steroids or immunosuppressives; fatal if untreated
Bullous pemphigoid	Vesicles, ulcers, or erosion; painful gingival involvement; pain, bleeding on brushing	Oral lesions rare—20%, usually skin lesions; gingiva demonstrate desquamative edema, inflammation, and desquamation; Nikolsky's sign negative	Attached and marginal gingiva demonstrate desquamative gingivitis; buccal mucosa also involved	60+ years; autoimmune antibasement membrane; no sex or racial predilection	Biopsy and immunofluorescence	Not life-threatening; chronic course; local oral care, steroids
Mucous membrane pemphigoid	Vesicles or, if broken, erosion and ulceration; pain	Oral lesions in most cases >85%; eye involvement common (50%)—symblepharon; also genital, urethral, larynx, pharynx, anal areas may be affected	Buccal mucosa, palate, and gingiva	40–50; female > male, 2:1; autoimmune cause; antibasement membrane antibody	Biopsy and immunofluorescence	Ophthalmology consult in cases of eye involvement; systemic and/or topical steroids; local oral care
Erythema multiforme	Drug intake; recent viral or bacterial infeciton; allergies; pain	Mouth-mucosa hemorrhagic, bullae, crusting often involving lips; may have ocular and genital lesions; may have skin lesions → target lesions	Mucosal surfaces, labial mucosa frequent; gingiva may be involved	Children to young adults most common but any age; cause multiple producing symptom complex; slight male sex predilection	Biopsy	Short course with steroids; palliative and supportive care; self-limiting
Bullous lichen planus	Skin lesions; stressful event	Vesiculobullous lesions, ulcers or erosions affecting any area; gingiva often involved; may have concurrent keratotic striae	Buccal mucosa, ventral tongue, attached gingiva	Middle age; no sex predilection	Biopsy	Self-limiting course, but chronic; palliation, steroids in severe cases

CHAPTER

38

Pigmented Lesions

Pigmented lesions of the oral cavity are not infrequent. They are caused by the deposition of pigment that may originate from endogenous or exogenous sources. Endogenous areas of pigmentation are most frequently attributable to melanin but may also be caused by bilirubin or iron. A number of systemic disorders are associated with increased intraoral or perioral pigmentation. Although rare, intraoral pigmented malignancies may occur. Exogenous pigmentation may be caused by deposits of foreign material in tissue, by the overgrowth of chromophilic bacteria or fungi, or by the ingestion of metals that are deposited in oral tissues. The approach to diagnosis of a pigmented area of the mouth should include an initial differentiation between vascular lesions and true pigmented lesions, followed by an analysis of the pigmented area (Fig. 38–1). In many cases, definitive diagnosis of a pigmented lesion can be made only by histologic tissue evaluation.

The easiest technique to differentiate a vascular area of pigmentation clinically from a true pigmented lesion is to examine the area for blanching. A vascular lesion blanches when a mirror handle is placed with firm pressure against the lesion, whereas an area of true pigmentation is unaffected.

LESIONS CAUSED BY ENDOGENOUS PIGMENTATION

Abnormalities of melanin pigmentation are classified into three groups of conditions that affect the oral mucosa: increased melanin deposition as a normal variation; pigmented nevi; and endocrine or metabolic disturbances.

Normal oral tissue may demonstrate wide variations in melanin deposition. Not infrequently, the attached gingiva of black patients may demonstrate significant normal blue-black color caused by melanin (Fig. 38–2). Such pigmentation may also be noted on other areas of oral mucosa including the palatal area. Generally, pigmentation resulting from normal variations of melanin deposition tends to be symmetric.

A number of metabolic and endocrine diseases cause abnormal melanin deposition of the oral mucosa, including Addison's disease, Peutz-Jeghers syndrome, McCune-Albright syndrome, and von Recklinghausen's disease.

Addison's Disease

Addison's disease, or primary adrenocortical deficiency, is rare. It is caused by progressive

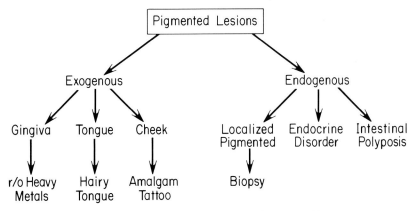

Figure 38–1. Approach to the diagnosis of pigmented lesions.

383

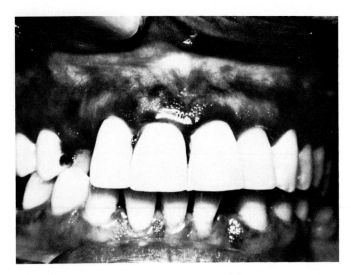

Figure 38–2. Gingival pigmentation resulting from melanin distribution, a variant of normal.

adrenocortical destruction resulting from a variety of agents including tuberculosis and fungal infections (Chap. 15). About 90% of the adrenal gland must be destroyed before clinical signs of the disease are present. Patients have a history of a progressively debilitating illness and complain of malaise, weakness, anorexia, nausea, vomiting, and weight loss. Also included in the classic signs and symptoms of the disease are cutaneous and mucosal pigmentation. Oral pigmentation is an early sign of Addison's disease and is characterized by bluish-black to dark brown areas that are most commonly present on the buccal and labial mucosae but that may occur on the gingival mucosa (Fig. 38–3). There is no unique pattern or distribution to the pigmentation. The hyperpigmentation, which is caused by mela-

nin, is also seen on skin and is nonspecific. Diagnosis requires the demonstration of decreased adrenal cortisol production and cannot be based solely on the presence of hyperpigmentation.

Peutz-Jeghers Syndrome

Peutz-Jeghers syndrome is a rare hereditary syndrome that consists of intestinal polyposis and oral and perioral pigmentation. The perioral lesions consist of numerous discrete melanin spots on the lips and around the mouth (Fig. 38–4). Similar pigmentation may be noted on the oral mucosa. Although intestinal polyposis is generally not of significance in terms of undergoing malignant transformation, it frequently results in intestinal symptoms and pathology, including obstruction. Ovarian neoplasms are noted in 5% of women with the syndrome.

McCune-Albright Syndrome

McCune-Albright syndrome is a rare disease characterized by fibrous dysplasia, areas of pigmentation, and endocrine dysfunction. The cause of McCune-Albright disease is unknown, although it does not appear to be hereditary. The unilateral distribution of the fibrous dysplasia has led to speculation that the disease represents a congenital anomaly. The fibrous dysplasia tends to be of the polyostotic form (Chap. 44). As with the fibrous changes, the pigmentation changes in McCune-Albright disease tend to be unilateral. The lips are most

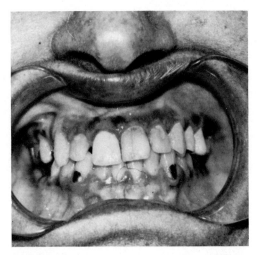

Figure 38–3. Oral pigmentation as a consequence of Addison's disease.

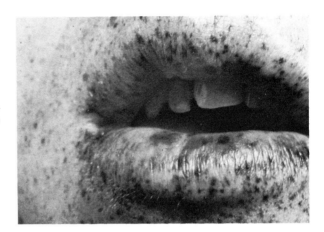

Figure 38–4. Perioral pigmentation as seen in Peutz-Jeghers syndrome. Patients have intestinal polyposis in addition to pigmentation.

commonly involved, but any area of mucosa may show hyperpigmentation. Commonly, irregular skin pigmentation is also present, and patients demonstrate precocious puberty.

Von Recklinghausen's Disease

Von Recklinghausen's disease, or neurofibromatosis, is a rare hereditary disorder that has been in the public eye as a result of the play "The Elephant Man." Von Recklinghausen's disease is caused by a mendelian dominant gene. Clinically, patients develop numerous neurofibromas, which develop from the neurilemmal sheath and fibroblasts of peripheral nerves. The tumors are most frequently distributed over the trunk and extremities. The pigmented lesions that accompany the tumors are brownish in color and are described as being café-au-lait spots (Fig. 38–5). On the skin, the pigmented areas have the same distribution as the tumors. They may occur on the lips or around the mouth and, on rare occasions, on the buccal mucosa. A significant percentage of neurofibromas (5 to 10%) may undergo malignant transformation.

Bilirubin

Abnormally high levels of serum bilirubin (greater than 1.5 mg/dl) result in a clinical state of jaundice. A variety of diseases, such as hepatitis, blockage of the common bile duct, and degenerative changes of the liver, result in a yellowish discoloration of the skin, sclerae, and oral mucosa (Chap. 23). Most commonly, oral manifestations of jaundice are noted on the ventral surface of the tongue, the buccal mucosa, and the soft palate.

Hemochromatosis

Hemochromatosis (bronze diabetes) is an iron storage disease in which excess amounts of iron are deposited in body tissues. Clinical signs of the disease include hepatomegaly, pigmentation, diabetes, arthropathy, cardiac disease, and hypogonadism. The disease may occur as a consequence of the patient's inability to control iron absorption (idiopathic hemochromatosis), as a manifestation of a disorder of erythropoiesis (erythropoietic hemochromatosis), in alcoholics with liver disease, or as a result of excessive iron intake. Oral manifestations of hemochromatosis include pigmentation (bluish-black) of the oral mucosa, which occurs in 10 to 15% of patients.

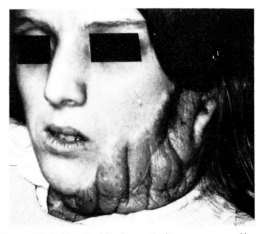

Figure 38–5. Von Recklinghausen's disease, or neurofibromatosis. This is often accompanied by café-au-lait pigmentation.

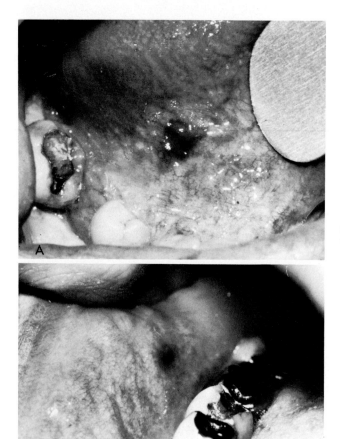

Figure 38–6. *A, B,* Amalgam tattoos resulting from the deposition of submucosal pigmentation following the placement of a restoration. Note the proximity of the pigmented areas to the restorations.

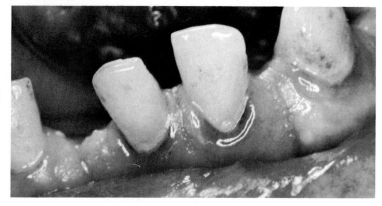

Figure 38–7. Deposition of lead in the marginal gingiva of a patient exposed to lead-based paint.

LESIONS CAUSED BY EXOGENOUS SOURCES OF PIGMENTATION

Amalgam Tattoo

Occasionally, small bits of amalgam are incorporated into tissue following the placement of a restoration. The material becomes impregnated into tissue, giving the appearance of a flat, bluish-black area that is usually adjacent to the restoration (Fig. 38–6). These lesions are totally asymptomatic and are of no clinical significance.

Heavy Metals

High systemic levels of some heavy metals, notably lead and bismuth, result in the deposition of metallic pigmentation along the gingival margin (Fig. 38–7). Clinically, these areas appear as dark blue-black areas affecting the marginal gingiva. Such pigmentation is usually bilateral and involves the mandibular and maxillary arches equally. Although the areas of pigmentation are of little clinical significance in themselves, they are of importance in the diagnosis of heavy metal toxicity.

Discoloration of the Tongue

Not infrequently, the papillae on the dorsal surface of the tongue become discolored (Fig. 38–8). Although classically referred to as black hairy tongue, pigmentation of the papillae may be white, yellow, brown, or green. Black hairy tongue is thought to be the result of antibiotic intake, which results in local proliferation of melanogenic bacteria. Other sources of black hairy tongue include pipe smoking, heavy cigarette smoking, certain foods, and fungal infections. Hyperplasia of the filiform papillae may occur simultaneously. This results in a hair-like appearance of the papillae caused by their overgrowth. Occasionally, glossodynia may be noted. Elimination of the source of pigmentation usually reverses the condition.

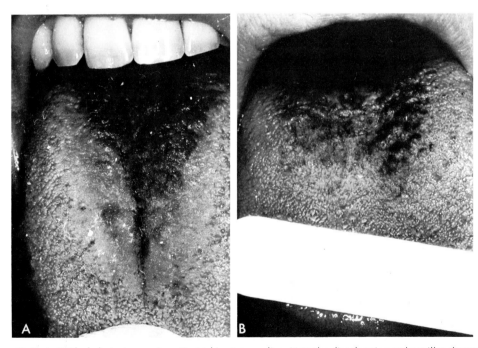

Figure 38–8. *A, B,* Black, hairy tongue in patient taking tetracycline. Note the discoloration and papillary hyperplasia.

Common Developmental Anomalies of Oral Soft Tissues

A number of developmental anomalies commonly affect the oral cavity. Most are of little or no pathologic or clinical significance and require no treatment. Frequently, the patient notices the presence of one of these conditions and becomes alarmed. The role of the dental practitioner is to identify these lesions and inform and reassure the patient. The exceptions are anomalies that affect function or appearance, such as clefts. In the discussion that follows only the most common anomalies are discussed. Clearly, a multitude of developmental disturbances affect the head and neck. The reader is referred to the excellent texts in this field that discuss these problems in detail.

LIP PITS

Lip pits are unilateral or bilateral indentations noted at the commissures of the mouth (Fig. 39–1). They have been considered hereditary in origin. They are of no clinical significance unless they represent the extension of a soft tissue fistula, in which case drainage may be present. Treatment is generally not re-

quired unless infection occurs; surgery is curative.

ANKYLOGLOSSIA

An absent or short lingual frenum results in partial or complete ankyloglossia (Fig. 39–2). Partial ankyloglossia is more common. Lingual motion may be limited; the degree is dependent on the extent of the frenum. Speech may be compromised, especially the ability to pronounce consonants. Surgical separation of the frenum is curative. Because speech development may be affected, early recognition and treatment are important.

CLEFTS

Facial and palatal clefts are relatively common congenital anomalies that occur with a frequency of 1 in 800 to 1000 births. Despite

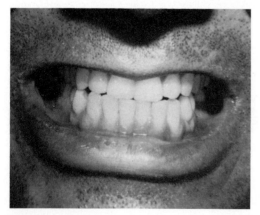

Figure 39–1. Congenital lip pits noted as indentations at the corners of the mouth.

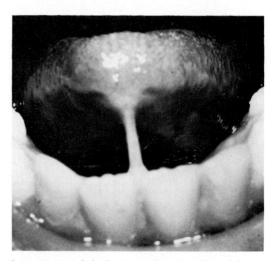

Figure 39–2. Ankyloglossia resulting from lingual frenum, which severely inhibits motion of the tongue.

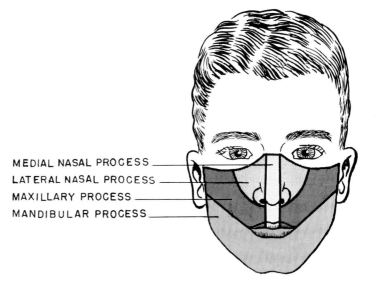

Figure 39–3. Developmental processes of the face. (From Shafer, W. G., Hine, M. G., and Levy, B. M.: Textbook of Oral Pathology, 4th ed. Philadelphia, W. B. Saunders, 1983.)

MEDIAL NASAL PROCESS

LATERAL NASAL PROCESS

MAXILLARY PROCESS

MANDIBULAR PROCESS

their frequency, much is unresolved regarding the mechanisms by which these defects occur, or their cause. Fortunately, patients with clefts are being treated more aggressively and at earlier ages than in the past.

Cleft lip (harelip) is most common in the maxilla and is thought to be the consequence of a failure of fusion of the maxillary and median nasal processes (Fig. 39–3). Whether this failure is the result of a true failure of the processes to join or a breakdown of fused tissue is unresolved. Clinically, cleft lips of the maxilla may be unilateral (81%) or bilateral (19%) (Fig. 39–4) and they may be partial (40%), extending only partway up the lip, or complete, extending to the nostrils. Because of the position of the median nasal and maxillary processes, midline cleft lips of the maxilla do not occur. Cleft lips of the mandible are extremely rare. Unlike maxillary cleft lips, these do occur in the midline.

Surgical repair of cleft lips is now so sophisticated that excellent cosmetic results can be achieved (Fig. 39–5). To minimize psychologic trauma to parent and child and to achieve a maximum esthetic and functional result, cleft lips are usually repaired during the first month of life, generally by a plastic surgeon or otolaryngologist who has had special training in this area.

Cleft palate may occur with cleft lip, or each condition may occur independently. Palatal clefts are the result of lack of fusion or breakdown of fused elements of the embryonic components of the hard palate (Fig. 39–6). If the palatal shelves elevate and then fail to fuse or break down, a midline cleft results. This may involve all or part of the hard palate and may extend posteriorly to involve the soft palate and uvula. If the palatal processes fail to fuse with the nasal process, a cleft extends into the base of the nose. This then deviates from the midline. Clefts involving the maxillary process affect the alveolar ridge and may be unilateral or bilateral. These may extend to involve soft tissue and result in a cleft lip.

Cleft palate creates both immediate and long-range problems for newborns. The most acute problems involve adequate nutrition. Infants having a palatal cleft may be unable to suck sufficiently to nurse. In these cases, obturation with a stint is helpful in providing the ability to suck as well as providing guidance for

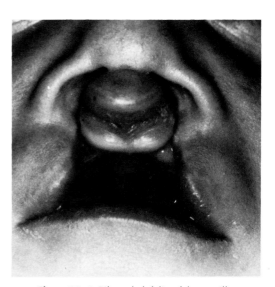

Figure 39–4. Bilateral cleft lip of the maxilla.

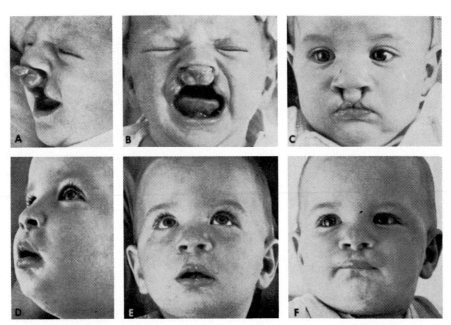

Figure 39–5. *A–F,* Postoperative result following surgical repair of a cleft lip. (From Converse, J. M.: Reconstructive Plastic Surgery, Vol. 4. Philadelphia, W. B. Saunders, 1964.)

the developing maxillary processes. Patients who also have a cleft lip usually have these repaired within the first month. Repair of the palate is usually deferred until the child is older.

Patients with cleft palate present a multitude of clinical problems that require close cooperation and interaction among the plastic surgeon, otolaryngologist (these patients have a high incidence of otitis media because of their inability to clear their eustachian tubes), general dentist, orthodontist, oral surgeon, and speech pathologist. A psychologist should also be included in the team caring for these patients. Care is longitudinal.

The cause of clefts is unresolved and the focus of much controversy. There appears to be a genetic component, in that children of parents having clefts have a higher incidence of the same problem. Nutritional deficiencies and hormonal imbalances have been implicated as causative agents in animal models. Toxic substances, including drugs and gaseous anesthetics such as nitrous oxide, have also been mentioned as having a causative role in the development of clefts.

BIFID UVULA

Bifid uvula results from an incomplete fusion of the posterior portion of the soft palate.

The major significance of bifid uvula is that it may indicate incomplete closure of the posterior border of the hard palate, which results in a submucosal cleft palate (Fig. 39–7). This defect can be diagnosed by having the patient say "ahh" to constrict the muscles over the posterior hard palate, allowing the dentist to visualize the underlying bony architecture. The major clinical significance of submucosal cleft palate is in the potential difficulty of the patient to clear the eustachian tubes. This may result in frequent middle ear infections, which, if undiagnosed and untreated, can result in deafness.

TORUS PALATINUS AND TORUS MANDIBULARIS

Tori are relatively common bony protuberances that occur most often on the lingual surfaces of the mandible and on the midline of the palate. They represent bony exostoses that are developmental malformations and are non-neoplastic. The overlying mucosa is normal but may at times be traumatized. Torus palatinus occurs in approximately 20% of the population. There are wide variations in clinical presentations, ranging from subtle bony enlargements of the midline of the hard palate to large, knob-like protuberances occurring in the same area (Fig. 39–8).

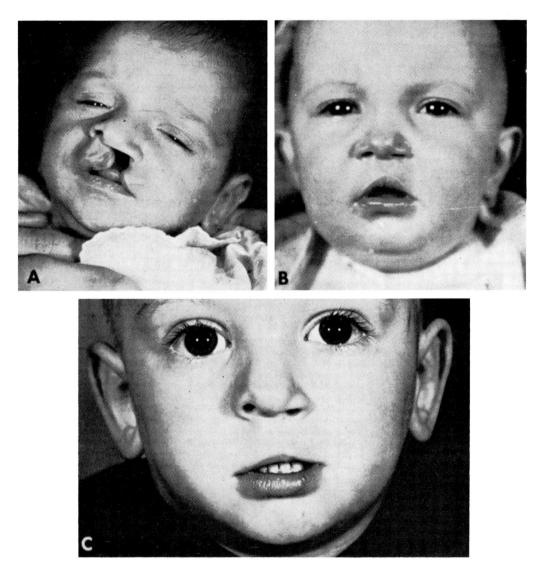

Figure 39–6. *A,* Complete cleft lip with associated cleft palate. *B, C,* Postoperative result in same patient. (From Converse, J. M.: Reconstructive Plastic Surgery, 2nd ed., Vol. 4. Philadelphia, W. B. Saunders, 1977.)

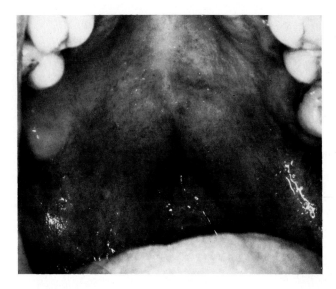

Figure 39–7. Submucosal cleft palate. Constriction of the palatal musculature reveals a submucosal cleft palate in an individual with a bifid uvula.

Torus mandibularis is less common and occurs in only 6% of the population. Mandibular tori usually present as bilateral, symmetric enlargements on the lingual surfaces of the mandibular canines or premolars. Mandibular tori range in clinical presentation from subtle, small, nodular areas to large, knob-like, hard lobules (Fig. 39–9).

Neither anomaly is of clinical significance unless the patient requires a prosthesis, in which case the tori may require surgical removal.

GLOSSITIS AREATA MIGRANS (GEOGRAPHIC TONGUE)

Geographic tongue is an inflammatory form of glossitis of unknown cause. In this condition, localized areas of filiform papillae are rapidly lost and replaced by uneven areas of smooth dorsal surface lingual mucosa that is often erythematous because of hyperemia (Fig. 39–10). The most common area of involvement is the dorsal surface of the tongue, although the lateral borders may be involved. The fungiform papillae are exaggerated. The borders of the lesions are uneven, giving a "geographic" appearance, and may appear raised and whitish.

The lesion shows no apparent age or sex predilection. Involved areas may appear suddenly, usually remaining in one area for 1 or 2 weeks and then disappearing and arising in another region of the tongue, giving an impression that the lesion migrates. Usually these lesions are asymptomatic, although they may result in burning, especially in response

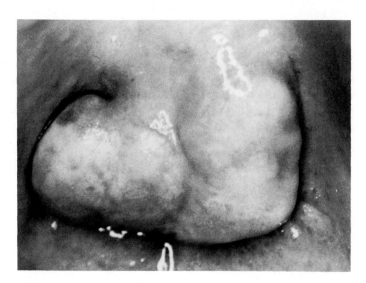

Figure 39–8. Torus palatinus. This is represented here by a large, bulb-like, pedunculated bony exostosis found in the palatal midline.

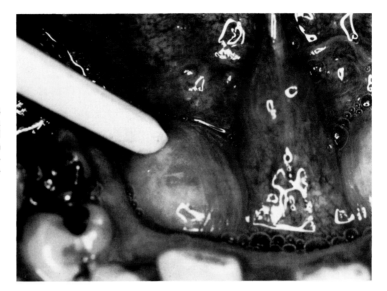

Figure 39–9. Torus mandibularis. This is demonstrated at the tip of the pointer. Mandibular tori are generally bilateral and occur as knob-like projections on the lingual surfaces of the mandible opposite the mandibular canines or premolars.

to spicy or acidic foods. Frequently, lesions go unnoticed by the patient. Approximately 50% of patients with geographic tongue also have a fissured tongue. Diagnosis of geographic tongue is made clinically. There is no specific therapy, although palliation in the form of sprays, ointments, or rinses may be helpful in symptomatic cases.

FISSURED TONGUE

Fissuring of the tongue is a relatively common occurrence and involves congenital deep furling or fissures running trench-like on the dorsal surface of the tongue (Fig. 39–11). Frequently, fissured tongue is associated with geo-

graphic tongue. Fissures vary significantly in their depth. The major clinical significance of fissuring is that debris can collect in the depths and create a chronic slight inflammatory condition that may manifest itself clinically as sensitivity to certain spicy foods. There is no specific therapy indicated.

FORDYCE'S GRANULES

Fordyce's granules are common congenital "lesions" that are caused by the presence of ectopic sebaceous glands on the buccal mucosa. Most commonly, the lesions are bilateral. They are generally asymptomatic and appear as raised, papillated, yellowish, clumped,

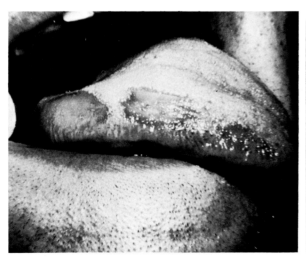
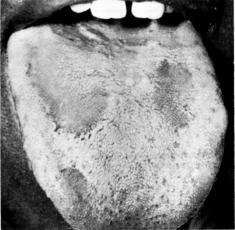

Figure 39–10. *A, B,* Geographic tongue. Irregular areas of lost filiform papillae are noted on the dorsal surface of the tongue. A surrounding band of erythema is often seen.

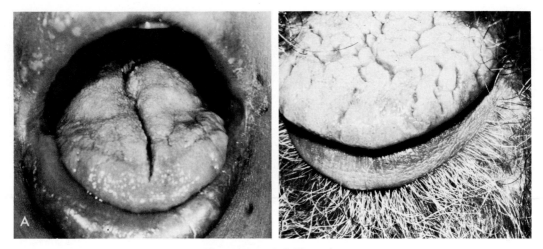

Figure 39–11. *A, B,* Fissured tongue.

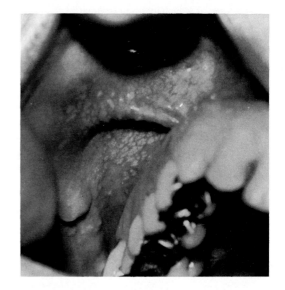

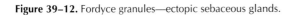

Figure 39–12. Fordyce granules—ectopic sebaceous glands.

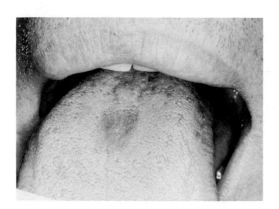

Figure 39–13. Median rhomboid glossitis.

spotty areas on the mucosa (Fig. 39–12). They are of no clinical significance and there is no treatment.

MEDIAN RHOMBOID GLOSSITIS

Median rhomboid glossitis is a benign congenital defect thought to represent remnants of the tuberculum impar, which remains on the posterior midline of the tongue (Fig. 39–13). Two clinical variations of median rhomboid glossitis have been described, one that appears as a slightly depressed oval or rhomboid-shaped reddish area on the posterior midline of the tongue, and the other that appears as a raised, tumor-like mass that is often pebbly and pinkish. Median rhomboid glossitis is reported to occur more frequently in men than in women. The lesion is totally asymptomatic and is frequently recognized incidentally by the patient, who then seeks consultation. Although *Candida* organisms often colonize the defect, their elimination does not result in resolution of the lesion. No treatment is required once the diagnosis is made.

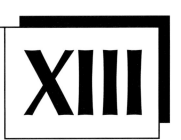
Evaluation and Management of the Patient with Neoplastic Disease

Squamous Cell Carcinoma of the Head and Neck

Cancer is the second leading cause of death in the United States. If not detected and treated early, oral cancer has both high morbidity and high mortality. It represents approximately 3% of all cancers in the United States and is much more common in some Asian societies. Although the impact of the disease is somewhat minimized by describing its frequency in terms of percentages, examination of the actual numbers of patients affected is more startling. In 1992, there were 30,300 new cases of oral cancer in the United States. This number represents an increase of 13% in the frequency of the disease since 1982. Deaths attributable to oral cancer in 1992 were projected at 7,950. Improvements in early detection and treatment have reduced the death rate from oral cancer by almost 12% in the past 10 years. Incidence and mortality statistics do little, however, to describe the tremendous impact on the quality of life caused by oral carcinoma. The patient's appearance and ability to communicate, eat, and be accepted by family, friends, and colleagues is often altered by the disease.

Morbidity and mortality of oral cancer can be minimized by early detection and treatment.

More than 90% of oral cancers are epidermoid or squamous cell carcinomas. The discussion that follows is thus confined to this form of cancer. Other less common oral malignancies are discussed elsewhere.

ETIOLOGY AND EPIDEMIOLOGY

Cancer incidence varies according to age, sex, race, occupation, geographic location, nutrition, and tobacco and alcohol use. Oral cancer is most common among older males; the average age of diagnosis is 60 years. While the male:female ratio for the disease is 2:1, this represents a significant increase in the number of cases in women. In 1950, this ratio was 6:1.

Differences in the incidence of oral cancer by race are dramatic, as demonstrated by the average annual age-adjusted incidence rates per 100,000 in the United States for oral cancer from 1975 to 1985: white males, 11.8; white females, 5.2; black males, 20.5; black females, 6.2; Hispanic males, 5.2; and Hispanic females, 1.7.

Of the causes of oral cancer, tobacco use (particularly cigarette smoking) and alcohol consumption are the most readily identified. The risk of oral cancer for smokers is at least double that for nonsmokers. This effect is dose related; heavy smokers are at higher risk. Also, the length of time a person has smoked influences risk. Fortunately, it appears that smoking cessation has a favorable impact on reducing the risk of oral cancer. In addition to cigarettes, use of smokeless tobacco, especially snuff, may lead to oral cancer. Snuff dipping, a practice that is relatively common among women in the southeastern United States, increases the risk of oral and pharyngeal cancer by four and increases the risk of gingival and buccal mucosal cancer by 50. Alarmingly, snuff dipping has found increasing popularity among teenagers.

Heavy alcohol consumption is strongly associated with the development of oral cancer. Day and colleagues recently reported that, after adjusting for smoking, heavy drinking (as defined by 30 or more drinks per week) resulted in a 9-fold increase in risk in whites and a 17-fold increase in risk in blacks. The type of alcohol consumed did not affect the result. Cigarette and alcohol used together are thus very strong cofactors in the development of oral cancer.

The complex origin or oral cancer is suggested by findings that implicate genetic, viral, and immunologic factors in the development of the disease. A familial tendency to develop oral cancer and its association with certain syndromes suggest a genetic component. Perhaps a genetic factor predisposes one to, rather than causes, the condition. Point mutations in the p53 gene have been associated with oral cancer development. This may represent a final common pathway in carcinogenesis that can be initiated by a variety of environmental or infectious agents. Herpes simplex, Epstein-Barr virus, and papillomavirus have been mentioned in this regard. Finally, immunosuppressed patients are at increased risk for the development of a number of malignancies, including oral cancer.

CLINICAL CHARACTERISTICS

Squamous cell carcinoma of the mouth may take on a variety of clinical presentations, including ulcers, leukoplakia, and exophytic forms. The former two are the most common. Oral carcinoma may present as an asymptomatic, nonhealing ulceration with borders that are raised, firm, and indurated. The base of the ulcer may appear as an uneven, granule-like surface, or it may be necrotic (Fig. 40–1).

Approximately 10% of keratotic white lesions in the mouth demonstrate histologic evidence of dysplasia or malignant change. These lesions appear as nonscrapable, asymptomatic, somewhat raised, adherent plaques that may have erythematous areas interspersed among the areas of leukoplakia (erythroplasia; Fig. 40–2). Finally, carcinomas may present as exophytic, verrucose-like growths with a pebbly, papillary-like top on a broad stalk (Fig. 40–3). The base of this form of cancer may be erythe-

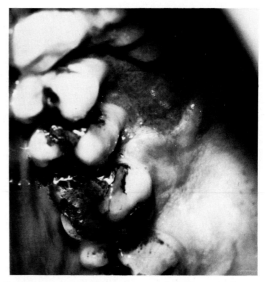

Figure 40–1. Clinical appearance of squamous cell carcinoma. Note the large palatal ulcer with raised borders.

matous and indurated. The lesion is firm and painless.

In scirrhous carcinoma, the majority of the lesion is submerged beneath the tissue. Frequently, a little of the tumor is visible in the mouth. The lesion can be detected only by palpation. This lesion is relatively common in the floor of the mouth and, because of its innocuous clinical presentation, can often spread to involve bone or the musculature of the tongue before being detected. Like other forms of carcinoma, it is asymptomatic, although restriction in lingual motion may be noted if the tongue musculature is involved.

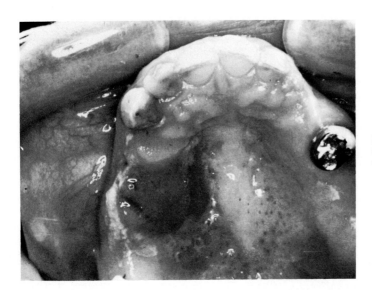

Figure 40–2. Squamous cell carcinoma presenting as a broad erythematous ulceration with keratotic borders.

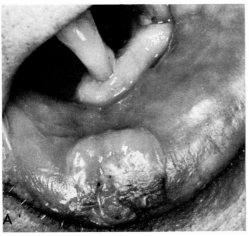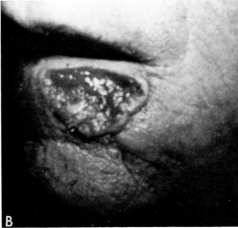

Figure 40–3. *A, B,* Verrucous carcinoma.

Location

The most common site of oral carcinoma is the mucosa of the lower lip (Table 40–1). Cancers at this site account for 38% of all oral carcinomas. Leukoplakia is a common presentation for such cancers, although other clinical forms are not uncommon. Cancer of the lower lip has been associated with both pipe and cigarette smoking, as well as with actinic rays from the sun.

The tongue, most frequently the posterior lateral border, is the second most common site for oral cancer. Its location makes it crucial for the dentist to be able to visualize this area during examination. The most frequent clinical appearance of carcinoma in this area is an indurated, firm, nonhealing ulceration. However, scirrhous and verrucous forms of the disease may also occur in this site. Carcinoma of the dorsal surface of the tongue, which may be seen freestanding or in association with Plummer-Vinson disease or syphilitic glossitis, appears as leukoplakia superimposed on an atrophic surface.

Carcinoma of the floor of the mouth, the third most common site for oral cancer, presents in a variety of forms, including ulcerations, papillary enlargement, and speckled leukoplakia. If the tumor invades tissue, the mandible and tongue may be involved. If the tongue is involved, fixation of the lingual musculature may result in limitation of motion. On palpation, the clinician notes a rock-hard mass in the floor of the mouth.

Other areas of the mouth, including the gingiva and palate, may be sites of oral carcinoma. In these cases, lesions take on a variety of appearances. Thus, nonhealing ulcerations, papillary masses, and areas of leukoplakia should always be viewed with suspicion.

Behavior

Squamous cell carcinomas of the mouth spread by local invasion and metastasize to regional lymph nodes through lymphatic channels. The severity of invasion and metastasis depends on the degree of anaplasia. Distant metastases are rare.

Recent data suggest that retinoids may play a role in the chemoprevention of oral carcinogenesis.

Table 40–1. DISTRIBUTION OF ORAL CARCINOMA

Anatomic Site	Number of Patients	Percentage
Lower lip	5399	38
Tongue	3117	22
Floor of mouth	2479	17
Gingiva	923	6
Palate	786	5.5
Tonsil	673	5
Upper lip	553	4
Buccal mucosa	245	2
Uvula	78	0.5

From Krolls, S. O., and Hoffman, S.: Squamous cell carcinoma of the oral soft tissues: A statistical analysis of 14,253 cases by age, sex, and race of patients. J. Am. Dent. Assoc., 92:571, 1976. Reprinted by permission of ADA Publishing Co., Inc.

DIAGNOSIS OF ORAL CANCER

Three techniques are currently available for routine diagnosis of a suspected oral carcinoma: biopsy, cellular smear, and toluidine blue staining. The merits and techniques of biopsy and cytologic examination have been discussed elsewhere (Chap. 2). Biopsy offers the most definitive and consistent information leading to diagnosis. Although cytologic smears are valuable for mass screening, they are associated with a high frequency (15%) of false-negative results. Toluidine blue staining purportedly has a preference for malignant tissue, and some individuals advocate its use as a screening device for oral cancer. As with cytologic examination, false-negatives are a disadvantage of this screening technique. It seems likely that a thorough clinical examination can expose most lesions that would be stained with toluidine blue. This technique has not gained widespread popularity or acceptance.

PROGNOSIS

The prognosis for oral cancer (Fig. 40–4) depends on a number of factors, including size, extent, and location of the lesion and nodal involvement. Generally, the earlier a lesion is diagnosed, the more favorable the prognosis. In addition, the morbidity associated with surgical resection of an oral lesion is minimized when the lesion is detected at an incipient stage. Disfigurement and functional problems can be significantly reduced by early diagnosis and treatment.

Response to cancer treatment is usually expressed as a survival rate over 5 years. In the case of carcinoma of the lip, the overall survival rate is 84% for all forms of disease. The importance of early diagnosis is clearly illustrated when one compares the 5-year survival rate for patients with localized lip cancer (87%) with the 5-year survival rate for patients in whom the disease has spread to involve lymph nodes (66%).

Unfortunately, the overall prognosis for men with other forms of oral cancer is not as bright as for lip cancer. Only 54% of patients with oral cancer survive 5 years. The prognosis for cancer of the tongue, which has the greatest likelihood of metastasis, is worse.

STAGING

In dealing with carcinomas, it became apparent that some system was needed to provide

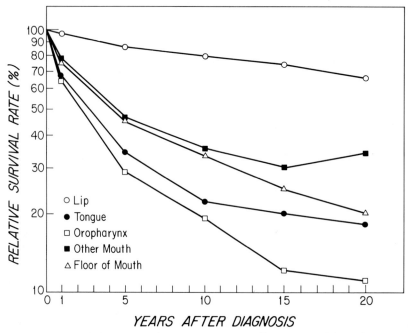

Figure 40–4. Relative survival rates for squamous cell carcinoma of the oral cavity.

a consistent method of defining the clinical status of a lesion. Such a system not only allowed individuals who had never seen the patient to appreciate the extent of the disease immediately, but it also correlated with the clinical behavior of the lesion and, hence, treatment and prognosis. The system by which carcinomas are clinically defined is called staging and, in the case of oral carcinoma, involves three parameters: the size and extent of the tumor (T), the presence and extent of lymphadenopathy (N), and the presence or absence of metastases (M). The current staging system was developed in 1942. The specific designations for each category are presented in Table 40–2. The system is referred to as the TNM system.

Once the tumor has been classified within the TNM system, the individual prognostic elements of the system can be brought together to "stage" the tumor (Fig. 40–5). Thus, the stage of a tumor gives the practitioner significant information relative to the projected course of the patient's disease. Generally, the higher the stage, the poorer the prognosis. For example, for cancers of the hard palate, the prognosis is 75% for patients with stage I disease compared to 11% for patients with stage IV disease.

Table 40–2. TNM CANCER STAGING SYSTEM

T	*Tumor size*
TX	Primary tumor cannot be assessed
T0	No evidence of primary tumor
Tis	Carcinoma in situ
T1	Tumor ≤ 2 cm in greatest dimension
T2	Tumor > 2 cm but ≤ 4 cm in greatest dimension
T3	Tumor > 4 cm in greatest dimension
N	*Regional lymph nodes*
NX	Regional lymph nodes cannot be assessed
N0	No clinically palpable cervical lymph nodes, but metastasis not suspected
N1	Clinically palpable cervical lymph nodes that are not fixed on same side as tumor; metastasis suspected
N2	Clinically palpable contralateral or bilateral cervical lymph nodes that are not fixed; metastasis suspected
N3	Clinically palpable lymph nodes that are fixed; metastasis suspected
M	*Distant metastasis*
MX	Presence of distant metastasis cannot be assessed
M0	No distant metastasis
M1	Clinical or radiographic evidence of metastasis other than to cervical lymph nodes

Modified from American Joint Committee on Cancer. Manual for Staging of Cancer, 3rd ed. Philadelphia, J.B. Lippincott, 1988, p. 27.

MEDICAL MANAGEMENT

Treatment for oral cancer may involve single or multimodality therapy consisting of surgery, radiation, and chemotherapy. The location and extent of the primary tumor, as well as the presence of nodal involvement, are key factors in the choice of treatment. For many early lesions (stage I), radiation and surgery are equally effective for treatment. For example, the overwhelming majority of early lip cancers are treated exclusively with surgery. If surgical excision might functionally compromise the patient, radiation therapy may be used. In contrast, lesions in which there is nodal involvement, but in which the primary tumor is manageable, may be treated with both radiation and surgery. In some instances in which the tumor is large, accessibility is difficult, and the projected surgical morbidity is high, radiation alone may be used to treat the primary tumor, and surgery may be employed for nodal resection. Generally, neck dissection of nodes is not indicated unless palpable lymph nodes are present. In the past, chemotherapy was used mostly for palliation or as an adjunct for radiation. However, results with techniques using multiple agents suggest that chemotherapy may have a role in the primary treatment of head and neck carcinoma.

Surgical therapy for oral cancer is intended to resect the primary tumor while leaving adequate margins of normal tissue, resect bone involved with tumor, and remove lymph nodes into which the cancer has spread. The major advantages of surgical treatment are that the therapy is specific for the neoplasm and that, in most instances, histologic confirmation of resection can be achieved. The major disadvantages of surgical therapy relate to its consequences, which, in the case of head and neck cancers, often are cosmetic and functional defects (Fig. 40–6).

Surgical removal of oral carcinoma can be accomplished using conventional "cold steel" surgery, cryosurgery, or laser surgery. In cryosurgery, liquid nitrogen is used to freeze a probe that is placed into the tumor, causing tumor death. The technique has the advantage of reducing tissue removal, but it does cause postoperative swelling and sometimes scarring. It appears that the technique is most effective for surface lesions. Laser surgery can be used in the treatment of oral carcinoma (Fig. 40–7). The laser actually causes thermal lysis of the tumor. One disadvantage is that it does not

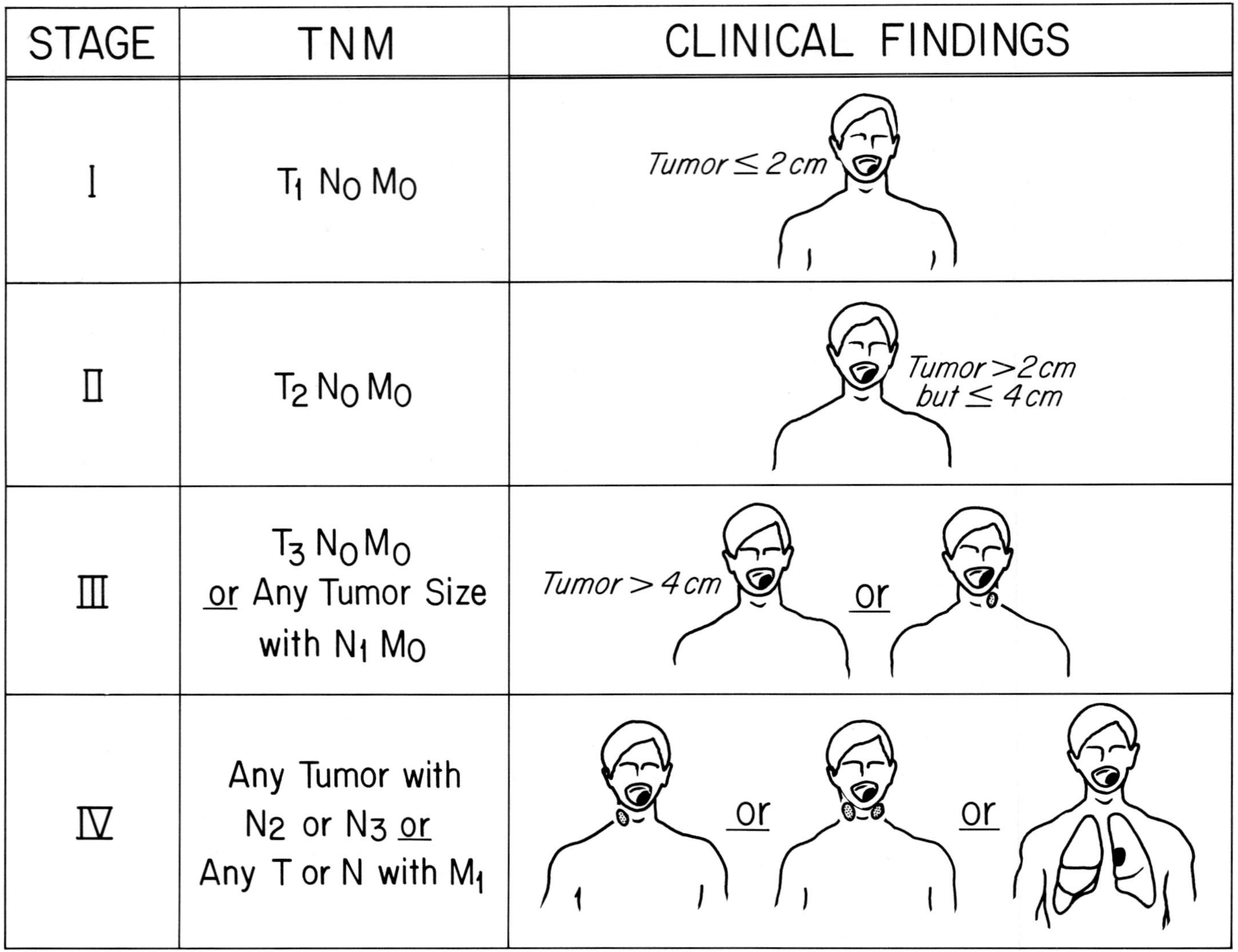

STAGE	TNM	CLINICAL FINDINGS
I	$T_1 N_0 M_0$	*Tumor $\leq 2cm$*
II	$T_2 N_0 M_0$	*Tumor $>2cm$ but $\leq 4cm$*
III	$T_3 N_0 M_0$ or Any Tumor Size with $N_1 M_0$	*Tumor $>4cm$* or
IV	Any Tumor with N_2 or N_3 or Any T or N with M_1	or or

Figure 40–5. TNM staging system (T, tumor size; N, extent of lymphadenopathy; M, presence or absence of metastases).

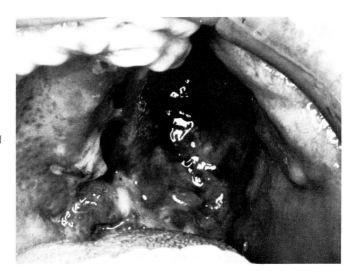

Figure 40–6. Postoperative result after surgical resection of tumor in Figure 40–2.

allow for histologic assessment of the success of resection.

Radiotherapy is used frequently in a number of different modes for the treatment of oral cancer. Many oral carcinomas appear to respond reasonably well to high dosages of radiation given in a repeated number of small increments. The more exposed the lesion, the more radiosensitive it is. Thus, deep penetrating lesions are most radioresistant. Furthermore, the inclusion of tumor in bone reduces its radiosensitivity. Radiation may be delivered through an external source or through radioactive needles, which may be implanted in and about the tumor bed. The side effects of external source radiotherapy have been markedly

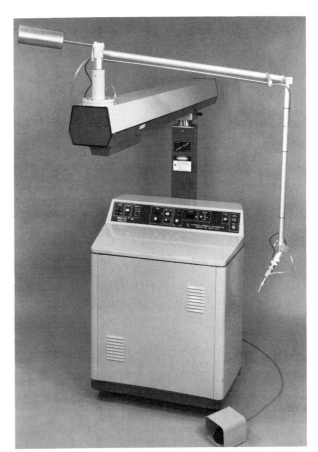

Figure 40–7. Laser of the type used for the treatment of head and neck carcinoma. (Courtesy of Advanced Biomedical Instruments.)

reduced through the use of high-energy therapy, which spares the surface tissue and penetrates to the tumor. At present, energies above 1 MeV (most common is 4–8 MeV) are used with both cobalt-60 and linear accelerator sources. The total dosage to a lesion varies but may be in the range of 4500 to 7000 cGy, given in divided doses over a period of up to about 8 weeks. Patients receiving conventional radiotherapy are usually not hospitalized. In contrast, patients in whom radioactive needles are implanted are hospitalized and isolated to limit the effects of radioactivity on others.

The role of chemotherapy in the treatment of oral cancer has traditionally been palliative. However, advances in multiagent therapy may produce effective chemotherapeutic treatment for head and neck carcinoma. Among chemotherapeutic agents available, methotrexate, bleomycin, and cisplatin are used most often. All these agents are extensively stomatotoxic (Chap. 42).

Clearly, the treatment of oral cancer is often a complicated task that requires the cooperation of a number of disciplines. A team approach in which individuals in general surgery, otolaryngology, plastic surgery, general dentistry, maxillofacial prosthetics, oral surgery, radiotherapy, and chemotherapy are represented is ideal. Support services of nutritionists, speech pathologists, and social workers are also often necessary in the complete management of the patient with head and neck cancer.

DENTAL MANAGEMENT

Dentists play three major roles in dealing with head and neck cancer. First, they are frequently responsible for making the initial diagnosis. Second, they should play a critical role in minimizing undesirable side effects of treatment. Third, during the reconstructive and rehabilitative phase, they are often responsible for replacing resected parts.

The diagnosis of oral lesions has already been discussed (Chap. 2). Dentists are frequently the practitioners from whom patients seek advice regarding oral lesions, and they should respond to this trust by being diligent in the diagnosis of suspicious oral lesions. Any keratotic white lesion has a significant chance of being a carcinoma and warrants biopsy. Similarly, any ulceration that does not heal within 14 days should be biopsied. Although there are rare exceptions, it is better to be overaggressive in biopsying lesions than to miss a carcinoma.

As noted, patients with head and neck cancer may be treated with radiotherapy and/or chemotherapy. Both these modalities have significant oral side effects, and the dentist is frequently called on to manage these problems.

The oral complications of radiotherapy are a function of dosage, timing, and field of radiation exposure. Although there tends to be a somewhat linear relationship between dose and complications, fragmenting the dose so that patients receive small doses of radiation spread over a 6-week period often reduces the severity of problems. Generally, the smaller the area receiving radiation, the fewer the complications associated with treatment. Thus, for the patient with Hodgkin's disease who is receiving radiation of the neck and submandibular areas, the effect of the treatment to the parotid glands is minimized. Problems that occur following radiotherapy include mucositis, xerostomia, loss of taste, radiation caries, and osteoradionecrosis (see later).

DENTAL EVALUATION AND EFFECTS OF RADIOTHERAPY

All patients who are to receive radiotherapy to the head and neck should receive a dental evaluation. Unfortunately, it is not uncommon for the dentist to see the patient after treatment has started. Initial evaluation of the patient is the same in either case and should include dental and medical histories, radiographs (full-mouth periapical series with bitewings or panoramic radiograph with bitewings), and comprehensive clinical examination.

Mucositis

The oral mucosa may break down following radiotherapy. This usually begins as a generalized mucosal erythema soon after the initiation of treatment. If radiotherapy is maintained, progressive breakdown of the mucosa may occur, resulting in desquamation and ulceration (Fig. 40–8). During this period, the mucosa is extremely painful, making eating nearly impossible. Similarly, functional movements of the mouth are compromised. The buccal, labial, and lingual mucosae are most affected by these changes. Healing of these lesions rapidly follows the cessation of radiotherapy, although mucosal atrophy may become permanent. The objectives of therapy for radiation mucositis are palliation and re-

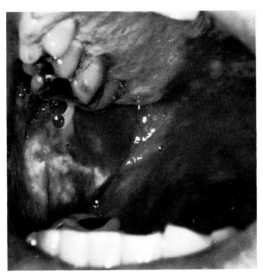

Figure 40–8. Radiation therapy-induced mucositis.

duction of secondary infection. Candidiasis is the most common infection. A variety of palliative mouth rinses are available, including lidocaine (Xylocaine Viscous), dyclonine hydrochloride (Dyclone), benzocaine in Orabase, benzocaine liquid, tetracaine, and diphenhydramine hydrochloride (Benadryl) in Kaopectate. The use of milk of magnesia or other such vehicles for topical anesthetics is to be avoided, because these materials produce desiccation of the mucosa. Patients who receive tetracaine should receive only limited doses and should be monitored, because this medication is readily absorbed and has systemic toxicity. Systemic analgesics should be used as needed. In severe cases, hospitalized patients may require intravenous opiate analgesics.

Candidiasis prophylaxis may be accomplished with nystatin suspension (400,000 to 600,000 units qid). More frequent exposures of smaller doses may also be used. Patients should swish as long as possible and then swallow. Alternatively, clotrimazole troches may be used (10-mg tablets five times per day); they seem to have good patient acceptance. Historically, gentian violet has been used effectively as an antifungal agent. Its unpleasant taste and purple staining of the mucosa are undesirable.

Salivary Gland Changes

Shortly after the initiation of external beam radiotherapy, fibroblast proliferation is noted in the interlobular areas of salivary glands. This follows the appearance of lymphocytes and plasma cells and precedes an eventual, progressive degeneration of the acinar epithe-

lium. There is increased fibrosis of both interlocular and intralocular areas. Serous portions of glands tend to be most involved. Because the parotid gland is entirely serous, it tends to be the most affected by radiation. Although fibrosis is reversible for some time after the start of therapy, eventually complete fibrosis occurs, and no regeneration is possible. Regeneration of salivary function is related to the dose and field of radiation and the age of the patient; younger patients recover better than elderly patients.

Xerostomia

The major clinical effects of radiation on salivary glands are related to xerostomia. Normally, this condition is first observed at doses of 1000 to 1500 cGy and occurs toward the end of the first week of treatment. Two major changes occur in the saliva. First, the consistency becomes thick, ropy, and mucus-like. This may be a consequence of the elimination of serous function in salivary glands, which then produce only mucus. Second, the pH drops significantly from a normal of about 6.75. Xerostomia affects the patient's ability to function, especially to eat, and the ability to resist bacterial colonization of the teeth. Saliva is critical in permitting normal deglutition and bolus formation. It also affects the taste of food. Patients with xerostomia have difficulty swallowing and managing foods. Normal saliva serves a number of bacteriostatic functions, including mechanical clearance of bacteria and prevention of bacterial adherence to teeth. Thus, patients with xerostomia are prone to plaque formation and debris accumulation, which results in a predisposition to caries. The condition may be further exaggerated by diets designed to compensate for decreased intake and that are high in cariogenic elements.

Little can be done to prevent the effects of radiation on salivary glands totally. Proper port design and shielding are helpful in minimizing effects. If xerostomia develops, various local and systemic agents can be used to reduce its effects. Mouth moisturizers such as Xero-Lube or Oralube are available for patient rinsing. Lemon-glycerin swabs are sometimes helpful for symptomatic relief. Patients should be instructed to be well hydrated. Systemic administration of the cholinergic antagonist pilocarpine HCl has recently been shown to be efficacious in stimulating residual salivary function. Pilocarpine HCl is dispensed as a 5-mg tablet three times per day. Because patients have a reduced ability to resist caries, reduction in sucrose intake is critical.

Radiation Caries

Radiation caries is characterized by the appearance of rampant caries in individuals receiving radiotherapy and is the result of a combination of factors, including xerostomia, accelerated decalcification of irradiated teeth, and reduced oral hygiene. Caries characteristically forms at the cervical margins (Fig. 40–9) and incisal edges of teeth. Radiation caries is not age-dependent. In addition to destruction of hard tissue, a major concern with respect to radiation caries is subsequent pulpal degeneration and infection. Fortunately, much can be done to reduce the frequency and severity of this form of caries. Of primary use in the prevention of radiation caries is fluoride.

Fluoride should be made available in a variety of forms. Daily topical application of a fluoride gel supplemented with fluoride rinses is not excessive in the patient with xerostomia. Topical application of fluoride gels is most easily accomplished through the use of customized trays. Trays should be constructed of a soft, fairly rigid material that loosely adapts to the teeth. Mouth guard material (0.150 mm thick) for use with vacuum-forming units (Omnivacs) is ideal. If such a unit is not available, a laboratory can construct the appliance. The borders of the tray should extend to the gingival margins (Fig. 40–10). Patients are instructed to use the trays daily by placing six to eight drops of an acidulated fluoride gel (such as Thera-Flur) into each tray and then spreading them around with the tip of the bottle. Maxillary and mandibular trays are placed into the mouth simultaneously, and patients are instructed to close on them for 6 minutes. Fol-

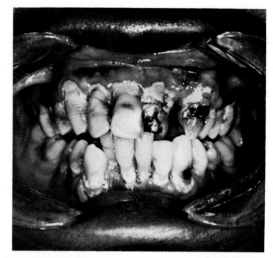

Figure 40–9. Extensive caries in a patient with xerostomia secondary to radiation therapy.

lowing application, the trays and mouth are rinsed with cold water. Gel application is repeated daily, usually at bedtime. Patients should be instructed not to eat or drink for 30 minutes after application.

Fluoride rinses are also helpful supplements and can be used in the morning. Initially, an acidulated fluoride rinse may be recommended for rinsing for 1 minute after breakfast. If patients develop erythema or mucositis following radiotherapy, acidulated rinses may be irritating and a neutral fluoride rinse can be substituted. Once the irritation disappears, acidulated rinses can again be resumed. Similarly, a neutral gel may be necessary for use in the custom trays (e.g., Thera-Flur-1-N).

Patients should be counseled regarding the importance of a low-sucrose diet while on ra-

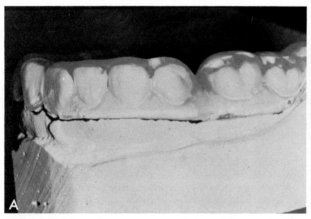
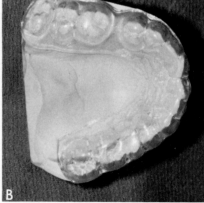

Figure 40–10. A, B, Customized tray used for the delivery of topical fluoride gel for the prevention of radiation-induced caries.

diotherapy. Interestingly, with alterations of taste buds and xerostomia, some patients lose their desire for sweet foods.

Prior to starting radiotherapy, or soon thereafter, patients should receive dental evaluation and prophylaxis. Incipient caries should be restored. At the same visit, patients should receive oral hygiene instruction and diet counseling. Impressions should be obtained for the construction of custom trays for topical fluoride gels. The patient should be immediately placed on acidulated fluoride rinses.

Patients undergoing radiotherapy should be followed closely. Recall visits at 6- to 8-week intervals are not excessive. Aggressive management of caries is recommended. Patients who are receiving systemic and regional radiotherapy and chemotherapy may have alterations in their bone marrow status that requires special management consideration for dental treatment (Chap. 42).

Special consideration must be given to the patient wearing orthodontic bands. In view of the severe consequences of radiation caries, the removal of bands is recommended until the return of normal salivary gland function. Although few patients with head and neck carcinoma fall into this category, it is not uncommon in patients with Hodgkin's disease.

Osteoradionecrosis and Extractions

Osteoradionecrosis, a serious sequela of radiation therapy, occurs when there is fibrotic thickening of blood vessels, replacement of marrow with connective tissue, subsequent lack of new bone formation, and consequent bone death. The bone becomes susceptible to infection and has a compromised ability to repair. The morbidity associated with osteoradionecrosis may include loss of the affected bone. Of cases of osteoradionecrosis, 90% occur in the mandible.

The reported incidence of osteoradionecrosis varies. Whereas some centers have reported frequencies as low as 4%, other authors have reported that as many as 35% of patients receiving head and neck irradiation develop the condition. It appears that the use of higher-energy radiation sources reduces the likelihood of this problem.

A number of risk factors have been identified with the development of osteoradionecrosis. Identification of such factors in a particular patient, followed by an aggressive prevention protocol, can do much to reduce the frequency of osteonecrosis. For example,

introduction of a prevention protocol at one cancer center resulted in a decrease in incidence of osteonecrosis from 35% to 24.5%.

The three major risk factors in the development of osteoradionecrosis appear to be the anatomic site of the tumor, dose of radiation, and dental status of the patient. Patients receiving radiation for tumors anatomically related to the mandible develop necrosis five times more frequently than patients with tumors at other sites (Table 40–3). Osteoradionecrosis of the maxilla is rare. There appears to be a nonlinear relationship between osteonecrosis and radiation dose (Fig. 40–11). For example, the risk of developing osteonecrosis is twice as great if a patient receives greater than 8000 cGy as compared with 5000 to 6000 cGy, and the risk is almost five times as great than if the patient receives 4000 to 5000 cGy. A number of studies have shown that patients with teeth are more likely to develop osteonecrosis than edentulous patients. Furthermore, it is clear that patients with dental disease are at significant risk compared with dentulous patients without disease (Table 40–4). The radiation source also affects frequency. Patients receiving radiation by implants are more susceptible to developing necrosis than patients receiving radiotherapy from an external source. The likelihood of developing necrosis appears to be greatest 3 to 12 months after the initiation of treatment (Fig. 40–12).

It is important to note that edentulous patients who wear prostheses may also develop serious sequelae from radiation therapy. Because osteoradionecrosis of irritated denture-bearing areas may occur, it is imperative to ensure the atraumatic fit of existing dentures. Construction of new dentures, especially of the mandible, should not be contemplated while the patient is receiving radiation therapy and

Table 40–3. INCIDENCE OF OSTEORADIONECROSIS BY SITE OF TUMOR IN RELATION TO THE MANDIBLE AND TEETH

Site	Incidence of Necrosis	
	No.	(%)
Tumor related to bone	9/16	56.3
Tumor adjacent to bone	30/104	28.8
Other (not related to bone)	38/284	13.4
Total	77/404	19.1

Reprinted from International Journal of Radiation Oncology, Biology, Physics, Vol. 6, Murray C. G., Herson, J., Daly, T., et al.: Radiation necrosis of the mandible: A 10-year study, p. 543, copyright 1980, with kind permission from Pergamon Press Ltd, Headington Hill Hall, Oxford OX3 0BW, UK.

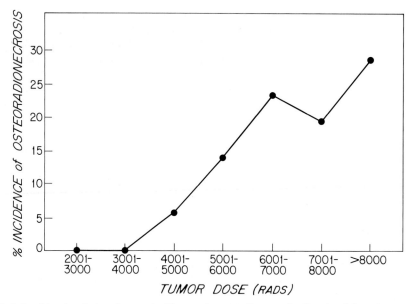

Figure 40–11. Relationship of radiation dose to incidence of osteoradionecrosis. (Reprinted from International Journal of Radiation, Oncology, Biology, Physics, Vol. 6, Murray, C. G., Herson, J., Daly, T., et al. Radiation necrosis of the mandible: A 10-year study, p. 543, Copyright 1980, with kind permission from Pergamon Press Ltd, Headington Hill Hall, Oxford OX3 OBW, UK.)

is best delayed until 6 months to 1 year after treatment.

There seems to be universal agreement that patients with clean mouths are less likely to have oral problems associated with cancer therapy than patients with poor oral hygiene. Thus, a major objective must be to ensure a high level of oral hygiene. This should be accompanied by reduced sucrose intake and the frequent use of topical fluorides.

The issue of whether and when extractions should be performed is less clear. The approach to extractions in patients undergoing head and neck radiation has undergone a variety of changes. In the earliest dental protocols, all teeth in the primary beam were extracted prior to radiation therapy. With less sophisticated types of radiation, this often involved full-mouth extraction. The rationale was that without teeth present during radiation therapy, there could be no odontogenic source of infection to cause osteoradionecrosis.

Improvements in the types of radiation used, smaller fields of radiation, and more selective application of radiation therapy have

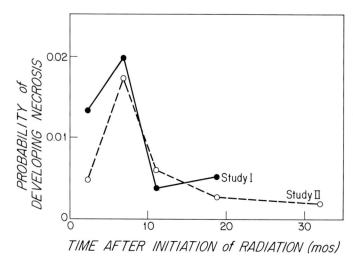

Figure 40–12. Relationship of time after treatment to development of osteoradionecrosis. (Reprinted from International Journal of Radiation, Oncology, Biology, Physics, Vol. 6, Murray, C. G., Herson, J., Daly, T., et al. Radiation necrosis of the mandible: A 10-year study, p. 543, Copyright 1980, with kind permission from Pergamon Press Ltd, Headington Hill Hall, Oxford OX3 OBW, UK.)

Table 40–4. RISK OF OSTEORADIONECROSIS

		Radiation Necrosis		
		+	−	Total
Dental disease	+	10	11	21
No disease	−	6	19	25
		16	30	46

From Murray, C. G., Daly, T. E., and Zimmerman, S. O.: The relationship between dental disease and radiation necrosis of the mandible. Oral Surg., 49:99, 1980.

coincided with increasing concerns for the patient's masticatory function and increasing knowledge of preventive dental protocols. A team management approach for the patient during radiation has evolved, using preradiation extractions of actively infected teeth and aggressive dental prevention during radiation therapy for the remaining dentition. With heavy emphasis still on the prevention of osteoradionecrosis from odontogenic infection during radiation therapy, even teeth at marginal risk (i.e., teeth with moderate periodontal disease and teeth with deep restorations) were sacrificed prior to radiation therapy. Some studies, however, have suggested a significant risk of osteoradionecrosis of sites associated with preradiation therapy extractions and a lesser risk associated with extractions done 12 months or more after radiation therapy.

It is suggested that extractions be limited to teeth demonstrating periapical pathology or severe periodontal infection. Nonrestorable teeth or teeth with deep caries with a significant risk of developing infection during radia-tion therapy should also be eliminated. Teeth at marginal risk (i.e., teeth with deep restorations or slight to moderate periodontal disease) that are unlikely to become infected during radiation therapy may be retained. This is a particularly important goal if these teeth are in the field of irradiation, where the risk of developing osteoradionecrosis is greatest. If possible, extractions should be postponed until 1 year after radiation therapy. At that time, antibiotic prophylaxis is recommended (potassium phenoxymethyl penicillin, 500 mg, every 6 hours for 10 days), largely on an empiric basis. Because there remains a risk of development of necrosis even 12 months after radiation therapy, extractions should be avoided if possible.

Teeth requiring extraction before radiotherapy should be removed as long as possible before the initiation of treatment. A minimal 2-week healing period is recommended, although one group of investigators found that extractions at the time of initiation of radiotherapy do not produce an increase in necrosis (minority view). The more extensive the surgery, the longer the necessary healing time. Although the 2-week period is ideal, it is not uncommon for the radiotherapist to feel an urgent need to proceed with treatment despite the need for dental care. Alternative approaches, including endodontics, should be considered.

Surgery should be performed as atraumatically as possible, with care being given to ensure minimal hard and soft tissue trauma. Alveolectomy is recommended. Bony prominences and edges should be eliminated. Where possible, primary closure is suggested.

Squamous Cell Carcinoma: General Information

Background and epidemiology
  90% squamous cell carcinoma
  5% of all cancers in men, 2% in women
  30,300 new cases per year (1992)
  Risk factors: alcohol, cigarette smoking, snuff dipping, urban living
  Race incidence per 100,000 males: whites 11.8, blacks 20.5

Clinical forms
  Ulcerative
  Keratotic white lesion
  Erythroplastic
  Scirrhotic

Staging: system for definition of clinical status of carcinoma based on tumor size, nodal involvement, and metastases; decreasing prognosis with increasing stage

Location: most common site is mucosa of lower lip followed by tongue and floor of the mouth

Treatment
  Surgery
  Radiation therapy
  Chemotherapy

Five-year survival
  Lip—84%
  Floor of mouth—45%
  Tongue—32%

Oral Complications of Head and Neck Radiation

Mucositis (secondary risk of candidiasis)

Xerostomia

Loss of taste

Radiation caries

Osteoradionecrosis

SUMMARY TABLE **40–III**

Factors Increasing Risk of Osteoradionecrosis

Location: tumors associated with mandible

Radiation dose greater than 5000 cGy

Dentulous patients with poor oral hygiene

Radiation source—implants greater than external beam

Ill-fitting prosthesis

Dentulous patients with pre-existing dental disease

SUMMARY TABLE **40–IV**

Fluoride Recommendation

Acidulated fluoride gel in custom tray* (brushing with stannous fluoride gel 0.4% is an alternative if trays are not tolerated)

Acidulated fluoride rinse*

*Note: if mucositis develops, a nonacidulated rinse is recommended.

SUMMARY TABLE **40–V**

Risk of Development of Osteoradionecrosis Relative to Timing of Extraction Only

Highest risk—extractions (in beam) during radiation therapy

Elevated risk—extractions just prior to radiation therapy

Lowest risk—12 mo or more after radiation therapy

SUMMARY TABLE 40–VI

Dental Management of the Patient Receiving Radiation Therapy

PRETREATMENT EVALUATION (ALL PATIENTS)
Full mouth radiographs or panoramic radiograph

Bitewing radiographs

Clinical examination

PREVENTION PROTOCOL (ALL PATIENTS)
Prophylaxis, scaling, and root planing

Oral hygiene instruction

Low-sucrose diet

Prescribe acidulated fluoride mouth rinse (neutral solution if mucosal irritation intervenes)

Construct custom trays for home fluoride treatment

Prescribe acidulated fluoride gel for daily use in trays (neutral gel if mucosal irritation intervenes)

Eliminate active caries

Repair or eliminate all potential sources of irritation and/or sharp cusps, fractured cusps, broken clasps, ill-fitting dentures, or orthodontic bands

Frequent recall examination and prophylaxis (every 6–8 wks) with restoration of incipient caries

Continue protocol for at least 12 mo after radiation therapy, or longer if xerostomia remains

EXTRACTION STRATEGY (ALL PATIENTS)
Eliminate seriously infected teeth demonstrating periapical pathology, severe periodontal infection, nonrestorable teeth, and teeth with deep caries

Retain teeth at marginal risk of infection (i.e., teeth with deep restorations or slight to moderate periodontal disease); if extraction necessary, delay procedure as long after end of radiation therapy as possible

Retain and restore dental health of as many teeth as possible, especially in field of radiation therapy

Postpone elective procedures with associated risk of iatrogenic result (i.e., prosthetic crown preparations with pulp encroachment risk or removable appliance insertion with risk of soft tissue insult)

Dental Management of the Patient Receiving Radiation Therapy
Continued

ANTIXEROSTOMIA PROTOCOL (ALL PATIENTS)
Salivary stimulation with sucrose-free lemon drops

Lemon-glycerin swabs

Salivary replacement with artificial saliva or mouth moisturizers (e.g., Xero-Lube, Oralube, Salivart)

Pilocarpine HCl 5 mg, if needed

MUCOSITIS PROTOCOL (IF NEEDED)
General (use as needed)
  Kaopectate:Benadryl, 1:1 suspension
  Viscous Xylocaine, 2% suspension
  Dyclone suspension
  Systemic analgesics, if needed

Localized (use as needed)
  Orabase and benzocaine
  Benzocaine solution (e.g., Hurricane)
  Orabase, plain
  Systemic analgesics, if needed

ANTIFUNGAL PROTOCOL (IF NEEDED)
Nystatin suspension (Mycostatin) 100,000 units/ml in 60-ml bottle (400,000–600,000 units), swish and swallow half for each side of mouth qid

Clotrimazole 10-mg troche, five times daily

If *Candida* is under a denture or corners of mouth, use nystatin cream (100,000 units/gm) in a 15- or 30-g tube; smear on affected area tid

For children or for those with concurrent mucositis use
  Nystatin suspension, 1/2–3/4 tsp/ice cube tray unit plus water, freeze and use as ice cube popsicle or as ice chips

41

Benign Tumors and Non–Squamous Cell Malignancies

BENIGN TUMORS OF THE ORAL MUCOSA

A wide variety of benign tumors affect the oral mucosa. It has been proposed that most of these lesions represent developmental anomalies rather than true neoplasms. In fact, the potential for malignant transformation for the majority of these lesions is minute. Clinically, these lesions may present a variety of appearances. They do, however, have some common features, including a generally raised appearance and well-circumscribed borders. When palpated, benign lesions are generally freely movable. In most instances, these lesions are asymptomatic and are noted only because they interfere with function or become irritated. Surgical excision is usually the treatment of choice and generally results in complete resolution of the problem. Some benign neoplasms have a tendency to recur, especially if excision is incomplete.

Pyogenic Granuloma (Granuloma Pyogenicum)

Pyogenic granuloma represents a proliferation of vascular granulation tissue in response to local irritation from rough restorations or prostheses, teeth, or calculus. The lesion appears as a bluish-red, raised, circumscribed mass that may be pedunculated (Fig. 41–1). Most frequently seen on any mucosal surface, including the tongue, cheek, and lip, the pyogenic granuloma varies in size from a few millimeters to 1 or 2 cm. The lesion is most common in adults. Treatment consists of removal of the source of irritation and excision and histologic evaluation of the lesion. Complete removal is curative.

Pregnancy Tumor

Pregnancy tumors are histologically identical to pyogenic granulomas and consist of vascular granulation tissue covered by stratified squamous epithelium. As the name implies, these lesions represent an exaggerated response to local irritation during pregnancy. As with pyogenic granuloma, pregnancy tumors appear as raised, reddish, smooth-surfaced masses. Unlike the pyogenic granuloma, however, they are usually confined to the interdental papillae (Fig. 41–2). These lesions usually arise rapidly following the first trimester of pregnancy. Patients with poor oral hygiene and pre-existing gingival inflammatory disease are at greater risk of developing these lesions than other patients. The size of pregnancy tumors is variable. Generally, no treatment is indicated until the pregnancy ends, at which time regression of the tumor may occur. If it does not, excision is required. If lesions be-

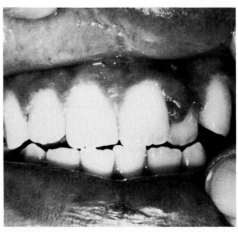

Figure 41–1. Pyogenic granuloma between the maxillary left central and lateral incisors presenting as a pedunculated enlargement of the interdental papillae.

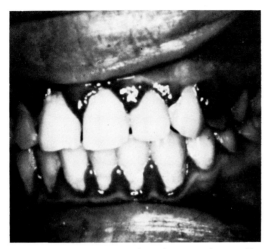

Figure 41–2. Pyogenic granuloma between the maxillary left canine and first premolar in a pregnant patient with pregnancy gingivitis.

come symptomatic during pregnancy, excision may be needed.

Giant Cell Granuloma (Giant Cell Epulis)

Although the cause is unknown, giant cell granulomas probably represent a tissue reaction to irritation or trauma. The mean age of occurrence is 30 years. Frequently, the onset of giant cell granuloma is rapid and may resemble a more serious neoplasm. The lesion appears as a large, smooth-surfaced pedunculated mass of the attached gingiva that seems to be arising from deep within the tissue (Fig. 41–3). Giant cell granulomas may have a predilection for the buccal or lingual attached gingiva and may become large enough to actually bury the teeth. Because of the underlying vascularity, the color of the lesion may vary from purple-red to pink, and bleeding may occur on provocation. Treatment consists of excision with curettage of the underlying bone. Additionally, it is recommended that appropriate laboratory studies be done to rule out the presence of hyperparathyroidism. These lesions do not undergo any malignant transformation.

Myoma

Tumors of smooth muscle (lyomyomas) and striated muscles (rhabdomyomas) are extremely rare intraoral lesions and, as with other lesions, probably represent developmental anomalies. Most commonly seen on the tongue, these lesions appear as raised, red, spongy nodules that respond well to surgery.

Papilloma

Papillomas are common benign tumors of the oral epithelium and occur on the tongue and buccal or labial mucosa, as well as the gingiva and palate. Clinically, they appear as white, exophytic, cauliflower-like lesions with a stalk penetrating into the mucosa (Fig. 41–4). Close examination reveals a pebbly surface. The lesions are generally firm and may vary in size, although they tend to be small. They may be present at any age. Treatment of papilloma involves surgical excision with confirmation by histologic diagnosis, because it is clinically impossible to distinguish a papilloma from a papillary carcinoma.

Lipoma

Lipomas are relatively common tumors occurring under the skin but are rare in the

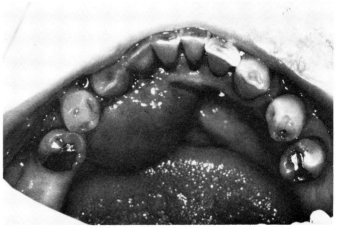

Figure 41–3. Giant cell granuloma on the left lingual surface of the attached gingiva.

mouth. They appear as pedunculated, soft, raised, smooth-surfaced masses and are composed essentially of adipose tissue (Fig. 41–5). Most commonly, intraoral lipomas involve buccal or lingual mucosa, but they also may be seen in the floor of the mouth and the gingiva. Initial coloration of the lesion is pinkish from the overlying mucosa, but as the lesion expands, a yellowish tinge may be observed. On palpation, lesions are soft and spongy and are generally freely movable. A diffuse form of lipoma also exists. Lipomas tend to be slow-growing and respond well to surgical excision.

Congenital Epulis (Congenital Myoblastoma)

Congenital epulides, as the name implies, are lesions congenitally found in the newborn, most typically on either the maxillary or mandibular alveolar mucosa, frequently at the midline. Clinically, the lesion appears as a pink, firm, raised mass that is often pedunculated and usually small. Treatment consists of excision.

Epulis Fissurata

Epulis fissurata usually arises as a result of irritation from a denture flange in the mucobuccal fold. These lesions are most commonly noted at the margins of the alveolar mucosa and edentulous ridges (Fig. 41–6). Growth of the lesions is usually progressive after denture insertion or may result, after prolonged wearing of dentures, from irritation as a consequence of decreased alveolar ridge height. Clinically, the lesions appear as a pinkish-red,

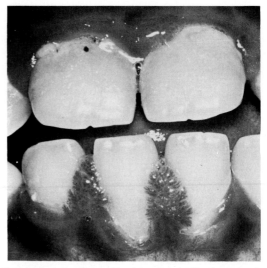

Figure 41–4. Papillomas involving the papillae between the mandibular incisors.

linear, elevated mass that may become ulcerated and painful. The size of these lesions is variable. Although epulis fissurata is totally benign, it is clinically impossible to rule out malignancy, and therefore excision and biopsy are mandatory. Reconstruction or relining of the denture is also required.

Mucocyst (Mucocele)

Mucoceles represent retention cysts, usually of the minor mucous salivary ducts of the labial mucosa, which become traumatized from frequent biting or chronic irritation. Although these lesions are most common in the mandibular labial mucosa, they are also noted on the palate and floor of the mouth. They are most

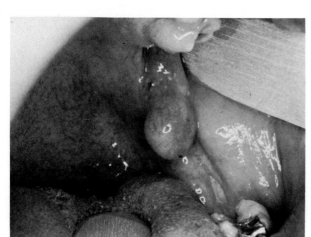

Figure 41–5. Lipoma.

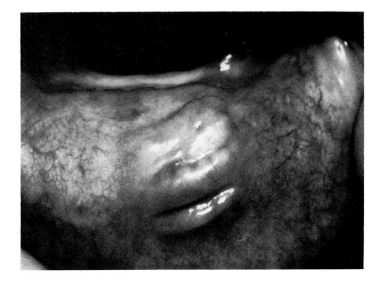

Figure 41–6. Epulis fissurata secondary to poorly fitting denture. Note the size of the alveolar ridge.

frequently seen in young adults. This lesion occurs often enough to cause the patient to seek professional consultation. Clinically, mucoceles appear as ovoid smooth swellings, often bluish (Fig. 41–7). Size is variable, with some mucoceles reaching 2 cm in diameter. Treatment consists of excision or marsupialization and removal of the source of irritation, where possible.

Ranula

Ranulas are large retention cysts in the ducts of the submandibular or sublingual glands or mucous glands of the floor of the mouth. The lesion takes its name from its clinical appearance—a large, submucosal, blue-purple-pink swelling of the floor of the mouth with prominent surface vascularity, which gives the lesion the appearance of the underside of a frog's belly (Fig. 41–8). These lesions can occur at any age and have a fairly rapid onset. They frequently attain a relatively large size, large enough that the tongue may be displaced. Treatment consists of excision or marsupialization.

Fibroma

Fibromas, dense collections of fibrous connective tissue, are the most common benign neoplasm of the oral cavity and generally represent a local tissue response to irritation. Fibromas can be seen anywhere on any mucosal surface but are most common on the buccal mucosa and tongue. These lesions have a var-

ied rate of growth but usually progress in size at a slow steady rate. Clinically, they appear as pinkish-white, firm, raised, ovoid lesions that are totally asymptomatic (Fig. 41–9). Fibromas may be seen at any age but are most common in the third to fifth decades. Congenital fibrous hyperplasia, which is histologically identical to fibroma, is characterized by bilateral fibroses that are most frequent in the maxillary tuberosity areas. Surgical removal is curative.

Neurofibroma

Neurofibromas may occur as single or multiple lesions (Fig. 41–10), usually of the skin. The multiple form is called neurofibromatosis or von Recklinghausen's disease.

The single oral neurofibroma is probably a developmental anomaly and is seen most fre-

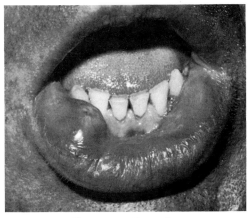

Figure 41–7. Mucocele.

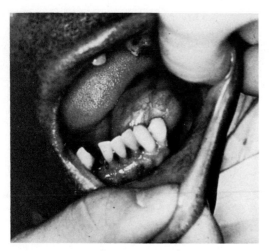

Figure 41–8. Ranula.

quently on the lingual mucosa of children as a raised pedunculated pink mass that may become large in size. The tumor responds well to excision.

Neurofibromatosis, or multiple neurofibroma, usually has its onset in childhood. There is no sex predilection. In addition to multiple skin lesions, the tongue, gingiva, and labial mucosa may also be involved. The lesions are hereditary and are usually accompanied by patches of deep brownish pigmentation called café-au-lait spots or areas. The lesions have a potential for malignant transformation and need to be followed closely for any change in their nature, in which case they should be biopsied. Clinically, the lesions appear as multiple raised masses that have a dull

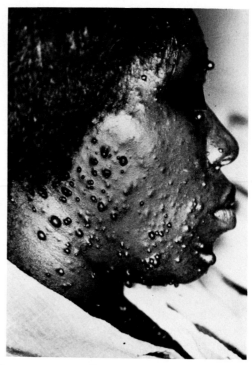

Figure 41–10. Neurofibromatosis characterized by multiple neurofibromas.

consistency or appear as flabby folds (Fig. 41–11). Neurofibromatosis presents a difficult management problem. Usually, large symptomatic lesions are excised, but there is no adequate treatment for a patient with multiple lesions.

Schwannoma (Neurinoma, Neurilemoma, and Perineural Fibroblastoma)

Schwannomas are tumors of the Schwann nerve cell sheath and appear as slowly developing submucosal masses. They generally acquire the color of the overlying mucosa (pink). Schwannomas appear at any age but are most common in young adults. The tongue is the most frequent site of these painless firm lesions, and excision is curative.

Neuroma (Traumatic Neuroma, Amputation Neuroma)

Neuromas usually develop after surgical severance of a nerve and result from the unsuccessful attempt by the body to create an anas-

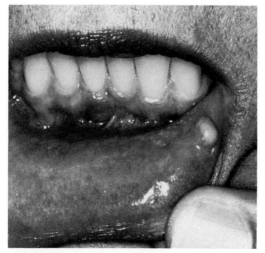

Figure 41–9. Fibroma resulting from chronic trauma of the labial mucosa.

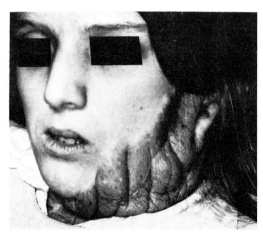

Figure 41–11. Neurofibromatosis with the presence of flabby folds and changes of pigmentation.

tomosis of the severed nerve. A tangled mass of nerve tissue ensues, resulting in a swelling that is most common in the mucobuccal fold in the area of the mental nerve. There is no sex or age predilection for these lesions. Unlike other benign lesions, these tend to be painful on palpation or pressure. However, they respond well to surgical intervention.

Keratoacanthoma

Keratoacanthomas are benign tumors that are most common in areas of the skin exposed to sunlight. Thus, the lips are the most frequent site of these lesions in and about the mouth, accounting for slightly less than 10% of all keratoacanthomas. The cause of keratoacanthomas is unresolved, although both genetic and viral causes have been suggested. Keratoacanthomas occur twice as frequently in males as in females and tend to develop during the fifth to seventh decades of life.

Clinically, keratoacanthomas are similar in appearance to squamous cell carcinomas. They appear as fast-growing, raised, nodular lesions with a central depression. The borders are firm and the central area may contain a plug of keratin. Lymphadenopathy may be present. Unlike squamous cell carcinomas, keratoacanthomas tend to be painful. Although these lesions tend to have a brisk initial growth period, the established lesion lasts only 1 to 2 months before regressing spontaneously.

Treatment of keratoacanthomas is surgical excision. Recurrence is rare.

Myoblastoma

Myoblastomas are derived from embryonic muscle tissue and probably represent a developmental anomaly (hamartoma) rather than a true neoplasm. The lateral border of the tongue is the most common intraoral site for these rare tumors. These neoplasms are asymptomatic, slow-growing, and well circumscribed. Myoblastomas are firm and feel somewhat nodular. They are usually deep to the surface and therefore the overlying mucosa is of normal appearance. A punch biopsy is effective for providing tissue for diagnosis. Myoblastomas respond well to wide surgical excision.

VASCULAR TUMORS OF THE ORAL MUCOSA

Hemangioma

Vascular tumors or angiomas are developmental abnormalities rather than true neoplasms and fall into two major categories, hemangiomas and lymphangiomas. Based on histologic criteria, hemangiomas are further classified into capillary and cavernous forms. They are more frequent in females than in males.

The clinical appearance of hemangiomas is varied. Some appear as diffuse, flat, bluish lesions referred to as port-wine stains. These are most commonly present on the buccal mucosa. Other lesions are discrete and raised, with a pebble-like surface texture. The raised pedunculated capillary hemangiomas occur most frequently on the tongue and have a soft but firm consistency. They often appear to be berry-like (Fig. 41–12). In either case, blanch-

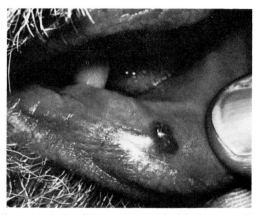

Figure 41–12. Small hemangioma of the labial mucosa. The lesion is raised. Its surface gives a berry-like appearance.

Table 41–1. SYNDROMES WITH ANGIOMAS AS A COMPONENT

Syndrome	Features
Osler-Weber-Rendu syndrome	Hereditary hemorrhagic telangiectasia, usually of the lips, oral and nasal mucosa, pharynx, conjunctiva, and face; neurofibromatosis, elliptocytosis, arteriovenous aneurysm
Sturge-Weber syndrome (encephalotrigeminal angiomatosis)	Angiomatosis of skin and mucosa, usually unilateral; port wine stain, usually to area supplied by trigeminal nerve; leptomeninges may have hemangiomatous areas; may cause neurologic symptoms: convulsions, retardation, spastic hemiplegia
Maffuci's syndrome	Hemangiomas of skin and mucosa (labial mucosa and palate); dyschondroplasia may cause deformity or pathologic long bone fracture; chondrosarcomas may occur secondarily to bone lesions

ing on pressure can be noted. Several discrete lesions may coalesce to form a more dramatic one.

Usually, hemangiomas arise as congenital abnormalities and tend to be asymptomatic. The broad port-wine cavernous lesions do not normally disappear with time and thus may present a significant esthetic problem for the patient. The more discrete form of hemangioma may resolve as patients grow older, although increases in the size of hemangiomas are not unusual during puberty. The diagnosis of hemangioma may usually be made clinically. A number of syndromes include hemangiomas as a component (Table 41–1; Figs. 41–13 and 41–14).

Treatment of hemangiomas depends on the site and size of the lesion, as well as the patient's age. Small lesions can be excised using conventional surgery, electrosurgery, or cryosurgery. Large lesions may not be suited to surgical therapy. Sclerosing agents, such as sodium morrhuate or invert sugar, may be used for large lesions. Radiation has been used for the treatment of radiosensitive superficial lesions. Because these lesions may disappear spontaneously, however, the efficacy of radia-

tion is unresolved. Steroids, given locally or systemically, may be helpful.

Hemangiomas may be deep to the mucosa. Aspiration is recommended before excision of any fluctuant lesion to rule out the presence of these lesions and to prevent the risk of hemorrhage.

Lymphangioma

Lymphangiomas are usually congenital and develop soon after birth. They appear as soft, spongy, somewhat fluctuant papillary masses that appear to be deep to the superficial tissue. Because of their size and submucosal location, they can cause deformity, such as macroglossia. The tongue, in fact, is the most common intraoral site of lymphangioma. Cystohygromas are large lymphangiomas of the neck. Deep lymphangiomas appear as smooth-surfaced elevations that usually acquire the color of the overlying mucosa but may be somewhat erythematous. They tend to be fairly soft and rubbery. Lesions may spontaneously regress after puberty. Surgical excision is the treatment of choice. The importance of wide mar-

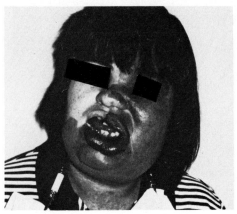

Figure 41–13. Extraoral port-wine hemangioma in patient with Sturge-Weber syndrome.

Benign Tumors and Non–Squamous Cell Malignancies

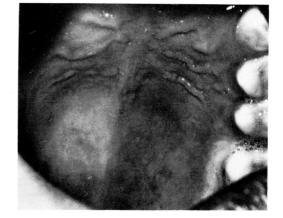

Figure 41–14. Intraoral cavernous hemangioma. Unilateral involvement of the palate can be seen.

gins of the excision is underscored by a 41% recurrence rate. Sclerosing agents, which may be effective in the treatment of hemangiomas, are not effective in the treatment of lymphangiomas. There is no malignant potential for these lesions.

Non–Squamous Cell Malignant Neoplasm

Of malignant neoplasms of the mouth, a maximum of 5% are not squamous cell carcinomas. Nonetheless, because these lesions have such a high degree of virulence, the prudent dentist always considers their possibility in the assessment of an oral lesion. Non–squamous cell malignant neoplasms of the mouth are of two varieties: primary lesions, which originate in the mouth, and lesions metastatic to the oral cavity.

Primary non–squamous cell malignancies are most often of mesenchymal origin and include fibrosarcomas, lymphomas, chondrosarcomas, rhabdomyosarcomas, and melanomas. Fibrosarcoma and chondrosarcoma are most often seen in or about the jaws rather than in soft tissue. Patients complain of a unilateral, progressive, painless enlargement, frequently accompanied by paresthesia. Clinical evaluation demonstrates a rock-hard localized enlargement of the jaws (Fig. 41–15). The overlying mucosa is usually intact, although it may be ulcerated. The tumor is generally nonmovable. Radiographic evaluation may demonstrate changes in the bone such as radiolucency or mixed radiolucency and radiopacity, depending on the nature of the lesion (Fig. 41–16). Diagnosis is based on histologic examination of biopsied material.

Lesions that involve only soft tissue demonstrate similar clinical findings. Examination demonstrates an increasing rock-hard mass

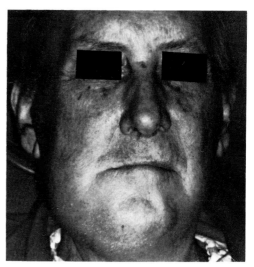

Figure 41–15. Clinical presentation of osteogenic sarcoma at the right side of the mandible. The patient complained of a painless enlargement of his jaw and paresthesia.

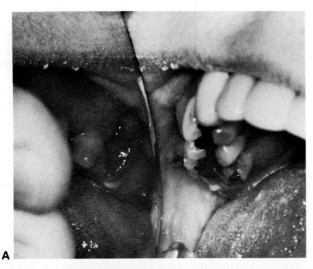

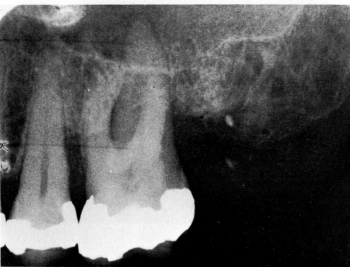

Figure 41-16. *A,* Clinical and radiographic appearance of a diffuse histiocytic lymphoma of the maxillary ridge and overlying mucosa. *B,* Destruction of the alveolar ridge extending to the first molar. The lesion presented as a nonhealing ulceration.

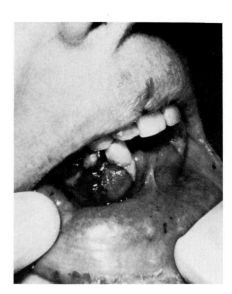

Figure 41-17. Metastatic lesion of the gingiva from a primary adenocarcinoma of the breast.

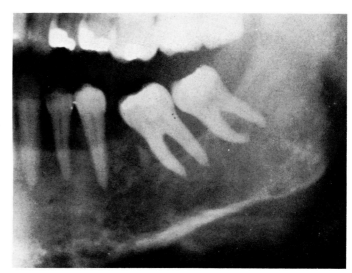

Figure 41–18. Radiolucency of the mandible caused by metastases from adenocarcinoma of the breast.

usually beneath the mucosa. Non–squamous cell malignancies may occur anywhere. Rhabdomyosarcomas, as expected, demonstrate a predilection for the tongue. Lymphomas often involve gingiva. Metastases to both near and distant sites may occur early. Spread of tumor cells is generally hematogenous as compared with squamous cell carcinoma, which often spreads through lymph channels.

Treatment depends on the form of tumor. Lymphomas are treated by chemotherapy and radiotherapy (Chap. 27). Surgical resection with adjuvant chemotherapy and radiotherapy may be the treatment of choice for other forms of malignancies.

Metastases of malignancies to the oral cavity are unusual. Most of these lesions metastasize to the mandible, but soft tissue lesions may also arise. A number of studies have agreed that tumors of breast, lung, and kidney are the most likely to metastasize to the mouth. Clinically, lesions resulting from metastatic spread often present as ulcerations of the mucosa or radiolucencies of the jaws (Figs. 41–17 and 41–18). Neither form is especially symptomatic, although expanding mandibular lesions may result in paresthesia. Certainly, any new oral lesion must be viewed with suspicion in patients with known malignancies. Diagnosis is based on histologic examination.

Oral Complications of Cancer Chemotherapy

Malignant neoplastic diseases represent one of the major causes of morbidity and mortality. Unfortunately, the frequency of these diseases does not appear to be on the wane. Rather, a number of cancers (such as in the lung) are on the rise. It is likely that well over 1,000,000 new cases of cancer will have been diagnosed in Americans in 1994. Much progress has been made in understanding the biology of cancer, leading to new forms of therapy. Whereas a diagnosis of cancer was once associated with certain death, new treatment modalities now offer prolonged survival and, in many cases, a chance for cure.

Three major modalities are currently used to treat malignant neoplasms: surgery, radiotherapy, and chemotherapy. Other forms of treatment, such as immunotherapy, are still largely in the investigational stages. Surgical treatment for cancer has two major objectives: resection of the cancerous mass and other involved tissues such as lymph nodes, and removal of endocrine organs that may modify the spread of the disease. An example of the latter is the oophorectomy or adrenalectomy performed for certain forms of breast cancer. Of the forms of cancer treatment currently available, only surgery is tissue-specific. In contrast, both radiotherapy and chemotherapy function by destroying or prohibiting the growth of rapidly dividing cells by interfering with cell replication (Tables 42–1, 42–2, and 42–3). Neither form of therapy differentiates between rapidly dividing neoplastic cells and rapidly proliferating normal cells such as those of the oral mucosa or bone marrow. Consequently, both chemotherapy and radiotherapy often produce a number of side effects manifested in the oral cavity. In addition, because the mouth harbors massive accumulations of bacteria, it becomes a major portal of entry for infectious organisms in the myelosuppressed host.

FACTORS AFFECTING FREQUENCY OF DEVELOPMENT OF ORAL PROBLEMS

A number of variables affect the frequency with which patients receiving chemotherapy develop oral problems. These may be divided into variables that are patient-related and those that are therapy-related. Patient-related factors include age, diagnosis, and the condition of the patient's mouth preceding and during therapy. Therapy-related variables include the type of drug, dose and frequency of treatment, and the use of concomitant therapy.

Patient-Related Variables

The younger the patient, the more likely it seems that chemotherapy affects the mouth. Whereas about 40% of all patients receiving chemotherapy develop oral side effects, this number jumps to more than 90% in children under the age of 12. Although patients in this age group tend to have malignancies that lend themselves to oral problems, it also seems likely that the high mitotic index of oral mucosal cells in this age group is a contributing factor.

As mentioned, the type of malignancy may have a bearing on the development of oral problems associated with therapy. In general, hematologic malignancies such as leukemia and lymphoma, which themselves cause myelosuppression, tend to be associated with the highest frequency of oral complications. Neoplasms of the gastrointestinal tract are also associated with a high frequency of oral complications.

Patients with poor oral hygiene and preexisting odontogenic or periodontal infection

Table 42–1. ANTINEOPLASTIC DRUGS—
MYELOSUPPRESSIVE TOXICITY POTENTIAL

Markedly myelosuppressive	Moderately myelosuppressive
Vinblastine	Taxol
Dactinomycin	Vindesine
Doxorubicin	VP-16
Daunorubicin	VM-26
Idarubicin	Fludarabine
Mitomycin C	Cyclophosphamide (po)
Methotrexate	Ifosfamide
5-Fluorouracil	Melphalan (po)
6-Mercaptopurine	Chlorambucil
6-Thioguanine	Azridinylbenzoquinone (AZQ)
Cytarabine	Procarbazine
5-Azacytidine	Mitoxantrone
Hydroxyurea	Mildly myelosuppressive
Melphalan (IV)	Vincristine
Cyclophosphamide (IV)	Mithramycin
Busulfan	Bleomycin
CCNU	5-Fluorodeoxyuridine
BCNU	Deoxycoformycin
Carboplatin	Streptozocin
	Dacarbazine

are at high risk for developing oral infection during periods of chemotherapy-induced myelosuppression. In patients with periodontitis, bacteria that are usually successfully confined by host defenses are free to invade following the elimination of white cells. Similarly, the cleaner a patient's mouth during therapy, the less likely are oral problems associated with chemotherapy. Both factors are important considerations for the dentist trying to maintain good oral health in a patient during chemotherapy. Patients should receive specific oral hygiene instruction, and the dentist should work with the oncologist to optimize the patient's oral health.

Therapy-Related Variables

Not all chemotherapeutic agents are equally stomatotoxic or cause the same effects on oral tissues (Table 42–4). Antimetabolites such as

Table 42–2. ANTINEOPLASTIC DRUGS WITH
HIGH DIRECT STOMATOTOXIC POTENTIAL

Vincristine	Cisplatin
Vinblastine	Etoposide
Dactinomycin	Doxorubicin
Idarubacin	Mithramycin
Methotrexate	Mitomycin
5-Fluorouracil	Hydroxyurea
Cytarabine	Procarbazine
5-Azacytidine	

methotrexate, which inhibit DNA synthesis, tend to produce mucositis. A similar effect is noted with alkylating agents such as 5-fluorouracil, a drug commonly used in treatment of cancers of the gastrointestinal tract. Antibiotics such as adriamycin may cause direct problems in the mouth or side effects as a consequence of their effects on minor salivary glands. The plant alkaloids rarely cause direct breakdown of oral mucosa but may create oral problems because of their neurotoxic potential.

In general, side effects tend to be directly related to the dose of drug administered at a given time. The timing of drug administration is probably more important than the total dose of the drug. For example, if a given dose may cause significant oral problems if it is given as a single dose (bolus), the same dose may not cause any side effects if it is given in smaller doses over a longer period. This also holds true for a number of other complications associated with chemotherapy. In addition, because not all cancer cells are in the same division cycle, prolonged administration of anticancer drugs optimizes the likelihood of destroying neoplastic cells.

Radiotherapy given at the same time a patient is receiving chemotherapy tends to potentiate the oral side effects of the chemotherapy. This is especially true for patients receiving treatment for head and neck malignancies.

FORMS OF ORAL COMPLICATIONS OF CANCER CHEMOTHERAPY

There are two major forms of oral complications of cancer chemotherapy. Problems that are a result of the drug's directly affecting oral tissues are termed forms of direct stomatotoxicity. In contrast, oral problems caused by modification of other tissues, such as bone marrow, are termed forms of indirect stomatotoxicity (Fig. 42–1).

Direct Stomatotoxicity

Mucositis

The most common form of direct stomatotoxicity is mucositis, a diffuse ulcerative condition, generally of nonkeratinized oral mucosa. Direct stomatotoxicity is noted within 5 to 7 days following administration of the drug. The

Text continued on page 436

Table 42–3. DRUGS USED FOR DIFFERENT TYPES OF CANCER IN WHICH CHEMOTHERAPY HAS MINOR ACTIVITY

Cancer	Drugs of Choice	Some Alternatives
Acute lymphocytic leukemia (ALL)[1]	*Induction:* vincristine + prednisone + asparaginase ± daunorubicin	*Induction:* Same ± high-dose methotrexate ± cytarabine
	CNS prophylaxis: intrathecal methotrexate + systemic high-dose methotrexate with leucovorin ± intrathecal cytarabine ± intrathecal hydrocortisone	Teniposide or etoposide High-dose cytarabine
	Maintenance: methotrexate + mercaptopurine	Same + periodic vincristine + prednisone
	Bone marrow transplant[2, 3]	
Acute myelogenous leukemia (AML)[4]	*Induction:* cytarabine + either daunorubicin or idarubicin	Cytarabine + mitoxantrone High-dose cytarabine
	Post Induction: Combined chemotherapy with high-dose cytarabine and other drugs such as etoposide	
	Bone marrow transplant[2]	
Adrenocortical carcinoma*	Mitotane Cisplatin	Doxorubicin
Bladder*	*Local:* Instillation of BCG or thiotepa	Instillation of thiotepa, doxorubicin, mitomycin, or interferon alfa
	Systemic: Methotrexate + vinblastine + doxorubicin + cisplatin (MVAC)	
	Cisplatin + methotrexate + vinblastine (CMV)	Fluorouracil, mitomycin, cyclophosphamide
Brain*		
anaplastic astrocytome	Procarbazine + lomustine + vincristine	Carmustine, cisplatin
anaplastic oligodendroglioma	Procarbazine + lomustine + vincristine	Carmustine, cisplatin
glioblastoma	Carmustine or lomustine	Procarbazine, cisplatin, etoposide
medulloblastoma	Vincristine + carmustine ± mechlorethamine ± methotrexate	Etoposide
	Mechlorethamine + vincristine + procarbazine + prednisone (MOPP)	
	Vincristine + cisplatin ± cyclophosphamide	
Breast cancer[5]	*Adjuvant:*[6] Cyclophosphamide + methotrexate + fluorouracil (CMF); Cyclophosphamide + doxorubicin ± fluorouracil (AC or CAF); Tamoxifen	
	Metastatic: Cyclophosphamide + methotrexate + fluorouracil (CMF) or Cyclophosphamide + doxorubicin ± fluorouracil (AC or CAF) for receptor negative and/or hormone refractory; Tamoxifen for receptor positive and/or hormone sensitive[7]	Thiotepa + doxorubicin + vinblastine; mitomycin + vinblastine; mitomycin + methotrexate + mitoxantrone; fluorouracil by continuous infusion; paclitaxel
		Bone marrow transplant[2]
Cervix*	Cisplatin	Cyclophosphamide, vincristine, mitomycin, fluorouracil, doxorubicin, vinblastine
	Ifosfamide with mesna	Vinblastine + ifosfamide with mesna + cisplatin
Choriocarcinoma	Methotrexate ± leucovorin Dactinomycin	Methotrexate + dactinomycin + cyclophosphamide (MAC)
		Etoposide + methotrexate + doxorubicin + cyclophosphamide + vincristine (EMA-CO)

Table 42–3. DRUGS USED FOR DIFFERENT TYPES OF CANCER IN WHICH CHEMOTHERAPY HAS MINOR ACTIVITY *Continued*

Cancer	Drugs of Choice	Some Alternatives
Chronic lymphocytic leukemia*	Chlorambucil ± prednisone Fludarabine	Cladribine, cyclophosphamide, pentostatin, vincristine, doxorubicin
Chronic myelogenous leukemia (CML)		
Chronic phase	Bone marrow transplant[2, 8]	Busulfan, hydroxyurea, interferon alfa
Acute phase[9]	Daunorubicin + cytarabine ± vincristine ± prednisone ± thioguanine High-dose cytarabine ± daunorubicin Vincristine + prednisone for lymphoid variant	Amsacrine,‡ azacitidine,‡ vincristine ± plicamycin
Colorectal*	*Adjuvant:* Fluorouracil[10] + levamisole *Metastatic:* Fluorouracil + leucovorin	*Hepatic metastases:* intra-arterial floxuridine Mitomycin
Embryonal rhabdomyosarcoma[5]	Vincristine + dactinomycin (or doxorubicin) + cyclophosphamide (or ifosfamide with mesna)	Same ± doxorubicin ± cisplatin ± etoposide
Endometrial*	Megestrol or another progestin Doxorubicin, cyclophosphamide, cisplatin	Fluorouracil, tamoxifen, altretamine
Ewing's sarcoma[5]	Cyclophosphamide (or ifosfamide with mesna) + doxorubicin + vincristine (CAV) ± dactinomycin	Same + etoposide
Gastric**	Fluorouracil + leucovorin	Doxorubicin, cisplatin, methotrexate, etoposide, mitomycin
Hairy cell leukemia	Pentostatin or cladribine	Interferon alfa, chlorambucil
Head and neck, squamous cell*[11]	Cisplatin + fluorouracil Methotrexate	Bleomycin, carboplatin, paclitaxel
Hodgkin's disease[12]	Doxorubicin + bleomycin + vinblastine + dacarbazine (ABVD) ABVD alternated with MOPP Mechlorethamine + vincristine + procarbazine (± prednisone) + doxorubicin + bleomycin + vinblastine (MOP[P]-ABV)	Mechlorethamine + vincristine + procarbazine + prednisone (MOPP) Chlorambucil + vinblastine + procarbazine + prednisone (CVPP) ± carmustine Etoposide + vinblastine + doxorubicin (EVA) Bone marrow transplant[2]
Islet cell carcinoma	Streptozocin + doxorubicin	Streptozocin + fluorouracil; chlorozotocin‡
Kaposi's sarcoma* (AIDS-related)	Etoposide or interferon alfa or vinblastine Doxorubicin + bleomycin + vincristine (ABV)	Cyclophosphamide, vincristine, doxorubicin, bleomycin
Liver**	Doxorubicin Fluorouracil	Intra-arterial floxuridine or cisplatin
Lung, small cell (oat cell)	Cisplatin + etoposide (PE) Cyclophosphamide + doxorubicin + vincristine (CAV) PE alternated with CAV Cyclophosphamide + etoposide + cisplatin (CEP) Doxorubicin + cyclophosphamide + etoposide (ACE)	Ifosfamide with mesna + carboplatin + etoposide (ICE) Daily oral etoposide

Table continued on following page

Table 42–3. DRUGS USED FOR DIFFERENT TYPES OF CANCER IN WHICH CHEMOTHERAPY HAS MINOR ACTIVITY *Continued*

Cancer	Drugs of Choice	Some Alternatives
Lung (non-small cell)**	Cisplatin + etoposide Cisplatin + mitomycin + vinblastine	Cisplatin + fluorouracil + leucovorin Methotrexate + doxorubicin + cyclophosphamide + lomustine (MACC) Carboplatin, paclitaxel
Lymphoma, non-Hodgkin's Burkitt's lymphoma	Cyclophosphamide + vincristine + methotrexate Cyclophosphamide + high-dose cytarabine ± methotrexate with leucovorin rescue Intrathecal methotrexate or cytarabine	Ifosfamide with mesna Cyclophosphamide + doxorubicin + vincristine + prednisone (CHOP)
Diffuse large-cell lymphoma	Cyclophosphamide + doxorubicin + vincristine + prednisone ± methotrexate with leucovorin rescue (CHOP or M-CHOP) Prednisone + methotrexate with leucovorin + doxorubicin + cyclophosphamide + etoposide + cytarabine + vincristine + bleomycin + prednisone (ProMACE CytaBOM) Bleomycin + doxorubicin + cyclophosphamide + vincristine + prednisone + procarbazine (COP-BLAM) Etoposide + doxorubicin + cyclophosphamide + vincristine + prednisone + bleomycin (VACOP-B)	Bone marrow transplant[2] Cytarabine, teniposide, high-dose cytarabine, mitoguazone,‡ ifosfamide with mesna Dexamethosone sometimes substituted for prednisone
Follicular lymphoma	Cyclophosphamide or chlorambucil	Same ± vincristine and prednisone, ± etoposide Interferon alfa, cladribine, fludarabine Bone marrow transplant[2] Cyclophosphamide + doxorubicin + vincristine + prednisone (CHOP)
Melanoma**	Aldesleukin Dacarbazine ± tamoxifen	Dactinomycin, interferon alfa, cisplatin
Mycosis fungoides*	Combination chemotherapy as in Hodgkin's disease or non-Hodgkin's lymphoma Mechlorethamine (topical)	Carmustine (topical) Photopheresis (psoralen + extracorporeal or lesional ultraviolet light) Vinblastine, methotrexate, interferon alfa, pentostatin, etretinate
Myeloma*	Melphalan (or cyclophosphamide) + prednisone Melphalan + carmustine + cyclophosphamide + prednisone Dexamethasone + doxorubicin + vincristine (VAD)	Lomustine, interferon alfa Bone marrow transplant[2] High-dose dexamethasone
Neuroblastoma*	Doxorubicin + cyclophosphamide + cisplatin + teniposide Doxorubicin + cyclophosphamide Cisplatin + cyclophosphamide Bone marrow transplant[2]	Carboplatin, etoposide

Table 42–3. DRUGS USED FOR DIFFERENT TYPES OF CANCER IN WHICH CHEMOTHERAPY HAS MINOR ACTIVITY *Continued*

Cancer	Drugs of Choice	Some Alternatives
Osteogenic sarcoma[5]	Doxorubicin + high-dose methotrexate with leucovorin rescue ± cisplatin ± bleomycin ± cyclophosphamide ± dactinomycin	Ifosfamide with mesna, etoposide
Ovary	Cisplatin (or carboplatin) + cyclophosphamide ± doxorubicin (CP)	Altretamine, fluorouracil, chlorambucil, thiotepa, ifosfamide with mesna, leuprolide, paclitaxel, etoposide, tamoxifen
	Cisplatin (or carboplatin) + paclitaxel	
Pancreatic**	Fluorouracil	
Prostate	Leuprolide (or goserelin) + flutamide	Cyclophosphamide ± fluorouracil, estramustine ± vinblastine, megestrol, cyproterone,‡ aminoglutethimide + hydrocortisone, diethylstilbestrol
Renal**	Aldesleukin	Vinblastine
	Interferon alfa	
Retinoblastoma[5]	Doxorubicin + cyclophosphamide ± cisplatin ± teniposide ± vincristine	Cisplatin, etoposide, ifosfamide with mesna
Sarcomas, soft tissue, adult	Doxorubicin + dacarbazine, ± cyclophosphamide (or ifosfamide with mesna)	Cisplatin, methotrexate
Testicular	Cisplatin + etoposide ± bleomycin (PEB)	Vinblastine (or etoposide) + ifosfamide with mesna + cisplatin (VIP)
		Carboplatin, cyclophosphamide, methotrexate, dactinomycin
		Bone marrow transplant[2]
Wilms' tumor[5]	Dactinomycin + vincristine ± doxorubicin ± cyclophosphamide	Cisplatin, ifosfamide with mesna, etoposide

From Drugs of choice for cancer chemotherapy. Med. Lett. Drugs Ther., 35(897):43–50, 1993.

*Chemotherapy has only moderate activity.

**Chemotherapy has only minor activity.

‡Available in the USA only for investigational use.

1. High-risk patients (e.g., high counts, cytogenetic abnormalities, adults) may require additional drugs for induction and maintenance, "intensification" (GK Rivera et al, Lancet, 337:61, 1991), and radiotherapy for CNS prophylaxis. Additional drugs include cyclophosphamide and mitoxantrone.

2. After high-dose chemotherapy ± total body radiation (Medical Letter, 34:79, 1992).

3. Patients with a poor prognosis initially or those who relapse after remission.

4. Some patients with acute progranulocytic leukemia have had complete responses to tretinoin (RP Warrell, Jr et al, N Engl J Med, 324:1385, 1991), but such treatment can cause a toxic syndrome characterized by fever and respiratory distress (SR Frankel et al, Ann Intern Med, 117:292, 1992) or severe hyperhistaminemia with intestinal ulceration and shock (T Koike et al, N Engl J Med, 327:385, 1992).

5. Drugs have major activity only when combined with surgical resection, radiotherapy, or both.

6. The choice of adjuvant drugs for different categories of patients with breast cancer was discussed in The Medical Letter, 32:49, 1990. Tamoxifen with or without chemotherapy is generally recommended for postmenopausal estrogen-receptor-positive, node-positive patients and chemotherapy with or without tamoxifen for premenopausal node-positive patients. Many oncologists also recommend adjuvant treatment for some node-negative patients, especially those with larger tumors or other adverse prognostic indicators.

7. Megestrol and other hormonal agents may be effective in some patients when tamoxifen fails.

8. Allogeneic sibling-matched bone marrow transplantation can cure 40% to 50% of patients with chronic CML. Chemotherapy alone is palliative.

9. If a chronic phase is achieved with any of these combinations, high-dose therapy followed by allogeneic bone marrow transplantation should be considered.

10. For rectal cancer, postoperative adjuvant treatment with fluorouracil plus radiation, preceded and followed by treatment with fluorouracil alone.

11. The vitamin A analog isotretinoin *(Accutane)* can control pre-neoplastic lesions (leukoplakia) and decreases the rate of second respiratory primaries (WK Hong et al, N Engl J Med, 323:795, 1990).

12. Limited-stage Hodgkin's disease (stages 1 and 2) is curable by radiotherapy. Disseminated disease (stages 3b and 4) requires chemotherapy. Some intermediate stages and selected clinical situations may benefit from both.

Table 42–4. SOME COMMERCIALLY AVAILABLE ANTICANCER DRUGS AND HORMONES

Drug	Acute Toxicity†	Delayed Toxicity†
Aldesleukin (interleukin-2; *Proleukin*—Cetus Oncology)	**Fever; fluid retention; hypotension; respiratory distress**; rash; anemia; thrombocytopenia; nausea and vomiting; diarrhea; capillary leak syndrome; nephrotoxicity; myocardial toxicity; hepatotoxicity; erythema nodosum	Neuropsychiatric disorders; hypothyroidism; nephrotic syndrome; possibly acute leukoencephalopathy; brachial plexopathy
Altretamine (hexamethylmelamine; *Hexalen*—US Bioscience)	Nausea and vomiting	**Bone marrow depression:** visual disturbances (reversible); CNS depression; peripheral neuritis; visual hallucinations; ataxia; tremors; alopecia; rash
Aminoglutethimide (*Cytadren*—Ciba)	Drowsiness; nausea; dizziness; rash	Hypothyroidism (rare); bone marrow depression; fever; hypotension; masculinization
Asparaginase (*Elspar*—Merck; *Kidrolase*—Rhône-Poulenc Rorer)	Nausea and vomiting; fever; chills; headache; hypersensitivity, anaphylaxis; abdominal pain; hyperglycemia leading to coma	CNS depression or hyperexcitability; acute hemorrhagic pancreatitis; coagulation defects; thrombosis; renal damage; hepatic damage
BCG (*TheraCys*—Connaught; *Tice BCG*—Organon)	Bladder irritation; nausea and vomiting; fever; sepsis	Granulomatous pyelonephritis; hepatitis; urethral obstruction; epididymitis; renal abscess
Bleomycin (*Blenoxane*—Bristol-Myers Oncology)	Nausea and vomiting; fever; anaphylaxis and other allergic reactions; phlebitis at injection site	**Pneumonitis and pulmonary fibrosis**; rash and hyperpigmentation; stomatitis; alopecia; Raynaud's phenomenon; cavitating granulomas; hemorrhagic cystitis
Busulfan (*Myleran*—Burroughs Wellcome)	Nausea and vomiting; rare diarrhea	**Bone marrow depression; pulmonary infiltrates and fibrosis**; alopecia; gynecomastia; ovarian failure; hyperpigmentation; azoospermia; leukemia; chromosome aberrations; cataracts; hepatitis; seizures and veno-occlusive disease with high doses
Carboplatin (*Paraplatin*—Bristol-Myers Oncology, DBL in Canada)	Nausea and vomiting	**Bone marrow depression**; peripheral neuropathy (uncommon); hearing loss; transient cortical blindness; hemolytic anemia
Carmustine (BCNU; *BiCNU*—Bristol-Myers Oncology)	Nausea and vomiting; local phlebitis	**Delayed leukopenia and thrombocytopenia** (may be prolonged); pulmonary fibrosis (may be irreversible); delayed renal damage; reversible liver damage; leukemia; myocardial ischemia
Chlorambucil (*Leukeran*—Burroughs Wellcome)	Seizures; nausea and vomiting	**Bone marrow depression**; pulmonary infiltrates and fibrosis; leukemia; hepatic toxicity; sterility
Cisplatin (Cis-DDP; *Platinol*—Bristol-Myers Oncology, DBL in Canada)	Nausea and vomiting; anaphylactic reactions	**Renal damage**; ototoxicity; bone marrow depression; hemolysis; hypomagnesemia; peripheral neuropathy; hypocalcemia; hypokalemia; Raynaud's disease; sterility; hypophosphatemia; hyperuricemia
Cladribine (2-chloro-deoxyadenosine; CdA; *Leustatin*—Ortho)	Fever; nausea and vomiting; rash	**Bone marrow depression**
Cyclophosphamide (*Cytoxan*—Bristol-Myers Oncology, *Procytox*—Horner, and others)	Nausea and vomiting; Type I (anaphylactoid) hypersensitivity; facial burning with IV administration; visual blurring	**Bone marrow depression**; alopecia; hemorrhagic cystitis; sterility (may be temporary); pulmonary infiltrates and fibrosis; hyponatremia; leukemia; bladder cancer, inappropriate ADH secretion
Cytarabine HCl (*Cytosar-U*—Upjohn, and others)	Nausea and vomiting; diarrhea; anaphylaxis; sudden respiratory distress with high doses	**Bone marrow depression**; conjunctivitis; megaloblastosis; oral ulceration; hepatic damage; fever; pulmonary edema and central and peripheral neurotoxicity with high doses; rhabdomyolysis; pancreatitis when used with asparaginase

Table 42–4. SOME COMMERCIALLY AVAILABLE ANTICANCER DRUGS AND HORMONES *Continued*

Drug	Acute Toxicity†	Delayed Toxicity†
Dacarbazine (*DTIC-Dome*— Miles, and others)	Nausea and vomiting; diarrhea; anaphylaxis; pain on administration	**Bone marrow depression**; alopecia; flu-like syndrome; renal impairment; hepatic necrosis; facial flushing; paresthesia; photosensitivity; urticarial rash
Dactinomycin (*Cosmegen*— Merck)	Nausea and vomiting; diarrhea; severe local tissue damage and necrosis on extravasation; anaphylactoid reaction	**Stomatitis; oral ulceration; bone marrow depression**; alopecia; folliculitis; dermatitis in previously irradiated areas
Daunorubicin HCl (*Cerubidine*—Wyeth-Ayerst, Rhône-Poulenc Rorer)	Nausea and vomiting; diarrhea; red urine (not hematuria); severe local tissue damage and necrosis on extravasation; transient EKG changes; facial flushing; anaphylactoid reaction	**Bone marrow depression; cardiotoxicity** (may be delayed for years); alopecia; stomatitis; anorexia; diarrhea; fever and chills; dermatitis in previously irradiated areas; skin and nail pigmentation
Doxorubicin HCl (*Adriamycin*— Adria, and others)	Nausea and vomiting; red urine (not hematuria); severe local tissue damage and necrosis on extravasation; diarrhea; fever; transient EKG changes; ventricular arrhythmia; anaphylactoid reaction	**Bone marrow depression; cardiotoxicity** (may be delayed for years); alopecia; stomatitis; anorexia; conjunctivitis; acral pigmentation; dermatitis in previously irradiated areas; acral erythrodysesthesia; hyperuricemia
Estramustine phosphate sodium (*Emcyt*—Kabi Pharmacia)	Nausea and vomiting; diarrhea	Mild gynecomastia; increased frequency of vascular accidents; myelosuppression (uncommon); edema; dyspnea; pulmonary infiltrates and fibrosis; decreased glucose tolerance
Etoposide (VP16-213; *VePesid*— Bristol-Myers Oncology)	Nausea and vomiting; diarrhea; fever; hypotension; anaphylactoid reactions; phlebitis at infusion site	**Bone marrow depression**; rashes; alopecia; peripheral neuropathy; mucositis and hepatic damage with high doses; leukemia
Etretinate (*Tegison*—Roche)		Dryness of mucous membranes; chapped lips; hair loss; bone and joint pain; eye irritation; peeling skin; pseudotumor cerebri; premature epiphyseal closure; hepatic injury; major teratogenic effects
Floxuridine (*FUDR*—Roche, and others)	Nausea and vomiting; diarrhea	**Oral and gastrointestinal ulceration, bone marrow depression**; alopecia; dermatitis; hepatic dysfunction with hepatic infusion
Fludarabine (*Fludara*—Berlex)	Nausea and vomiting	**Bone marrow depression**; CNS effects; visual disturbances; renal damage with higher doses; pulmonary infiltrates; tumor lysis syndrome
Fluorouracil (5-FU, *Adrucil*— Adria, and others)	Nausea and vomiting; diarrhea; hypersensitivity reaction (rare)	**Oral and GI ulcers; bone marrow depression**; diarrhea (especially with fluorouracil and leucovorin); neurological defects, usually cerebellar; cardiac arrhythmias; angina pectoris; alopecia; hyperpigmentation; palmar-plantar erythrodysesthesia; conjunctivitis; heart failure
Flutamide (anti-androgen; *Eulexin*—Schering, *Euflex* in Canada)	Nausea; diarrhea	Gynecomastia; hepatotoxicity; CNS effects
Goserelin (*Zoladex*—Zeneca)	Transient increase in bone pain and ureteral obstruction in patients with metastatic prostate cancer; hot flashes	Impotence; testicular atrophy
Hydroxyurea (*Hydrea*— Immunex, Squibb in Canada)	Nausea and vomiting; allergic reactions to tartrazine dye	**Bone marrow depression**; stomatitis; dysuria; alopecia; rare neurological disturbances
Idarubicin (*Idamycin*—Adria)	Nausea and vomiting; tissue damage on extravasation	**Bone marrow depression**; alopecia; stomatitis; myocardial toxicity
Ifosfamide (*Iflex*—Bristol-Myers Oncology)	Nausea and vomiting; confusion; nephrotoxicity; metabolic acidosis and renal Fanconi's syndrome; **cardiac toxicity** with high doses	**Bone marrow depression; hemorrhagic cystitis** (prevented by concurrent mesna); alopecia; inappropriate ADH secretion; neurotoxicity (somnolence, hallucinations, blurring of vision, coma)

Table continued on following page

Table 42–4. SOME COMMERCIALLY AVAILABLE ANTICANCER DRUGS AND HORMONES *Continued*

Drug	Acute Toxicity†	Delayed Toxicity†
Interferon alfa-2a, alfa-2b (*Roferon-A*—Roche, *Intron A*—Schering)	Fever; chills; myalgias; fatigue; headache; arthralgias; hypotension	Bone marrow depression; anorexia; neutropenia; anemia; confusion; depression; renal toxicity; possible hepatic injury; facial and peripheral edema; cardiac arrhythmias
Leuprolide acetate (LHRH-analog; *Lupron, Lupron Depot*—TAP)	Transient increase in bone pain and ureteral obstruction in patients with metastatic prostate cancer; hot flashes; nausea and vomiting; constipation	Impotence; testicular atrophy; CNS effects
Levamisole (*Ergamisol*—Janssen)	Nausea and vomiting; flu-like symptoms; dizziness; metallic taste	Agranulocytosis; myalgias; arthralgias
Lomustine (CCNU; *CeeNU*—Bristol-Myers Oncology)	Nausea and vomiting	**Delayed (4 to 6 weeks) leukopenia and thrombocytopenia** (may be prolonged); transient elevation of transaminase activity; neurological reactions; pulmonary fibrosis; renal damage; leukemia
Mechlorethamine HCl (nitrogen mustard; *Mustargen*—Merck)	**Nausea and vomiting**; local reaction and phlebitis	**Bone marrow depression**; alopecia; diarrhea; oral ulcers; leukemia; amenorrhea; sterility; hyperuricemia
Melphalan (*Alkeran*—Burroughs Wellcome)	Mild nausea; hypersensitivity reactions	**Bone marrow depression** (especially platelets); pulmonary infiltrates and fibrosis; amenorrhea; sterility; leukemia
Mercaptopurine (*Purinethol*—Burroughs Wellcome)	Nausea and vomiting; diarrhea	**Bone marrow depression**; cholestasis and rarely hepatic necrosis; oral and intestinal ulcers; pancreatitis; allopurinol and azathioprine increase overall toxicity
Mesna (*Mesnex*—Bristol-Myers Oncology; *Uromitexan*, Bristol Canada)	Nausea and vomiting; diarrhea; allergic reactions	
Methotrexate (MTX; *Folex*—Adria, and others)	Nausea and vomiting; diarrhea; fever; anaphylaxis; hepatic necrosis	**Oral and gastrointestinal ulceration**, perforation may occur; **bone marrow depression**; hepatic toxicity including cirrhosis; renal toxicity; **pulmonary infiltrates and fibrosis**; osteoporosis; conjunctivitis; alopecia; depigmentation; menstrual dysfunction; encephalopathy; infertility
Mitomycin (*Mutamycin*—Bristol-Myers Oncology)	Nausea and vomiting; tissue necrosis; fever	**Bone marrow depression** (cumulative); stomatitis; alopecia; acute pulmonary toxicity; pulmonary fibrosis; hepatotoxicity; renal toxicity; amenorrhea; hemolytic-uremic syndrome; bladder calcification (with intravesical administration)
Mitotane (o,p'-DDD; *Lysodren*—Bristol-Myers Oncology)	Nausea and vomiting; diarrhea	**CNS depression**; rash; visual disturbances; adrenal insufficiency; hematuria; hemorrhagic cystitis; albuminuria; hypertension; orthostatic hypotension; cataracts; prolonged bleeding time
Mitoxantrone HCl (*Novantrone*—Lederle)	Blue-green pigment in urine; blue-green sclera; nausea and vomiting; stomatitis; fever; phlebitis	**Bone marrow depression**; cardiotoxicity; alopecia; white hair; skin lesions; hepatic damage; renal failure; extravasation necrosis
Octreotide (*Sandostatin*—Sandoz)	Nausea and vomiting; diarrhea	Steatorrhea; gallstones
Paclitaxel (*Taxol*—Bristol-Myers Squibb)	Anaphylaxis, dyspnea, hypotension, angioedema, urticaria (probably due to vehicle)	**Bone marrow depression**; peripheral neuropathy; alopecia; arthralgias; myalgias; heart block; mild GI disturbances
Pentostatin (2'-deoxyco-formycin; *Nipent*—Parke-Davis)	Nausea and vomiting; rash	**Nephrotoxicity; CNS depression**; bone marrow depression; respiratory failure; hepatic toxicity; arthralgia; myalgia, photophobia; conjunctivitis

Table 42–4. SOME COMMERCIALLY AVAILABLE ANTICANCER DRUGS AND HORMONES *Continued*

Drug	Acute Toxicity†	Delayed Toxicity†
Plicamycin (*Mithracin*—Miles)	Nausea and vomiting; diarrhea; fever; facial flushing	**Hemorrhagic diathesis; bone marrow depression** (thrombocytopenia); coagulation abnormalities; hepatic damage; hypocalcemia and hypokalemia; stomatitis; renal damage; CNS depression
Procarbazine HCl (*Matulane*—Roche, *Natulan* in Canada)	Nausea and vomiting; CNS depression; disulfiram-like effect with alcohol	**Bone marrow depression**; stomatitis; peripheral neuropathy; pneumonitis; leukemia
Streptozocin (*Zanosar*—Upjohn, and others)	Nausea and vomiting; local pain; chills and fever	**Renal damage**; hypoglycemia; hyperglycemia; liver damage; diarrhea; bone marrow depression (uncommon); fever; eosinophilia; nephrogenic diabetes insipidus
Tamoxifen citrate (*Nolvadex*—Zeneca, *Tamofen*—Rhône-Poulenc Rorer, and others)	Hot flashes; nausea and vomiting; transient increased bone or tumor pain; hypercalcemia	Vaginal bleeding and discharge; rash; thrombocytopenia; peripheral edema; depression; dizziness; headache; decreased visual acuity; corneal changes; retinopathy; purpuric vasculitis
Teniposide (VM-26; *Vumon*—Bristol-Myers Squibb)	Nausea and vomiting; diarrhea; phlebitis; anaphylactoid symptoms	Bone marrow depression; alopecia; peripheral neuropathy; leukemia
Thioguanine (Burroughs Wellcome, *Lanvis* in Canada)	Occasional nausea and vomiting; diarrhea	**Bone marrow depression**; hepatic damage; stomatitis
Thiotepa (Lederle)	Nausea and vomiting; rare hypersensitivity reaction	**Bone marrow depression**; menstrual dysfunction; interference with spermatogenesis; leukemia; mucositis with high doses
Vinblastine sulfate (*Velban, Velbe*—Lilly, Horner, and others)	Nausea and vomiting; local reaction and tissue damage with extravasation	**Bone marrow depression**; alopecia; stomatitis; loss of deep tendon reflexes; jaw pain; muscle pain; paralytic ileus
Vincristine sulfate (*Oncovin*—Lilly, and others)	Tissue damage with extravasation	**Peripheral neuropathy**; alopecia; mild bone marrow depression; constipation; paralytic ileus; jaw pain; inappropriate ADH secretion; optic atrophy

From Drugs of choice for cancer chemotherapy. Med. Lett. Drugs Ther., 35(897):43–50, 1993.

†Dose-limiting effects are in bold type. Cutaneous reactions (sometimes severe), hyperpigmentation, and ocular toxicity have been reported with virtually all nonhormonal anticancer drugs. For adverse interactions with other drugs, see *The Medical Letter Handbook of Adverse Drug Interactions*, 1993).

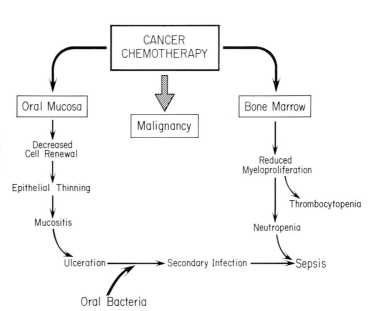

Figure 42–1. Mechanisms by which cancer chemotherapy causes oral problems. (From Peterson, D., and Sonis, S.: Oral Complications of Cancer Chemotherapy. Amsterdam, Martinus Nijhoff, 1983.)

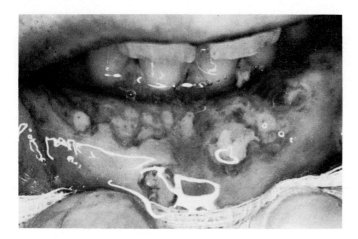

Figure 42–2. Mucositis of the labial mucosa caused by methotrexate. Note the severe disruption of epithelial integrity.

most consistent symptom of mucositis is extreme pain. Examination usually demonstrates erythema and ulceration of some or all mucosal surfaces (Figs. 42–2 and 42–3). Typically, the gingiva, dorsal surface of the tongue, and hard palate are not involved. Ulcerative areas may appear grayish-white with central areas of necrosis (Figs. 42–4 and 42–5). If the patient's bone marrow is relatively unaffected by the chemotherapy, the mucositis is self-limiting and tends to heal spontaneously in about 14 days.

The major objective in the treatment of stomatitis is palliation. A variety of agents are available for this purpose, including lidocaine (Xylocaine Viscous) and dyclonine hydrochloride (Dyclone). A simple and effective rinse may also be made by the pharmacist by combining Benadryl and Kaopectate in equal proportions. The use of milk of magnesia as a vehicle for palliating medicaments is to be discouraged, because it frequently causes mucosal desiccation. For limited areas of ulceration, benzocaine in Orabase or lidocaine

ointment may be helpful. Because cold is often soothing, ice chips and popsicles can be routinely recommended. Systemic analgesics may be prescribed, as needed.

Xerostomia

Some agents, such as adriamycin, may produce xerostomia. If xerostomia occurs concurrently with other forms of direct stomatotoxicity, it may promote ulceration and increase symptoms. In addition, lack of saliva results in increased accumulation of bacteria and other debris.

Little can be done to prevent chemotherapy-induced xerostomia. However, once present, artificial saliva substitutes, such as Xero-Lube or Salivart, may be prescribed. Lemon-glycerin swabs, routinely available at hospital pharmacies, may be helpful. Sucrose-free lemon drops can be recommended to stimulate salivary flow. Fluoride mouth rinses (Chap. 40) are helpful in preventing bacterial accumulation on teeth. Although acidulated rinses are most

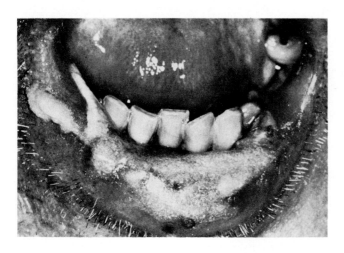

Figure 42–3. Severe breakdown of the labial mucosa as a result of direct stomatotoxicity. Note the lack of involvement of nonmucosal surfaces.

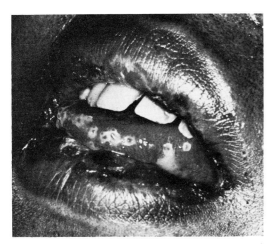

Figure 42–4. Ulceration with secondary hemorrhage resulting from direct stomatotoxicity. A line of demarcation is apparent at the mucocutaneous junction.

effective, mucosal sensitivity may preclude their use, in which case neutral rinses should be used.

Neurotoxicity

Plant alkaloids may produce neurotoxicity. This problem is of special significance to the dentist, because involvement of oral nerves may produce odontogenic pain. Although this problem tends to be relatively rare, accounting for about 6% of all oral complications, it is disturbing for patients who complain of tooth-related discomfort. Such pain is pulpitis-like,

constant, and usually of acute onset. Mandibular molars tend to be most frequently affected. Clinical examination is generally unremarkable. Radiographic examination may demonstrate widening of the periodontal ligament space in vital teeth. Treatment consists of palliation. Symptoms usually disappear with the discontinuance of the drug.

Indirect Stomatotoxicity

The major oral problems associated with indirect stomatotoxicity are infection and hemorrhage. Both of these problems result from the chemotherapy-induced myelosuppression that produces leukopenia and thrombocytopenia.

Infection

Bacterial, fungal, and viral infections may occur in the mouths of patients myelosuppressed as a result of cancer chemotherapy. In each case, infection must be recognized, properly diagnosed, and treated quickly and aggressively, because systemic involvement in these individuals is frequently fatal. *The most frequently documented source of sepsis in the granulocytopenic cancer patient is the mouth* (Table 42–5).

Bacterial Infection. Bacterial infections of the mouth may involve the teeth, gingiva, or mucosa. In all cases, the normal signs of infec-

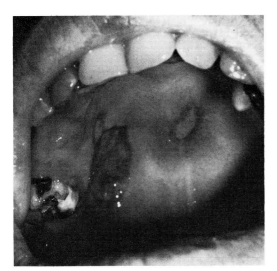

Figure 42–5. Unusual case of localized ulcerations of the hard palate as a consequence of direct stomatotoxicity. The large ulcer is healing. Note the lack of erythema.

Table 42–5. SITES OF MICROBIOLOGICALLY AND CLINICALLY DOCUMENTED INFECTIONS IN GRANULOCYTOPENIC PATIENTS WITH CANCER

Site	Percentage of All Recognized Sites
Oral cavity*	19
Skin/soft tissue	14
Lung†	13
Urinary tract	11
Trachea/bronchus	8
Anus/rectum	9
Intestine/esophagus	5
Nose/sinus	3
Intravenous site/catheter	2
Other	10
Bacteremia (no primary site identified)	7
Total sites	100

The EORTC International Antimicrobial Therapy Project Group: Three antibiotic regimens in the treatment of infection in febrile granulocytic patients with cancer. J. Infect. Dis. 137:14, 1978.
*Mouth, pharynx, and tonsil.
†Parenchymal infection (pneumonia).

tion may be obscured by the myelosuppressed state of the patient. The patient's inability to mount a normal inflammatory reaction means that the classic signs of infection are often absent. *The most consistent signs and symptoms of oral infection in the myelosuppressed patient are pain, fever, and the presence of some form of lesion.* Generally, patients describe localized discomfort of varying severity. Fever associated with infection usually exceeds 100° F (38° C). Lesions may involve teeth or mucosal or gingival surfaces.

Odontogenic Infection. Odontogenic infection in myelosuppressed patients is frequently diagnosed based on the presence of tooth-related pain, deep caries, tooth sensitivity to percussion, or thermal changes.

In keeping with the general principles of treating localized sites of identifiable infection in myelosuppressed patients, the source of the odontogenic infection should be eliminated. In approaching the myelosuppressed patient, the dentist should determine the extent of leukopenia and thrombocytopenia (Fig. 42–6). Consultation with the patient's oncologist is mandatory. Generally, patients with white blood cell counts greater than 3,500 cells/mm³

and platelet counts greater than 100,000 cells/mm³ may be treated as normal patients, assuming that the percentage of neutrophils is greater than 50%. In this group, extraction or definitive endodontic therapy is indicated. Extraction is the treatment of choice for teeth that cannot be treated by definitive endodontic therapy in a single visit. Antibiotic therapy, using oral penicillin 500 mg, qid, is suggested during and 1 week following treatment.

Patients with white blood cell counts between 1,000 and 3,500 cells/mm³ and platelet counts over 100,000 cells/mm³ may be treated with special consideration for the prevention of sepsis. Extraction or endodontic therapy may be performed in this group with antibiotic coverage (oral potassium phenoxymethyl penicillin, 500 mg, qid, for 2 weeks). If possible, cultures should be obtained before the initiation of antibiotic therapy (Chap. 46). Patients should be monitored closely for any signs of advancing infection.

Patients with white blood cell counts under 1000 cells/mm³ and signs of infection require hospitalization. In no instance should individuals in this category be managed on an ambulatory basis. Management of oral infection in this group requires close cooperation between

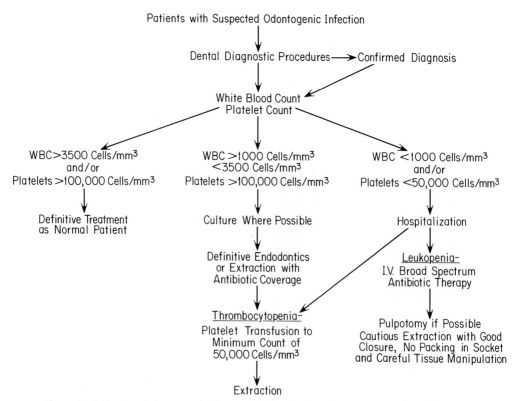

Figure 42–6. Treatment of suspected odontogenic infection in patients receiving chemotherapy.

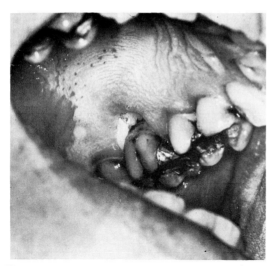

Figure 42–7. Necrotizing gingivitis in a patient with pre-existing periodontitis who then received chemotherapy.

the dentist and oncologist, because oral infection may lead to sepsis. Once the patient is hospitalized, appropriate intravenous antibiotic therapy should be started. Although gram-positive organisms, especially *Streptococcus viridans*, are the most common pathogens causing infection in granulocytopenic cancer patients, increases in the frequency of oral gram-negative organisms mandates use of broad-spectrum antibiotic coverage (penicillin and an aminoglycoside). In keeping with the principles of infection management, however, elimination of the infected focus is the treatment of choice. Extraction may be performed given appropriate antibiotic coverage and platelet support. Platelet transfusions given to patients to a level of 50,000 cells/mm³ imme-

diately before extraction are desirable. Tissue should be treated carefully, with extractions performed as atraumatically as possible. No sharp edges of bone should remain. The area should be débrided, but the socket should not be packed with hemostatic agents. The wound edges should be approximated as well as possible and sutured with nonresorbable sutures.

Soft Tissue Infection
Gingiva. Soft tissue infections in the myelosuppressed patient may occur anywhere in the mouth. In patients with pre-existing periodontal disease, the marginal, papillary, and attached gingivae are frequent sites of infection. In these sites, the initial infectious lesion appears as a localized necrotic area of gingiva, similar in appearance to acute necrotizing ulcerative gingivitis (ANUG) (Fig. 42–7). The lesion then tends to spread laterally and apically, and large areas of gingiva and mucosa may become involved (Fig. 42–8). Patients complain of pain and a bad taste in the mouth. Clinical examination reveals gingival necrosis that may be contiguous with adjacent mucosa. At times, underlying bone may be exposed. Bleeding may occur but is not a uniform finding, unlike in conventional ANUG.

Gingival infection most frequently occurs during periods when the white count is significantly depressed (nadir) (Fig. 42–9). Patients are usually febrile. The treatment of gingival infection with systemic involvement requires hospitalization. Parenteral antibiotic therapy should include a combination of agents with activity against spirochetes, fusiform bacteria, and gram-negative organisms. The frequency of gingival involvement in myelosuppressed patients may be significantly reduced with ef-

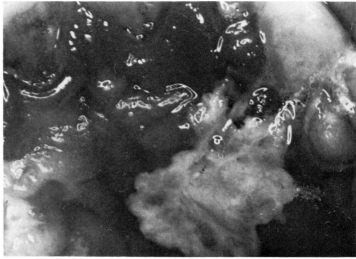

Figure 42–8. Spreading gingival infection in a patient made neutropenic by chemotherapy.

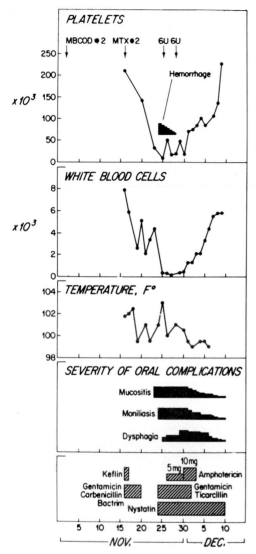

Figure 42–9. Temporal relationship between white blood count and infection in a patient receiving chemotherapy for lymphoma. (From Lockhart, P. B., and Sonis, S. T.: Relationship of oral complications to peripheral blood leukocyte and platelet counts in patients receiving cancer chemotherapy. Oral Surg., 48:21, 1979.)

Patients with white blood cell counts greater than 1,000 cells/mm^3 and platelet counts greater than 50,000 cells/mm^3 may brush with a soft brush and floss routinely. Acidulated fluoride mouth rinses used for 1 min daily help reduce the accumulation of tooth-borne bacteria. The efficacy of 0.12% chlorhexidine gluconate rinses in reducing the frequency of mucositis is unresolved. The rinse may be helpful in reducing plaque formation, but its alcohol content may cause local tissue irritation. Alternatively, povidone-iodine rinses may be used. Patients with counts lower than these should continue to clean their mouths; rather than a toothbrush, moist 2- × 2-inch sponges wrapped around the forefinger can be used to débride the teeth. This is at least as effective as using commercially available sponge-type tooth wipes. Fluoride rinses should be continued. Professional prophylaxis with antibiotic coverage should be performed prior to administration of chemotherapy if at all possible.

Mucosal Infection. Whereas the mucosa of normal individuals readily tolerates routine traumatic insult, chemotherapy predisposes to mucosal breakdown, ulceration, and in many cases, secondary infection. Mucosal lesions are ulcerative in nature. Usually, the center is deeply punched out and contains a grayish-white necrotic center (Fig. 42–10). The borders of the ulcer may be raised but lack the erythematous border characteristic of many other oral ulcers because of the absence of an inflammatory response in the myelosup-

fective oral hygiene supplemented with professional prophylaxis.

Oral hygiene in myelosuppressed patients has, in many instances, been curtailed because of a fear of evoking gingival hemorrhage in the presence of thrombocytopenia. Consequently, it is not unusual for patients receiving chemotherapy to be instructed to discontinue brushing and flossing. Clearly, this leads to many more problems than it prevents. A modified regimen of aggressive oral hygiene is an imperative part of treatment in the cancer patient receiving chemotherapy.

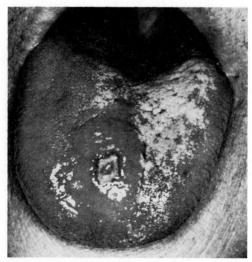

Figure 42–10. Infected ulceration on the dorsal portion of the tongue. A necrotic center with raised borders is apparent. Note the lack of erythema.

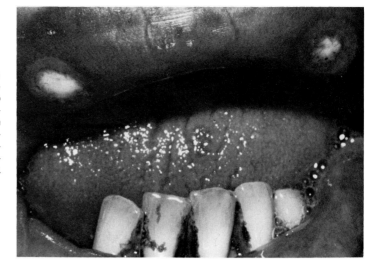

Figure 42–11. Bilateral infected ulcers in a patient made neutropenic by chemotherapy. The patient traumatized the lip with a biting habit and subsequently developed these unusual lesions. (From Lockhart, P. B.: Dental management of patients receiving chemotherapy. In Peterson, D., and Sonis, S. [eds.]: Oral Complications of Cancer Chemotherapy. Amsterdam, Martinus Nijhoff, 1983.)

pressed individual (Figs. 42–11 and 42–12). It is often difficult to determine whether the ulcerative area is secondarily infected. However, in the absence of another identifiable focus of infection, an oral ulceration must be presumed to be the source of sepsis until definitively proven otherwise. Symptomatically, patients complain of discomfort. Infection is suggested by fever. As with other infections in myelosuppressed patients, the bacterial cause of mucosal infections should be considered to be mixed—both gram-positive and gram-negative (*Klebsiella, Proteus, Pseudomonas, Enterobacter,* and *Escherichia coli*). Patients who are leukopenic (white blood cell count less than 1000

cells/mm^3) should be admitted to the hospital and treated with intravenous antibiotics. Because virally induced ulcers may be similar in clinical presentation, it is critical to obtain both viral and bacterial cultures to establish a correct diagnosis.

Traumatic insult to the mucosa should be minimized by the elimination of removable prostheses during periods of myelosuppression, elimination of sharp restorations or cusps, and care in the choice of food.

Salivary Gland Infection. Any patient debilitated over a long period of time is susceptible to developing infections of the major salivary glands. The parotid glands are most frequently affected (Chap. 43). Salivary stasis and the spread of bacteria up the duct are the most likely causes. *Staphylococcus aureus* is the most frequently identifiable source of infection, although other organisms including streptococci have also been implicated.

Clinically, patients complain of pain of sudden onset. Almost all cases are unilateral. The parotid gland may be enlarged and erythematous. If the patient is not sufficiently leukopenic, pus may be milked from the parotid duct. Fever is a consistent finding, and the mouth may appear dry.

The prevention of parotid infection is aimed at ensuring good hydration and adequate salivary flow. If the patient is unable to eat normally, ice chips, popsicles, or sucrose-free lemon drops may provide stimulation for salivary gland function. Myelosuppressed patients suspected of having salivary gland infection require hospitalization. Management of infection requires the cooperation of the dentist, oncologist, and infectious disease specialist.

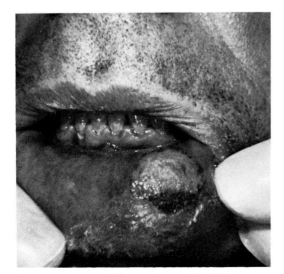

Figure 42–12. Large infected ulcer of the labial mucosa. This lesion is actually in a healing phase. The patient, who was being treated for lymphoma, initiated the ulcer by biting his lip.

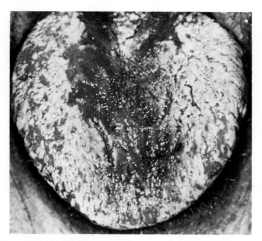

Figure 42–13. Candidiasis in a neutropenic patient receiving chemotherapy. Infection appears as raised white curdy areas, which can be scraped off.

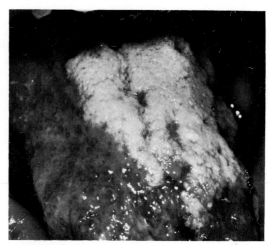

Figure 42–14. Candidiasis. Note the mixed clinical appearance of the infection, which includes classic raised white areas and atrophic erythematous regions.

Exudate from the parotid duct should be cultured and the patient started on an intravenous antibiotic regimen that includes activity against penicillin-resistant staphylococci (Chap. 46). Steps should be taken to ensure that the patient is adequately hydrated by oral or intravenous fluids.

Fungal Infections. The most common causative organism of oral infection in the myelosuppressed host is *Candida albicans*. Although this organism is normally inconsequential in the 40% of the population in which it is a normal inhabitant of the oral flora, in the leukopenic individual the organism may overgrow and invade local tissue, spread to the esopha-

gus or lungs, or produce generalized sepsis through hematogenous spread. A British study has suggested that oral candidiasis develops in all patients whose white blood cell counts drop below 200 cells/mm^3.

The clinical appearance of oral candidiasis is varied. Classically, infections are described as raised, white, curdy-looking areas involving any part of the mouth. These superficial white necrotic areas may be scraped off, revealing a raw, bleeding base (Figs. 42–13 to 42–15). Microscopic examination of smears stained with Gram's stain (Chap. 48) or prepared with potassium hydroxide reveals epithelial cells with numerous hyphae. It is not unusual for oral

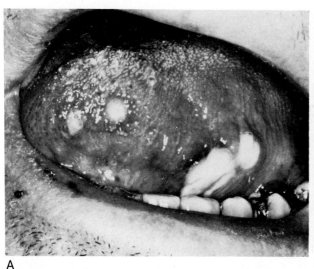

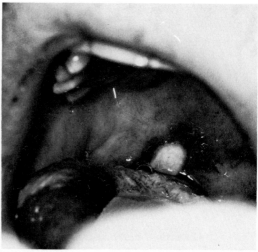

A   B

Figure 42–15. *A, B,* Localized *Candida* infections of the tongue and palate in a patient receiving chemotherapy. Note the discrete lesions and surrounding erythema.

candidiasis to appear as a broad area of painful erythema. This is frequently the case under removable prostheses. In patients taking oral antibiotics or other staining substances, candidiasis may take on the pigmentation of the staining material. Any area of mucosa, palate, or tongue may be involved.

Oral *Candida* infections may spread to the esophagus or lungs. Esophageal or pulmonary involvement may also occur in the absence of obvious oral infection. Patients with esophageal candidiasis complain of dysphagia and are frequently febrile. These symptoms in the myelosuppressed cancer patient require a thorough workup, including a radiographic assessment of the esophagus by barium esophagram (Fig. 42–16).

Controversy exists as to whether the prophylactic use of nystatin in myelosuppressed patients reduces the frequency or severity of oral candidiasis. Because this drug does not pose a threat to the patient and may offer some degree of protection by postponing the onset of oral candidiasis, it is recommended (nystatin oral suspension 200,000 to 400,000 units, qid, swish and swallow). The degree and duration of oral candidiasis are related to the severity and length of myelosuppression. Thus, patients who receive prophylaxis as their white

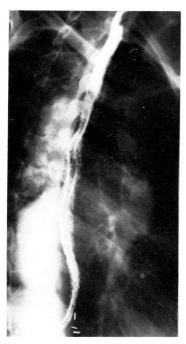

Figure 42–16. Typical shaggy, irregular, finely nodular appearance of the esophageal mucosa in moniliasis. (Courtesy of Department of Radiology, Boston City Hospital, Boston, MA.)

blood cell counts drop have a reduced risk of developing extended candidal infections. Nystatin is also supplied in lozenge form as vaginal suppositories. The advantage of the lozenge over the suspension is a prolonged presence of the drug in contact with mucosa.

An antifungal troche, clotrimazone, may be used. This medication is pleasant-tasting and offers the advantage of prolonged mucosal contact. It is supplied in 10-mg tablets that are taken five times per day for 2 weeks. Its efficacy in myelosuppressed cancer patients seems to be comparable to that of nystatin. Alternatively, nystatin oral suspension can be diluted with water to the desired concentration and poured into ice cube trays. Patients find the nystatin ice cubes soothing and pleasant-tasting, and the mucosal contact is prolonged.

Ketoconazole tablets may be given instead of topical medication. Gentian violet applied to the mucosa is an effective antifungal agent; however, its taste and color are often displeasing to patients. In addition, the mucosal discoloration that accompanies the use of gentian violet makes longitudinal clinical assessment of lesions almost impossible.

A new antifungal agent, fluconazole, has been introduced. This agent is administered as an oral tablet and has documented efficacy in the treatment of mucocutaneous candidiasis associated with HIV infection.

Esophageal or systemic fungal infections in the myelosuppressed patient require aggressive therapy. Patients require hospitalization and intravenous medication. Amphotericin B is usually the drug of choice in these patients. Unfortunately, nephrotoxicity may occur with the use of this medication. Careful and constant evaluation of patients' renal function is required.

Other types of oral fungal infections are relatively unusual (Chap. 49).

Viral Infection. Herpes simplex virus (HSV) and herpes zoster infections are not uncommon in myelosuppressed patients.

Recurrent herpes infection, a reactivation of the virus from its latent state, is not uncommon (Chap. 48). Although the appearance of recurrent herpes simplex infection is most common in extraoral sites in healthy patients, intraoral manifestations also occur in the myelosuppressed patient. Patients who demonstrate antibodies to HSV are at significantly higher risk of reactivation during periods of myelosuppression than are patients who are seronegative. Hence, the determination of HSV antibody status prior to the initiation of myelosuppressive therapy may be prudent. Intraoral lesions appear as croppy vesicular lesions that may ulcerate rapidly (Fig. 42–17). The lesions are frequently noted on the palate and are often unilateral. Erythema may be present, depending on the degree of myelosuppression. If ulcerated, lesions have a grayish-white necrotic center that may become secondarily infected.

Extraoral herpes simplex infection is often noted at the commissures of the lips, at the mucocutaneous junction of the lip and skin, or just under the nose (Chap. 48). These lesions present as painful crops of vesicles that may coalesce. In the thrombocytopenic patient, intralesional hemorrhage may be noted. Secondary infection with staphylococci may occur.

In both intraoral and extraoral infections, patients may have lymphadenopathy and fever. They may also exhibit systemic signs of viremia, including malaise and anorexia. Smears of the lesion demonstrate nuclear viral inclusions within cells.

Intraoral herpes simplex infection is best palliated. The normal course of infection is about 1 to 2 weeks, although the state of the patient's marrow affects the rapidity of recovery. Extraoral herpetic lesions heal best when kept lubricated. Viral infections that occur during myelosuppression are best treated with acyclovir. Acyclovir is available as an ointment, tablet, or IV solution. Parenteral administration is indicated for the treatment of HSV

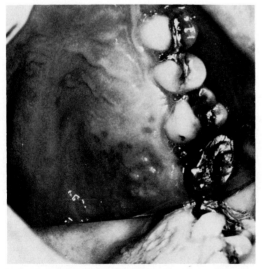

Figure 42–17. Viral stomatitis in a patient receiving chemotherapy. Note the croppy collection of ulcerations of the palate, which characterizes ruptured vesicles in viral infection.

infection in the compromised patient. If superficial secondary infection is suspected, Neosporin or bacitracin ointment can be applied topically. In patients in whom systemic secondary bacterial infection is suspected, aggressive intravenous antibiotic therapy is required during periods of myelosuppression.

Herpes zoster infections (Chap. 48) are caused by the varicella zoster virus and are extremely contagious in individuals who have not been exposed to chickenpox as children. In the patient who undergoes prolonged myelosuppression or immunosuppression, this virus can be activated from posterior root ganglion. Clinically, patients note an extremely painful vesicular eruption that, in the head and neck region, most frequently follows the distribution of a branch of the trigeminal nerve. The vesicular stage of the lesions may be short-lived, and lesions may degenerate into ulcers. Treatment is usually palliative.

A variety of nonspecific viral infections may affect the mouths of myelosuppressed patients. In almost all cases, lesions appear as painful, crop-like vesicular eruptions, most frequently affecting palatal mucosa. Patients often have a prodrome of fever, malaise, and anorexia or cold- or flu-like symptoms that precede the development of oral lesions. Lesions persist during periods of myelosuppression but then disappear within 10 to 14 days. Treatment of the lesions is palliative with systemic support, including bed rest, hydration, control of fever, and attention to possible secondary infection. The prophylactic administration of acyclovir has demonstrated efficacy in preventing HSV infection in markedly myelosuppressed cancer patients.

Oral Bleeding Caused by Thrombocytopenia

Thrombocytopenia is a frequent side effect of cancer chemotherapy and is a result of nonspecific myelosuppression. The implications of thrombocytopenia to the dentist are threefold: spontaneous gingival bleeding, spontaneous submucosal bleeding, and postoperative hemorrhage. Although "thrombocytopenia" refers to a quantitative assessment of platelets, it should also be remembered that qualitative characteristics in platelet function are also altered by chemotherapy.

Spontaneous oral bleeding usually does not occur unless thrombocytopenia is relatively profound. It is unlikely for patients to experience spontaneous gingival hemorrhage with platelet counts greater than 20,000 cells/mm³.

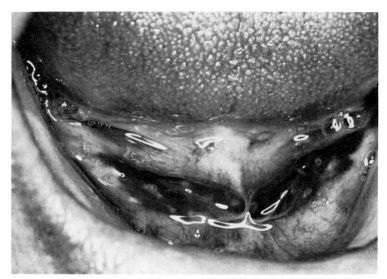

Figure 42–18. Submucosal hematoma in a patient made thrombocytopenic by chemotherapy.

Patients with pre-existing periodontal disease are more prone to gingival bleeding than periodontally healthy individuals. Submucosal hemorrhage is similarly rare, although mucosal trauma may produce hematoma formation with counts under 50,000 cells/mm³.

The effects of thrombocytopenia on postoperative hemorrhage have been previously discussed (Chap. 26). Essentially, platelet counts of less than 100,000 cells/mm³ may result in prolonged postoperative bleeding. Platelet counts of less than 50,000 cells/mm³ probably require platelet transfusion before a procedure can be performed.

Submucosal bleeding is of special concern when it occurs sublingually (Fig. 42–18). Extensive hemorrhage can result in superior and posterior elevation of the tongue and produce respiratory embarassment. Thus, patients who are profoundly thrombocytopenic require careful and daily oral evaluation to determine the presence of hemorrhage. Appropriate instruments for emergency intubation should be readily available. Platelet transfusion should be considered in conjunction with the physician who is managing the patient.

Spontaneous gingival hemorrhage can be a significant management problem (Fig. 42–19). Patients who experience continuous oozing from the gingival margins find their mouths constantly full of blood. Subsequently, they are unable to sleep, eat, or communicate. In some cases, significant amounts of blood can be lost by the gingival route, resulting in a drop in the hematocrit and the production of anemia. Because pre-existing periodontal disease predisposes to gingival bleeding, prechemotherapy evaluation and dental prophylaxis are of value, as is scrupulous oral hygiene during therapy.

Local measures for treating gingival bleed-

Figure 42–19. Spontaneous gingival hemorrhage in a patient receiving chemotherapy for leukemia. Note the lack of oral hygiene and the presence of gingival disease, which predisposes to bleeding. (From Lockhart, P. B.: Dental management of patients receiving chemotherapy. In Peterson, D., and Sonis, S. [eds.]: Oral Complications of Cancer Chemotherapy. Amsterdam, Martinus Nijhoff, 1983.)

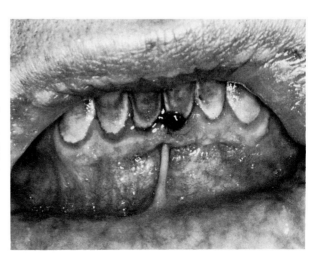

ing include the application of pressure with gauze soaked in topical thrombin solution. The use of acrylic stents to control bleeding has not met with great success, because these tend to irritate an already compromised gingiva and prevent adequate oral hygiene. Periodontal pack also does not function well, because this material tends to float off in the presence of constant oozing. The most definitive form of therapy is platelet transfusion. However, because platelets carry HLA surface antigens, their use may result in sensitization of the patient so that future platelets are lysed by circulating anti-HLA antibodies and complement. Indeed, one of the most frustrating situations that can occur in the myelosuppressed patient is gingival hemorrhage along with high titers of antiplatelet antibody. In this case, palliation until the patient's marrow function returns is the only treatment available short of bone marrow transplantation.

Avoidance of trauma from prostheses, restorations, or sharp teeth helps minimize the likelihood of hemorrhage.

Patients who require extraction or other surgical dental procedures (including block anesthesia) and who have received chemotherapy should have a qualitative and quantitative assessment of their platelets (Chaps. 1 and 26). This includes a platelet count and measurement of bleeding time. Patients with platelet counts between 50,000 and 100,000 cells/mm³ may be treated as outpatients if they are readily accessible to follow-up. Block local anesthesia into areas in which large vessels are present should be avoided. Extractions should be as atraumatic as possible. Any areas of sharp bone should be smoothed. The wound should be closed with nonabsorbable sutures to approximate primary closure as closely as possible. A hemostatic agent such as Gelfoam may be used in patients having white blood cell counts *greater* than 2,500 cells/mm³ with an adequate number of neutrophils. Antibiotic coverage, as discussed, should be prescribed. Patients should be observed for 2 hours after the procedure to ensure adequate hemostasis.

Patients with platelet counts less than 50,000 cells/mm³ require hospitalization for surgical dental procedures. Clearly, any elective treatment should be deferred. The most common reason for dental treatment in this group is to eliminate a source of infection. In addition to platelet considerations, adequate protection against infection must be considered, as already discussed. The platelet count should be brought up to 50,000 cells/mm³ by platelet transfusion given immediately before the ex-

Table 42–6. PREVENTION PROTOCOL IN PATIENTS RECEIVING CANCER CHEMOTHERAPY

Pretreatment evaluation
  Oral examination
  Radiographs
  Consultation
Pretreatment therapy
  Oral hygiene instruction
  Elimination of infected teeth
  Elimination of faulty or sharp restoration or prostheses
  Dental prophylaxis
Prevention during therapy
  Oral hygiene
    Brushing, flossing, rubber tip when WBC greater than 1,000 cells/mm³ and platelets greater than 50,000 cells/mm³
    Débridement of teeth with moistened 2- × 2-inch gauze sponge during periods of profound myelosuppression
    Acidulated fluoride mouth rinse daily for 1 min
    Avoid mouthwashes containing alcohol or undiluted hydrogen peroxide
  Mycostatin oral suspension, 300,000 units qid, swish and swallow
  Removal of prostheses
  Soft foods during periods of myelosuppression or during periods of stomatotoxicity
  Limit sucrose intake
  Periodic oral evaluation

traction. Generally, an increase of 10,000 cells/mm³ is observed following the administration of one unit of platelets. The techniques described earlier should be followed.

GENERAL PRINCIPLES OF PREVENTION

The primary goal of oral management of the cancer patient should be the prevention of complications of chemotherapy (Table 42–6). Ideally, patients should receive a thorough dental evaluation, including radiographs, prior to the initiation of chemotherapy. If the patient's blood counts and overall condition permit, hopeless teeth should be extracted and the rest restored to reduce the chance of infection. Endodontic therapy should be considered as an alternative to extractions for patients who can maintain their dentition and hygiene at a high level of care. Endodontic therapy is fraught with risk, however, in those patients who are expected to demonstrate granulocytopenia and thrombocytopenia before the endodontic treatment can be completed. Temporary restorations may have to be placed in teeth to "buy time" until the patient's blood and fluid counts return to acceptable levels and time is available for more permanent restorations. Patients too ill or whose counts are too low and who have unresolved carious lesions should be started on a fluoride rinse in an effort to slow the progression of the caries. Sharp teeth and appliances should be smoothed. In addition, if time and blood counts permit, the patient should have thorough oral prophylaxis to remove all local irritants from the teeth. At this time, the relationship between the mouth and the patient's overall health during chemotherapy should be discussed with the patient.

The systemic and local effects of chemotherapy also predispose these patients to nutritional disorders. Careful consideration of the patient's diet, including sucrose and refined carbohydrate intake, should be made on a continuing basis. Reduced nutritional intake may result as a consequence of stomatitis and oral pain or overall debilitation. Nausea and vomiting also inhibit nutritional intake and increase the loss of proteins and water soluble vitamins necessary for epithelial cell structure. Foods that are rough (e.g., toast) and may abrade the mucosa, those too thick for the minimal saliva present, foods that are too spicy, seasoned, or hot, or foods that sting or burn the oral mucosa such as citric juices and alcoholic beverages should be avoided. Cold foods and fluids are well tolerated and often soothing.

ORAL COMPLICATIONS OF BONE MARROW TRANSPLANTATION

Bone marrow transplantation (BMT) is becoming increasingly popular in the treatment of a number of forms of cancer. The rationale for the use of BMT is that it permits the patient to receive extremely high doses of che-

motherapy, which normally would be fatal, by providing a mechanism whereby the marrow can be rescued. Two forms of BMT are used most commonly. Allogeneic transplants involve the transfer of marrow from a genetically matched donor to the recipient. In autologous transplants, marrow is harvested from the patient, treated and preserved, and then reinfused after the patient is treated with chemotherapy. In both cases, patients receive their marrow transplants about 5 to 9 days after they begin their chemotherapy.

In addition to being at risk for the direct and indirect effects of chemotherapy (see earlier), patients who receive allogeneic transplants are at risk for another condition, graft-versus-host disease. This disorder is the result of the effects of immunocompetent donor cells reacting against the anergic cells of the recipient. Four major tissues are affected in this reaction—the mouth, skin, liver, and lungs. Of these, oral changes are the most common.

The typical oral mucosal manifestations of graft-versus-host disease clinically resemble those of lichen planus. White, lacy, keratotic lesions occur, often in conjunction with erosive or bullous lesions, which produce great discomfort for the patient. The degree of patient symptoms is directly related to the extent of the lesions. The oral lesions of graft-versus-host disease are generally responsive to steroid therapy. The intensity of treatment (topical or systemic) varies according to the severity of the patient's lesions.

Changes in the major and minor salivary glands often occur as a consequence of graft-versus-host disease. Patients often develop xerostomia (Chap. 40). Because of the frequency of these changes, biopsy of the minor salivary glands of the lip is often helpful in making the diagnosis.

Common Complications of Chemotherapy

PROBLEM	TIME SEEN FOLLOWING CHEMOTHERAPY	CLINICAL SIGNS AND SYMPTOMS	LABORATORY FINDINGS	TREATMENT	COURSE
Xerostomia	Variable, Adriamycin predisposes	Dry mouth, thick ropy saliva; diminished taste sensation; metallic taste in mouth; difficulty with speech and nutrition	Noncontributory	Lemon drops (artificial sweeteners); lemon-glycerine swabs; sugarless gum; ice chips; saliva substitute; fluoride (Fl⁻) rinses—acidulated Fl⁻ rinse qd × 1 min at hs until mucositis, nonacidulated Fl⁻ rinse as above if acidulated burns; check vertical dimension of teeth; Mycolog ointment, Vaseline	Resolves following treatment
Angular cheilitis	Anytime, but increases with xerostomia; infectious cause (fungal) in compromised host	Cracking, bleeding; possible exudate and pain in corner of mouth	Smear demonstrates fungi if *Candida*		Watch for secondary infection
Mucositis and ulceration	Direct stomatotoxicity: methotrexate: 5–7 days; indirect stomatotoxicity: 10–14 days	Broad shallow to deep ulceration on mucosa Poorly defined borders; may be hemorrhagic; mucosal erythema; distinct ovoid deep ulceration with white necrotic centers and dense surrounding band of erythema; may involve keratinized tissue; often at gingival margin, especially in neutropenic patient	Early leukopenia, but precedes nadir; neutropenia	Palliation—Xylocaine Viscous, Benadryl and Kaopectate, dyclone, or cocaine rinses; benzocaine in Orabase for discrete lesions; systemic analgesics; ice chips; if secondary infection, parenteral antibiotics to cover gram-negative organisms in addition to conventional flora (gram-positive); hemorrhage: topical thrombin, soft bland diet, as tolerated	Resolves following chemotherapy
Gingival bleeding	Variable, 10–14 days; increases with thrombocytopenia	Marginal hemorrhage from gingiva; may be spontaneous; may be presenting sign	Thrombocytopenia; usually not spontaneous if platelets >15,000/mm³	Platelets; topical thrombin soaked 2- × 2-inch gauze; aminocaproic acid; avitene; do not disturb clot; D/C mechanical hygiene	Resolves as platelets increase

Complication	Timing	Clinical features	Diagnosis	Treatment	Resolution
Mucosal bleeding	10–14 days	Hematoma or bleeding area, especially mucosal sites commonly traumatized; in case of neutropenic patient, likely chance of secondary infection	Thrombocytopenia; blast crisis with functional decrease in platelets	Remove partial and full dentures; eliminate orthodontic bands or retainers; as above, cover for secondary infection	Resolves with increased platelets; resolving hematoma may extrude granulation plug from healing base—do not disturb
Odontogenic infection in myelo-suppressed host	Anytime	secondary infection; beware of sublingual or pharyngeal extension → airway obstruction; variable, may present with fever of unknown origin, swelling, pain, lymphadenopathy; swelling not consistent finding with neutropenia; may be subclinical until increase PMNL	Neutropenia; positive blood culture	Parenteral broad-spectrum antibiotics to cover for opportunistic organisms and normal flora; remove source in presence of adequate cells (WBC >1,000/mm^3 and reasonable PMNL and >25,000/mm^3 platelets)	Variable: depends on organism, counts, location
Odontogenic pain of neurotoxic origin	Following neurotoxic agent (for example, vincristine)	Spontaneous, constant, dental pain often mimicking infective pulpitis, difficult to localize; may be bilateral; afebrile; no swelling, lymphadenopathy, no significant caries, periodontitis	Pulpal infarct (?)	Systemic pain medications; if pulpal necrosis (localized), may require extraction	Resolves following discontinuation of neurotoxic agent
Salivary gland infection	Anytime: most common in debilitated patient with diminished oral intake and dehydration	Swelling (may be unilateral or bilateral); pain; suppuration from duct when no myelosuppression; xerostomia; fever	Variable, bacterial cultures → Staphylococcus sp; may be viral; cytomegalovirus most common	Antibiotics (parenteral) to cover staph if bacterial; rehydrate; watch for possible airway obstruction	Resolution depends on host status and treatment
Moniliasis	Anytime; more likely with prolonged neutropenia, antibiotics, or steroid use	White curds, plaques, ulcerations, tender; affects buccal and palatal mucosa most frequently; corners of mouth may be affected, especially in edentulous patients (see angular cheilitis)	Neutropenia, smear → organisms; positive barium swallow with esophageal involvement (watch for false-negative)	Prophylactic nystatin swish-swallow, vaginal suppositories if tolerated; amphotericin if esophageal or systemic involvement suspected; nystatin ointment	Resolves with antifungal treatment or with increased PMNL
Herpes labialis	Anytime	Crops of vesicular lesions that are at or beyond mucocutaneous junction; frequently extraoral with no anatomic distribution	Smear of base of vesicle—increased nuclear:cytoplasmic ratio; viral inclusion bodies	Prevention: keep lubricated; often secondary infection in neutropenic host; local treatment: neosporin; acyclovir for failure to heal	10–14 days, depending on host resistance

Modified from Lockhart, P. B.: Dental management of the patient receiving chemotherapy. In Peterson, D., and Sonis, S. [eds.]: Oral Complications of Cancer Chemotherapy. Amsterdam, Martinus Nijhoff, 1983.

Formulary of Medications for Specific Oral Problems

Antibacterial

Neosporin (polymyxin B, bacitracin, neomycin)

Use:	Antibacterial against most commonly occurring bacteria known to be topical invaders
Action:	Antibacterial as above, activity against many bacteria resistant to other antibiotics (e.g., *Pseudomonas* and *Staphylococcus*)
Availability:	1- or 1/2-oz tubes, and foil packet of 1/32 oz
Dose/timing:	Apply to circumoral lesions two to five times daily, depending on severity of condition
Route:	Topical use only
Precautions:	Sensitivity to any of its components; watch for overgrowth of nonsusceptible organisms, including fungi
Manufacturer:	Burroughs-Wellcome Co., Research Triangle Park, NC 27709

Acidulated phosphate fluoride (Phos-Flur); (APF)

Use:	Prevention of dental caries
Action:	Hardening of dental enamel through incorporation into enamel matrix, antibacterial effects
Availability:	250- and 500-ml plastic bottles
Dose/timing:	Children age 6 and over and all adults rinse vigorously with 1 or 2 tsp (5 to 10 ml) for 1 min and expectorate; should be done once per day after last meal of the day and following oral hygiene measures
Route:	Oral
Precautions:	Do not swallow; switch to neutral fluoride solution if acidulated fluoride irritates mucosa
Manufacturer:	Colgate Oral Pharmaceuticals, Canton, MA 02021

Neutral sodium fluoride

Use:	Fluoride uptake lower and more shallow than with acidulated phosphate fluoride; less likely to irritate mucosal lesions
Action:	Same as APF, above
Dose:	Same as APF, above

Brush-on fluorides (Stannous fluoride 0.4% Gel-Kam; sodium fluoride 1.1% PreviDent)

Use:	Prevention of dental caries and reduction of bacterial adhesion to teeth
Action:	Same as APF, above
Availability:	4.3-oz bottles or 2-oz plastic tubes
Dose/timing:	Brush liberally onto all tooth surfaces for 1 min, then swish for 1 min; use at bedtime; do not eat for 30 min after use
Route:	Oral topical
Precautions:	Do not use in children under 6 years of age; do not swallow; rare allergic reactions
Manufacturer:	Colgate Oral Pharmaceuticals, Canton, MA 02021

Chlorhexidine gluconate 0.12% (Peridex)

Use:	Antibacterial rinse
Action:	Microbicidal
Availability:	1-pt bottles
Dose/timing:	Rinse for 30 sec twice daily; expectorate after use
Route:	Oral rinse
Precautions:	May cause irritation of mucosal surfaces; in pregnancy and nursing mothers, children under age 18; may cause staining of tooth surfaces and tongue
Manufacturer:	Procter & Gamble, Cincinnati, OH 45201

Antifungal

Mycolog (nystatin, neomycin sulfate, gramicidin, triamcinolone acetonide)

Use:	Angular cheilitis where candidal infection is suspected
Actions:	Anti-inflammatory, antipruritic, vasoconstrictive, anticandidal, antibacterial
Availability:	Tubes of 15, 30, and 60 g
Dose/timing:	Cream: rub into affected area bid or tid; ointment: apply thin film to affected area bid or tid

Formulary of Medications for Specific Oral Problems
Continued

Route:	Topical only
Precautions:	Not for use in viral diseases of skin (e.g., herpes); hypersensitivity to any component; prolonged use may result in overgrowth of nonsusceptible organisms
Manufacturer:	Squibb & Sons, Princeton, NJ 08540

Nystatin (Mycostatin oral suspension)

Use:	Antifungal antibiotic
Action:	Polyene antibiotic that is fungistatic and fungicidal against wide variety of yeasts and yeast-like fungi, binds to yeast and fungi and alters membrane permeability
Availability:	60-ml bottles, 100,000 U/ml; vaginal tablets, 100,000 U
Dose/timing:	1–4 ml (100,000 to 400,000 U) tid or qid, swish for several minutes if possible and swallow, continue until white count rises and for 2 days after lesions disappear; hold vaginal suppository in mouth until dissolved
Route:	Oral
Precautions:	Hypersensitivity to any component, solution contains 50% sucrose; may initiate or accelerate dental caries
Manufacturer:	Squibb & Sons, Princeton, NJ 08540

Mycelex (clotrimazole)

Use:	Antifungal antibiotic for topical use
Action:	Antifungal
Availability:	Bottles of 70 tablets, 10 mg each
Dose/timing:	1 tablet five times daily for 14 days, used as a troche
Route:	Oral
Precautions:	Increased values of liver function tests have been reported in 15% of patients
Manufacturer:	Miles Pharmaceuticals, West Haven, CT 06516

Ketoconazole (Nizoral)

Use:	Oral candidiasis, histoplasmosis
Action:	Antifungal
Availability:	200-mg tablets
Dose/timing:	200 mg once per day (400 mg in severe cases)
Route:	Oral
Precautions:	Do not give with antacids
Manufacturer:	Janssen Pharmaceutica, Inc., New Brunswick, NJ 08903

Fluconazole (Diflucan)

Use:	Treatment of oropharyngeal candidiasis
Action:	First of a new class of synthetic antifungal agents that is a highly selective inhibitor of fungal cytochrome demethylation
Availability:	Tablets of 50 mg, 100 mg, and 200 mg and as a solution for injection
Dose/timing:	200 mg on day 1, then 100 mg for subsequent days, usually for 2 weeks
Route:	Oral or intravenous
Precautions:	In pregnancy, nursing mothers, children; liver and skin toxicity, renal disease, and drug interactions may occur
Manufacturer:	Roerig Division, Pfizer Inc., New York, NY 10017

Amphotericin B (Fungizone intravenous)

Use:	Progressive and potentially fatal fungal infections
Action:	Antifungal antibiotic, fungistatic or fungicidal; probably acts by binding to sterols in fungus cell membrane with resultant change in membrane permeability
Availability:	Vials of 50 mg amphotericin B, 41 mg sodium desoxycholate, 25.2 mg sodium phosphate as a buffer
Dose/timing:	Slow intravenous infusion; dosage depends on nature of infection
Route:	IV; not available in United States for oral use
Precautions:	Hypersensitivity; possible life-saving benefit must be balanced against its untoward and dangerous side effect of nephrotoxicity
Manufacturer:	Apothecon, a Bristol-Myers Squibb Company, Princeton, NJ 08540

Table continued on following page

Formulary of Medications for Specific Oral Problems
Continued

Bleeding

Thrombin, topical

Use:	Surface bleeding from capillaries and small venules
Action:	Clots fibrinogen directly
Availability:	Package of one 5,000 US (NIH)-unit vial of thrombin, topical, and one 5-ml vial of isotonic saline with Phemerol as preservative Package of 10,000 or 1,000 U.S. (NIH) unit vials
Dose/timing:	Sponge (not wipe) recipient surface and apply 2- × 2-inch sponge soaked in topical thrombin to bleeding mucosa and hold with moderate pressure for several minutes; do not wipe clotted area; repeat as necessary; sponge may be left in place for extended period of time, if necessary; do not disturb clot that forms with rinsing or manipulation
Route:	Surface bleeding only; do not inject
Precautions:	Sensitivity to any of its components or material of bovine origin; use solution the day it is prepared; refrigerate if not used for several hours
Manufacturer:	Parke-Davis, Morris Plains, NJ 07950

Microfibrillar collagen hemostat (Avitene)

Use:	Surface mucosal bleeding
Action:	In contact with bleeding surface, Avitene attracts platelets that adhere to the fibrils and triggers platelet aggregation; usually effective in presence of heparinization and in most patients taking aspirin
Availability:	1- and 5-g sterile jars in sealed can
Dose/timing:	Compress site with dry sponge immediately prior to applying dry Avitene with smooth dry forceps; apply pressure over area with dry sponge for 1 to 5 min depending on severity of bleeding; can be reapplied if bleeding recurs
Precautions:	Not to be used in closure of mucosal incisions; may potentiate infection; for surface use only; do not resterilize; not for injection; do not moisten with saline or thrombin; should be used dry; use only enough to produce hemostasis; carefully remove excess material after several minutes
Manufacturer:	Avicon, Inc., Forth Worth, TX 76134

Aminocaproic acid (Amicar)

Use:	Excessive bleeding
Action:	Inhibition of fibrinolysis by inhibition of plasminogen activator substances and antiplasmin activity
Availability:	20-ml vial with 5.0 g aminocaproic acid; 25% syrup; 250 mg/ml; tablets—500 mg
Dose/timing:	5 g orally or intravenously followed by 1- to $1\frac{1}{4}$-g doses at hourly intervals
Route:	Intravenous or oral; benefit from topical use on bleeding mucosa is unknown
Precautions:	Not for use if evidence of active intravascular clotting processes; use caution in patients with cardiac, hepatic, or renal disease; should be used in situations where benefits outweigh hazards
Manufacturer:	Lederle Laboratories, Pearl River, NY 10965

Gelfoam (absorbable gelatin sponge)

Use:	Hemostasis postextraction
Action:	Serves as matrix for clot formation
Availability:	Gelfoam dental packs (size 2 or 4)—each measures 10 × 20 × 7 mm or 20 × 20 × 7 mm, respectively, packaged in jars of 15 packs
Precautions:	Question of increased incidence of infection in granulocytopenic patients
Manufacturer:	Upjohn Company, Kalamazoo, MI 49001

Pain: topical agents

Xylocaine Viscous (lidocaine HCl)

Use:	Topical anesthetic for mucous membranes
Action:	Stabilizes neuronal membrane, blocks peripheral nerve conduction
Availability:	2% solution in 100-ml and 450-ml polyethylene squeeze bottles
Dose/timing:	1 tbsp (15 ml; 300 mg) as needed for pain, not to exceed q3h, or 120 ml in a 24-hr period

Formulary of Medications for Specific Oral Problems
Continued

Route:	Swish for 30 sec and expectorate
Precautions:	Increased uptake by traumatized mucosa; watch for central nervous system (CNS) toxicity
Manufacturer:	Astra Pharmaceutical Products, Worcester, MA 01606

Diphenhydramine hydrochloride (Benadryl)

Use:	Mixed with Kaopectate 1:1 as topical anesthetic for mucous membranes
Action:	Antihistamine with anticholinergic (drying) and sedative side effects
Availability:	Mixed with Kaopectate 1:1 by pharmacy
Dose /timing:	1 tbsp as needed for pain
Route:	Swish for 30 sec and expectorate
Precautions:	Concurrent monoamine oxidase inhibitor therapy, narrow-angle glaucoma, peptic ulcer, additive effects with other CNS depressants; watch for excitation or sedation with systemic uptake
Manufacturer:	Upjohn Company, Kalamazoo, MI 49001

Dyclonine hydrochloride (Dyclone)

Use:	Topical anesthetic for mucous membranes
Action:	Prevents depolarization of nerve fibers
Availability:	0.5% and 1% solutions
Dose /timing:	1 Tbsp as needed for pain
Route:	Swish for 30 sec and expectorate
Manufacturer:	Dow Pharmaceuticals, Indianapolis, IN 46268

Cocaine

Use:	Topical anesthetic for mucous membranes
Action:	Anesthesia and vasoconstriction, mucous membrane shrinkage; inhibition of uptake of catecholamines by adrenergic nerve terminals (?)
Availability:	Liquid
Dose /timing:	2 1/2–5% applied to mucous membranes; total dose should be limited
Route:	Swish and expectorate or apply to area
Precautions:	CNS toxicity, euphoria, addiction

Benzocaine (with Orabase)

Use:	Topical anesthetic for localized areas of pain
Action:	Benzocaine held to site by Orabase; prevents depolarization of nerve fibers
Availability:	5- and 15-g tubes
Dose /timing:	Dry mucosa; apply small dab over area as needed for pain
Precautions:	PDR warns against use in presence of infection
Manufacturer:	Colgate-Hoyt Laboratories, Canton, MA 02021

Sialorrhea

Atropine

Use:	Antisialogogue
Action:	Inhibition of smooth muscle and glands innervated by postganglionic cholinergic nerves, CNS excitation, or depression, depending on dose
Availability:	Vials: 20 ml (0.4 mg/ml); tablets: 0.4 mg
Dose /timing:	Adults: 0.4–0.6 mg as needed for sialorrhea
Route:	By mouth or intramuscular
Precautions:	Glaucoma, asthma, bradycardia
Manufacturer:	Knoll Pharmaceutical Co., Whippany, NJ 07981

Xerostomia

Salivart synthetic saliva

Use:	Mouth moisturizer, caries inhibition
Action:	Remineralization of surface enamel, replacement of lubricating action of missing saliva
Availability:	50-ml spray cans

Table continued on following page

Formulary of Medications for Specific Oral Problems
Continued

Dose /timing:	As needed for xerostomia
Manufacturer:	Westport Pharmaceuticals Inc., Westport, CT 06881
Xero-Lube	
Use:	Mouth moisturizer; caries inhibition
Action:	Remineralization of surface enamel, replacement of lubricating action of missing saliva, fluoride incorporation into surface enamel
Availability:	As supplied by manufacturer or as prepared by local pharmacy
Dose /timing:	As needed for xerostomia
Manufacturer:	Scherer Laboratories, Inc., Dallas, TX 75234

Modified from Lockhart, P. B.: Dental management of the patient receiving chemotherapy. In Peterson, D., and Sonis, S. [eds.]: Oral Complications of Cancer Chemotherapy. Amsterdam, Martinus Nijhoff, 1983.
The use of product names in this table is for informational purposes only.

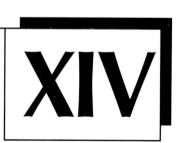
Evaluation and Management of the Patient with Disease of the Salivary Glands

CHAPTER 43

Diseases of the Salivary Glands

SALIVARY GLANDS

Anatomy

The salivary apparatus consist of three pairs of major symmetric glands located adjacent to the mandible: the parotid, the submandibular, and the sublingual glands (Fig. 43–1). In addition, there are numerous unnamed minor salivary glands distributed in the palatal, buccal, and sublingual mucosae.

Whereas the minor salivary glands are almost entirely mucous glands, the parotid is entirely serous. The nature of the gland determines the form of the secretion. For example, the clear consistency of normal saliva is a function of the serous nature of the parotid gland. Elimination of serous function as a consequence of radiation of the gland or the intake of certain drugs results in significant changes in the composition, function, and consistency of saliva. The gland lies over the masseter muscle and extends to the inferior border of the mandible and posteriorly. The duct to the pa-

rotid (Stensen's duct) opens at the level of the maxillary second molar (Fig. 43–2).

The submandibular gland is a mixed mucous and serous gland located in the floor of the mouth and extending forward about halfway down the mandible. The duct of the submandibular gland (Wharton's duct) enters the floor of the mouth just behind the mandibular incisors (Fig. 43–3).

The sublingual glands, lying anterior to the submandibular glands, are wholly mucous. Unlike the other major salivary glands, the sublingual glands do not have a large single excretory duct. Rather, they drain through a series of small ducts in the floor of the mouth.

Clinical Evaluation

The patient's history frequently provides useful clues to the diagnosis of salivary gland disease. The nature and duration of onset, as well as symptomatology, should be noted. In

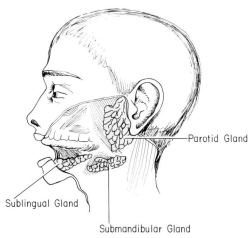

Figure 43–1. Anatomic relationships of the major salivary glands.

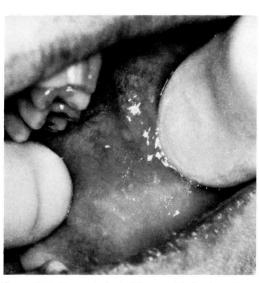

Figure 43–2. Stensen's duct of the parotid gland opening at the level of the maxillary secondary molar.

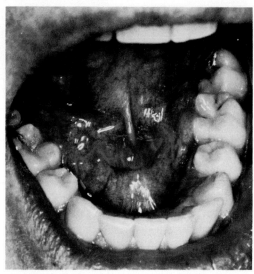

Figure 43–3. Wharton's duct. This enters the floor of the mouth behind the mandibular incisors and appears here as raised, bilateral, fleshy areas at the base of the lingual frenum.

patients who complain of salivary gland enlargement of acute onset or of periods of exacerbation followed by return of the gland to normal size, some form of inflammatory condition should be suspected. In contrast, the patient who notices progressive chronic enlargement of the gland may well have a tumor. As with other diseases, the medical history may provide clues associated with salivary gland disease. For example, xerostomia may be related to certain medications such as the phenothiazines or may represent a localized component of a systemic disease, such as Sjögren's syndrome.

Examination of the quality and quantity of saliva can be performed by observation. Saliva is normally clear and relatively free-flowing. Cloudy saliva may indicate infection. Occasionally, particulate elements can be noted in saliva, representing small sialoliths. Destruction of parotid gland function by radiation will eliminate many of the serous components of the saliva. As a result, the saliva appears thick and ropy. Chemical analysis of saliva might be helpful in diagnosing inflammatory diseases of the glands, although in most cases standard clinical and radiographic techniques provide adequate diagnostic information.

Each gland should be palpated to determine the presence of masses and the consistency of the gland. For the submandibular and sublingual glands this is best done using a bimanual technique (Fig. 43–4). Salivary function can be determined by applying pressure to the gland

to actually milk the glands. If the cheek is retracted and Stensen's duct visualized, extraoral pressure on the parotid gland permits clear visualization of the salivary flow. Definitive milking of the submandibular and sublingual glands is more difficult, but observation of the duct of the submandibular gland while stimulating function by talking about spices or food usually results in detectable flow.

Radiographic Evaluation

Radiographic techniques are frequently helpful in evaluating patients with suspected salivary gland disease. Conventional radiographs are of little value in observing the salivary glands or duct system except to demonstrate solid objects, such as sialoliths, in the ductal systems of either the sublingual or submandibular gland (Fig. 43–5). The most useful radiographic studies are either contrast studies, in which a radiopaque dye is injected into the ducts (sialography), or radionucleotide studies, in which the glands are labeled with an isotope (salivary scintigraphy).

Sialography is accomplished by the injection of radiopaque dye into a salivary gland duct. Blockages of ductal flow may be easily noted. Parenchymal abnormalities, such as inflammatory or neoplastic disease, are inferred from ductal changes (Fig. 43–6). Sialography is generally performed by oral surgeons or otolaryngologists.

Scintigraphy requires patient referral to a radiologist. The major indication for this pro-

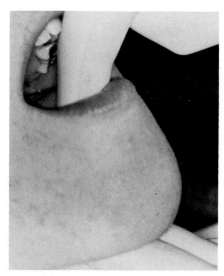

Figure 43–4. Bimanual palpation technique used for the examination of the submandibular and sublingual glands.

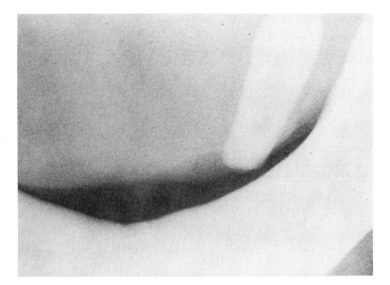

Figure 43–5. Tooth-shaped sialolith in the duct of the submandibular gland demonstrated by conventional radiography with the patient biting on an occlusal film.

cedure is suspected inflammatory or neoplastic disease. Scanning permits imaging of the glandular parenchyma and an assessment of functional status. The procedure relies on the ability of the salivary glands to concentrate isotope before it is secreted. Thus, the procedure involves a (sequential) visual recording of isotope uptake concentration and secretion using a gamma scintillation camera (Fig. 43–7). The sequential nature of the images produced provides functional data as well as information relative to pure anatomic changes. The technique is reasonably accurate, although a 22% false-negative rate has been reported.

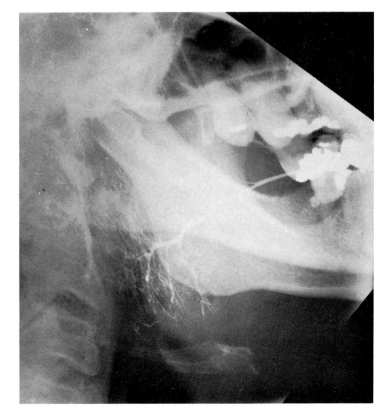

Figure 43–6. Sialogram of the parotid gland. (From Stafne, E. C., and Gibilisco, J. A.: Oral Roentgenographic Diagnosis, 4th ed. Philadelphia, W. B. Saunders, 1975.)

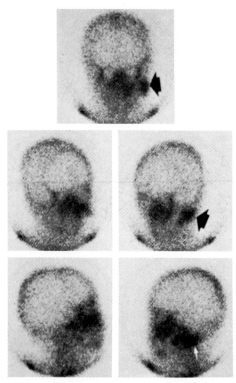

Figure 43–7. Left parotid accumulation of ⁶⁷Ga in a child who had radiation therapy to the left maxillary sinus and contiguous facial areas for fibrosarcoma. The arrow points to the parotid, which was irradiated; there was no neoplastic disease in the area. (From Gates, G.: Radionuclide diagnosis. In Laskin, D. M.: Oral and Maxillofacial Surgery, Vol. I. St. Louis, C. V. Mosby, 1980.)

INFLAMMATORY DISEASES

Inflammation of the salivary glands (sialadenitis) is usually the result of bacterial or viral infection. The glands are enlarged and painful and salivary flow is frequently disrupted. Often, the quality of saliva is also altered. Sialadenitis is clinically classified into acute and chronic forms.

Sialothiasis

Acute bacterial infections are frequently the result of stone formation within the salivary ducts. The stones, called sialoliths, are laminated calcified structures of a mineralized matrix or proteins and lipopolysaccharides calcified with calcium phosphate. The cause of sialolith formation is unresolved but may involve some disturbance in calcium balance, dehydration, stasis, and obstruction.

Stones may vary in size and therefore can produce a variety of symptoms (Fig. 43–8). Patients with stones are generally in some degree of pain. They may experience unilateral swelling of one of the major salivary glands, often at times of stimulation of salivary flow, such as mealtimes. When milked, flow from the duct is often intermittent and may be cloudy. Symptoms are related to the size of the stones. Small stones may pass unimpeded through the duct. Larger stones can result in complete obstruction. If saliva backs up, infection may occur and may cause systemic signs of infection.

Diagnosis of sialoliths is based on clinical history, examination, and radiographic examination. Treatment varies with the size of the stones. Stimulation of salivary flow with lemon drops and hydration of the patient is helpful. Antibiotic therapy should be considered when there has been evidence of stasis of salivary flow and of systemic involvement such as fever, malaise, or lymphadenopathy. Dilatation of the duct may be required to remove stones. Large stones that cannot be removed conservatively may necessitate surgical elimination.

Acute Bacterial Sialadenitis

Acute bacterial sialadenitis (acute parotid sialadenitis, ascending parotitis, suppurative parotitis, surgical mumps) is an acute infection

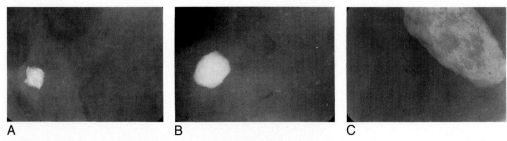

A   B   C

Figure 43–8. A–C, Salivary calculi of different sizes seen in the ducts of parotid glands. These are demonstrated by standard dental film placed on the inside of the cheek. (From Stafne, E. C., and Gibilisco, J. A.: Oral Roentgenographic Diagnosis, 4th ed. Philadelphia, W. B. Saunders, 1975.)

of the parotid gland originally seen almost exclusively in debilitated, elderly, dehydrated, or postoperative patients. It may also be associated with drugs that cause xerostomia or conditions associated with xerostomia (Sjögren's syndrome).

The major causative factor associated with acute bacterial sialadenitis seems to be a decrease in salivary flow. It is believed that parotitis results from a retrograde infection caused by stasis of saliva within the salivary duct, thereby producing a bacterially induced inflammatory state in the gland. Ductal trauma and hematogenous spread have also been cited as possible etiologies.

Acute bacterial parotitis is usually (80%) characterized by the sudden onset of unilateral firm erythematous swelling and localized pain and tenderness at the angle of the mandible, which then spread to involve the parotid gland. The gland increases in size so that the overlying skin becomes shiny and tense. A purulent discharge may be expressed from the parotid duct (Fig. 43–9). Simultaneously, the patient experiences systemic signs of infection characterized by fever, leukocytosis, chills, and malaise.

The organism most commonly isolated from the infected gland is penicillin-resistant *Staph-ylococcus aureus*. Other organisms may be isolated, however, including opportunistic and gram-negative organisms in patients who have been hospitalized for relatively long periods or who have become myelosuppressed as a result of malignancy or chemotherapy.

Management of the patient with acute bacterial parotitis is aimed at eliminating the infecting organism, rehydrating the patient, and eliminating purulent material, if needed. Discharge from the parotid duct in a patient suspected of having acute bacterial parotitis should be immediately cultured and analyzed for antibiotic sensitivity. After a culture is obtained, the patient should be empirically started on an antistaphylococcal semisynthetic penicillin, because most infections are caused by penicillin-resistant staphylococci (Chap. 46). The penicillin-allergic patient can be placed on clindamycin. Generally, patients should be hospitalized and should receive antibiotics by the intravenous route. Supportive care should be aimed at stimulation of salivary flow, application of moist heat to the affected area, rehydration, pain medication, and bed rest. Patients on antisialogogic drugs (Table 43–1) should have them discontinued. Surgical drainage may be required, depending on the involvement of the capsule of the gland.

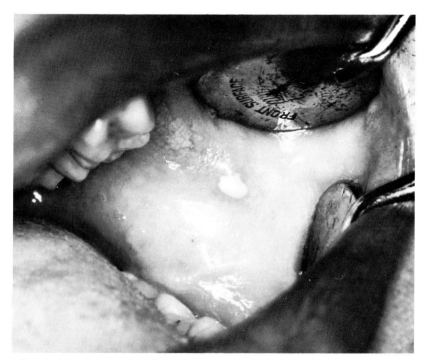

Figure 43–9. Purulent discharge from Stensen's duct. (From Topazian, R. G., and Goldberg, M. H.: Management of Infections of the Oral and Maxillofacial Regions, 3rd ed. Philadelphia, W. B. Saunders, 1993.)

Table 43–1. PARTIAL LIST OF DRUGS WITH ANTISIALOGOGIC PROPERTIES

Triprolidine HCl (Actifed)
Methyldopate HCl (Aldomet)
Atropine
Diphenhydramine HCl (Benadryl)
Chlorpheniramine maleate (Chlor-Trimeton)
Prochlorperazine (Compazine)
Chlorthiazide (Diuril)
Brompheniramine maleate, phenylephrine HCl, phenyl propanolamine HCl (Dimetapp)
Phenobarbital, atropine sulfate, hyoscine hydrobromide (Donnatal)
Dephenoxylate HCl with atropine sulfate (Lomotil)
Hydrochlorothiazide
Guanethidine monosulfate (Esimil)
Sinus tablets (Novahistine)
Simethicone, butabarbital sodium, belladonna alkaloids, atropine sulfate, and scopolamine hydrobromide (Sidonna)
Promethazine HCl (Phenergan)
Guaifenesin NF codeine phosphate (Robitussin)
Diazepam (Valium)
Meclizine HCl (Antivert)
Propantheline bromide (Pro-Banthine)
Dextroamphetamine sulfate (Dexedrine)
Reserpine
Acetaminophen and phenylpropanolamine (Sinubid)

Chronic Bacterial Parotitis

Unlike acute bacterial parotitis, chronic bacterial parotitis is most common in nondebilitated children and adults and is usually a sequela of chronic duct obstruction. The condition may also occur secondary to acute bacterial parotitis or as a consequence of Sjögren's syndrome. Because of its chronic nature, degeneration of the gland may result.

Chronic bacterial parotitis is characterized by a recurrent unilateral swelling of the parotid gland. Each episode is usually of rapid onset, but unlike acute bacterial parotitis, pain is not a consistent symptom. Similarly, because of the low-grade nature of the infection, fever, leukocytosis, and pus are not always present. The swelling may last for periods ranging from days to months, during which the infection seems to go through periods of remission. If pus is present, culture generally produces streptococci in children and a mixed streptococcal-staphylococcal flora in adults. As evidenced by sialography, a sialectatic pattern of the gland is present in which multiple cystic cavities occur instead of the normal glandular parenchyma.

Initially, conservative treatment of chronic bacterial parotitis is recommended. The ducts may be carefully dilated and irrigated with an antibiotic solution (15 mg/ml) of either eryth-romycin or tetracycline for 5 to 7 days. Systemic antibiotics may be administered.

For persistent cases, parotidectomy is the definitive therapy.

Viral Infection

Mumps

One of the most common forms of acute sialadenitis is that associated with mumps. Mumps is a communicable viral disease; the virus is transmitted in saliva. Although most common in children, the disease is not unusual in adults. Mumps is most frequently seen as an epidemic episode occurring in the winter or spring. The disease is caused by a paramyxovirus. Following an incubation period of about 2 to 3 weeks after exposure to the virus, patients develop fever, malaise, periauricular pain, headache, and chills for about 2 to 4 days. Bilateral enlargement of the parotids then occurs, with one parotid swelling before the other. The parotid duct may be enlarged and tender.

Parotid enlargement is maximal in about 3 days and then gradually subsides. Occurrence of the disease usually confers lifelong immunity. The submandibular and sublingual glands may also be involved. Orchitis and oophoritis are commonly mentioned complications of mumps. If bilateral, the infection can result in sterility. Nervous system, kidney, and pancreatic involvement may also occur.

The diagnosis of mumps is made largely on history, patient age, and bilateral distribution (usually) of parotid enlargement. The disease runs about a 1- to 2-week course, after which it resolves spontaneously. Treatment is palliative. It is important to ensure adequate levels of hydration.

Coxsackie A Virus

Coxsackie A virus may cause a parotitis. The virus, which also causes herpangina (Chap. 48), is most frequently seen in children during the summer and fall.

Following a 2- to 4-day incubation period, the patient becomes febrile, with a high fever. A sore throat usually develops, and intraoral examination demonstrates vesiculation of the posterior third of the oral pharynx. A bilateral parotitis may follow within 2 to 3 days. Lymphadenopathy, coated tongue, and gingivitis may occur simultaneously. Treatment is palliative. In young patients, adequate fluid intake may be difficult because of the patient's unwillingness to take food by mouth, because the pain on swallowing is great. Popsicles and flavored ice chips may be tolerated more easily. Patients should be closely monitored to ensure adequate hydration.

Cytomegalovirus

Cytomegalovirus may affect the salivary glands. Usually, the virus is disseminated and occurs almost universally in newborn or premature infants. Cases have also been reported in patients who are functionally myelosuppressed by diseases such as leukemia or individuals receiving immunosuppressive medication. Clinically, patients may present with salivary gland enlargement. The disease is usually fatal.

NONINFLAMMATORY, NONNEOPLASTIC SWELLINGS OF THE SALIVARY GLANDS

Sialadenoses

Noninflammatory swellings of the salivary glands are predominantly caused by drugs, endocrine disturbances, or nutritional deficiencies.

A number of drugs have been reported to cause salivary gland enlargement. Among these are sympathomimetic drugs such as isoproterenol. These drugs markedly increase secretion of the salivary glands and are thought to produce hyperplasia of the glands. Other drugs that interfere with autonomic nerve function may also affect gland size. Included among these are guanethidine and imidazolamine.

Enlargement of the salivary glands, especially the parotids, has been associated with some endocrine disturbances. The most consistent parotid changes have been noted in patients with diabetes mellitus. Less frequent are salivary gland changes associated with gonadal disturbances and hypothyroidism.

Nutritional deficiencies may result in salivary gland changes. Some investigators believe that vitamin A deficiency affects specialized epithelium such as that found in salivary glands and results in squamous metaplasia. Functionally, salivary retention follows, which results in inflammation of the gland. Deficiencies of niacin clinically produce pellagra, in which salivary gland changes have been reported. The role of thiamine deficiency in causing salivary gland enlargement is unresolved. Severe protein deficiency has also been associated with mumps-like swelling of the parotid glands. Interestingly, salivary gland enlargement has also been reported in patients with chronic alcoholism and Laennec's hepatic cirrhosis. Parotid gland enlargement has been reported in a number of cases of anorexia nervosa. This disease, usually seen in young women initially seeking weight control, results in functional nutritional deficiencies. It seems likely that the salivary gland changes ascribed to the condition are a result of these deficiencies.

SYSTEMIC GRANULOMATOUS DISEASES

Tuberculosis

Tuberculosis may affect the salivary glands and lymph nodes that lie in proximity to them (Chap. 20). The parotid gland is most commonly affected by this disease, usually secondary to pulmonary involvement. Patients present with firm, unilateral, nontender parotid swelling. Culture of drainage may yield acid-fast organisms. Chest film and skin testing also provide diagnostic information.

Sarcoidosis

Sarcoidosis may involve the parotid gland. When such involvement occurs, together with fever, lacrimal adenitis, and uveitis, the condition is termed uveoparotid fever. If there is also paralysis of the facial nerve, the condition is called Heerfordt's syndrome (10% of cases).

Sarcoidosis is a systemic granulomatous disease of unresolved cause that predominantly affects the heart, lungs, muscles, eyes, central nervous system, and liver. Infection, chemicals, and autoimmune reactions are all suggested causes of sarcoidosis. Cutaneous lesions, consisting of multiple (croppy) raised erythematous areas, may be ulcerated and occur in 50% of patients. The disease usually develops in blacks in the third or fourth decade of life. Sarcoidosis has been reported concomitant with HIV infection.

The clinical presentation of sarcoidosis is often subtle. Symptoms vary with the severity of disease but may include malaise, fever, and weight loss. Lymph node biopsy is used for definitive diagnosis. Laboratory tests, particularly showing increased levels of angiotensin converting enzyme, are also important. A skin test for sarcoidosis is the Kveim reaction. The test, which is positive in 50 to 80% of patients with the disease, consists of the intracutaneous injection of heat-sterilized human tissue from lymphoid tissue of patients with sarcoid. A positive reaction is noted if patients develop a histologically evaluated nodule 4 to 6 weeks after testing. Additional diagnostic tests include imaging studies with gallium-67.

The extent of parotid involvement is unresolved; the reported frequency varies from 5 to 60%. Parotid involvement usually is demonstrated by bilateral asymptomatic enlargement. Other salivary glands may also be affected. Chronic salivary gland enlargement is eventually followed by decreased function. Generally, there is no pus present.

Therapy is symptomatic, with corticosteroid treatment used as needed. Chloroquine, an antimalarial drug, has been shown to produce symptomatic improvement of skin and mucosal lesions.

SJÖGREN'S SYNDROME

Sjögren's syndrome is a chronic autoimmune disorder that affects the salivary glands and eyes. The condition may occur in the absence of connective tissue diseases (primary Sjögren's syndrome) or in association with them (secondary Sjögren's syndrome). Xerostomia is a consistent and prominent feature of the syndrome. Bilateral parotid involvement occurs in about 50% of cases. Lymphocyte infiltration of the salivary glands with replacement of the normal acinar anatomy accounts for the functional salivary changes. Dry eyes are the sequelae of keratoconjunctivitis sicca, which is caused by atrophy of the secretory epithelium of the eyes. Rheumatoid arthritis occurs in about half of the cases of Sjögren's syndrome; other connective tissue diseases, including systemic lupus erythematosus, polyarteritis, dermatomyositis, and scleroderma, may also be associated with the syndrome.

Sjögren's syndrome is seen predominantly in women of about 50 years of age. Women with the syndrome outnumber men by about 10%. Although unusual, Sjögren's syndrome has been reported in children and young adults. In patients with secondary Sjögren's syndrome, connective tissue disease precedes eye or salivary gland involvement. However, 10% of patients demonstrate dry eyes and xerostomia prior to the onset of connective tissue disease.

Although an autoimmune mechanism is now well established for Sjögren's syndrome, the exact cause of the condition is not as clear. There may be a genetic predilection for primary Sjögren's syndrome because specific tissue transplantation antigens are associated with the condition. However, some evidence suggests that an infectious etiology, probably viral, exists. In all cases, autoantibodies are produced and are directed against SSA/Ro antigens, which are nuclear and cytoplasmic polypeptides. Indirect immunofluorescence has demonstrated antisalivary gland antibody in a significant percentage of patients with the syndrome. The frequency of antibody demonstration seems to correlate with the severity of the disease. Additional evidence for an autoimmune etiology is suggested by the presence of lymphocytes infiltrating into the parenchyma of the salivary glands and the finding that these lymphocytes secrete IgG, IgM, and rheumatoid factor.

Although Sjögren's syndrome was originally considered a totally benign entity, there is now evidence to suggest an association of the syndrome with the development of lymphoreticular malignancies in a relatively small percentage of cases. Among the malignancies reported are lymphoma, reticulum cell sarcoma, and Waldenström's macroglobulinemia.

Diagnosis. The diagnosis of Sjögren's syndrome can usually be made clinically and confirmed by a variety of supplemental tests (Table 43–2). Biopsy of the minor salivary glands demonstrates focal sialadenitis. Autoantibodies can be demonstrated in serum.

Oral Findings. The most prominent oral manifestations of Sjögren's syndrome include xerostomia, bilateral parotid enlargement, and atrophy of the filiform and fungiform lingual papillae. As a consequence of the papillary atrophy, the lingual mucosa may appear red. Because of the lack of secretions, patients may experience oral bleeding and dysphagia. Angular cheilitis has also been reported.

Treatment of the oral problems associated with Sjögren's syndrome is palliative. The recommended regimen for other forms of xerostomia may be followed (Chap. 40). Artificial saliva, stimulation of salivary flow, and an anticaries protocol may be helpful. There is no satisfactory treatment for the overall syndrome.

Table 43–2. DIAGNOSIS OF SJÖGREN'S SYNDROME

Diagnostic Aid	Findings
Clinical	Usually women, around 50 years of age, 90% have connective tissue disease first; xerostomia; dry eyes; connective tissue disease (50% rheumatoid arthritis); atrophy of papillae of tongue; 50% salivary gland enlargement (parotids)
Immunofluorescence	Indirect immunofluorescence demonstrates presence of antisalivary duct antibody in about 25–70% of cases, depending on extent of disease
Salivary flow rate	Reduced (compared with normal of 1.0 ml/6 min/parotid gland when stimulated with lemon juice)
Secretory sialography	Injection of dye into salivary ducts may demonstrate abnormal patterns in glandular anatomy
Scintigraphy	Concentration of injected ^{99m}Tc-pertechnetate in salivary glands reduced as severity of disease increases
Biopsy	Biopsy of minor salivary gland of lower lip; salivary glands of lip classified to the extent of lymphocyte infiltration (0–3+)

DRY MOUTH

Dry mouth caused by xerostomia is a distressing problem for the patient and frequently a frustrating problem for the dentist. Unfortunately, it is relatively common. In evaluating the patient with xerostomia, the major differentiation to be made is in the determination of the underlying cause of the condition. There are three major factors that produce clinical manifestations of dry mouth: local conditions that produce drying of the mucosa, inherent diseases of the salivary glands or their ductal systems, and systemic conditions that affect salivary gland function.

Local factors that cause dry mouth are most common in younger individuals. Mouth breathing is a major cause of dryness in this group. Generally, this is most notable the morning after the patient sleeps with the mouth open. Gingival enlargement and inflammation, especially of anterior areas, may be noted in conjunction with this problem. Malocclusion (anterior open bite) and blockage of the nasal passages by a deviated septum or enlarged adenoids are frequent causes of mouth breathing. Patients may also note dryness of the throat and may snore. A cephalometric radiograph is often helpful in demonstrating enlarged adenoids. Treatment is aimed at rectifying the underlying problem.

Pipe smoking and, rarely, cigarette and cigar smoking may cause dry mouth. Although nicotine usually stimulates salivary flow, excessive smoking, especially of hot smoke (e.g., from pipe smoking), may result in dryness. Restoration of normal mucosal moisture usually occurs following elimination of smoking.

A number of medical conditions of the salivary glands, discussed elsewhere in this chapter, produce xerostomia. These fall into two major categories—conditions that cause obstruction of salivary flow, and conditions that actually affect the gland. Overall, xerostomia produced by salivary gland duct obstruction is not as dramatic as that caused by nonsalivary gland causes or inflammatory disease of the glands, because multiple ducts are rarely blocked simultaneously. In contrast, systemic inflammatory diseases such as mumps affect both glands. Resolution occurs with elimination of the source of ductal blockage or after recovery from the underlying inflammatory disease. Irradiation of the salivary glands produces fibrosis of the gland and causes xerostomia (Chap. 40).

A number of systemic factors affect the ability of salivary glands to respond to stimuli. It is well known that anxiety states may produce dryness of the mouth. For most individuals, this is a transient condition. If the patient is chronically anxious, however, psychiatric evaluation and treatment may be required.

A large number of drugs cause dryness of the mouth (Table 43–1). Among the most common are antihypertensive drugs (Chap. 4), sympathomimetics such as amphetamines, antihistamines, tricyclic antidepressants, and antiparkinsonian agents. There are many other medications that can also cause the condition. Thus, it is important to establish the medication history of the patient with dryness. Consultation with the product insert or a pharmacology text generally provides information as to whether xerostomia is a drug side effect. Usually, elimination of the medication reverses the condition.

Other systemic conditions may produce reduced salivary flow. In many cases, the dryness noted is dramatic. Some diseases of the central nervous system, such as multiple sclerosis or neoplasms, can result in xerostomia. Inexplicably, xerostomia is often associated with menopause. Atrophic changes of the salivary glands may cause reduced function in the elderly. Autoimmune diseases such as Sjögren's syndrome may also produce dry mouth.

Treatment. The treatment of dry mouth is aimed at elimination of the cause of the dryness, stimulation of remaining salivary gland function, and palliation. Salivary function may be stimulated by having the patient use sucrose-free lemon drops, which are commonly available at pharmacies or the dietetic section of markets. Some patients also respond well to lemon-glycerin swabs. Sugar-free gum may be of benefit.

Palliation can be most easily achieved through the use of a saliva substitute or mouth moisturizer (Chap. 40). For patients in whom dry mouth becomes a chronic problem, topical fluoride applications on a daily basis should be considered to prevent caries.

Recent studies suggest that pilocarpine, a cholinergic agonist, is effective as a sialagogue. Systemic administration of the drug to patients with Sjögren's syndrome or radiation-induced xerostomia has resulted in significant saliva production with few side effects. Typical dosage is 5 mg given three to four times daily.

MALIGNANT TUMORS OF THE MAJOR SALIVARY GLANDS

Tumors of the major salivary glands are rare. Most of these tumors (80%) occur within the parotid gland; 30% are malignant. Tumors of the sublingual (1%) and submandibular glands (10%) tend to have a greater tendency toward malignancy.

Malignancies of the major salivary glands are characterized by rapid growth and invasion of other anatomic structures. Much of the symptomatology associated with these tumors is a consequence of local invasion. Thus, pain, facial paralysis, paresthesia, and weakness of the tongue may be presenting symptoms in a patient with salivary gland malignancy. Lymphadenopathy may be noted. The gland itself usually demonstrates unilateral, nontender, firm, fixed swelling.

Clinical signs and symptoms are frequently helpful in differentiating benign from malignant salivary gland neoplasms (Table 43–3). As expected, the rate of growth of malignant neoplasms is greater than that of benign tumors. Although pain and seventh nerve paral-

Table 43–3. SALIVARY GLAND TUMORS

Feature	Benign	Malignant
Growth	Slow, steady	Rapid
Pain	Rare	May be present
Seventh nerve paralysis	None	May be present
Consistency	Rubbery	Firm
Attachment	None, mobile	Fixed
Trismus	None	May be present
Nodes	None	May be present

Adapted from Bales, H. W., and Norante, J. D.: Head and neck tumors. In Rubin, P. (ed.): Clinical Oncology for Medical Students and Physicians. Rochester NY, University of Rochester, 1974.

ysis are inconsistent findings, they are more likely to occur with malignancies. Whereas malignant neoplasms are board-hard and fixed, benign lesions tend to be rubbery and freely movable. Trismus and nodal involvement are rarely noted with benign lesions but may be present with malignancies. As with any neoplasm, clinical signs and symptoms are suggestions at best and must be supplemented with histologic studies for definitive diagnosis.

The diagnosis of salivary gland neoplasia is based on biopsy. Generally, patients suspected of having a salivary gland tumor should be referred to an oral surgeon, otolaryngologist, or head and neck surgeon. A consideration in obtaining the biopsy specimen is that only part of the salivary gland may be involved with tumor. Thus, it is possible that a limited biopsy site might miss the involved area. To avoid this, many surgeons advocate complete excision of the involved gland as part of the biopsy procedure of a potentially malignant lesion. Needle aspiration of multiple sites of a gland suspected of having tumor has also been suggested. Imaging with computed tomography or magnetic resonance imaging may be helpful in evaluating the extent of a particular lesion but should be used selectively.

Treatment and Prognosis. Treatment of parotid malignancies has relied heavily on surgical resection. However, because of the relationship of the facial nerve to the body of the gland, such surgery was often disfiguring. In an attempt to minimize this complication, surgical techniques have been modified to include resection of the superficial portion of the gland, in which 90% of the malignant parotid tumors are found. Radiation therapy has been used as an adjunct to surgery and to treat recurrent disease.

Malignancies of the submandibular gland tend to be more aggressive than those of the parotid. Hence, any nontender submandibular mass should be regarded as cancer until proven otherwise. As with parotid tumors, excision of submandibular tumors must be comprehensive and involves dissection of the submandibular triangle. Because of its proximity to the area, the lingual nerve is frequently resected. Radiation therapy may also be used.

Prognosis. Prognosis of salivary gland neoplasms is most dependent on the clinical stage of the tumor. As with oral squamous cell carcinoma, staging is based on the extent of the tumor and the presence or absence of nodal involvement and metastases (Table 43–4). Survival is significantly better with Stage I and Stage II tumors than with Stage III and Stage IV tumors (Fig. 43–10). Whereas the 10-year predicted cumulative survival rate is 74% for Stage I tumors, it is only 10% for patients with Stage IV disease. The clinical stage of the tumor is more predictive of outcome than is the histologic diagnosis. This finding demon-

strates the importance of early detection and treatment of salivary gland tumors. Older patients seem to have a worse prognosis than younger patients.

Specific Malignant Neoplasms

Mucoepidermoid Carcinoma

Mucoepidermoid carcinoma (Fig. 43–11) is one of the more frequent malignancies of salivary glands and affects both the major salivary glands, predominantly the parotid, and also the minor salivary glands, usually of the palate, tongue, and retromolar pad. Mucoepidermoid carcinoma generally occurs in patients between the third and sixth decades of life. Slightly over 30% of cases of mucoepidermoid carcinoma occur in patients between the ages of 21 and 30 years, although it may be seen in younger individuals. There is no sex predilection.

The clinical features of mucoepidermoid carcinoma depend largely on the grade of malignancy of the tumor. Whereas low-grade mucoepidermoid carcinomas tend to be slow, progressively growing, painless masses, high-grade malignancies grow at a faster rate, with pain as an early symptom. Of mucoepidermoid tumors involving the parotid gland, seventh nerve paralysis is common. Mucoepidermoid tumors that involve the retromolar pad may present with the same clinical appearance as a mucocele.

Mucoepidermoid carcinomas metastasize locally to regional nodes and distally to lung, bone, and brain. Subcutaneous metastases may also be observed.

Surgery is the treatment of choice for low-grade mucoepidermoid carcinomas; surgery combined with radiotherapy may be used for high-grade malignancies. The prognosis for mucoepidermoid carcinoma varies from 20% to over 90% depending on the stage of the tumor.

Cylindroma or Adenoid Cystic Carcinoma

These tumors are relatively common malignancies occurring within the parotid and submandibular salivary glands and also in the minor glands of the palate and tongue. Although the tumor can be seen at earlier ages, it is most commonly observed during the fifth and sixth decades of life. Clinically, the lesion feels semifirm, because it is cystic. There may be

Table 43–4. TNM CLASSIFICATION

T: Primary tumor
  TX: Minimum requirements to assess the primary tumor cannot be met
  T0: No evidence of primary tumor
  T1: Tumor ≤ 2.0 cm in greatest diameter, without significant local extension*
  T2: Tumor 2.0–4.0 cm in greatest diameter without significant local extension
  T3: Tumor 4.0–6.0 cm in greatest diameter without significant local extension
  T4a: Tumor > 6.0 cm in greatest diameter without significant local extension
  T4b: Tumor of any size with significant local extension*
N: Nodal involvement
  NX: Minimum requirements to assess the regional nodes cannot be met
  N0: No evidence of regional lymph node involvement
  N1: Evidence of regional lymph node involvement
M: Distant metastasis
  MX: Minimum requirements to assess the presence of distant metastasis cannot be met
  M0: No (known) distant metastasis
  M1: Distant metastasis present
Stage I
  T1, N0, M0
  T2, N0, M0
Stage II
  T3, N0, M0
Stage III
  T1, T2; N1, M0
  T4a, T4b; N0, M0
Stage IV
  T3, N1, M0
  T4a, T4b; N1, M0
  Any T, any N, M1

*Significant local extension is defined as evidence of tumor involvement of skin, soft tissues, bone, or the lingual or facial nerves.

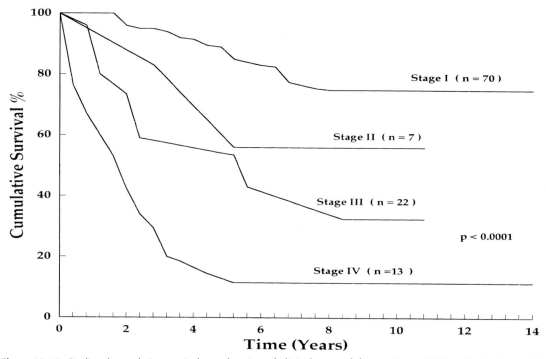

Figure 43–10. Predicted cumulative survival as a function of clinical stage of disease. (From O'Brien, C. J., Soong, S. J., Herrera, G. A., et al.: Malignant salivary tumors—analysis of prognostic factors and survival. Head Neck. Surg., 9[2]:82–92, 1986. Reprinted by permission of John Wiley & Sons, Inc.)

local pain and overlying fixation of the skin in the presence of continued swelling. Occasionally, the skin surface may be ulcerated. In the case of parotid involvement, seventh nerve paralysis may occur. Treatment consists of surgery and radiotherapy. Survival rate for cylindroma is stage-dependent.

Malignant Pleomorphic Adenoma

Malignant pleomorphic adenoma is relatively rare in comparison with benign pleomorphic adenoma. Although these lesions

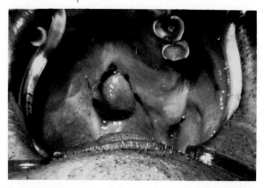

Figure 43–11. Mucoepidermoid carcinoma on the palate.

may appear benign histologically, they may metastasize. The malignant variety of pleomorphic adenoma is clinically similar to the benign lesion, although it tends to be faster growing and larger. It presents fixed to the tissue and may have surface ulceration. Pain appears to be a more frequent complaint with the malignant lesion than with the benign type.

Treatment consists of complete surgical excision, with the occasional use of radiotherapy. There is a high degree of local recurrence and local metastases. Distant metastases generally appear in the lung, bone, viscera, and brain.

Miscellaneous Malignant Tumors

Other types of malignancies may affect the salivary glands, including a variety of adenocarcinomas and epidermoid carcinomas. Generally, these tumors manifest themselves as progressive, firm, dense swellings of the glands, which are usually fixed to underlying tissue. When there is parotid involvement, there may be seventh nerve paralysis. These lesions tend to be painful. Regional lymphadenopathy is commonly noted.

Specific Benign Tumors

Pleomorphic Adenoma

Pleomorphic adenoma, also called benign mixed tumor, occurs frequently in both the major and minor salivary glands. It is the most common of all the tumors of the major and minor salivary glands, accounting for more than 50% of the tumors observed and about 90% of benign tumors. The most common site for pleomorphic adenoma among the major salivary glands is the parotid. Pleomorphic adenoma may also be observed in the submandibular glands, but only rarely in the sublingual glands. The chief intraoral sites for pleomorphic adenoma are the palate and upper lip. There is a question as to whether there is some sex predilection for these tumors, because some reports have suggested that women tend to develop these tumors more frequently than men by a 3:2 ratio. Although these lesions can occur in children and young adults, they are most commonly observed during the fourth through sixth decades of life.

Clinically, pleomorphic adenomas begin as painless, small, circumscribed, unilateral parotid swellings that slowly and intermittently increase in size. There is generally no fixation to the underlying tissue. The tumors feel rubbery to firm, with irregular margins. Although they are generally not painful, there may be local discomfort. Pleomorphic adenomas of the intraoral minor salivary glands clinically present the same findings, although they tend to be smaller. Patients usually become aware of them at an early stage because of interference with function.

Surgery is the treatment of choice for pleomorphic adenoma, with wide excision of the tumor. If there is not adequate excision, recurrence is inevitable. The extent of surgery varies with the size and extent of the tumor. Generally, these tumors are radioresistant and are therefore not amenable to radiotherapy.

Papillary Cystadenoma Lymphomatosum (Mikulicz's Disease, Adenolymphoma)

This rare and unusual condition combines both inflammatory and neoplastic features. It is thought to represent a process similar to Sjögren's syndrome but is more localized. The lesion is characterized by unilateral or bilateral swelling of the major salivary glands, predominantly the parotid. Although the swelling is usually asymptomatic, it may sometimes be accompanied by mild local discomfort or pain. Occasionally, xerostomia is observed. The swelling may proceed for months or years and may be associated with some other type of systemic inflammatory process such as upper respiratory infection, another oral infection, or oral manipulation. The cause of this condition is unknown. The disease tends to occur in late middle age. Sex predilection is uncertain. Clinically, there is an ill-defined enlargement of the involved gland. The enlargement tends not to be nodular. The lesion may not progress uniformly, but may have intermittent periods of growth and regression.

Treatment consists of surgical excision and radiotherapy. The prognosis is excellent.

TUMORS OF THE MINOR SALIVARY GLANDS

Tumors of the minor salivary glands are relatively rare (Tables 43–5 and 43–6). However, these structures are affected by both benign and malignant neoplasms. Minor salivary gland neoplasms are noted over a wide age range, from the early teens to the late seventies. In contrast to carcinoma of the oral cavity, malignancies of the minor salivary glands tend to occur in the early to mid- to late forties. A similar finding is true with respect to benign tumors of these glands. An interesting trend has been noted by some investigators, which suggests that tumors of the lip are more than twice as frequent in males than females and that the opposite trend is true for minor salivary gland tumors of the buccal mucosa.

The most common benign tumor of the minor salivary glands is benign mixed tumor. Of these, the majority occur on the posterior hard palate and the soft palate. The upper lip and buccal mucosa are the next most common sites (Table 43–6).

The most frequent malignant tumor of the minor salivary glands is cylindromatous adenocarcinoma. There is some controversy over the most frequent site for these tumors. Although most studies have indicated the palate as the predominant location, other investigators have reported that the retromolar pad is the most frequent site. The tongue is the next most common site for these malignancies, followed by the upper lip. Mucoepidermoid carcinoma, adenocarcinoma, and pleomorphic adenomas also occur fairly frequently.

There is little clinical difference between be-

Table 43–5. MALIGNANT TUMORS OF THE MINOR SALIVARY GLANDS AND THEIR LOCATION (1927–1960)

Tumor Type	Palate	Lip U	Lip L	Lip NS*	Cheek	Tongue	Jaws	Others	NS*	Total
Cylindromatous adenocarcinoma	104	6	1	5	17	62	12	2	6	215
Mucoepidermoid tumor	43	0	0	2	15	23	22	0	2	107
Adenocarcinoma	69	2	0	12	15	19	4	0	8	129
Pleomorphic adenoma	13	1	0	0	5	0	5	0	2	26
Papillary cystadenocarcinoma	3	0	0	0	0	1	1	0	0	5
Mucus-producing adenocarcinoma	0	1	0	0	0	0	0	0	2	3
Serous cell adenocarcinoma	1	0	0	0	0	0	2	0	0	3
Acinic cell adenocarcinoma	1	0	0	0	0	0	0	0	0	1
Squamous cell carcinoma	1	0	0	0	2	0	0	0	0	3
Unclassified	7	1	0	0	2	6	0	0	2	18
Undifferentiated	1	0	0	0	0	0	1	0	1	3
Unstated	0	0	0	0	0	0	0	0	7	7
Total	243	11	1	19	56	111	47	2	30	520

From Chaudhry, S. P., Vichers, R. A., and Gorlin, R. J.: Intraoral minor salivary gland tumors. Oral Surg., 14:1194, 1961.
*NS, not specified.

nign and malignant neoplasms of the minor salivary glands. These lesions usually present as nontender swellings of the glands. Pain may be a variable symptom, especially in association with advanced malignant lesions. Ulcera-tion of the surface of the lesions is rare. In the case of malignant disease, spread to regional lymph nodes must be evaluated.

Treatment of neoplasms of the minor salivary glands consists of local excision.

Table 43–6. BENIGN TUMORS OF THE MINOR SALIVARY GLANDS AND THEIR LOCATION (1927–1960)

Tumor Type	Palate	Lip U	Lip L	Lip NS*	Cheek	Tongue	Jaws	Others	NS*	Total
Pleomorphic adenoma	476	105	13	15	38	18	40	22	6	733
Adenoma	15	2	0	0	0	4	0	0	0	21
Myoepithelial adenoma	12	1	0	0	4	0	0	0	0	17
Papillary cystadenoma	9	1	0	0	4	1	0	1	0	16
Canicular adenoma	1	0	0	2	1	0	0	0	0	4
Fibroadenoma	3	0	0	0	0	0	0	0	0	3
Cystadenoma	1	0	0	0	0	0	1	0	0	2
Oncocytoma	0	0	0	0	0	1	1	0	0	2
Mucocyst adenoma	2	0	0	0	0	0	0	0	0	2
Total	520	108	13	17	47	24	42	23	6	800

From Chaudhry, S. P., Vichers, R. A., and Gorlin, R. J.: Intraoral minor salivary gland tumors. Oral Surg., 14:1194, 1961.
*NS, not specified.

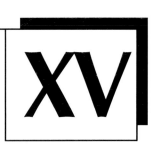

SECTION

XV

Evaluation and Management of the Patient with Disease of the Jaws

CHAPTER 44

Diseases of Bone

Bone is a complex tissue that is susceptible to a wide variety of disease processes. Bone frequently reflects metabolic disturbances and may also become a primary or secondary site for neoplastic diseases.

Bone and calcium metabolism are closely linked (Table 44–1). Thus, factors that affect calcium metabolism also affect the status of an individual's bone. Three major hormones influence calcium metabolism; parathyroid hormone (PTH), calcitonin, and vitamin D.

Parathyroid hormone, produced by the four parathyroid glands in response to low levels of serum calcium, has three major actions: it increases intestinal absorption of calcium; it increases renal reabsorption of calcium; and it stimulates bone resorption. Synthesis of activated vitamin D in the kidney is also stimulated. PTH is the most important regulator of the extracellular concentration of calcium.

Calcitonin is produced by the C cells of the thyroid gland. Despite much speculation, the lack of clinical disease associated with low levels of calcitonin places its physiologic significance in question. It has been suggested that calcitonin may play a role in bone resorption.

Vitamin D has been shown to play an important role in skeletal growth and maintenance. The vitamin undergoes a series of steps to become fully active. These take place in the skin, liver, and kidney. The activated compound then works in the gut to increase calcium absorption. Other functions include increasing absorption of phosphate by the gut, increased renal reabsorption of calcium and phosphate, and production of a bone-resorbing substance.

In addition to the preceding, a number of other compounds have significant effects on bone metabolism, growth, and absorption. Prostaglandins, which can themselves be produced by bone cells, may function as local regulators of bone growth. Depending on concentration, prostaglandins, mostly of the E class, may act as stimulators of bone resorption, causing osteolysis and hypercalcemia, or conversely they may stimulate bone formation.

Lymphocyte-derived factors (lymphokines) may cause changes in bone. Osteoclast-activat-

Table 44–1. REGULATION OF BONE METABOLISM

Regulator	Function
Glucocorticoids	Excess → ↓ skeletal growth and ↓ bone mass, ↓ bone formation; excess → ↓ intestinal absorption of calcium and phosphate and ↑ renal excretion
Insulin	Diabetes mellitus → osteoporosis
Parathyroid hormone	Most important regulator of extracellular calcium concentration; serum calcium → PTH → stimulates calcium from bone, renal tubular reabsorption of calcium, and synthesis of calcitriol (vitamin D function)
Vitamin D (calcitriol)	↑ mineral supply by stimulating calcium and phosphate transport systems in intestine
Prostaglandins	Stimulators of bone resorption; may cause osteolysis and hypercalcemia in neoplasia; local regulators of bone growth; also stimulators of bone formation; effect may be concentration-dependent; produced by bone cells
Osteoclast-activating factor (OAF)	Lymphocyte-derived, stimulates bone resorption and bone-collagen synthesis; can stimulate bone resorption in vitro; PTH and calcitriol can mobilize bone mineral; → ↓ impaired mineralization in children (rickets) and adults (osteomalacia)
Bone-derived growth regulators	Factors may have stimulatory effects on bone cell replication and matrix synthesis
Ions	Calcium may affect bone formation by controlling secretion of calcium-regulating hormones, by accelerating mineralization, and by ↑ matrix formation and cell proliferation Phosphate → effects in skeletal growth rate
Androgens and estrogens	Estrogens may ↓ osteoporosis by ↑ intestinal calcium absorption

ing factor (OAF) is released from sensitized lymphocytes on exposure to the sensitizing antigen and may result in osteoclast-mediated bone resorption. Other lymphokines that affect macrophages may result in bony changes through the release of enzymes or prostaglandins. Bone deposition may be stimulated by bone morphogenic protein and protein of the transforming growth factor (TGF)–β superclass.

Endocrine gland–derived hormones also seem to affect bone. Osteoporotic changes may be noted in patients with diabetes mellitus or increased adrenal function. Estrogens may reduce osteoporosis by increasing intestinal calcium absorption.

Clearly, the balance between bone deposition and resorption represents a complex interaction of many factors (Fig. 44–1). Alteration of any of these factors may produce disease.

DISEASES OF BONE METABOLISM

Osteoporosis

Osteoporosis is the most common disease of bone metabolism. It has been estimated that between one-quarter and one-third of patients over 60 years of age have osteoporosis. More than 1.5 million women in the United States are said to be affected by the disease. Osteo-

porosis is about twice as common in women as in men. This may relate to the finding of increased bone loss in postmenopausal women and in women whose ovaries have been removed.

The cause of osteoporosis is still not completely resolved, because a number of conditions appear to be related to the disease. Hormonal changes, notably reduction in estrogen production, seem to be significant and are thought to cause primary osteoporosis. Steroids and thyroid hormone may produce osteoporotic changes. Osteoporosis has been reported in patients following organ transplant, but this may be related to steroids administered for immunosuppression. Other causes of osteoporosis include high levels of heparin intake, prolonged immobilization, osteogenesis imperfecta, and other inherited disorders. In addition to hormone-mediated effects on bone, age-related bone loss has been described in men and women. This type of osteoporosis is referred to as type II or involutional osteoporosis.

Clinically, the most frequent manifestation of osteoporosis occurs in the vertebrae, which undergo spontaneous fracture and produce severe, acute-onset back pain. This may cause the patient to seek medical attention. Fracture of the long bones spontaneously, or in response to minimal trauma, may also occur. Healing usually occurs, although the bones never return to their normal form or strength.

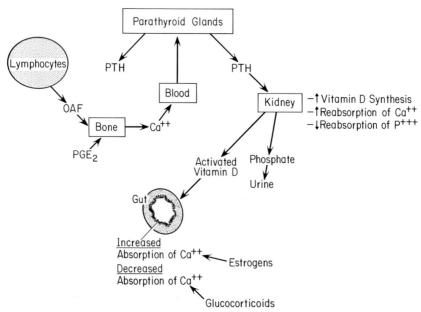

Figure 44–1. Some factors that regulate bone metabolism. These include parathyroid hormone (PTH), lymphocyte-produced osteoclast-activating factor (OAF), vitamin D, prostaglandins, and glucocorticoids.

In cases of osteoporosis in which a definitive cause can be established, elimination of the underlying cause generally cures the disease. For example, in cases of osteoporosis resulting from an overt endocrine cause, surgery is usually curative. However, therapy for primary osteoporosis is less clear-cut and includes mobilization, physical therapy, calcium and vitamin supplements, estrogens, and perhaps fluoride.

The oral findings of osteoporosis are not unlike the findings in other bones. Thinning of the cortical plate and loss of trabeculation are noted. It has been suggested that edentulous patients with osteoporosis are more likely to demonstrate increased resorption under dentures. Other clinical considerations include increased risk of fracture during extraction, delayed healing of extraction sites, and an increase of referred pain to teeth from thinned maxillary sinuses. The role of osteoporosis in the development of periodontal disease is not clear.

Laboratory findings are shown in Table 44–2.

Disorders of Vitamin D Metabolism

Disorders of vitamin D metabolism produce rickets in children and osteomalacia in adults. Vitamin D plays an important role in bone and calcium metabolism by increasing calcium and phosphate absorption from the intestines and increasing calcium and phosphate reabsorption in the kidneys.

Vitamin D metabolism consists of a complex series of events that involves the skin, liver, kidney, and intestine. Any disease that modifies action of these organs or the patient's ability to absorb the vitamin may produce disease. The major causes of osteomalacia are dietary vitamin D deficiency and lack of exposure to sunlight. Generally, dietary vitamin D deficiency is extremely rare, because many foods are fortified with the vitamin. Osteomalacia may occur in elderly, homebound adults or in strict vegetarians.

Drug-induced osteomalacia may result from the interference of drugs with vitamin D metabolism. Anticonvulsant drugs, specifically diphenylhydantoin and phenobarbital, are most frequently implicated as causing this condition. The incidence of rickets or osteomalacia has been reported to range from 4 to 75% and seems attributable to the relatively ubiquitous finding of alterations in hepatic enzyme activity.

A variety of gastrointestinal malabsorption syndromes, including sprue, regional enteritis, prolonged biliary obstruction, and chronic pancreatic insufficiency, may also result in osteomalacia because of inadequate vitamin D absorption. Additionally, patients with chronic renal failure and, to a lesser extent, patients who have received renal transplants may have bony changes as a consequence of altered vitamin D metabolism.

Clinically, retarded skeletal growth, bowing of the legs, and other skeletal deformities are the signs of rickets. Teeth developing during periods of rickets show hypoplastic enamel. Osteomalacia in adults may produce weakness, ataxia, and skeletal pain.

Laboratory findings in osteomalacia include normal or reduced calcium, reduced phosphorus, and elevated alkaline phosphatase and parathyroid hormone levels (see Table 44–2).

The oral findings associated with vitamin D deficiency are not uniform and may not be dramatic. Enamel hypoplasia, delayed tooth eruption, and abnormal dentin may be noted in children with rickets during odontogenesis and eruption. Both patients with rickets and patients with osteomalacia may demonstrate widened trabecular patterns of bone and indistinct lamina dura. It has been reported that patients with osteomalacia are prone to chronic periodontal disease.

Table 44–2. LABORATORY FINDINGS IN METABOLIC BONE DISEASE

Disease	Calcium	Phosphorus	Alkaline Phosphatase	Parathyroid Hormone
Osteoporosis	N or ↓	↓	↑	↑
Osteomalacia	T, N, or ↓	N	↑	N
Hyperparathyroidism (primary)	↑	↓	↑	↑
Osteitis deformans	N	N	N	N

N, normal; ↓, decreased; ↑, increased.

Hyperparathyroidism

Parathyroid hormone (PTH) is probably the single most important regulator of extracellular calcium. Hyperparathyroidism occurs by one of two major mechanisms, depending on whether it is primary or secondary. Primary hyperparathyroidism is the consequence of excess secretion of PTH by the gland. In most cases (about 75%), primary hyperparathyroidism is the result of the presence of a single parathyroid adenoma. Other causes include hyperplasia of the gland and carcinoma. Secondary hyperparathyroidism develops in response to hypocalcemia and in most cases is a reflection of renal disease in which there is increased calcium loss. Laboratory examination in patients with hyperparathyroidism demonstrates significant increases in serum calcium levels. Alkaline phosphatase levels may also be elevated (see Table 44–2).

Clinically, the manifestations of hyperparathyroidism vary significantly, depending on the severity of the disease. Mild forms may be completely asymptomatic. Renal colic of chronic onset tends to occur in moderate forms of the disease. Patients with more severe disease may note bone pain, debility, weight loss, weakness, and renal colic. Bone, renal, and gastric disturbances may also be manifestations of hyperparathyroidism.

Generally, oral changes associated with hyperparathyroidism occur when the disease is fairly advanced. It is unusual for oral changes to be the presenting sign of the disease. As expected, the oral changes of hyperparathyroidism reflect alterations in calcium metabolism. Classically, loss of the lamina dura is cited as a significant oral finding. Additionally, patients may demonstrate an altered trabecular pattern of bone characterized as having a ground-glass appearance (Fig. 44–2). Intrabony and extrabony giant cell tumors may form.

Treatment of hyperparathyroidism is aimed at elimination of the underlying causal factors. Surgery is generally the treatment of choice for primary hyperparathyroidism. Clearly, subsequent management of calcium levels is important. Other forms of the disease are treated medically.

Fibrous Dysplasia

Fibrous dysplasia is a disorder in which fibrous connective tissue replaces the normal bone. Although the precise cause is unknown,

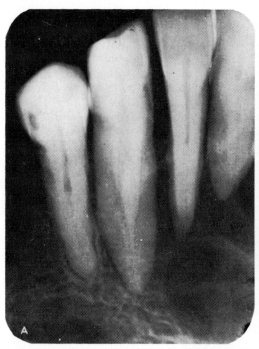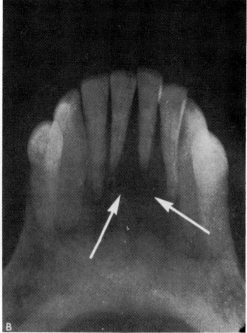

Figure 44–2. *A, B,* Hyperparathyroidism. The absence of the lamina dura and the ground-glass appearance of bone can be noted. The arrows demonstrate PTH-induced radiolucencies. (From Shafer W. G., Hine M. G., and Levy B. M.: A Textbook of Oral Pathology, 3rd ed. Philadelphia, W. B. Saunders, 1974.)

the process is thought to be developmental. There are two forms of the disease: monostotic fibrous dysplasia, in which a single bone is involved, and polyostotic fibrous dysplasia, in which there is multiple bone involvement. The former is more common than the latter by a ratio of about 4:1. The condition demonstrates a female predilection by a ratio of about 2:1.

Monostotic fibrous dysplasia generally begins when patients are in their twenties or early thirties, whereas the polyostotic form presents about 15 years earlier. Monostotic fibrous dysplasia may affect any bone. The jaws are involved in about 20% of cases, with the maxilla affected about twice as frequently as the mandible.

Monostotic fibrous dysplasia of the jaws generally begins as a painless, progressive swelling. Usually the buccal or labial plate demonstrates expansion. Patients may note changes in the position of their teeth and occasional sensitivity within the bone. Maxillary involvement, especially in children, may lead to facial deformities or malocclusions.

The radiographic manifestations of monostotic fibrous dysplasia are variable (Figs. 44–3 to 44–5) but basically fall into one of three patterns. Radiographs may demonstrate unilocular or multilocular patterns. Alternatively, the former appearance may be noted with an increase in trabeculation, which gives the film a mottled appearance. Finally, like other conditions of bone, a ground-glass pattern may be noted. In some instances, roots of teeth may be displaced, but it is unusual to observe external root resorption.

Treatment of monostotic fibrous dysplasia is aimed at surgical resection of the involved tissue, if possible. If the area of involvement precludes total removal because of the potential

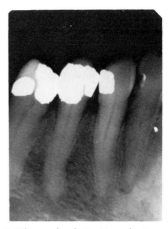

Figure 44–3. Fibrous dysplasia. Note the increased radiodensity.

of a significant postoperative deformity, a block resection of the area (shell-out procedure) may be attempted.

There have been a number of reports of spontaneous transformation of fibrous dysplasia to osteosarcoma or chondrosarcoma. However, it has been suggested that such changes might be related to treatment of fibrous dysplasia with radiotherapy.

There are two forms of polyostotic fibrous dysplasia. The first type involves more than one bone, although most bones are normal. Café-au-lait skin pigmentation often occurs simultaneously, in which case the disease bears a strong resemblance to neurofibromatosis. The most significant clinical problem is a predisposition to fracture. In the second form, almost all bones are affected. In addition, patients demonstrate disturbances of pigmentation and endocrine function. The triad of fibrous dysplasia and disturbances of pigmen-

Figure 44–4. A, B, Fibrous dysplasia. Note the locular radiopacity.

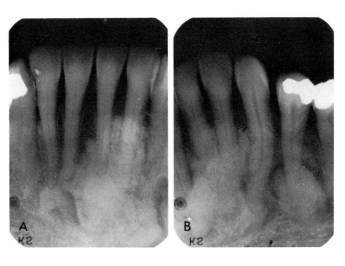

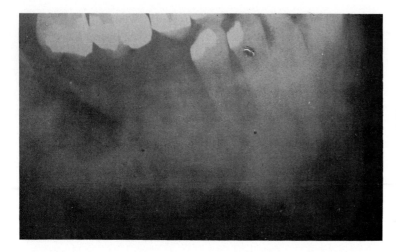

Figure 44–5. Fibrous dysplasia involving the mandible.

tation and endocrine function make up Mc-Cune-Albright syndrome.

McCune-Albright syndrome is a relatively rare condition that is usually first noted at an early age. Fibrous dysplasia affects most bones and produces aching bone pain, the most common symptom. Deformity of the facial bones may occur, and spontaneous fracture is not uncommon. Skin lesions, characterized by café-au-lait pigmentation, and manifestation of precocious puberty as well as other endocrine problems are noted.

The oral lesions of McCune-Albright syndrome are relatively common. About one-third of patients demonstrate mandibular involvement, which consists of expansion and deformity of the jaw. Inevitably, the tooth eruption pattern is altered. Radiographs of mandibular lesions demonstrate a multilocular cystic appearance with a reduction in bone density and an altered trabecular pattern. Serum alkaline phosphatase may be elevated.

Treatment may consist of surgery or radiotherapy.

Cherubism

Cherubism is a rare hereditary (autosomal dominant) disease that affects the maxilla and mandible. The condition presents as a progressive symmetric swelling of the mandible and/or the maxilla that is usually present by 3 or 4 years of age. The mandible is more often involved than the maxilla. There are no systemic features. The child often presents with a roundish mandible, giving a chipmunk-like appearance.

On examination, patients present with rock-hard bilateral swelling of the jaws. Lymphade-nopathy may be present but is not a universal finding. Premature loss of the deciduous teeth may be noted with possible defects in the permanent dentition. Radiographic examination demonstrates severe destruction of the jaws as manifested by extensive bilateral radiolucencies. There is thinning and expansion of the cortical plates. There are no significant laboratory findings.

It appears that cherubism may be self-limiting and undergo spontaneous remission during puberty. Corrective surgery may be considered to improve esthetics after that period.

Osteitis Deformans (Paget's Disease)

Osteitis deformans, or Paget's disease, is a chronic, slowly progressing disease in which there is an abnormality of bone remodeling characterized by both osteoblastic activity and osteolysis, the former being more prevalent. The cause of Paget's disease is unknown, but a possible circulatory disturbance has been suggested. The disease may involve one bone or many. Paget's disease occurs in individuals over the age of 40 and increases in prevalence with age. Men tend to be affected at a slightly greater frequency than women.

Patients with osteitis deformans may experience bone pain, headache, deafness, blindness, Bell's palsy, dizziness, changes in mental status, joint pain, and postural changes. On examination, bony enlargement may be appreciated in bones of the skull (Fig. 44–6). Changes in gait may be noted as a result of bowing of the legs. Spontaneous fracture is relatively common. It has been suggested that the increased osseous vascularity may be felt by

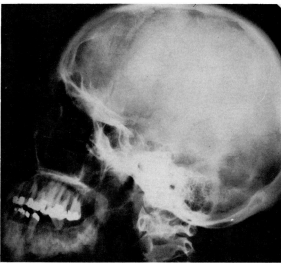

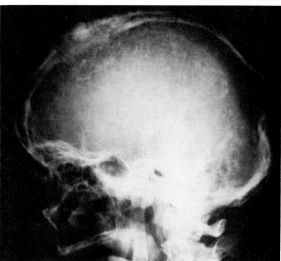

Figure 44–6. Paget's disease characterized by changes in the skull *(A)* and mandible *(B)*.

the examiner as increased heat over bony areas.

Paget's disease is characterized by marked elevations in alkaline phosphatase levels in the presence of normal calcium and phosphorus levels (see Table 44–2).

Involvement of the jaws is noted in about 20% of patients with osteitis deformans. The maxilla is more often involved than the mandible. The maxilla enlarges, causing an increase in the size of the ridge, flattening of the palate, and increased spacing between teeth. Increased tooth mobility is often reported. Edentulous patients who wear dentures complain of improper fit of their prostheses.

Radiographic examination demonstrates variable findings, depending on the stage of the disease. Radiographs show a characteristic ground-glass appearance.

There is no specific treatment for Paget's disease. The thrust of treatment is palliative and consists of analgesics and mild nonsteroidal anti-inflammatory drugs (NSAIDs). Patients with Paget's disease should be followed closely, because they are predisposed to develop osteosarcoma.

HISTIOCYTOSIS X

Histiocytosis X is a collective term used to describe three nonlipid reticuloendothelioses, which include a localized form (eosinophilic granuloma), a chronic disseminated form (Hand-Schüller-Christian syndrome), and an acute disseminated form (Letterer-Siwe disease). The cause of histiocytosis X is unclear, although a number of investigators have suggested that the disease represents a reactive process and is not a true neoplasm. At one time, histiocytosis X was thought to be a disorder of lipid metabolism. There is a lack of histiologic evidence to support this theory. Among the causes suggested for the disease are an immune hypersensitivity reaction to a virus, intestinal malabsorption, smoking, pituitary dysfunction, autoimmunity, and viral infection. The disease is not hereditary and there is no sex predilection. The frequency of reported oral involvement is variable, ranging from 10 to 77%.

The mildest form of histiocytosis X is eosinophilic granuloma, in which solitary (monostotic) or multiple (polyostotic) lesions are found in bone. There is no nonskeletal involvement. The ribs, pelvis, flat bones, and skull are most frequently involved. The disease primarily affects children and young adults. The lesions are composed of large numbers of reticuloendothelial and eosinophilic cells. Mandibular involvement is common and generally occurs in the posterior region of the jaw (Fig. 44–7). Radiographically, there is evidence of a destructive process of bone that may also affect roots of teeth. Definitive diagnosis is made by biopsy.

Clinically, a tender swelling or mass is the most common complaint. Other signs and symptoms may include gingivitis, tooth mobility, oral ulceration, poor healing, and a bad taste in the mouth.

Although lesions of eosinophilic granuloma may heal spontaneously, treatment is usually surgical and consists of curettage of the bony defects. Lesions may heal even with incomplete removal of diseased tissue. Radiation at low doses (700 to 1500 cGy) has been used to treat disseminated forms of the disease, as has

chemotherapy. The prognosis for patients with eosinophilic granuloma is good.

Hand-Schüller-Christian (HSC) syndrome is the chronic disseminated form of histiocytosis X. As with eosinophilic granuloma, this syndrome generally affects children over 3 and young adults. The syndrome refers to a triad of findings, which includes bony lesions of the skull, exophthalmos, and diabetes insipidus. However, it is rare for a patient to demonstrate all three signs. Generally, lesions are found outside bone, the most common oral location being the gingiva, where lesions usually appear in an ulcerative form. Histologically, lesions demonstrate masses or sheets of foamy reticuloendothelial cells. Radiographically, destructive lesions of bone are noted, particularly in the mandible. Diagnosis is made by biopsy.

Clinical signs or symptoms include precocious exfoliation of teeth, tooth mobility, or an enlarged painful mass. Probably because of the severe bony defects around the teeth, patients may also complain of bad breath or a foul taste. Treatment for Hand-Schüller-Christian syndrome includes surgical curettage or excision of accessible lesions. Chemotherapy using a variety of agents including vinblastine sulfate, prednisone, etoposide, and cyclophosphamide has reportedly been effective in reducing the progression of the disease. Extraskeletal involvement and young age are both negative factors in determining prognosis. Generally, there is a chronic, increasingly severe course.

The most severe form of histiocytosis X is the acute disseminated form, Letterer-Siwe disease. The age of onset for Letterer-Siwe disease is usually under 3, but infants are commonly affected. Jaw lesions are less common than in other forms of histiocytosis X. Clinical

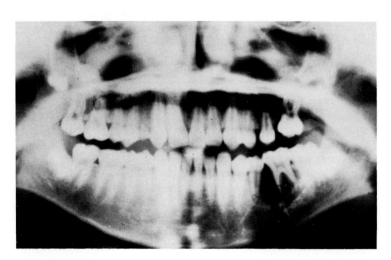

Figure 44–7. Histiocytosis X. The eosinophilic granuloma is affecting the mandibular left first molar. Note the floating appearance of the tooth.

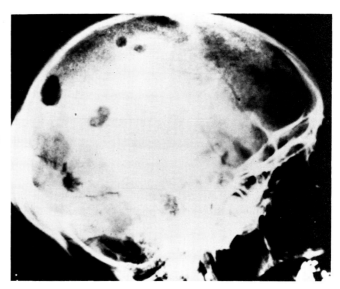

Figure 44–8. Punched-out lesions of multiple myeloma.

findings are varied and include fever, otitis media, hepatomegaly, anemia, lymphadenopathy, bleeding, seborrhea, and eczema, in addition to bony lesions. The course of the disease is usually rapid and fatal as a result of organ involvement and bleeding and infection. There is no satisfactory treatment.

MULTIPLE MYELOMA

Multiple myeloma is a plasma cell neoplasm originating in bone marrow that causes widespread bone destruction with subsequent hypercalcemia, immunosuppression, anemia, and thrombocytopenia.

There is some controversy relative to sex predilection of the disease; a more frequent involvement of men has been suggested by some, whereas others have claimed equal distribution between the sexes. The disease is most commonly observed in patients in their mid-fifties, although multiple myeloma occurs between the ages of 40 and 70.

Patients most often present with skeletal pain. It is unknown how long the disease is present before symptoms appear. However, a prodromal period of up to 20 years has been reported in some patients. Generally, the disease affects many bones. Untreated, multiple myeloma progresses to cause severe skeletal pain. Pathologic fractures may occur. Radiographically, multiple myeloma presents a characteristic picture of punched-out lesions in bone (Fig. 44–8).

Oral involvement in multiple myeloma is common and involves the presence of lesions in the mandible or maxilla or both. About 80% of patients with the disease develop jaw manifestations, which are characterized as radiolucent ovoid lesions. Patients may also experience symptoms frequently associated with malignancies, including paresthesia, swelling, tooth mobility, and tooth movement. Soft tissue involvement has been reported. In these cases, the lesions appear as gingival enlargements.

Because multiple myeloma is a malignancy involving plasma cells, characteristic laboratory findings associated with plasma cell function are a unique feature of the disease. Light chains called Bence Jones proteins are found in the urine in about 75% of patients with multiple myeloma. Anemia is also a feature of the disease.

Chemotherapy, radiation therapy, and bone marrow transplantation are the current modes of treatment to control the disease.

45

Temporomandibular Joint Disorders

Facial pain is the most common acute problem presenting to the dentist. Most often, the cause is an odontogenic infection of endodontic or periodontal origin. Routine tests of tooth percussion and palpation, pulp testing, intraoral soft tissue examination, periodontal probing, and periapical radiographs typically yield the appropriate diagnosis. The diagnosis of nonodontogenic facial pain, however, may be more perplexing. Basal bone pathology, sinus pathology, trigeminal neuralgia, other localized neurologic disorders (e.g., tic douloureux), or systemic disease (e.g., multiple sclerosis), although important diagnostic considerations, are relatively uncommon disorders.

Second in incidence to odontogenic infection as a source of facial pain are disorders of the temporomandibular joint (TMJ). Classically, a patient with TMJ disease presents with pain and tenderness, joint noises, and limitation of mandibular motion. The vast majority of TMJ disorders are functional in character and are the result of a complex interaction of several variables, including psychologic stress, bruxism, muscle spasm, occlusal disharmony, and iatrogenic insult. This syndrome is variously known as TMJ pain dysfunction syndrome, TMJ syndrome, and myofacial pain dysfunction syndrome.

DIAGNOSIS

Diagnosis of TMJ disorders is the result of an analysis of the history and physical and radiologic examinations (Fig. 45–1). The dentist first considers the general diagnosis when the patient reports a syndrome of pain, tenderness, joint noises, and limitation of motion in the absence of odontogenic infection.

In patients with TMJ pain in which anxiety is an important causative factor, the history may provide the most significant source of information leading to a functional diagnosis. Patients should be queried specifically about the longevity of symptoms, time of day when symptoms are most severe, and factors precipitating the onset of symptoms.

Pain and limitation of motion are the two most important symptoms. Muscle tenderness may be elicited by clinical examination but not reported by the patient, whereas the presence or absence of joint noise, either clicking or crepitus, may be a false-positive or false-negative sign. The most common muscles involved in spasm are those of mastication: the masseter muscle, the pterygoids, and temporalis muscle. Other head and neck muscles including the sternocleidomastoid and trapezius may also be affected. Limited opening occurs with multiple masticating muscle involvement, or deviation on opening implicates dominant spasm of the lateral pterygoid muscle on the side of the deviation. A history of bruxism and psychologic stress is common.

Pain may also be localized to the temporomandibular joint. Here the cause can often be the result of a functional discrepancy in the joint head–articular disk relationship. Once a TMJ disorder is suspected, the essential diagnostic consideration is to rule out organic pathology. Trauma, arthritis, tumor, and ankylosis may account for classic TMJ signs and symptoms. A detailed history regarding acute trauma, such as a blow to the chin, may suggest fracture or ankylosis. The presence of a mass on the condylar region suggests a tumor, whereas dominant symptoms directly related to the joint may result from arthritic pathology, particularly for those patients with a history of generalized arthritis. Such case histories require a high index of suspicion for organic pathology and extraordinary diagnostic procedures may be advisable.

Radiographic Evaluation

Because of its anatomy and orientation, the temporomandibular joint is not easy to radiograph. The approach to radiographic evalua-

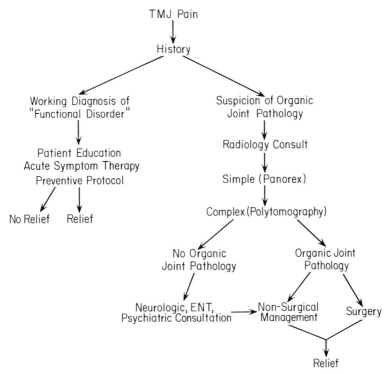

Figure 45–1. Clinical approach to patients presenting with temporomandibular pain.

tion should be one of logical sequence of increasing complexity. Radiographs are not necessary for many patients whose TMJ symptoms are of a functional nature. Rather, radiographic diagnosis is of significance in degenerative joint disease, neoplasia, and trauma.

A variety of projections are available for radiographic evaluation of the temporomandibular joint. The panoramic radiograph offers the advantages of easy availability and bilateral projection of the TMJ and condyles. Although the resolution of the TMJ is not exceptional, trauma and neoplasms are usually easy to visualize. Thus, the panoramic radiograph is often a good screening device for TMJ pathology. Its disadvantages are its poor resolution of detail and lack of functional assessment.

Standard radiographic technique can be used in the dental office for visualization of the TMJ. The transpharyngeal projection is a relatively simple technique, requiring only an intraoral cassette with an intensifying screen. A standard dental x-ray machine is used.

For many years, computed tomography has provided the best data for radiographic evaluation of the TMJ. This technique offers the advantage of functional assessment of the joint. It is generally ordered from hospital radiology departments.

Functional assessment of soft tissue pathology of the TMJ may be obtained with the use of arthrography. In this technique, a water-soluble contrast medium is injected into the synovial spaces of the joint. By placing medium into the spaces above and below the articular disk, the disk may be visualized.

Generally, the technique is performed with the patient going through a series of movements so that the position of the disk and its relationship to the joint spaces may be dynamically assessed. Arthrography requires thorough knowledge of anatomy of the temporomandibular joint. Placement of the dye into the joint space is technically difficult but usually is accomplished by a radiologist experienced in this technique. There is a low complication rate associated with arthrographic examinations.

Interpretation of Results

As mentioned, history and clinical examination generally yield more information about the nature of TMJ disorders than extensive radiographic evaluation. The major role of radiographs is thus to determine the presence of organic pathology as the cause for TMJ symptoms.

Radiographic studies provide data regarding

the hard and soft tissues of the TMJ. Films should be evaluated for condylar shape, condylar surface erosion, ankylosis, integrity of the articular disk, position of the articular disk and condyles during movement, and neoplasia.

DENTAL MANAGEMENT

Once the initial diagnosis of a functional TMJ disorder is made, the dentist must elect a therapeutic regimen. In order of approach, this should include patient education, acute symptomatic relief, a preventive protocol, and the consideration of secondary consultations.

Patient Education

All patients, but particularly those with TMJ disorders, must understand the cause of their disorder. The most successful clinician is one with patience and understanding who informs the patient and does not offer a panacea but rather an approach to the chronic control of TMJ symptoms. A discussion of the interaction of stress, bruxism, muscle spasm, and occlusion variables is crucial. The clinician should never lose sight of studies that report significant therapeutic success with patient education and placebo therapy only.

Acute Symptomatic Relief

Detailed strict orders regarding rest, soft diet, and moist heat application are essential. Anti-inflammatory medications and analgesia may also be necessary. Therapeutic choices range from prescribing simple aspirin or aspirin and codeine preparations to the use of nonsteroidal anti-inflammatory drugs (NSAIDs) with analgesic properties such as ibuprofen (Motrin). Muscle relaxants may also be an integral part of initial acute symptomatic relief.

Depending on the severity of the case, the clinician may choose maximum muscle relaxant therapy by prescribing diazepam (Valium) for adults, in doses ranging from 2 to 10 mg tid or qid. The disadvantages are dose-dependent mental impairment and reflex slowing, which may preclude daytime use. The potential drug interaction of diazepam with other central nervous system depressants such as the narcotic analgesics must also be considered. Alternative choices are less potent muscle relaxants with less prominent mental impairment and no interaction with narcotic analge-

sics. In the less severe case, the primary advantage of these drugs is to allow a patient to continue normal daytime activities (with variable drowsiness) while taking therapeutic doses of the medication. These alternative drugs may also allow the concomitant use of potent analgesics when pain predominates. There is little to choose from among the alternative muscle relaxants to diazepam. The choice is often based on familiarity and individual preference. Examples include methocarbamol (Robaxin), carisoprodol (Soma), cyclobenzaprine HCl (Flexeril), orphenadrine citrate (Norflex), and various combinations with aspirin, acetaminophen, and codeine (Robaxisal, Norgesic, Soma compound with codeine, Parofon Forte).

When such a protocol fails, the use of steroids injected into the joint capsule for pain relief must be considered. This therapy is generally delegated to the oral surgeon or other clinician experienced in intrajoint injection techniques.

Preventive Protocol

The primary concern of the preventive protocol involves the construction of removable appliances of various designs with the common effect of disarticulating the occlusion and stretching the overcontracted muscles of mastication in spasm. The rigid acrylic full-maxillary night guard is recommended. Indeed, such an appliance may also be an integral part of the relief of acute symptoms. Its advantage as part of a preventive protocol is that the therapy is reversible. The appliance can be discarded, altered, or restructured without permanent change to the dentition. The theory of breaking the pattern of periodontal ligament proprioception, bruxism, muscle fatigue, overcontracture, and spasm seems reasonable.

The appropriate use of occlusal adjustment is controversial. Many clinicians have suggested occlusal adjustment as an integral if not paramount consideration in the relief of acute symptoms, particularly when lateral pterygoid muscle spasm dominates. Although we consider minor occlusal adjustment of gross discrepancies as reasonable, the irreversible major alteration of cusp-fossae relationships during the period of acute symptoms seems inadvisable. Such an occlusal approach should be relegated to a role in the preventive protocol after the acute episode is terminated. Because of its irreversible character, caution is also advised in the use of therapeutic occlusal adjustment for the relief of low-grade symptomatology after acute episode relief.

After acute symptom relief, restoration to an appropriate intact dentition and vertical dimension is in order. Complete occlusal prosthetic rehabilitation of a reasonably intact dentition should rarely be prescribed, however, and must be considered a radical approach to therapy.

Secondary Consultations

At all times the dentist must consider the possibility of successful therapy for functional TMJ disorders outside the general dental realm, as well as the possibility of misdiagnosed organic pathology. Indeed, the role of psychiatric, neurologic, otolaryngologic, radiologic, or surgical consultation becomes increasingly important in the functional TMJ case that is unresponsive to therapy. Similarly, aggressive dental therapy, including major prosthetic rehabilitation and joint surgery, have their place in the treatment of appropriate TMJ disorders, but both carry significant risks of complication and should be considered only when conditions inappropriate or unresponsive to such aggressive therapy have been meticulously ruled out.

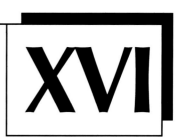

SECTION

XVI

Evaluation and Management of the Patient with Oral Infection

46

Bacterial Infection and the Use of Antibiotics

The recognition and management of infection is one of the most frequently encountered clinical problems in dental practice. Few conditions present the dentist with the systemic ramifications of untreated oral infection. Historical analysis of causes of death in the 18th century has demonstrated that oral bacterial infection was a major problem. Fortunately, since the discovery of antibiotics, the morbidity and mortality associated with infection have been markedly reduced. However, over-reliance on antimicrobial medication does not replace the principles of a sound systematic approach to the evaluation and treatment of the patient with oral infection.

GENERAL CONSIDERATIONS

Three factors must be considered in the overall assessment and management of infection: extent of the infectious process, status of the host, and virulence of the organism.

Assessment of the Extent of Infection

The first point in the assessment of the patient with infection involves the determination of whether the practitioner is confronted with a localized condition or one that is spreading.

Local infection may present as one of two forms, localized inflammation or abscesses. Redness, swelling, heat, and pain are the cardinal signs of inflammation. An example of frequently encountered localized oral inflammation is a dry socket. An abscess presents as a localized suppurative process that is usually in proximity to the source of infection. Pus forms as a result of toxin-induced necrosis and vascular injury (Figs. 46–1 and 46–2). A hypertonic center absorbs fluid from surrounding tissue until the abscess increases in size, at which time ingress of leukocytes and serum is impaired. Patients with abscess formation may exhibit systemic signs of reaction to the local process, including malaise, fever, and lymphadenopathy.

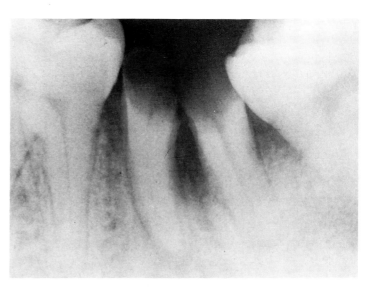

Figure 46–1. Dentoalveolar abscess near the source of infection.

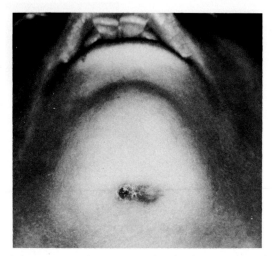

Figure 46–2. Fistula opening to the skin from an infected mandibular incisor.

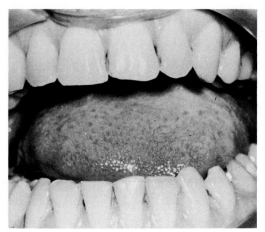

Figure 46–3. Elevated tongue as a consequence of Ludwig's angina.

Although local infections are common in dentistry, spreading infection is also frequently encountered. These infections, if uncontrolled, can pose a major physiologic threat to the patient, in the form of either septicemia or extension into an anatomic area that can compromise function. The patient with a spreading infection, known as a cellulitis, often complains of a variety of symptoms including fever, chills, malaise, nonlocalized swelling, anorexia, and lymphadenopathy. Tachycardia may be noted in these patients and is often proportional to the level of fever (an increase of 10 beats/min for each degree Fahrenheit increase in temperature). Because infection may spread by way of tissue planes, by septic embolization, or along lymphatic channels, the anatomic site of infection is critical.

In assessing the patient with cellulitis, it is incumbent to ascertain whether the infection is life-threatening. Four specific questions should be considered:

1. Is the airway obstructed and does the patient have difficulty swallowing?
2. What is the patient's mental status—is there confusion, delirium, or stupor?
3. Are the eyes closed?
4. Is the nasolabial fold intact?

The first question is easily answered by history and physical examination. A positive answer may suggest retropharyngeal spread of infection or Ludwig's angina (cellulitis of submandibular and sublingual spaces; Fig. 46–3).

The second question may be answered by querying patients about their surroundings and by determination of a clinical history.

The spread of infection through the facial veins could proceed to involve the cavernous sinus, resulting in neurologic signs and symptoms. Similarly, direct spread of infection may result in formation of a brain abscess (Fig. 46–4). This is most frequently reported after extraction of infected teeth but may also occur as the result of severe chronic suppurative periodontitis.

Periorbital edema and loss of the nasolabial fold are indicative of localized cellulitis (Fig. 46–5). Because this occurs in the anterior facial area, the potential for spread to the central nervous system by way of the valveless facial veins must be considered.

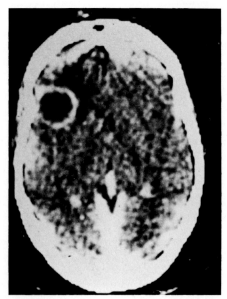

Figure 46–4. CT scan demonstrating brain abscess as an ovoid area. This infection resulted from direct spread from periodontally involved maxillary teeth.

Systemic Conditions (Host Factors) Influencing the Course of Infection

Many systemic conditions and medications can affect the body's response to infection. These may affect the ability of the patient to localize bacteria, to provide leukocytes to an area of infection, or to eliminate the infecting agent. Infection in individuals with compromised host defenses must be dealt with aggressively.

Patient age may affect ability to deal with infection. As with many conditions, patients at either age extreme handle infection less well than patients in their middle years. Patients with diabetes mellitus, especially if it is not well controlled, are at major risk for poor response to bacteria. Similarly, the patient who is malnourished or has liver, renal, or cardiovascular disease should be considered to be at risk for infection. Clearly, patients with blood dyscrasias such as agranulocytosis, leukemia, or aplastic anemia are unable to mount a reasonable acute inflammatory response. The first indication of such a disease is often the patient's inability to handle a seemingly minor local inflammatory reaction.

A number of medications may impair host defenses. Chemotherapeutic drugs used in cancer are frequently mentioned. Patients on long-term antibiotic therapy may be susceptible to superinfection by resistant organisms. It is also important to note that many drugs can cause neutropenia as a transient or permanent side effect.

Virulence of the Organism

Laboratory Evaluation

The most consistent laboratory findings in patients with infection are leukocytosis and an increase in the number of neutrophils (especially immature forms). Hematologic examinations for these problems are easily obtained and are inexpensive (Table 46–1). These tests should be performed if there is a question of infection or if there is persistent infection for no apparent cause following treatment.

Identification of the microorganism is frequently not made in oral infections. The overwhelming susceptibility of oral pathogens to penicillin often makes isolation of the causative organism unnecessary. There are, however, a number of cases in which culture, identification, and antibiotic susceptibility testing should be done (Table 46–2). If the patient

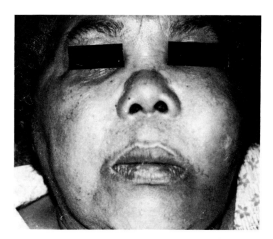

Figure 46–5. Spreading cellulitis involving the left side of the patient's face. Note the lack of the nasolabial fold, swelling of the cheek, and suborbital edema.

fails to respond to the initial course of antibiotic therapy, culture should be attempted *before* a new antibiotic is prescribed. Similarly, if the patient presents with systemic signs of infection, a blood culture should be obtained for both aerobic and anaerobic organisms *before* the initiation of treatment. Patients who present with lesions involving the pharynx should be cultured for beta-hemolytic streptococci. Culture should be done in patients with underlying diseases, especially those who are myelosuppressed and who are receiving immunosuppressive therapy.

Smears may be helpful in diagnosing *Candida*, but Gram's staining of oral suppurative infections generally shows mixed and nonspecific flora (Tables 46–3 and 46–4).

Table 46–1. LABORATORY EVALUATION OF INFECTION

White blood cells
   Number of white blood cells in peripheral blood elevated
   Percentage of neutrophils in peripheral blood increases with more immature forms noted (shift to the left)

Sedimentation rate: measures the amount of serum protein by determining its ability to retard the sedimentation of formed blood elements; increased in infection

Each of these tests is performed with peripheral blood.
   To order the above tests,
   1. Call the laboratory or hospital (ask for outpatient laboratory, give the patient's name, age and address, and identify ourself).
   2. Specify the test(s) to be performed.
   3. Indicate when the patient will be in.
   4. Ask for results to be telephoned. The laboratory can also mail results.

Table 46–2. CULTURING BACTERIAL INFECTION

When to culture:
  Ideally, always; however, from practical standpoint with oral infection, not always possible
  The following are cases when culture of local lesion and/or peripheral blood should not be delayed:
    Nonresolving infection in spite of appropriate treatment
    Patients in whom atypical flora may be expected: patients on long-term antibiotics, patients at age extremes (under 2
      or older than 65 years), patients with malignancies
    Infections in which there is life-threatening systemic involvement
    Patients who are at risk from infection and who cannot be expected to deal with infection normally, such as
      immunocompromised or myelosuppressed individuals
How to culture (Fig. 46–6):
  Most cultures are obtained from purulent infections. The easiest technique is to take a sterile swab after incising the
    abscess and place the specimen into a sterile tube with either sterile saline solution or broth.
  Promptness of specimen to laboratory is important. If there is a question of the presence of an anaerobic organism,
    withdraw fluctuant material into a 2-ml syringe with a 22-gauge needle and plunge into a blood culture bottle.
    Syringes and needle are available at the hospital pharmacy. Blood culture bottles may be obtained from the
    hospital microbiology laboratory or commercially. The shelf life ranges from several weeks up to a year, depending
    on the source.
Data obtained:
  Usually takes 1–3 days to obtain laboratory report
  Types of bacteria present
  Quantitation of bacteria—may be specific or estimate (Fig. 46–7)
  Sensitivity of organisms to specific antibiotic in case of culture and sensitivity (Fig. 46–8)

Microbiology of Oral Infections

Most oral infections are caused by a mixture of organisms. The streptococci are the most frequent isolates of oral soft tissue infections. Of these, *Streptococcus viridans* is the most common. One study has demonstrated that all streptococcal isolates are sensitive to ampicillin, cephalothin, or penicillin. *Staphylococcus aureus* is sometimes found in oral infections as a pure isolate or as a component of mixed infection. Of staphylococci (isolated from oral infections), 20% appear to be resistant to penicillin and 50% to erythromycin. Gram-negative anaerobes may contribute to infections of periodontal origin.

Effectiveness of Antibiotics

Antibiotics are indicated in dental practice in two areas, the treatment of bacterial infec-

tions and the prophylaxis of specific bacterial infections in susceptible patients.

The ideal antibiotic has five properties. First, it should be specific in its antibacterial action. Second, it should kill organisms (bactericidal) rather than delaying their replication (bacteriostatic). Third, it should have a high therapeutic index with few side effects. Fourth, few patients should develop sensitivity to the drug. Finally, it should be effective in body fluids. Because almost no antibiotics satisfy all these criteria, it is incumbent on the clinician to select an appropriate antibiotic for a specific clinical situation.

Table 46–4. PROPERTIES OF COMMON BACTERIAL ORGANISMS

Organism	Gram-Negative (−) or Positive (+)
Streptococci	+
Enterococci	+
Staphylococci	+
Other species	
Neisseria	−
Veillonella	−
Bacillus	+
Clostridium	+
Corynebacterium	+
Escherichia coli	−
Enterobacter	−
Klebsiella	−
Proteus	−
Pseudomonas	−
Bacteroides	−
Serratia	−
Hemophilus	−

Table 46–3. PREPARATION OF MATERIAL FOR GRAM'S-STAIN EXAMINATION

Examination reveals
  Approximation of density of bacteria in specimen
  Classification of organism type

Preparation of Gram's-stained smear:
  Smear: with sterile swab, make a *thin* film of material of glass slide; let dry in air and then fix by passing through flame a few times (Note: Once fixed, smear can remain for up to 14 hr before staining; smears can thus be prepared in office and transported to laboratory for staining and interpretation)

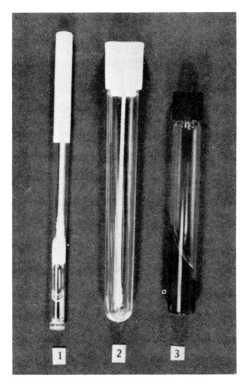

Figure 46–6. Sample tubes for bacteriologic specimens: *(1)* culture tube with rayon-tipped swab and crushed ampule containing moisture; *(2)* conventional culture tube with cotton swab; *(3)* tube containing slant solid medium for anaerobic growth. (From Doku H, C.: Basic clinical bacteriologic techniques of importance to dentistry. Dent. Clin North Am., 18:209, 1974.)

Five important considerations in the selection of an appropriate antibiotic are

1. Knowledge of the infectious agent and its sensitivity
2. Status of the patient (clearly, tablets would not be suitable for a very young or unconscious patient, nor would an intramuscular injection be appropriate in a patient with a bleeding dyscrasia)
3. The dose of drug needed and duration of therapy
4. Patient sensitivity to particular drugs
5. Cost of the drug

These issues are discussed specifically later in this chapter.

MANAGEMENT

Three objectives in treating the patient with infection are the preservation of life functions, elimination of the infecting agent, and establishment of patient comfort. Maintenance of

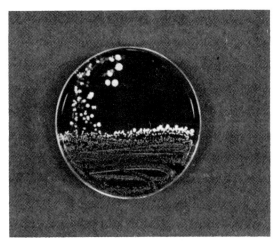

Figure 46–7. Various configurations of growing bacterial colonies. There are areas of heavy growth and areas of no growth. (From Doku, H. C.: Basic clinical bacteriologic techniques of importance to dentistry. Dent. Clin. North Am., 18:209, 1974.)

vital functions is, of course, the first principle of patient management. A patient with a dental infection must be assessed for a patent airway, systemic spread of infection, and cerebral complications. Supportive care is indicated in any patient with the potential for life-threatening complications as a result of infection. Patients who have an actual or potential inabil-

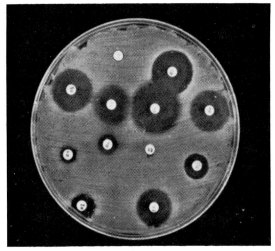

Figure 46–8. Determination of sensitivity of microorganisms to antibiotics using the disk method. Numbered filter paper disks containing antibodies are placed with a dispenser on the surface of solid medium. The clear zone around the disk indicates that the microorganisms in this culture are sensitive to that particular antibiotic. Areas that show no inhibition or a small clear zone around the disk indicate that the microorganisms are resistant to the particular antibiotic in the disk. (From Doku, H. C.: Basic clinical bacteriologic techniques of importance to dentistry. Dent. Clin. North Am., 18:209, 1974.)

ity to deal with infection physiologically must be approached more aggressively than normal individuals. Thus, patients with an underlying disease that may affect the ability to deal with infection must have the secondary problem managed if the infection is to be treated successfully. Good communication between physician and dentist is critical. For example, the insulin needs of a patient with well-controlled diabetes may be significantly altered in the presence of infection.

To treat a local infection peripherally with only antibiotics does little to remedy the long-range course of the illness. An attempt should be made to localize the infection to allow appropriate incision and drainage. Fortunately, many infections of the oral cavity lend themselves well to local treatment. Clearly, if there are signs of nonlocalized infection, appropriate antibiotic therapy must be instituted.

Finally, the patient's symptoms need to be addressed. Pain, fever, and dehydration should all be treated.

Types of Infection

Localized Infection

The treatment of localized oral infection is a routine clinical problem. Complicating secondary disease must be considered (see later). In the absence of systemic disease, the first consideration is to remove the infectious material. Depending on the clinical circumstances, this may include extraction of an infected tooth, pulpotomy and root canal débridement, or incision and drainage. The patient should be advised to maintain normal fluid and food intake. Appropriate analgesics (Chap. 50) should be prescribed as needed. Finally, antibiotic therapy is generally advisable.

Spreading Infection

For non–life-threatening spreading infections, an attempt to localize the infection must be made. Warm rinses may produce a focus so that incision and drainage can be accomplished. The application of heat to the skin should be avoided, because it could lead to fistula formation. In the case of endodontic pathology, the tooth should be opened and instrumented, when possible. Activity should be limited and hydration and food intake ensured. Antibiotic therapy is mandatory, as is 24- to 48-hour follow-up for definitive treatment such as incision and drainage or extraction. If constitutional symptoms are marked, blood cultures for aerobic and anaerobic organisms are advisable before beginning antibiotic therapy.

Life-threatening infection requires hospitalization. Examples include spreading infections significantly involving the floor of the mouth or those causing impaired mental status or airway obstruction of the otherwise healthy patient. For the medically debilitated patient, any infection may require hospitalization. Consultation with medical specialists in infectious disease is appropriate. Every effort to culture the infecting organisms should be made and followed by the initiation of high-dose intravenous antibiotics. Precautions should be undertaken to prevent life-threatening consequences of infection. For instance, in the case of Ludwig's angina, in which elevation of the tongue might cause airway obstruction, the possible necessity of a tracheotomy must be considered. Localization of the infection and removal of its source should be attempted when the patient is stabilized. Appropriate follow-up operative and preventive dental care can then be planned.

Antibiotic Selection

Selection of the appropriate antibiotic depends on the type of infection, the status of the patient, and the organisms involved in the infection. Although it is beyond our scope here to discuss each antibiotic in detail, a general outline of common therapeutic agents used in oral infection can be presented (Fig. 46–9). The clinician is advised to be thoroughly familiar with any agent prior to prescribing it and is referred to manufacturers' directives and pharmacologic textbooks.

Penicillins and Related Drugs

Penicillin is the drug of choice in the absence of specific cultures for the treatment of oral infection. When a choice exists between penicillin and other antimicrobials, the former should be used. Phenoxymethyl penicillin (penicillin V) is acid-stable and is, therefore, an excellent drug that can be taken by mouth. The potassium salt of the drug is the best absorbed oral preparation. It is a bactericidal agent for infections caused by gram-positive cocci (e.g., *Streptococcus viridans,* group A streptococci, anaerobic streptococci) and for strains of bacteroides and other gram-negative rods

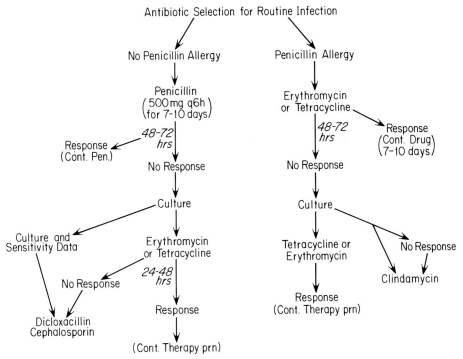

Figure 46–9. Rationale for antibiotic selection.

often implicated in acute periodontal pathology. Many but not all staphylococci are susceptible to penicillin. Therapeutic doses range from 250 to 500 mg, qid, daily for 7 to 14 days. Anaphylactic reactions are as frequent as 1 in 10,000 cases when penicillin is administered parenterally but are exceedingly rare when the oral form is used.

Dicloxacillin is the best available oral penicillin V substitute when penicillinase-producing staphylococci are present. Dicloxacillin is effective against other penicillin V–sensitive gram-positive organisms, but not as effective as penicillin V. The dose most commonly prescribed is 250 mg given by mouth qid. The counterparts to dicloxacillin for parenteral use are nafcillin, methicillin, and oxacillin. Oxacillin as an oral agent is variably effective.

The most common extended-spectrum penicillin is ampicillin. It is not as effective as penicillin V against gram-positive cocci and is ineffective against penicillinase-producing staphylococci. The extended spectrum of ampicillin is sensitive to gram-negative organisms rarely involved in oral infection. Even when gram-negative organisms are suspected in the debilitated patient with malignancy (see later), for instance, the intravenous alternative, carbenicillin, may be used. Such an antibiotic is

particularly useful when *Pseudomonas* infection is a problem. Ampicillin is used in dentistry as an intramuscular alternative to the amoxicillin oral regimen for prophylaxis of subacute bacterial endocarditis.

Amoxicillin is the oral form of an extended-spectrum penicillin recommended by the American Heart Association instead of conventional penicillin preparations. Amoxicillin has a more rapid and reliable uptake from the gastrointestinal tract. Nevertheless, penicillin-VK prophylaxis is still acceptable (see Chap. 11).

Augmentin is an amoxicillin preparation compounded with clavulanate potassium. This combination enhances the spectrum of microbiota susceptibility. *Staphylococcus aureus* strains are susceptible to Augmentin, as are several of the organisms associated with rapidly destructive periodontitis.

Crystalline (aqueous) penicillin G and procaine penicillin G are penicillins given by the intramuscular or intravenous route and have antimicrobial activity equivalent to that of penicillin V. Their use is often dictated by convenience (e.g., in the hospital setting), operator experience, or the requirement for predictable blood levels. Crystalline penicillin provides a rapidly peaking blood level 15 to 30 minutes after intramuscular administration. Procaine penicillin peaks more slowly but provides detectable blood levels for 8 to 12 hours.

Benzathine penicillin G gives low detectable blood levels for 4 weeks following a single injection. Its primary use is as a rheumatic fever antibiotic prophylaxis regimen in patients with a pre-existing history of rheumatic fever and in the treatment of syphilis. Single-dose therapy does not protect the susceptible patient from subacute bacterial endocarditis.

Other Antimicrobial Agents

Erythromycin is a bacteriostatic agent with an antibiotic spectrum similar to that of penicillin V. It is the first alternative to penicillin V for oral infection if the patient has a penicillin allergy but is generally less effective. As noted earlier, more than 50% of oral staphylococci are resistant to erythromycin. Doses are generally 250 to 500 mg by mouth, qid, for 7 to 14 days. Gastrointestinal upset is a common side effect of erythromycin. It can significantly affect patient compliance with prescribed regimens. Gastrointestinal intolerance must be distinguished from true allergy, which is rare. Some clinicians recommend administration of the drug with food to minimize the risk of gastrointestinal upset. Unfortunately, the absorption of erythromycin stearate, the generic form of the drug, is compromised by the presence of food. The stearate form should be administered in the fasting state or immediately before meals. Enteric-coated erythromycin preparations (E-MYCIN and ERY-TAB), erythromycin ethylsuccinate, and delayed-release capsules (ERYC) are all well absorbed and may be given without regard to meals.

In addition, these preparations are themselves "kinder" to the stomach, causing significantly fewer adverse reactions. The delayed-release capsule form is absorbed in the small intestine. Adequate blood levels are slightly slower to develop, but the bioavailability of the drug is sustained for longer periods of time. For this reason, 500 mg bid is acceptable for the delayed-release capsules as an alternative to 250-mg qid regimens. Improved patient compliance with bid dosage regimens can be anticipated. The estolate form of the drug gives higher and more reliable blood levels but carries a significant (but rare) risk of idiosyncratic hepatic dysfunction. Except for rare circumstances, other forms of erythromycin are generally preferred for oral infection therapy.

Two newer preparations of erythromycin are clarithromycin (Biaxin) and azithromycin (Zithromax). Their major advantage over the other preparations is that *Staphylococcus aureus* strains are susceptible to both. Bid and qid dosages, respectively, provide improved patient compliance. Both drugs are significantly more expensive than other preparations.

Specific contraindications for erythromycin use do exist. These include concurrent use of theophylline (Chap. 18), cyclosporine (Chap. 29), terfenadine (Seldane), and astemizole (Hismanal). Additionally, patients taking birth control pills should be cautioned to seek an alternative method of birth control when taking antibiotics.

Clindamycin (Cleocin) is an oral antibiotic similar in antimicrobial activity to erythromycin with good results against *Staphylococcus aureus* and with particular effectiveness against most anaerobes, including bacteroides. Oral doses are generally 150 to 300 mg given by mouth tid.

Refractory endodontic infections or deep-seated soft tissue infections unresponsive to penicillin are often treated empirically with clindamycin. In addition, clindamycin has a role in the treatment of a rapidly destructive form of periodontitis. Clindamycin therapy is associated with a risk for pseudomembranous colitis, a severe colitis that may be fatal. Therefore, it should be reserved for serious infections when less toxic antimicrobial agents are inappropriate.

The cephalosporins are similar in spectrum to the extended-spectrum penicillins (e.g., amoxicillin) with the added feature of being excellent agents for the treatment of *Staphylococcus aureus* infections. Penicillin itself, however, is generally more effective against susceptible organisms. Furthermore, 10 to 15% of patients allergic to penicillin also demonstrate hypersensitivity to cephalosporins. Use in oral infection, therefore, is generally limited to patients in whom specific drug sensitivity has been demonstrated. Cephalexin (Keflex) and cefadroxil (Duricef) are bactericidal. These common preparations are given by mouth as 250 mg qid or 500 mg bid. Diarrhea is a common adverse side effect. Several parenteral preparations are also used (Keflin, Mandol).

Vancomycin is a bactericidal agent active against gram-positive cocci only. It must be administered intravenously and has several adverse side effects associated with its administration. Its primary use in dentistry is as part of an alternate regimen in the prophylaxis for subacute bacterial endocarditis in the patient who is penicillin-allergic.

The tetracyclines are true broad-spectrum antibiotics that are active against both gram-negative and penicillin-sensitive organisms. Tetracyclines are the first alternative drugs of choice to penicillin when mixed infection or bacteroides-related periodontal infection is suspected. As the incidence of gram-negative oral infection increases, the tetracyclines are replacing erythromycin as the usual second drug of choice in all oral infections treated empirically, except in those patients susceptible to subacute bacterial endocarditis. Adequate absorption of the drug can be a problem. Generic tetracycline is absorbed best on an empty stomach (1 hour before or 2 hours after meals); dairy products and commonly used antacids markedly interfere with uptake. Tetracycline hydrochloride is the least expensive and is most commonly prescribed in doses of 250 mg by mouth, qid.

Doxycycline (Vibramycin) is a slightly more expensive form of tetracycline given as a 200-mg initial dose, followed by 100 mg daily. It offers several advantages, including the once-daily dose for therapeutic levels and excellent absorption regardless of food intake. It is the only tetracycline allowable for patients with renal failure, because this form of tetracycline does not accumulate in the patient's serum.

All tetracycline therapy has associated risks, including superinfection (especially vaginal candidiasis), photosensitivity, and irreversible pigmentation of developing teeth. In addition, the use of tetracycline is contraindicated in patients on anticoagulant therapy or with other bleeding diatheses (Chap. 26). The metabolism of doxycycline is increased by concurrent use of the medications most commonly used for seizure disorders. These include phenytoin (Dilantin), carbamazepine (Tegretol), and all barbiturates. These drugs decrease the effectiveness of doxycycline, and the clinician should choose an alternative antibiotic.

Tetracyclines are the safest and least expensive of a group of antibiotics commonly used for rapidly destructive periodontitis syndromes. In addition to the tetracyclines Augmentin and clindamycin, other drugs used for aggressive periodontal pathogens include metronidazole (Flagyl) and ciprofloxacin (Cipro). The latter two drugs have significant potential side effects and are often prescribed only when specific culture data recommend them and when the benefit:risk ratio has been closely evaluated.

The aminoglycoside antibiotics are also broad-spectrum agents and include streptomycin, gentamicin, and tobramycin. They are bactericidal drugs for an assortment of gram-positive and gram-negative species. Because of poor gastrointestinal absorption, oral administration is not used. All have significant side effects, including nephrotoxicity producing renal tubular damage and ototoxicity causing eighth cranial nerve damage. The most common dental use for gentamycin is as part of an alternate regimen for the antibiotic prophylaxis of subacute bacterial endocarditis (Chap. 11). In this setting, as a single intramuscular dose, the risk of toxicity is small.

Gentamicin and tobramycin are often used in combination with a broad-spectrum penicillin or a cephalosporin in life-threatening infections of the hospitalized cancer patient. The aminoglycosides have no outpatient use in oral infection.

Use of Different Drugs

Localized and minimally spreading infection in the healthy patient is most often treated without culture. The drug of choice in this group is penicillin. In the presence of penicillin allergy, erythromycin or tetracycline may be used. The latter has most application in the treatment of periodontal abscess. If after 48 hours there is no response to the initial antibiotic therapy, every attempt must be made to culture the infecting organism. While awaiting culture and sensitivity data, the antibiotic therapy should be changed. The appropriate follow-up to penicillin is erythromycin or tetracycline. In the penicillin-allergic patient in whom erythromycin or tetracycline was used initially, the other drug should be the alternative choice. The overwhelming majority of oral infections respond to this approach. The most common exception is the infection from penicillinase-producing *Staphylococcus aureus*. Here, culture data most often suggest the use of penicillinase-resistant dicloxacillin or a cephalosporin. For the penicillin-allergic patient, clindamycin is often the drug of choice. The clinician must always consider the need for hospitalization and consultation with an infectious disease specialist for the spreading oral infection unresponsive to antibiotic therapy.

Patients with a number of systemic diseases often require special consideration relative to the treatment of infection and selection of an antibiotic. Within this group are patients in whom bacteremia subsequent to oral manifestation may complicate a pre-existing medical problem, as in the patient with valvular heart disease. The other group that requires special consideration are those patients with diseases known to compromise their ability to deal with infection.

Antibiotic Prophylaxis. As previously discussed (Chap. 11), almost any manipulation that results in gingival bleeding results in a significant bacteremia. The extent of the resultant bacteremia is a function of the degree of tissue manipulation and the status of oral health. Patients with pre-existing periodontal disease develop significantly greater bacteremias than do patients with clean healthy mouths.

Although bacteremias are of little clinical significance in the healthy patient, they may predispose to local bacterial colonization in patients with underlying pathology.

Subacute Bacterial Endocarditis. Patients with a number of cardiac abnormalities are at variable risk for developing subacute bacterial endocarditis. In this situation, blood-borne bacteria can multiply on the defective part of the heart and infection might then ensue, with subsequent extended cardiovascular damage. The most common source of the bacteremia is the mouth, and the most common organism involved is *Streptococcus viridans.*

Fortunately, the organisms that cause subacute bacterial endocarditis are generally susceptible to the penicillin class of antibiotics. Hence, the American Heart Association's recommended prophylaxis for patients susceptible to SBE is heavily dependent on these agents (e.g., amoxicillin). A detailed discussion of this subject can be found in Chapter 11.

Renal Disease. Two forms of treatment of chronic renal disease require consideration for prophylactic antibiotic therapy. These include those patients undergoing hemodialysis and those who have received renal transplants (Chap. 29).

The patient undergoing hemodialysis may have an arteriovenous shunt, fistula, or graft placed to facilitate adequate hook-up to the dialysis machine. The shunt, fistula, or graft is susceptible to bacterial infection secondary to a bacteremia. To prevent such an occurrence, antibiotic prophylaxis is recommended for this group. Although the standard regimen is usually sufficient, patients with severe local inflammatory disease or those requiring dental surgical procedures might receive an alternate regimen. Indeed, one common practice is the use of vancomycin as a single bolus for dental procedure prophylaxis. Vancomycin is excreted renally and is not dialyzable. Therefore,

a single dose of vancomycin can provide adequate antibiotic prophylaxis for several days. Vancomycin can be given slowly at the time of dialysis and is therefore reasonably convenient. This possibility should be discussed with the patient's physician, and vancomycin can be given with the dialysis treatment prior to dental therapy. The vancomycin given lasts about 4 to 7 days in such patients.

The use of antibiotic prophylaxis for dental treatment in renal allograft recipients is poorly defined. Although patients who receive immunosuppression are at increased risk for infection, the form and course of antibiotic prophylaxis in this group are largely empiric. The dentist should consult with the patient's physician. Generally, oral penicillin or erythromycin is used for prophylaxis. The dentist should remember that a seemingly innocuous oral infection can progress rapidly to a severe cellulitis in the immunocompromised host. Any frank infection must be treated aggressively, therefore, and any patient with a renal transplant who presents with a cellulitis should be hospitalized for infection control. An infectious disease specialist should be consulted.

Joint Prostheses. The use of joint prostheses in the treatment of degenerative joint disease has enjoyed increasing success. It has been suggested that an association exists between late streptococcal and staphylococcal infections of these joints and dental infection and manipulation. The evidence to support this association is still speculative and may be coincidental. However, until this issue is definitively resolved, the prudent practitioner provides antibiotic prophylaxis prior to dental treatment. The consequences of infection of the prosthesis far outweigh the risk of antibiotic prophylaxis.

The form of antibiotic prophylaxis is also controversial. Although penicillin in the doses used for endocarditis prophylaxis has been standard, other studies have suggested that some of the causative organisms are penicillin-resistant. Thus, penicillinase-resistant penicillin, clindamycin, and cephalosporins are recommended for prophylaxis.

Cancer. Patients being treated for malignancy present many management considerations with respect to antibiotics as a consequence of both the disease and the therapy used to treat it (Chap. 42).

Chemotherapy. Cancer chemotherapy influences antibiotic management in two ways—the patient's defense mechanisms are severely compromised as a consequence of epithelial destruction, and myelosuppression and the oral bacterial flora are altered.

Thus, oral infection in the myelosuppressed cancer patient results in a high degree of morbidity and mortality. The mouth is the most frequently identified source of infection in these patients. Because patients are unable to mount an inflammatory response, conventional signs and symptoms of infection are absent. Hence, any patient with fever and oral pain should be assumed to have infection until proven otherwise. Management of this group is complicated and involves hospitalization. Cooperation and communication between the dentist and the patient's physician are mandatory. Because the oral bacterial flora undergoes changes, broad-spectrum parenteral antibiotic therapy is required.

Any myelosuppressed patient with fever (temperature over 100° F or 38° C) should be hospitalized. The site and source of infection, as well as the causative organisms, should be identified and the patient started on broad-spectrum parenteral antibiotics. One must balance the effectiveness of coverage with the potential toxicity (usually renal) of these drugs. Examples of the antibiotics of choice for a patient with adequate renal function and without penicillin allergy are aminoglycoside (gentamicin or tobramycin) and semisynthetic penicillin (carbenicillin) for adequate anaerobic coverage. For patients with renal dysfunction or pre-existing auditory or vestibular problems, carbenicillin and cephalothin may be used. In patients with a penicillin allergy, an aminoglycoside (gentamicin) plus clindamycin may be used. Patients with documented infec-

tion should be covered for a full course of 1 to 2 weeks.

Radiotherapy. The major consideration with respect to oral infection in the patient receiving head and neck radiotherapy is the development of osteoradionecrosis. Much can be done to prevent this debilitating and painful complication by preradiation dental evaluation and aggressive removal of teeth that have the potential to develop infection (Chap. 40).

If extraction is required in patients receiving radiation to the head and neck, preoperative antibiotic coverage with penicillin is recommended. Although some depression of white blood cell counts is noted following radiation therapy (head and neck), the decrease is not of the same magnitude as noted in patients receiving chemotherapy. Thus, aggressive treatment of oral infection with standard antibiotic regimens is recommended for this group.

Antibiotics and Periodontal Disease. Refractory disease and rapidly destructive periodontal lesions are often treated in part by the use of adjunctive antibiotics. Tetracycline has usually been prescribed. With the current availability of in-office bacterial culturing and the retrieval of antibiotic sensitivity data, more drugs are now used for this purpose. These include amoxicillin with clavulanic acid (Augmentin), metronidazole (Flagyl), clindamycin (Cleocin), and ciprofloxacin (Cipro). Each drug has its own bacterial spectrum and side effects. Given the varied toxicities associated with each agent, a careful assessment of the benefit:risk ratio is mandated.

SUMMARY TABLE 46–I

Signs and Symptoms of Infection

Local infection—abscess or cellulitis; inflammation denotes process

Signs and symptoms of inflammation
  Redness
  Swelling
  Pain
  Heat
  Loss of function

Definitions
  Abscess: localized collection of pus
  Cellulitis: local spreading infection
  Bacteremia: presence of bacteria in normally sterile blood
  Septicemia: infection involving bloodstream, in which there is dissemination of organisms

Signs and symptoms of nonlocalized infection or infection with systemic involvement—includes preceding plus fever, malaise, lymphadenopathy, muscle aches, and chills

SUMMARY TABLE 46–II

Host Factors That Inhibit Patient's Ability to Deal with Infection Effectively

Age: patients at either extreme

Diabetes mellitus

Cardiovascular disease

Liver disease

Splenectomy

Malnutrition

Agranulocytosis

Malignancies

Immunodeficiencies

Drug therapy, including steroids, cancer chemotherapeutic agents, anti-inflammatory drugs, antibiotics

Renal disease

Common Microbiology of Oral Infection

Most infections are "mixed flora"

Streptococcus viridans most common single isolate

Staphylococcus aureus common as isolate or part of mixed flora (20% penicillin-resistant, 50% erythromycin-resistant)

Bacteroides-like gram-negative anaerobes are more common in infections of periodontal origin

Immunosuppressed hosts have dramatic shift to predominance of gram-negative anaerobic infection

Evidence of Spreading Infection

Airway obstruction or difficulty swallowing

Impaired mental status

Raised tongue

Closure of the eye

Loss of the nasolabial fold

Reasons to Culture

Failure to respond to initial course of antibiotic (culture before changing antibiotic)

Systemic signs of infection (blood culture before initiating antimicrobial therapy)

Pharyngeal lesions (culture to rule out beta-hemolytic streptococci)

Patient on immunosuppressive therapy or with significant underlying disease

Management of Nonspecific Infectious Processes

STAGE OF INFECTION	CLINICAL SIGNS AND SYMPTOMS	LABORATORY FINDINGS	TREATMENT
Local inflammatory response	Pain, redness, edema	None	Local palliation, elimination of irritants, reduce potential for infection
Abscess	Pain; fluctuant localized swelling in close relationship to source, suppuration, malaise, fever, lymphadenopathy, tooth sensitivity	May have leukocytosis, increase in polymorphonuclear leukocytes with shift to left, increased sedimentation rate	Elimination of suppurative material (incision and drainage) and source, antibiotic coverage, salt water rinses, pain medication
Cellulitis (spreading infection)	Fever, malaise, lymphadenopathy, pain, nonlocalized swelling, anorexia, myalgia, chills	Increased PMNL, increased WBC, increased sedimentation rate	Maintain vital functions, treat secondary disease, treat symptoms, antibiotics, localize

Infection Management: Specific Treatment

LOCAL INFECTION (e.g., dry socket, pulpitis)

Treat any complicating secondary disease

Remove infectious material and/or source of infection (incision and drainage, extraction, pulpotomy)

Treatment symptoms
    Pain medication, as needed (Chap. 50)
    Appropriate activity level
    Hydration
    Prescribe antibiotics

NON–LIFE-THREATENING SPREADING INFECTION

Attempt to localize infection—warm rinses

Treat symptoms
    Fever: aspirin, acetaminophen, nonsteroidal antiinflammatory drugs
    Pain: analgesics

Appropriate activity level, bed rest

Antibiotics

Re-evaluate in 24 hours

Treat secondary disease, consult physician

LIFE-THREATENING INFECTION

Hospitalize patient

Treat secondary disease, consult physician

High-dose antibiotics (IV)

Hydrate

Appropriate precautions

Localize infection and remove source

Appropriate follow-up care

Selection of Antibiotics

1. Be *specific.* Identify causative agent. If not possible, base selection on knowledge of likely pathogen. Do not use "shotgun" approach. Broad-spectrum antibiotics such as tetracycline should not be used routinely for oral infections.
2. Use antibiotic that is *compatible* with nature of illness (no PO antibiotic if patient vomiting; no IM antibiotic if patient has bleeding problem; IV antibiotic if rapid, high level of antibiotic required).
3. Be sure patient is not *allergic* to drug.
4. Select most *economical* antibiotic to do job. Prescibe generically.
5. Prescribe adequate dosage for adequate length of time.

Common Antibiotics in Oral Infection

ANTIBIOTIC	SPECIFICITY	USUAL DOSE	ROUTE OF ADMINISTRATION	USE IN DENTAL INFECTION	COMMENTS
Penicillin-VK	Predominantly gram-positive cocci and gram-negative bacter-oides common in periodontal in-fection (bacteri-cidal)	250–500 mg q6h	PO	Routine drug of choice	20% *S. aureus* are re-sistant
Amoxicillin	Extended-spectrum penicillin	250–500 mg q8h	PO	Rapid plus relia-ble GI uptake	Major indication: SBE prophylaxis
Penicillin G—aqueous (crystalline), procaine	Same as penicillin-VK	1,000,000 units 600,000 units	IM	SBE prophylaxis (Chap. 11)	Guarantees high blood level; aqueous peaks rap-idly, Procaine peaks slowly
Benzathine penicillin	Same as penicillin-VK	1,200,000 units monthly	IM	Rheumatic fever prophylaxis	Not effective SBE prophylaxis
Broad-spectrum peni-cillins: carbenicillin, ticarcillin	Same as penicillin-VK plus many gram-negative organisms, espe-cially *Pseudo-monas* (not *S. aureus* penicillin-ase-producing species)		IM, IV	Hospitalized de-bilitated pa-tients with se-vere infection	Immunosuppressed cancer patients with infection most common dental use
Dicloxacillin	Same as penicillin-VK plus penicil-linase-producing *S. aureus*	250 mg q6h	PO	Culture and sen-sitivity data for *S. aureus*	Less effective against other penicillin-sensitive organisms
Augmentin	Extended-spectrum penicillin plus *S. aureus*	250–500 mg q8h	PO	Rapidly destruc-tive periodon-titis	Expensive
Erythromycin	Similar to penicillin (bacteriostatic)	250–500 mg q6h	PO	Routine second choice to penicillin or first choice if penicillin al-lergy, espe-cially in SBE prophylaxis	50% *S. aureus* is re-sistant, GI intoler-ance common

Table continued on following page

SUMMARY TABLE | **46–IX**

Common Antibiotics in Oral Infection *Continued*

ANTIBIOTIC	SPECIFICITY	USUAL DOSE	ROUTE OF ADMINISTRATION	USE IN DENTAL INFECTION	COMMENTS
Biaxin	Erythromycin spectrum plus *S. aureus*	250 mg q12h	PO	Good GI tolerance	Should not be used in pregnant patients; expensive
Tetracycline HCl	Broad-spectrum (bacteriostatic)	250 mg qid	PO	Second or third choice to penicillin in routine infection	Vaginitis risk, GI flora modified, photosensitivity and tooth staining risk, variable absorption
Doxycycline	Same	100 mg at hs	PO		Better absorption, use in renal failure
Clindamycin (Cleocin)	Similar to erythromycin, plus especially effective against *S. aureus* and anaerobes (bacteriostatic)	150–300 mg q8h	PO	Culture and sensitivity data for *S. aureus* in penicillin allergy or for specific anaerobes	Significant risk of severe colitis
Cephalosporins	Comparable to extended-spectrum penicillins plus *S. aureus*	Keflex, 250 mg q6h Keflin, variable	PO IM, IV	Culture and sensitivity data for *S. aureus*, hospitalized debilitated patient with severe infection	10–15% cross-reaction sensitivity for penicillin allergy
Vancomycin	Gram-positive cocci (bactericidal)	1 g over 20 min	IV	Alternate-regimen SBE prophylaxis in patients with penicillin allergy	Significant risk of adverse reactions during administration
Aminoglycosides—streptomycin, gentamicin, tobramycin	Broad-spectrum	1 g Variable	IM IV	Part of alternate-regimen SBE prophylaxis, hospitalized debilitated patient with severe infection	Single dose, low toxicity—but multiple doses, significant nephrotoxicity and ototoxicty

Acquired Immunodeficiency Syndrome and Related Diseases

No disease in recent memory has raised the number of clinical, emotional, or ethical issues as has acquired immunodeficiency syndrome (AIDS). The infectious nature of the disease has created considerable concern among health care providers and patients. Universal precautions are now exercised routinely, and stringent infection control procedures have been put in place. Heightened public and professional consciousness about the disease has resulted in a deluge of regulatory guidelines that have a marked impact on dental practice. The cost of compliance is not insignificant.

Dentistry is involved at many levels in dealing with the problems associated with AIDS. These include initial diagnosis of the condition because of its oral manifestations, management of the oral problems associated with the disease, and providing dental care to patients with the disease. In many ways, AIDS has led to a rigid definition of universal precautions in every field of health care delivery, and dentistry is no exception.

AIDS was first recognized in 1977 following the presentation of a small group of young men with rare forms of pneumonia and cancers normally seen only in immunocompromised individuals. The disease was acknowledged as an entity by the Centers for Disease Control in 1982. Since its ominous beginning, the number of patients with the disease has grown at an alarming rate.

It is known that AIDS is caused by a retrovirus that has an affinity for CD4-bearing T-helper lymphocytes that has been named the human immunodeficiency virus (HIV). This virus invades the susceptible lymphocyte and renders it nonfunctional, thereby interfering with a large number of important immunologic functions. Such interference can result in opportunistic infections and in the occurrence of a variety of normally rare neoplasms. AIDS and related diseases can therefore have a myriad of presentations. It is important for the dentist to be familiar with the nature of HIV infection and its many consequences. Management of patients with HIV infection is challenging and complicated and requires an understanding of the clinical issues raised by this disease.

MEDICAL ASPECTS

The virus that causes HIV infection has been isolated from almost all bodily fluids, although it is found in highest concentration in blood and semen. The major routes of transmission of infection are through sexual contact, shared intravenous needles, transfusions with infected blood, needle sticks with infected blood, or vertical transmission from mother to infant. Groups of at-risk patients include intravenous drug users, homosexual or bisexual men, sexual partners of patients with HIV, infants of HIV-infected mothers, and hemophiliacs. The rate of seropositivity to HIV among homosexual men ranges from 4 to 50%. Intravenous drug abusers have a higher frequency of positive antibody status, between 50 and 60%. Fortunately, aggressive screening programs for blood donors and the use of recombinant products for blood factor replacement have decreased the frequency of HIV transmission by blood donation.

Unfortunately, HIV infection is not always limited to those in high-risk groups. Studies of individuals entering the military have indicated a seropositive rate of 0.15%. It is estimated that as of 1993, about 2.8 million people in the United States have been infected by the virus with over 250,000 cases of symptomatic HIV infection.

The virus can remain dormant in the lymphocyte for long periods. Thus, a patient can remain asymptomatic for years. However, these patients are infectious and can infect others. Actually, infectivity is high during this early period of disease because of rapid viral replication; during the first 6 weeks to 6 months, the patient may be antibody-negative and still be infectious. Even after patients have seroconverted to HIV-positive status, they can be totally asymptomatic and not be aware of their infectivity. Because of the clinical course of AIDS, it is not practical to believe that a potential carrier can be identified. Hence, universal precautions must be exercised to avoid the transmission of infection. After the initial phase of the disease, the viral titer decreases and the patient is usually not as infectious.

Of patients currently known to be infected with HIV, only 10% have overt disease, while the remainder have normal immune responses. It is estimated that, left untreated, 5 to 10% of the infected patients would develop overt disease in 3 years and 60% would develop overt disease in 5 years.

With clinical disease, patients have a wasting illness with many systemic manifestations; fatigue, night sweats, fevers, chills, anorexia, and weight loss are common. Laboratory evaluation reveals leukopenia, lymphopenia, and thrombocytopenia. Evaluation of the T-cell subsets reveals a decreased CD4 count. By definition, opportunistic infections and the occurrence of unusual neoplasms, such as Kaposi's sarcoma, herald the onset of the AIDS. Patients often have progressive wasting, diarrhea, depression, and apathy and can progress to dementia, culminating in a vegetative state.

As the disease progresses, multiple organ systems are involved, with cutaneous, oral, pulmonary, cardiac, renal, gastrointestinal, hematologic, and neurologic sequelae. Early experiences with the disease indicated that patients with clinical AIDS, left untreated, have a median survival of only 6.4 months. With current treatment and the prompt and aggressive management of opportunistic infections, the median survival is now estimated at 3.8 years. Patients usually die from infectious complications or from malignancies. Late in the disease, viral titers increase dramatically, and the patient is again highly infectious.

MEDICAL EVALUATION

Most patients with HIV infection are totally asymptomatic. These patients are usually diagnosed as having the infection on the basis of finding of antibodies on blood testing (Table 47–1). Screening for antibodies is usually through the test known as ELISA (enzyme-

Table 47–1. SCREENING TESTS FOR HIV INFECTION

Name of Test	Purpose
ELISA	Screening (98% specificity)
Western blot	Confirmation
Polymerase chain reaction	Identification of viral genome

linked immunosorbent assay). This test carries a 98% specificity, although its sensitivity has not been fully evaluated. In a patient with a positive ELISA, a Western blot test is usually performed to confirm the diagnosis. In special circumstances, polymerase chain reaction procedures may be used to identify the actual presence of the virus itself. As noted, because seroconversion can be delayed for as long as 6 months following exposure, absence of the antibodies does not indicate noninfectivity.

In the seropositive patient (HIV-infected or HIV-positive), evaluation is performed to rule out opportunistic infections and occult malignancies. Complete blood and platelet counts are usually obtained and a baseline CD4 count is often done. Individuals with high CD4 counts (greater than 600 cells/μl) are less prone to developing complications. As the disease progresses, the CD4 count falls and complications begin to set in.

The asymptomatic HIV-positive patient is then carefully followed clinically. Heightened awareness of the many opportunistic infections these patients can have and aggressive early intervention have dramatically influenced the median survival. Common opportunistic infections include *Pneumocystis carinii* pneumonia, toxoplasmosis (including cerebral infections), atypical mycobacterial, viral, parasitic, and fungal infections, and conventional bacterial infections. These patients are also at risk of developing Kaposi's sarcoma and lymphoma.

CD4 counts are usually followed serially to assess the potential risks of infection and occult malignancies. Complete blood counts are also monitored. Other tests, such as chest x-rays and cranial CT scans, are performed if warranted by the clinical situation.

MEDICAL MANAGEMENT

A number of drugs have been shown to be efficacious in the management of patients with AIDS (Table 47–2). The most frequently prescribed medications are zidovudine (AZT) and

Table 47–2. DRUGS COMMONLY USED BY PATIENTS WITH AIDS AND RELATED SYNDROMES

Name of Drug	Function
AZT	Inhibition of reverse transcriptase
DDI	Inhibition of reverse transcriptase
Trimethoprim-sulfamethoxazole	Treatment of *Pneumocystis carinii* pneumonia
Pentamadine	Treatment of *P. carinii* pneumonia
Aerosolized pentamadine	Treatment of *P. carinii* pneumonia

didanosine (DDI). These drugs interfere with a key enzyme, reverse transcriptase, that is unique to the retrovirus, and thus prevent viral replication. They have exceptional in vitro activity against HIV.

Clinical trials have indicated that AZT is more effective than a placebo in improving the CD4 count and in delaying death in subjects with AIDS, the development of AIDS in subjects with AIDS-related complex, and the development of AIDS or AIDS-related complex in subjects with asymptomatic HIV infection. DDI also displays anti-HIV activity in vitro. Clinical trials have indicated that DDI is effective in the treatment of HIV viral isolates resistant to AZT. DDI is often used to treat patients in whom AZT treatment has failed or who have become intolerant to AZT.

AZT and DDI are often prescribed to patients with AIDS and to patients with a CD4 count lower than 500 cells/μl because of the high predisposition of these patients for developing infections and malignancies. Some patients with seropositivity and a normal CD4 count have also elected to be on AZT or DDI, but the practice remains controversial. Clinical trials in these patients have indicated that early treatment delays progression to AIDS but is no different from late treatment in improving survival.

Unfortunately, these medications have side effects (Table 47–3). AZT can cause anorexia, nausea, vomiting, diarrhea, and fatigue. It can also cause bone marrow suppression, with resultant leukopenia and anemia. Some patients may develop abnormal liver function. DDI can cause pancreatitis, peripheral neuropathy, and mild leukopenia.

In addition to these drugs, which are designed to interfere with viral replication, the

most important principle in managing the HIV-infected patient is to be aware of possible complications and to treat such complications aggressively.

Pneumocystis carinii pneumonia can now be diagnosed early in the course of HIV infection. It is treated with trimethoprim-sulfamethoxazole or pentamadine. Some patients with AIDS develop an allergic rash on trimethoprim-sulfamethoxazole, and others develop leukopenia and granulocytopenia. Abnormal liver function and abnormal kidney function test results have also been ascribed to trimethoprim-sulfamethoxazole. In these patients, pentamadine can be used. In acute infections, pentamadine is given intravenously; for maintenance or prophylactic therapy, it can be given in an aerosolized form. Pentamadine can cause pancreatitis, hypoglycemia or hyperglycemia, hypotension, leukopenia, and nephrotoxicity. In selected cases, dapsone may be used to treat the infection. Patients with *P. carinii* pneumonia often have recurrent infection. Most of these patients can be managed with aerosolized pentamadine on an outpatient basis.

Many other opportunistic infections should also be addressed promptly because of a heightened index of suspicion. Central nervous system toxoplasmosis, atypical mycobacterial pneumonia, and parasitic infections of

Table 47–3. SIDE EFFECTS OF DRUGS COMMONLY USED BY PATIENTS WITH AIDS AND RELATED SYNDROMES

Name of Drug	Side Effects
AZT	Fatigue; gastrointestinal intolerance: nausea, vomiting, anorexia, diarrhea; leukopenia, granulocytopenia, anemia; abnormal liver function
DDI	Pancreatitis; peripheral neuropathy; mild leukopenia
Trimethoprim-sulfamethoxazole	Fever; rash; stomatitis; pruritis; headache; nausea, vomiting; leukopenia, granulocytopenia; abnormal liver function; nephrotoxicity
Pentamadine	Nephrotoxicity; pancreatitis; hypoglycemia, hyperglycemia; arrhythmia; hypotension; leukopenia
Aerosolized pentamadine	Bronchospasm; nephrotoxicity; hypoglycemia; pancreatitis

the gastrointestinal tract all are diagnoses that can be made early in the course of the disease. Aggressive management of these problems can result in an improved quality of life and lengthened survival for the patients with AIDS.

ORAL MANIFESTATIONS

There are a number of well-defined oral manifestations of HIV infection. It has been reported that 70% of patients with AIDS develop oral changes associated with the disease. Oral manifestations of HIV infection include fungal, viral (Fig. 47–1), and bacterial infections, periodontal disease, soft tissue lesions, and cancers.

Mucocutaneous candidiasis is a common finding among patients with AIDS. Not infrequently, this may be the first sign of AIDS. As in other immunosuppressed hosts, the clinical manifestation ranges from the classic "cottage cheese" presentation to areas of broad atrophic erythema. Although the palate is most often involved, no area of the oral mucosa is spared. Candidiasis is usually localized to the oropharynx and the mouth and can be controlled with nystatin rinses or Mycelex (clotrimazole) troches. Nystatin rinses should be prescribed as a swish-and-swallow rinse tid or qid. Mycelex troches (10 mg) should be used five times daily. Low-dose fluconazole (Diflucan) (100 mg/day) has been introduced and is effective in the management of mucocutaneous candidiasis.

Hairy leukoplakia occurs with significant frequency in patients with HIV infection. The lesions are believed to be viral in origin. Its presence has been reported to precede the development of active infection in about 35%

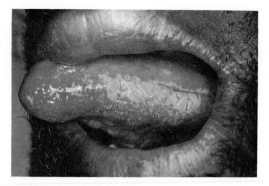

Figure 47–2. Hairy leukoplakia in a patient infected with HIV. Lesions usually present on the lateral borders of the tongue and are asymptomatic.

of patients. Patients present with nondescript keratotic lesions, usually on the lateral borders of the tongue (Fig. 47–2). The lesions are asymptomatic and require no active therapy. They should be biopsied, especially in individuals with undiagnosed disease.

Two forms of periodontal changes have been described in patients with AIDS. HIV gingivitis presents as an erythematous lesion that extends from the marginal gingiva to the alveolar mucosa. It is typically asymptomatic. It is important to be able to differentiate this lesion from Kaposi's sarcoma or thrombocytopenia-related hematoma. The second form of HIV-related periodontal disease is more dramatic. Its clinical presentation mimics that of acute necrotizing gingivitis in that there is a loss of papillary architecture, marginal necrosis, soft tissue cratering, and loss of gingival attachment. Often, lesions are painful and foul-smelling. Rapid loss of alveolar bone may accompany the soft tissue changes. It was proposed that this condition represents a unique form of acute necrotizing ulcerative gingivitis (ANUG), but bacteriologic analysis has shown that the organisms present are no different from those found in conventional periodontitis. Treatment of HIV-related periodontal disease consists of a combination of local and systemic therapy. Local mechanical débridement supplemented by good oral hygiene is helpful. Irrigation with chlorhexidine gluconate, 0.12% rinses, may be of benefit. During acute phases, antibiotic therapy with penicillin often alleviates symptoms (penicillin-VK, 500 mg, q6h).

Thrombocytopenia is not an uncommon finding among patients with symptomatic HIV infection. Consequently, petechiae may be noted on the palatal mucosa. Areas of minor

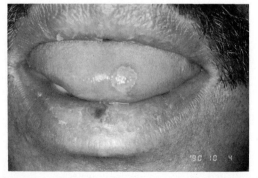

Figure 47–1. Herpes simplex infection in a patient infected with HIV. This tongue ulcer demonstrated herpes simplex virus by culture and responded to treatment with acyclovir.

oral trauma are susceptible to hematoma formation.

Aphthous-like ulcerations may be seen on any area of movable mucosa. The lesions present as severe, large painful ulcerations, with or without bands of surrounding erythema. Viral cultures are usually negative. Although these lesions are often dramatic in appearance, they are benign. However, unlike conventional canker sores, they often linger for long periods. Biopsy is recommended to rule out the possibility of cancer or tuberculosis.

Kaposi's sarcoma, a cancer that is seen frequently in patients with AIDS, is often found in the oral cavity. The clinical appearance of Kaposi's sarcoma in the mouth is frequently unimpressive. Typical lesions present as bluish-red or black macules that are usually asymptomatic (Fig. 47–3). However, more aggressive lesions of Kaposi's sarcoma may be raised. If the tumor involves the gingiva, the lesion may become hyperplastic and overgrow the tooth's crown. Alternatively, bony lesions of Kaposi's sarcoma may produce a swelling of overlying normal mucosa, so that the presentation might be confused with a periapical abscess. Biopsy is required for definitive diagnosis. In general, intraoral lesions of Kaposi's sarcoma need not be resected, except when the lesion becomes unesthetic or compromises patient function. Local infiltration of lesions with vinblastine, a chemotherapeutic plant alkaloid, has demonstrated efficacy. Individuals with extensive oral involvement may be treated with radiotherapy.

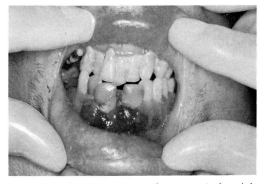

Figure 47–3. Kaposi's sarcoma. This tumor is found frequently in the oral cavity of patients with AIDS and is characterized by macular or raised pigmented lesions of the mucosa or gingiva. Small macular lesions usually do not require treatment. Lesions extending over teeth that are of esthetic concern may be excised. Direct injection of cancer chemotherapeutic agents into the tumor may be useful in some circumstances. (Courtesy of Dr. Sook B. Woo.)

Patients may have oral lesions of Kaposi's sarcoma without having skin lesions.

In addition to Kaposi's sarcoma, patients with AIDS have an increased frequency of intraoral lymphomas, which may present in various ways. The most common presentation is that of a rapidly enlarging mass. In some cases, the surface mucosa may be pigmented, but it is often intact. The lesions are firm to palpation but lack the rock-hardness seen in squamous cell carcinomas. Diagnosis is made by biopsy. If the lesion is large, an incisional biopsy is adequate. The tissue often resembles fish flesh in consistency. The treatment of intraoral lymphomas is usually chemotherapy.

DENTAL EVALUATION

In providing dental care to a patient known to be HIV-positive, it is important to assess the state of immunosuppression of the patient and to understand the possible side effects of the medications the patient is taking. The state of immunosuppression can usually be assessed by the clinical history. Asymptomatic patients generally are more immunoresponsive than patients with multiple opportunistic infections. Similarly, patients not requiring therapy are usually more immunocompetent than patients on multiple medications.

An objective guide to the state of immunocompromise is the CD4 count. Most patients are aware of their most recent CD4 count, but the patient's physician may have to be consulted. A CD4 count greater than 500 denotes reasonable immune response, a CD4 count less than 500 cells/μl signifies significant immunocompromise, and a CD4 count less than 200 cells/μl indicates severe immunocompromise. In addition to the CD4 count, it is important to review the patient's complete blood and platelet counts. Anemia, leukopenia, and thrombocytopenia are all common sequelae of AIDS that can complicate dental management and alter the dental treatment plan significantly.

A review of the patient's medications can alert the dentist to possible complications. Patients on AZT or trimethoprim-sulfamethoxazole may have leukopenia. Patients on pentamadine may develop hypoglycemia, which can complicate treatment. It is important to consult the patient's physician and discuss the treatment plan in detail, asking specifically about the need for antibiotic therapy after the dental procedures.

DENTAL MANAGEMENT

Dental management of patients with HIV infection requires consideration of their immunocompromised status, as well as their infectivity. Concern over becoming infected by a patient with AIDS has been a psychologic barrier that has limited access of AIDS patients to dental and medical care. The law is clear that a practitioner cannot deny a patient care based on the patient's HIV status. In fact, available data strongly support the concept that there is minimal risk to health care workers caring for patients with AIDS. The major concern involves parenteral exposure to blood products. In dentistry, almost every procedure involves some sort of sharp instrument. Thus, the major risk is that of a puncture wound from a contaminated instrument. The use of gloves provides some protection, but careful, attentive technique is probably more important. Fortunately, the rate of seroconversion of health care workers who have received needle sticks from known HIV carriers is low.

It has been estimated that the average dentist has a puncture wound related to practice at least once every 5 years. It is therefore important for the dentist to have a protocol for dealing with puncture wounds. The wound should be thoroughly cleansed with soap and water. If the HIV antibody status of the patient was recently determined to be negative, the patient should be asked to have a repeat test in 6 to 8 weeks. The injured individual should have an HIV antibody test immediately. If the patient is known to be HIV-positive, a baseline HIV antibody test should be done on the injured professional and consideration made for anti-HIV prophylactic treatment. Currently, prompt treatment with a course of AZT is available for individuals with a puncture wound, but the efficacy of such treatment remains controversial. The HIV antibody status should be determined again in the injured individual 6 to 8 weeks after exposure. However, the HIV status of the patient is usually unknown. The patient should be asked to have an HIV antibody determination. Patients are naturally hesitant to have the test, but if the dentist explains the rationale, patient compliance is usually high. As in the other situations, the injured individual should have a baseline HIV antibody screen and should be retested 6 to 8 weeks later.

It is not necessary to treat patients who are seropositive in an environment different from that of the standard operatory. The use of universal precautions, consisting of gloves, eye protection, a mask, and appropriate clinic attire, provides adequate protection. It may be advisable to use a surgical gown for especially bloody or messy procedures.

From a medical standpoint, there are two major considerations in providing dental treatment in patients with AIDS, their level of immunocompromise and their level of thrombocytopenia. Many patients with AIDS can tolerate routine dental care without difficulty. However, even if the patient is asymptomatic, immunosuppression may lead to infection after oral manipulation. Furthermore, both the disease and the medications the patient may be taking (e.g., AZT or trimethoprim-sulfamethoxazole) can cause leukopenia and granulocytopenia. Therefore, perioperative antibiotic prophylaxis is recommended for procedures that place the patient at risk for infection. Occasionally, patients with AIDS develop thrombocytopenia. It is therefore important to obtain a platelet count before initiating any treatment that might cause bleeding.

CHAPTER

48

Viral Infections

Viruses are microscopic complexes that contain single or double strands of nucleic acids, either DNA or RNA. Whether viruses are "alive" has not been resolved. However, viruses transmit genetic information and replicate, which ensures their survival. Unlike other microorganisms, viruses do not themselves divide. Rather, the synthesis of new viral nucleic acids is performed by the cells into which viruses penetrate.

Viral invasion of cells and the production of new viral particles is a six-stage process. The initial phase occurs when the virus attaches to the cell surface. Because viruses themselves are not mobile, attachment to the cell surface is mediated by receptors. Once attachment has occurred, the virus penetrates into the cell, and uncoating, or the functional release of nucleic acid from the protein and lipid covering, occurs. Subsequently, replication of the nucleic acids takes place. This is followed by reconstitution or assembly of the viral particle and its release from the cell. Viral invasion does not by itself destroy the infected cell. Host cell destruction is dependent on the mode of viral release from the cell, the effect of the virus on cell metabolism, and the release of viral toxins. Thus, viral infection may result in cytolysis, chronic metabolic dysfunction, or transformation of the cell, or there may be no pathologic effects.

There are two major forms of viral infection; classification is based on the extent of viral involvement. Viral infections may be confined to a specific entry site, as in the case of a respiratory viral infection. The incubation period is usually short, as is the duration of subsequent immunity, and there is no hematogenous phase. Immunity to such infections relies heavily on the secretory immune system (IgA) and on local cell-mediated immune reactions.

In contrast, systemic viral infections, such as measles, have a relatively long incubation period. Patients suffer from hematogenous spread of the infecting organism. When conferred, immunity is mediated by both the humoral and cellular immune systems, and is long-lasting.

Host defense mechanisms against viruses are specific and nonspecific. Specific defenses to viral infection are mediated by all components of the immune system. Nonspecific host defense is dependent on phagocytosis and inflammation. Clearly, any pathologic process or drug therapy that negatively alters host resistance can result in overwhelming, fatal viral infection.

VIRAL INFECTIONS OF THE ORAL MUCOSA

Virally induced infections of the oral cavity are common. A number of specific oral manifestations of viral infections have been described, and there are large numbers of viruses that produce oral changes.

In general, oral mucosal changes induced by viruses are relatively consistent. In addition to the systemic signs of viremia that include malaise, anorexia, fever, and myalgia, oral signs of viral infection include croppy vesicle formation and coated tongue. The distribution of these lesions varies, but ulceration because of ruptured vesicles usually produces clinical symptoms of pain.

The diagnosis of viral infection is usually a clinical one made on the basis of history and the appearance of oral lesions. Treatment is generally aimed at reducing fever and discomfort and ensuring hydration. In almost all cases, the oral lesions associated with viral infections spontaneously resolve in 10 to 14 days without scarring.

A number of specific viral infections are routinely encountered in dental practice. These include primary and recurrent herpes simplex infection, herpangina, herpes zoster, varicella, hand, foot, and mouth disease, and human immunodeficiency virus (HIV).

Viral infections of the salivary glands are discussed elsewhere (Chap. 43).

Herpes Simplex

Of the viruses that cause infections in the mouth, the most common is herpes simplex. There is more than one type of herpes simplex virus. In the oral cavity, herpes simplex type I commonly produces oral disease. Two forms of oral infection are produced by the virus: an acute form of stomatitis, which represents primary infection, and a chronic recurrent localized form, which represents secondary infection.

Primary herpetic gingivostomatitis represents the patient's initial exposure to the virus. Not surprisingly, this usually occurs during childhood but may also be noted during adolescence and early adulthood. It is not an uncommon occurrence in a college community. Clinically, the patient usually develops a classic viral prodrome consisting of malaise, arthralgia, and anorexia accompanied by fever and chills. Shortly thereafter (24 to 48 hours), the mouth erupts into a triad of lesions that generally affects the mucosa (Figs. 48–1 and 48–2), gingiva, and tongue. Vesicles on the mucosa do not remain intact for long and rupture into large, painful ulcerated areas. An acute gingivitis that demonstrates swelling, redness, and bleeding affects the marginal and papillary gingivae and is uncomfortable. Typically, the tongue has a white coating (Figs. 48–3 and 48–4). Submandibular and cervical lymphadenopathy are usually noted. The patient is febrile, uncomfortable, and generally miserable.

The diagnosis of primary herpes is clinically based on history and appearance of the lesions. The clinical picture must be differen-

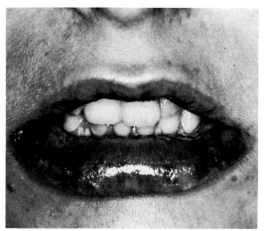

Figure 48–2. Acute herpetic gingivostomatitis. Note the swollen condition of the lips, with secondary hemorrhagic involvement.

tiated from acute necrotizing ulcerative gingivitis (ANUG). ANUG does not present with a prodrome, and oral involvement is limited to the gingiva. The diagnosis of herpes infection can be confirmed by viral culture of lesions or by obtaining a serum sample during the acute phase of the disease and again 6 weeks later (convalescent sample). If herpes infection has occurred, a rise in antibody titer is seen in the sample from the convalescing patient. Cytology can also help in diagnosis by the demonstration of giant cells with viral inclusion bodies (Fig. 48–5).

In healthy patients, primary herpes infections are self-limiting and the acute phase rarely lasts more than 1 week. Unless there are specific signs of secondary infection, patients need not be treated with antibiotics. Treatment should consist of bed rest, aspirin to control fever and pain, large fluid intake, and palliative mouth rinses. If the dentist is unable to ensure adequate fluid intake because of the age of the patient and/or oral pain, the patient may require intravenous fluid replacement. The ulcers heal completely without scarring.

Recurrent Herpes Simplex

Recurrent herpes simplex type I infections are common. These lesions, it is believed, result from reactivation of the herpes virus from a dormant state in the trigeminal ganglia in a previously infected host. The lesions produced by this reactivation are commonly referred to

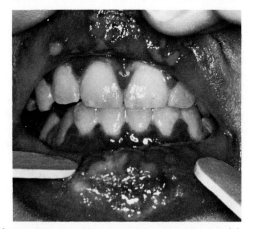

Figure 48–1. Acute herpetic gingivostomatitis. Painful vesicular lesions are present on the maxillary and mandibular labial mucosae. Note the swollen inflamed condition of the marginal and papillary gingivae.

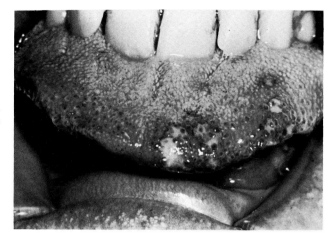

Figure 48–3. Tongue of a patient with acute herpetic gingivostomatitis. Note the vesicular lesions and coating on the tongue.

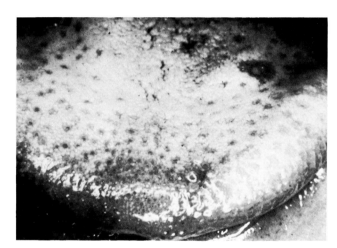

Figure 48–4. Coated tongue of a patient with acute herpetic gingivostomatitis.

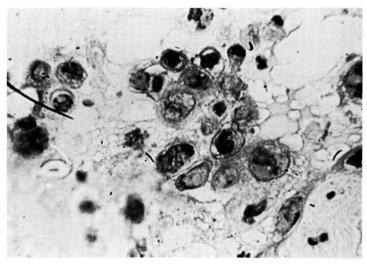

Figure 48–5. Multinucleated giant cell in a smear from a patient with a primary herpes infection.

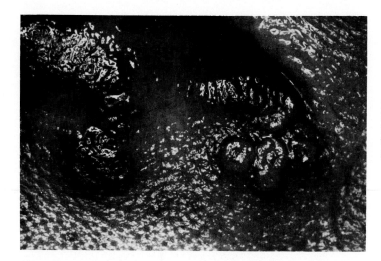

Figure 48–6. Typical appearance of herpes labialis prior to the rupture of vesicles. Note the croppy intact vesicles at the corner of the mouth. These lesions are generally restricted to the skin.

as cold sores or herpes labialis. The frequency of recurrence varies among patients, but 25% of patients affected by recurrent herpes labialis have one or more episodes per month.

Clinically, herpes labialis most often results in single or multiple small (2 to 4 mm in diameter) lesions on the lips at the mucocutaneous junction, at the corners of the mouth, or beneath the nose (Fig. 48–6). Patients may experience a prodrome often described as itchiness, drawing, or tingling. The vesicles appear shortly thereafter (about 12 hours), often surrounded by a small area of erythema. Frequently, patients are uncomfortable. Most discomfort is noted during the first 24 hours following vesicle formation. Lymphadenopathy can usually be detected and patients may complain of mild flu-like symptoms, depending on the severity of the infection and their level of immunization. Vesicles usually rupture in 36 to 48 hours, resulting in an ulcer that may be crusted. The viral titer is highest during the first 48 hours of infection and then falls off over time. Thus, it is during this period that the lesion is most infective. Over 7 to 10 days the vesicle dries up, leaving a crusting lesion that soon disappears.

The lesions of secondary herpes infections are recurrent, completely disappearing and then returning. It has been proposed that their appearance is seasonal and related to cold, sunlight, and stress. Indeed, some patients tend to develop fewer lesions if they continually wear a sunblock during periods of frequent exposure to the sun. However, there is no universally accepted preventive or treatment modality for herpes labialis. Dyes, ultraviolet light, ether, and alcohol have all been suggested, but their ability to control the infection is unsubstantiated. In healthy patients, application of acyclovir ointment may be of benefit.

Generally, it is best to keep the lesions lubricated to allow maximum healing. It should also be remembered that the vesicle harbors live virus particles. Thus, the dentist should avoid contact with the patient with active herpes to avoid infection (Fig. 48–7). Similarly, family members should be cautioned, especially if there is a youngster in the household who is at risk for primary herpes infection.

Secondary herpes simplex infections are particularly common in immunocompromised

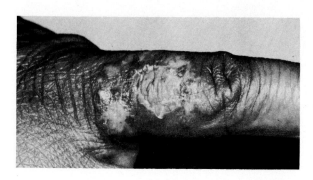

Figure 48–7. Herpetic infection (herpetic whitlow) of the skin secondary to contact with an active oral lesion.

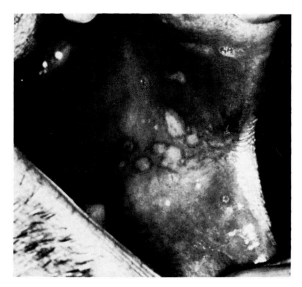

Figure 48–8. Herpes zoster. Note the somewhat linear distribution of the lesions, which are characteristically painful and unilateral.

patients who have antibody titers to the virus (Chap. 47). This group includes patients who are myelosuppressed as a consequence of cancer chemotherapy or immunosuppressed owing to disease (HIV infection) or medication. The presentation of oral lesions of secondary herpes simplex virus infection in these individuals are varied and often dramatic. Vesicles and bullae often give rise to large ulcerated areas. Aggressive culturing of lesions suspected of being viral in origin is mandatory. Systemic therapy with acyclovir is the treatment of choice.

Herpes Zoster

Herpes zoster is a painful viral infection of the posterior root ganglia caused by varicella-zoster virus. It is generally believed that the same virus causes chickenpox. Herpes zoster infection may affect all branches of the trigeminal nerve, in which case there is involvement on the face or in the oral cavity.

Herpes zoster infection is heralded by extreme unilateral pain. Approximately 3 to 5 days later, crops of small vesicles appear that usually have a somewhat linear distribution and are always unilateral (Figs. 48–8 and 48–9). If the vesicles rupture, ulcerative lesions remain, generally on an erythematous base. The lesions are usually uncomfortable. Oral lesions may occur on the buccal, labial, or palatal mucosa or on the lips. Healing is usually complete in 7 to 14 days.

Herpes zoster is a relatively frequent complication of immunosuppression related to cancer therapy, renal transplants, and HIV infection. In these individuals, viremias of potential

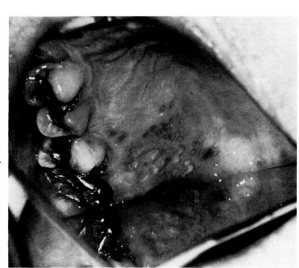

Figure 48–9. Herpes zoster infection of the palate.

systemic consequence may develop. Occasionally, severe complications of herpes zoster infection may develop, including neuralgia, facial paralysis, and corneal scarring.

As with many other viral infections, there is no satisfactory treatment for herpes zoster other than palliation. Because the infection is usually self-limiting, this is usually sufficient. In severe cases, or when the patient is immunosuppressed, intravenous acyclovir is the treatment of choice.

Herpangina

Herpangina, a viral disease that affects the mouth, is caused by a group A coxsackie virus. The disease, which is most common in young children under 4 years of age, demonstrates seasonal variation, being most frequent in the summer months.

Clinically, the initial manifestation of the disease is the acute onset of fever, usually greater than 100° F (38° C), in an otherwise healthy child. The patient may develop other flu-like symptoms including malaise, myalgia, runny nose, throat pain, and dysphagia. The predominant clinical lesions associated with herpangina occur in the mouth and are manifested as multiple, small, ovoid vesicular lesions occurring on the soft palate and oropharynx (Fig. 48–10). There is usually an erythematous base. The vesicles may rupture, leaving an ulcer. Usually there are multiple lesions, although solitary lesions have been reported. Typically, there is little or no involvement of the anterior two-thirds of the mouth. The lesions are painful. Lymphadenopathy may also be present. The acute symptoms of herpangina persist for about 3 days and the lesions heal without scarring in about a week.

Treatment of herpangina is palliative and supportive. Bed rest, aspirin, and fluids are recommended. Palliative rinses, such as Xylocaine Viscous or Benadryl and Kaopectate, may be helpful to control discomfort. A soft diet should be suggested.

The differential diagnosis of herpangina includes other viral infections, streptococcal and other bacterial pharyngitis, and aphthous stomatitis. The diagnosis can usually be made

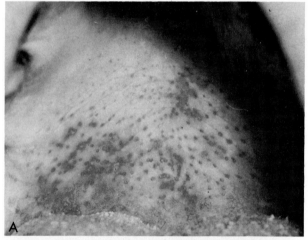

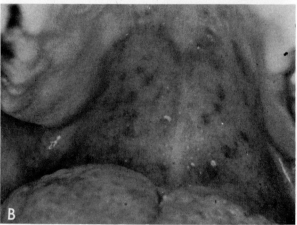

Figure 48–10. *A, B,* Two presentations of herpangina. Note the involvement of the soft palate.

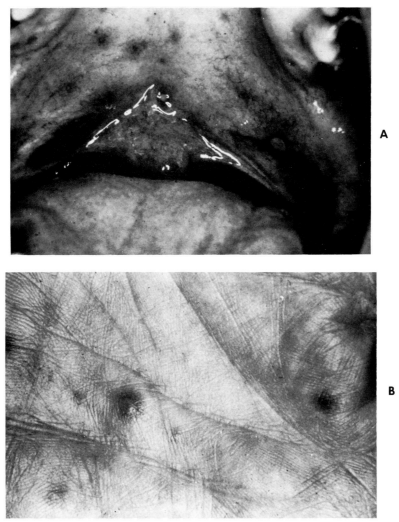

Figure 48–11. Hand, foot, and mouth disease. This infection, caused by a group A coxsackie virus, affects the oral mucosa (A) and skin of the palms and soles (B).

based on the history and clinical appearance. However, bacterial culture may be performed to rule out a bacterial cause.

Hand, Foot, and Mouth Disease

Hand, foot, and mouth disease is a relatively rare infection caused by a group A coxsackie virus. The clinical course of this disease is similar to that of herpangina. A typical prodromal phase of malaise is followed by the development of vesicles and erythema in the posterior soft palate. Additionally, small, ovoid, erythematous areas are noted on the palms and soles (Fig. 48–11). The disease resolves spontaneously in 7 to 14 days. Treatment is palliative.

CHAPTER 49

Fungal Infections

Fungal infections of the mouth are generally uncommon. Their appearance is most often associated with an underlying systemic disorder that adversely affects the patient's ability to deal with these organisms. A variety of fungal forms are normal inhabitants of the oral cavity, but are kept in balance by competing bacteria and the body's normal defense mechanisms. Alterations of either of these may result in the development of fungal infection. Thus, the presence of oral fungal infections should be viewed with suspicion, and the prudent workup requires not only diagnosis and treatment of the overt infection, but also investigation into the underlying cause. Among the systemic diseases that predispose to fungal infections are diabetes mellitus, leukemia, aplastic anemia, uremia, acquired immunodeficiency syndrome (AIDS), immunosuppression, and the ingestion of antibiotics.

The diagnosis of fungal infections is based on history, clinical appearance, and where possible, culture or biopsy.

CANDIDIASIS

Of fungal infections that affect the mouth, candidiasis is the most common. Approximately 50% of the population has *Candida albicans* as part of their normal oral flora. Usually, this organism is of no clinical significance. However, if changes occur in the oral environment, candidal organisms can proliferate and cause infection.

Candidiasis is most frequent in patients at either age extreme; in newborns the infection is called thrush. It has been reported that fungal proliferation is seen frequently under the palate of a maxillary prosthesis. Any patient who has a change in marrow status resulting from diseases such as aplastic anemia or drugs such as are used in chemotherapy is at high risk to develop candidiasis. Similarly, patients receiving immunosuppressive therapy such as steroids or debilitated individuals such as those

with diabetes may develop fungal infections of this type. Prolonged use of antibiotics, particularly those that are broad in spectrum, may produce candidiasis. Mucocutaneous candidiasis is a hallmark finding in patients with AIDS (Chap. 47).

Clinically, candidiasis has a wide variety of manifestations. Patients may be totally asymptomatic or may complain of pain or burning or of having a coated feeling in the mouth. Four clinical presentations of oral candidiasis have been described. Pseudomembranous candidiasis is the classic and most common appearance of the infection. In these cases, patients have raised, curdy, white areas, often of the palate and tongue (Fig. 49–1A). The white areas, which are necrotic, can usually be scraped off with a wet tongue blade, leaving a raw, bleeding surface (Fig. 49–1B). Hyphae can be easily demonstrated microscopically in the scraped debris after it is treated with potassium hydroxide (Fig. 49–2). Hyperplastic candidiasis is markedly less common and appears as raised, white, nonscrapable lesions that may appear in the commissures of the mouth or, in the case of patients with HIV, on the buccal mucosa. Erythematous candidiasis is most often present on the palate or dorsal surface of the tongue and is characterized by varying degrees of mucosal erythema. It is a frequent cause of burning mouth. Finally, candidiasis may cause angular cheilitis.

Candidiasis usually responds well to topical therapy if there is no significant underlying pathology. Nystatin oral suspension, given at a dose of 200,000 to 400,000 units tid or qid, daily with instructions to swish and swallow, is effective for most mucosal candidiasis. Alternatively, clotrimazole, 10-mg troches given five times daily for 14 days, may be used. Candidiasis beneath dentures can be treated with nystatin ointment applied to the prosthesis. Gentian violet suspension is also an effective topical antifungal agent, but its presence so discolors tissue that assessment is confounded. Systemic medications for mucosal candidiasis

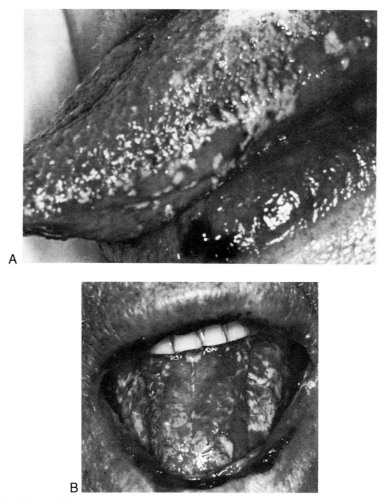

Figure 49–1. Candidiasis of the tongue presenting as raised white areas *(A)* with an underlying erythematous base *(B)*.

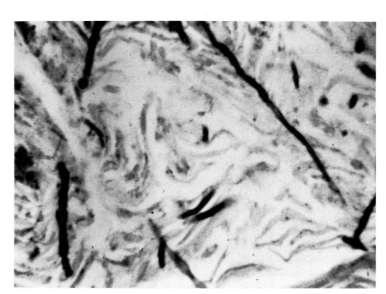

Figure 49–2. Smear from area infected with *Candida* demonstrating fungal hyphae.

include ketoconazole tablets and fluconazole (Diflucan). Fluconazole is extremely effective for persistent cases of oral candidiasis and has a dosing schedule that is easy for patients (200 mg on day 1, then 100 mg on subsequent days). However, the drug is expensive. For patients with systemic fungal involvement or esophageal or pulmonary candidiasis and who have compromised ability to deal with infection, amphotericin B must be considered. This medication requires intravenous administration and is *highly* nephrotoxic. Its use should be considered only after consultation with the patient's physician and administered in an inpatient setting.

ACTINOMYCOSIS

Actinomycosis is caused by an organism that has both fungal and bacterial properties. Although some have concluded that actinomycosis more closely resembles bacteria, others refer to the organism as a bacteria-like fungus. The organism is anaerobic. Five species of Actinomyces are present in the mouth; the majority are nonpathologic. For the most part, *Actinomyces israelii* is the most frequent pathogen causing cervicofacial infection.

Although actinomycosis may occur in other sites, cervicofacial infection is the most common and accounts for about two-thirds of the infections caused by this organism. Whereas the organism is present in the normal flora, infection is precipitated by its introduction into tissue. Typically, mandibular extraction or a compound mandibular fracture is mentioned as such a precipitating event. However, actinomycosis has also been reported as a sequela to endodontic and periodontal treatment and as a sequela to extraction in patients with HIV infection.

The infection has an insidious onset that progresses slowly. Manifestations of actinomyces may occur some time after the initiating event (2 weeks or more). Patients note the development of a rock-hard, tumor-like swelling. Reddish-purple discoloration of the skin overlying the area is common. As time progresses, the surface of the skin fistulates, and small sinus tracts develop and eventually drain a particulate fluid consisting of sulfur granules (Fig. 49–3). The infection site remains hard and demarcated, giving a "lumpy" feeling often associated with this condition.

Bony involvement, manifested as an osteomyelitis, may occur in the latter stages of the infection. Diagnosis is based on history, clini-

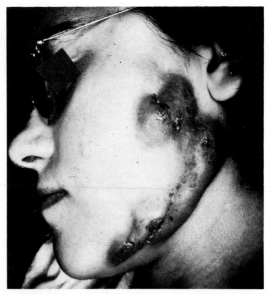

Figure 49–3. Actinomycosis. (From Ash and Spitz, *Pathology of Tropical Disease—An Atlas,* 1945, ARP/AFIP 98947.)

cal presentation, and culture of drainage. Actinomycosis must be differentiated from other forms of infection, including tuberculosis, and tumor. The infection is usually responsive to a prolonged antibiotic course; penicillin is the drug of choice (2 to 4 million units qid for 2 months). Surgical débridement of the infected region is often helpful.

HISTOPLASMOSIS

Histoplasmosis is a deep fungal infection that sometimes affects the mouth. The disease is caused by the fungus *Histoplasma capsulatum,* an organism endemic to certain parts of the world. In the United States, the Mississippi River Valley region is the most common location for the disease. Although there are an estimated 500,000 new cases of histoplasmosis in the United States annually, most cases are subclinical or restricted to respiratory tract involvement. Of the total, 5% of cases are disseminated, however, and it is in these cases that oral involvement has been reported.

The organism is found in spores in the soil that can be spread by birds in endemic areas, thus allowing urbanites to be exposed to the fungus. The spores enter the body by way of the respiratory tree to the lung. Most cases remain confined to the respiratory tract, although 5% of cases become disseminated. Clinical manifestations of histoplasmosis therefore include cough, dyspnea, and frequently weight loss.

Men are more frequently affected by the disease than women. Oral involvement has never been reported in a patient under 20 years of age. Whereas the infection used to be most common in elderly white people, it is now seen with increasing frequency as an opportunistic infection in HIV-infected individuals.

The oral manifestations of histoplasmosis are varied and include painful ulcerations, nodules, or vegetative processes. Most patients with oral lesions have more than one oral manifestation of the disease. Patients complain of pain, weakness, and the other symptoms. Fever is an infrequent complaint. The appearance of the lesions may also vary, and ulcers may be deep or shallow.

Oral lesions occur anywhere in the mouth but are most common on the oropharynx, buccal mucosa, tongue, and palate.

The clinical appearance of histoplasmosis is generally the same as that of epidermoid carcinoma. Thus, biopsy is mandatory and diagnostic when stained appropriately (Gomori-methenamine silver). Cultures of smears of lesions may give false-negative results. A skin test for histoplasmin may be effective for diagnosis, depending on when the patient was infected.

Treatment of histoplasmosis is reasonably successful with amphotericin B.

PHYCOMYCOSIS (MUCORMYCOSIS NECROSIS)

Mucormycosis is a rare fungal infection most commonly noted in debilitated patients. The infection is caused by organisms of the order Mucorales, especially *Mucor* and *Rhizopus.* Both are common in soil and decaying vegetable matter and can be cultured easily from normal individuals, in whom they are nonpathogenic. The organisms are most easily noted using periodic acid–Schiff (PAS) stain.

Mucormycosis has long been associated with poorly controlled diabetes mellitus. It is now noted with increasing frequency in myelosuppressed patients, notably those with leukemia or those receiving chemotherapy for other malignancies and patients with AIDS.

The most common form of disease is rhinocerebral, in which organisms normally present in the nasal passages produce infection. The infection may then spread to involve the lungs and gastrointestinal tract.

Oral manifestations of mucormycosis are relatively rare but when present include a nonhealing progressive necrotic ulcer (Fig. 49–4). Underlying bony destruction may occur. Tissue destruction associated with the disease is the result of vessel thrombosis caused by the organism. The organism has an affinity for blood vessel walls, where proliferation occurs, causing thrombosis and subsequent necrosis. Facial swelling, proptosis, and eye and facial symptoms may be noted in patients with disease extending to the orbit, paranasal sinuses, and cranial cavity.

The diagnosis of mucormycosis is based on the demonstration of the infecting organisms in tissue. Biopsy and PAS stain are diagnostic; cultures are also helpful. Patients with debilitating disease are at risk for developing this infection, and nonhealing ulcers must be dealt with aggressively in this group.

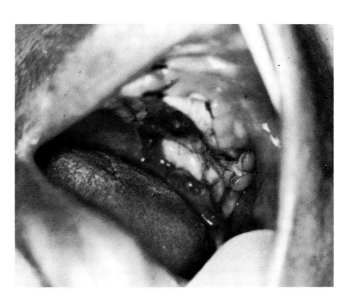

Figure 49–4. Mucormycosis.

Untreated, mucormycosis proceeds to a fatal conclusion. Treatment of the underlying disease should be undertaken. The fungal infection should be treated with a long course (months) of amphotericin B.

OTHER FUNGAL INFECTIONS OF THE HEAD AND NECK

A small number of other fungi may infect the head and neck. For the most part, these organisms are transmitted by the respiratory route, but underlying disease may predispose to the colonization of head and neck structures, sometimes including the mouth.

Aspergillosis is caused by airborne spores of *Aspergillus* species. Head and neck infection is most common in the debilitated patient, especially those with leukemia. Aspergillosis of the head and neck most frequently involves the paranasal and maxillary sinuses. Diagnosis is made on the basis of clinical and radiographic signs and culture (Fig. 49–5). Treatment consists of surgical débridement and drainage, which may be supplemented with antifungal medication.

North American blastomycosis is caused by the fungus *Blastomyces dermatitidis,* generally transmitted by the respiratory route. Infection may take one of three forms, pulmonary, cutaneous, or systemic. The cutaneous form rarely affects the mouth, but when it does it produces an oral ulceration that may be suppurative. Biopsy is of value for diagnosis. The fungus is recoverable from draining lesions. Systemic antifungal medication (amphotericin B) is the treatment of choice.

Coccidioidomycosis is caused by the dust and soil inhabitant *Coccidioides immitis.* Unlike many other fungal infections, coccidioidomy-

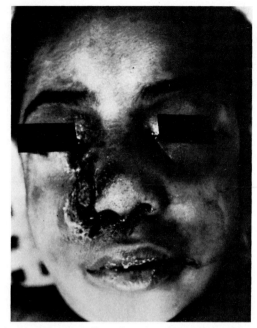

Figure 49–5. Aspergillosis demonstrating overlying skin necrosis extending from the paranasal sinuses.

cosis is relatively common, especially in certain geographic areas such as the southwestern United States. Coccidioidomycosis is generally manifested as an upper respiratory infection that is usually self-limiting. However, a disseminated form that is progressive and fatal may also occur. Oral manifestations of the latter include the formation of purplish nodules that may remain for up to 2 months. Diagnosis is usually made clinically or by laboratory evaluation. Treatment of the self-limiting form is generally symptomatic. Systemic antifungal agents (e.g., amphotericin B) may also be used.

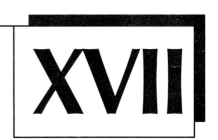
Selection and Clinical Pharmacology of Drugs Commonly Used in Dentistry

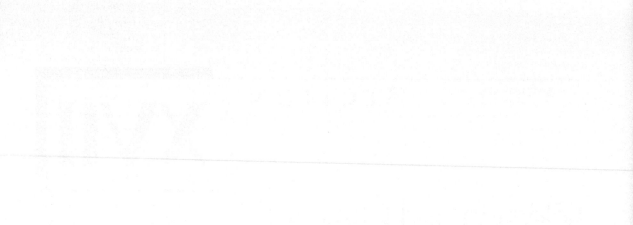

CHAPTER 50

Analgesics

The choice of an appropriate analgesic depends on the severity of pain elicited by a procedure, injury, or disease; the clinician's evaluation of the patient's reaction to the procedure; and a consideration of the attendant medical problems. The dentist must strike a delicate balance between providing the patient with adequate pain relief and overmedicating.

The dentist must also not underestimate the role of a patient's anxiety in contributing to the level of discomfort. An analgesic that would otherwise be adequate for the pain of a particular procedure may be ineffective in a patient whose anxiety has not been addressed. The informed, assured patient may be expected to require less analgesic medication than a patient with whom the provider does not communicate. When needed, increased pain relief may be accomplished not by adding analgesics but by using appropriate sedation techniques preoperatively, intraoperatively, or sometimes postoperatively (Chap. 51). The placebo effect of medications should not be underestimated. A patient who gives a past history of success with a particular pain medication can probably do well with the same medication for similar pain, because the initial experience has been a positive one, regardless of its potency relative to other medications.

An exhaustive discussion of analgesics is beyond the scope of this text. However, the following should offer a framework onto which medications may be added or subtracted based on training and experience. Before prescribing any medication, the dentist should be thoroughly familiar with its pharmacologic properties, its indications, and any precautions associated with its use.

NON-NARCOTICS: MILD TO MODERATE ANALGESIA

Salicylates

Aspirin is the most commonly recommended pain medication. The drug is often used in combination with others. There are more than 200 compounds containing aspirin. The primary advantage of aspirin is that it is an anti-inflammatory agent in addition to being analgesic and antipyretic. Its major disadvantages are the potential for gastrointestinal distress and its negative effect on platelet function. Most commonly in dentistry, therefore, aspirin is not recommended for patients with a history of gastrointestinal intolerance or patients who have had recent surgical procedures. The impact on platelet function, which is not dose dependent, is an alteration in platelet function lasting 7 to 10 days, or the half-life of platelet production. Aspirin or aspirin-containing compounds are strictly contraindicated in patients receiving anticoagulation therapy (e.g., warfarin, heparin); patients with known coagulation disorders (e.g., hemophilia; Chap. 26); aspirin-induced asthma (Chap. 18); peptic ulcer diseases or gastritis (Chap. 21); gout patients receiving probenecid (Chap. 28); patients with renal failure (Chap. 29); and patients receiving methotrexate.

Acetaminophen

Acetaminophen is the primary metabolite of phenacetin. Acetaminophen alone is the first drug of choice as an alternative to aspirin. It is frequently recommended in patients in whom postoperative bleeding is a concern. It is an analgesic and antipyretic but not an anti-inflammatory agent.

Nonsteroidal Anti-inflammatory Drugs

Nonsteroidal anti-inflammatory drugs (NSAIDs) are comparatively new to the analgesic armamentarium. Their primary advantage is to offer a non-narcotic alternative to codeine compounds for moderate pain relief without codeine's significant diminution of reflexes as a side effect. The contraindications are similar to those for aspirin. NSAIDs, therefore, should not be used for patients with known coagulopathies or patients on anticoagulant therapy because of their negative impact on platelet function. Unlike aspirin, NSAIDs cause reversible inhibition of platelet aggregation. Therefore, when the drug is eliminated, platelet function rapidly returns to normal. These agents are also contraindicated for patients with aspirin-sensitive asthma or a history of peptic ulcer disease or gastritis, patients afflicted with gout and receiving probenecid or methotrexate, or patients with renal failure. Also, these drugs should not be used concurrently with aspirin. Ibuprofen (Motrin) is the most commonly prescribed NSAID. Other, longer acting drugs in this class offer little advantage other than that of single-dose therapy.

Ketorolac (Toradol) is supplied in an oral and an intramuscular form. It is often used as an intramuscular alterative to narcotics in the hospitalized patient undergoing general anesthesia.

Non-narcotic Advanced Analgesics

Pentazocine (Talwin) is not a first-choice drug. Infrequently used, this agent offers an advanced analgesic alternative for narcotic contraindication. Adverse effects, including CNS disturbances, are more common. Also, this drug is a mild narcotic antagonist. Because pentazocine may cause elevation of cerebrospinal fluid pressure, its use in patients with head injury is not recommended.

Narcotic Analgesics

Most narcotic analgesics are used for relief of moderate to severe pain. In addition to their analgesic effect, some sedation can be anticipated. Gastrointestinal distress manifested by nausea, cramping, and vomiting is relatively common. The potential for respiratory and cardiovascular depression and psychologic and physiologic dependence must be considered when narcotics are prescribed. In addition, narcotics may impair mental and physical functions. Thus, patients must be cautioned about driving. Generally, narcotics are contraindicated in those with chronic obstructive pulmonary disease (Chap. 19) and in

psychiatric patients receiving phenothiazines, tricyclic antidepressants, and especially monoamine oxidase inhibitors (Chap. 36). Narcotics are also contraindicated in patients with head trauma and those with deficiencies in thyroid, adrenal, or pituitary function (Chaps. 15 and 16). If narcotics must be used in these cases, the dosage must be reduced, often to 25 to 50% of normal levels, in consultation with the physician.

Codeine. Codeine is the most commonly prescribed narcotic in dentistry for moderate to severe pain. It is most often prescribed in compound with aspirin (Empirin 3) or acetaminophen (Tylenol 3), as these drugs potentiate the effect of the codeine dose. When prescribed in noncompounded form (codeine sulfate or codeine phosphate), appropriate instructions for use with aspirin, acetaminophen, or NSAIDs offer the patient the ability to titrate the dosage of codeine, as needed. Gastrointestinal intolerance and headache are common side effects and may complicate therapy.

Codeine Analogues. Oxycodone is approximately 12 times as potent as codeine sulfate and is somewhat longer acting. Percodan and Percocet 5 have an oxycodone dose roughly equivalent to 60 mg of codeine derivative compounded with aspirin and acetaminophen, respectively.

Vicodin and Lorcet offer a hydrocodone combination with acetaminophen of similar potency to the oxycodone preparations.

Compounds of Codeine and Codeine Analogues. If anxiety is a significant problem and codeine is needed for analgesia, Fiorinal 3 might be used. This codeine-aspirin-caffeine combination has a barbiturate (butalbital) added, as well, therefore providing significant sedation. Fioricet-3 offers an acetaminophen substitution for the aspirin component.

Demerol. Meperidine hydrochloride (Demerol) offers a narcotic analgesic intermediate in potency between codeine and morphine. Nausea and vomiting are common side effects, and therefore the addition of promethazine may be recommended. This antihistamine is chemically a phenothiazine, which potentiates meperidine's analgesic effect. The effective dose of meperidine may therefore be reduced. In addition, the promethazine has an antiemetic and sedative action that may be beneficial.

Mild Narcotics

Propoxyphene (Darvon) is a controversial mild narcotic; some studies have suggested limited effectiveness. In combination with aspirin (Darvon Compound-65) or acetaminophen (Darvocet-N 100), propoxyphene proba-bly offers better analgesia than either aspirin or acetaminophen alone but is less effective than these agents in combination with the narcotic codeine. It is not a first-choice drug. Its use in dentistry is in situations in which moderate analgesia is needed but codeine intolerance or a strong narcotic contraindication is present.

SUMMARY TABLE **50–1**

Oral Non-narcotic Analgesics for Mild to Moderate Pain

CLASS	DRUG	DOSAGE	COMMENTS
Aspirin base	Anacin	2 tabs q4h up to 10 tabs/day	400 mg aspirin with 32 mg caffeine
	Bufferin	2 tabs q4h up to 12 tabs/day	Aspirin buffered with aluminum glycinate and magnesium carbonate
	Maximum Strength Anacin	2 tabs to start, 1 tab q3h or 2 q6h up to 8 tabs/day	500 mg ASA (acetylsalicylic acid) with 32 mg caffeine
	Bayer	2 tabs q4h up to 3900 mg/day	325 mg ASA
	Ascriptin	2–3 tabs qid	With magnesium-aluminum hydroxide
	Ecotrin	1–2 tabs q4h up to 12 tabs/day	Enteric-coated 325-mg tablets
	Sodium salicylate	600 mg, 4–6 times/day	300- or 600-mg tabs
Acetaminophen base	Tylenol	325–650 mg q4-6h up to a maximum of 3900 mg/day	325-mg tabs
	Datril	650 mg to 1 g q4h up to a maximum of 4 g/day	325- or 500-mg tabs
	Aspirin Free Anacin	2 tabs tid or qid up to a maximum of 8 tabs/day	Acetaminophen 500 mg, caffeine 32 mg

Oral Non-narcotic Analgesics for Moderate to Severe Pain

CLASS	DRUG	DOSAGE	COMMENTS
Nonsteroidal anti-inflammatory drugs (NSAIDs)	Ibuprofen (Motrin, Advil, Nuprin, Rufen, others)	200 mg, 400 mg, 600 mg qid PO	2400-mg maximum daily dose; 400 mg comparable to acetaminophen/60-mg codeine combinations
	Flurbiprofen (Ansaid)	50 mg, 100 mg q8–12h	300-mg maximum daily dose; chronic use may decrease peri-odontal disease progression
	Naproxen (Naprosyn)	500 mg initially, then 250 mg q6–8h	1250-mg maximum daily dose
	Naproxen sodium (Anaprox)	550 mg initially, then 275 mg q6–8h PO	1375-mg maximum daily dose
	Diflunisal (Dolobid)	1000 mg initially, then 500 mg q8–12h PO	Maintenance doses of higher than 2500 mg daily not recommended
	Kotorolac (Toradol)	10 mg q6h	40-mg maximum daily dose
Others	Pentazocine (Talacen)	1 tablet q4h PO	25 mg pentazocine with acetaminophen 650 mg; 6-tablet maximum daily dose
	Pentazocine (Talwin compound)	2 caplets tid or qid	12.5 mg pentazocine and 325 mg acetylsalicylic acid

Oral Narcotic Analgesics for Moderate to Severe Pain

CLASS	DRUG	DOSAGE	COMMENTS
Codeine base	Codeine sulfate	15–60 mg q4h	
	Codeine phosphate	15–60 mg q4h	360 mg/day maximum dose
	Empracet 3	1 or 2 tabs q4h	30 mg codeine with acetaminophen (maximum daily dose of acetaminophen: 4000 mg)
	Tylenol 3	1 or 2 tabs q4h	30 mg codeine with acetaminophen
	Empirin 3	1 or 2 tabs q4h	30 mg codeine with acetylsalicylic acid
	Phenaphen 3	1 or 2 tabs q4h	Acetaminophen with codeine (no. 2, 15 mg; no. 3, 30 mg; no. 4, 60 mg)
Codeine analogue base	Percodan	1 tab q6h	5 mg oxycodone equivalent of 60 mg codeine with 325 mg acetylsalicylic acid
	Percocet 5	1 tab q6h	5 mg oxycodone equivalent of 60 mg codeine with 325 mg acetaminophen
	Tylox	1 tab q6h	5 mg oxycodone equivalent of 60 mg codeine with 500 mg acetaminophen
	Vicodin	2 tabs q4–6h	5 mg hydrocodone bitartrate/500 mg acetaminophen (maximum daily dose 8 tabs)
	Vicodin ES	1 tab q4–6h	7.5 mg hydrocodone/750 mg acetaminophen (maximum daily dose 5 tabs)
	Lorcet	1 tab q4–6h	10 mg hydrocodone/650 mg acetaminophen maximum daily dose 6 tabs)
	Synalgos-DC	2 caps q4h	Dihydrocodeine bitartrate aspirin/caffeine

Table continued on following page

SUMMARY TABLE **50–III**

Oral Narcotic Analgesics for Moderate to Severe Pain
Continued

CLASS	DRUG	DOSAGE	COMMENTS
Other codeine or codeine analogue compounds	Fiorinal with Codeine	1–2 caps q4h up to a total of 6/day or 2 tid	30 mg codeine, butalbital, and aspirin/caffeine
	Fioricet with Codeine	1 cap q4h	30 mg codeine, butalbital, and acetaminophen/caffeine
Meperidine base	Meperidine HCl (Demerol)	50–150 mg q3–4h	Can use 25–50 mg promethazine (Phenergan) as an adjunctive antiemetic—will potentiate narcotic
Mild narcotics—propoxyphene	Darvocet-N 100	1 tab q4h	With acetaminophen
	Wygesic	1 tab q4h	With acetaminophen
	Darvon Compound 65	1 cap q4h	With aspirin and caffeine
Other	Hydromorphone HCl (Dilaudid)	2–4 mg q4–6h	1- to 4-mg tabs

SUMMARY TABLE **50–IV**

Parenteral Analgesics for Moderate to Severe Pain

CLASS	DRUG	DOSAGE	COMMENTS
Non-narcotic	Pentazocine lactate (Talwin)	30 mg IV, IM, or SC q3–4h up to 360 mg/day, not to exceed 30 mg/dose IV or 60 mg/dose IM or SC	Generally used for hospitalized patients
Narcotic	Codeine sulfate	15–60 mg IM or SC q4h	
	Meperidine hydrochloride (Demerol)	50–150 mg SC or IM q3–4h	
	Morphine sulfate	5–20 mg SC or IM q4h	
Adjunctive antiemetic for narcotic parenteral analgesics	Promethazine hydrochloride (Phenergan)	25 mg IM	

Drugs Used for Sedation

Sedation techniques in the dental office are an important adjunct to the delivery of optimal care. Their goal is to allay the apprehension of the patient. Some medical problems can be acutely exacerbated by the emotional and physical stresses of dental procedures. The decision to use adjunctive sedation techniques depends on several variables: the anticipated duration and stress of the procedure, the medical status of the patient, and the anticipated anxiety level that could be evoked in a particular individual.

There is no substitute for a good doctor-patient rapport to minimize stress to the patient. Sedation should not be a substitution for reassurance and patient education.

Sedation techniques should be used only after appropriate training. The dentist must fully understand the sedation techniques available and must be aware of and prepared to handle all possible complications of these techniques.

It is beyond our scope here to discuss exhaustively the range of sedation choices or the details of any one technique. However, it is our intention to outline a sedation protocol framework onto which the individual dentist may add or from which techniques may be subtracted based on the dentist's knowledge and training. One goal of this text is to discuss the variables of the planned procedure (types I to VI) as they relate to the variable severity of the attendant medical problem. The suggested or recommended use of sedation techniques often follows. The practitioner must modify these recommendations based on the clinical evaluation of the individual patient's potential for anxiety. Thus, for a given procedure with a known medical problem, the stoic patient may require simple sedation, whereas the baseline anxious patient may require advanced sedation.

SIMPLE SEDATION TECHNIQUES

Nitrous oxide (N_2O-O_2) inhalation sedation is probably the most commonly used, safest, and simplest of the sedation techniques. Among its advantages are the ability to titrate dosage and, therefore, to individualize therapy, the drug's quick and easy reversibility, the safety margin of the drug, the minimal preparation prior to the appointment, and the minimal follow-up afterward. Certain guidelines maximize the safety of N_2O-O_2. Nitrous oxide should never be administered in a preset dosage. Inhalation analgesia should begin with 100% oxygen flow and incremental nitrous oxide should be added. Studies have shown that 35% N_2O, 65% O_2 flow is the mean dosage that can accomplish maximum analgesia and still ensure proper patient cooperation and responsiveness. This desired level, however, may be reached with as little as a 10% N_2O mixture. Rarely does the required flow exceed 50% N_2O, and it should never exceed 65% N_2O.

Higher concentrations of N_2O may be required early in the procedure (i.e., while local anesthetic solutions are administered), but every attempt should be made to reduce the N_2O flow during extended procedures under profound local anesthesia.

When N_2O-O_2 analgesia administration is being stopped, the patient should be allowed to breathe 100% oxygen for several minutes to allow for the differential diffusion of O_2 and N_2O across the alveolar-blood barrier. The N_2O molecule remains intact without degradation and is eliminated almost totally during expiration within minutes of the cessation of N_2O delivery.

Occasionally there can be paradoxical excitation in response to N_2O-O_2 delivery. This may be a particular risk for those patients undergoing psychiatric therapy (Chap. 34). Chronic obstructive pulmonary disease (Chap. 19) may also contraindicate the use of N_2O-O_2, as may known hypersensitivity to the drug. The clinical sign of cyanosis as an indicator of hypoxia may be absent in a patient with severe anemia, so N_2O-O_2 sedation is contraindicated in this patient.

INTERMEDIATE SEDATION TECHNIQUES

The cornerstone of intermediate sedation techniques is the oral administration of various sedative-hypnotic drugs. Additional adjunctive N_2O-O_2 inhalation sedation or oral analgesic drugs broaden the spectrum of the intermediate sedation techniques. All patients receiving such sedation must be accompanied by an adult to and from the dental office.

The disadvantage of the orally administered agents is the inability of the doctor to titrate the dosage to the individual patient during the procedure. A clinical judgment mut be made prior to the appointment as to the appropriate dose.

Prior to administration, the dentist must assess the impact of the drug on several organ systems. The drug's potential for cardiovascular and respiratory depression and the site of detoxification or excretion (i.e., liver or kidney) must be evaluated. This is most important when there is systemic disease associated with any of these organs. Further, the potential drug interaction of sedative-hypnotics with analgesics (Chap. 50) and the drugs used in managing psychiatric disorders, particularly the phenothiazines (Chap. 34), must be considered. Finally, dosage adjustments must be considered in the elderly, in whom minimal dosages may be effective.

Diazepam (Valium)

The first drug of choice among the oral intermediate sedation drugs is diazepam (Valium). When it is administered orally, cardiovascular and respiratory depression is minimal. Diazepam also has additional benefits beyond the antianxiety effects. Amnesia and prominent muscle relaxant properties add to its advantage for dentistry, particularly for the longer, more traumatic type V and VI moderate to advanced surgical procedures. Peak blood levels are attained 1 to 3 hours following administration. A 2- to 10-mg dose taken 1 to 1½ hours prior to the appointment is a typical protocol. Diazepam is detoxified primarily in the liver. Contraindications include hypersensitivity and the rare disorder acute narrow-angle glaucoma. Patients with hepatic or renal impairment should be given the drug only with caution. Similarly, the elderly may respond significantly to small doses. If narcotic analgesics are used concomitantly, the nar-

cotic dosage should be reduced by one-third to one-half.

Barbiturates

Generally, the short- to intermediate-acting barbiturates are the best choices for dental use. The most commonly used are amobarbital (Amytal), pentobarbital (Nembutal), or secobarbital (Seconal) in a 100- to 200-mg oral dose 1 to 1½ hours prior to the appointment. These preparations are metabolized by the liver and are not as often associated with postadministration hangover as are the longer-acting preparations, which have a significantly higher incidence of hangover. Phenobarbital (Luminal) in a 100- to 200-mg oral dose is the most commonly used barbiturate drug. It may be considered when intermediate sedation is needed in a patient with suspected or known liver disease (Chaps. 23 and 24), because the long-acting barbiturates are primarily excreted by the kidneys. Barbiturates diminish the effectiveness of anticoagulation with warfarin (Chap. 26) and are contraindicated in patients with the rare condition acute intermittent porphyria. Barbiturate therapy acts synergistically with other central nervous system depressants. Caution must be exercised when prescribing barbiturates to patients with chronic lung disease, those with significant cardiovascular compromise, and the elderly.

Antihistamines

The antihistamine promethazine HCl (Phenergan) in a 25- or 50-mg oral dose is often used with 50 to 100 mg of the narcotic analgesic meperidine (Demerol) in combination therapy. In addition to the sedation effects of the promethazine, it is an antiemetic, counterbalancing the potential side effects of the meperidine, and because it is chemically a phenothiazine, the drug markedly potentiates the analgesic action of the meperidine. The advantage of using this combination is that it may easily be continued for postoperative analgesia every 4 to 6 hours, and the effective dose of meperidine can be reduced. The disadvantage is that the meperidine, as a narcotic, has a side effect of prominent respiratory depression. Because they may predispose the patient to an acute exacerbation, antihistamines are relatively contraindicated in patients with asthma (Chap. 18). Vistaril (50 to 100 mg orally) may be used in a fashion similar to that for promethazine.

Other Preparations

Several alternative drugs used for sedation are available. Two worth mentioning because of their occasional daily use by patients are chlordiazepoxide (Librium) and meprobamate (Equanil, Miltown). Patients may present to the dentist on daily maintenance doses of these drugs. In consultation with the physician, a larger than normal maintenance dose may be used prior to the dental appointment. In all circumstances, the interaction and synergistic effects of CNS depressants must be kept in mind.

ADVANCED SEDATION TECHNIQUES

Administration of intravenous medications for sedation constitutes an advanced sedation technique. The major advantages of all intravenous sedation techniques include the depth of sedation possible and the ability to titrate the dosage specifically to the individual's needs. The major disadvantages depend to a large extent on the drug used and the impact on cardiovascular and respiratory status. Clinicians using intravenous sedation must have appropriate training and experience as well as an office fully equipped for all major emergencies. The American Society of Anesthesiologists (ASA) has developed a short-hand Physical Status Scale to assess patient anesthetic risk (Summary Table 51–II). Class I patients are those free of systemic disease. Class II patients are those with mild systemic disease. Class III patients have severe systemic disease that is not incapacitating. Class IV patients have incapacitating systemic disease that is a constant threat to life. Class V patients are moribund. Only class I and class II patients should be considered for outpatient intravenous sedation. All other patients in need of intravenous sedation should be electively admitted to the hospital.

Several drugs are used for intravenous sedation in the dental office. Diazepam (Valium) is the most common. In addition to its antianxiety potential, diazepam has the advantage of being a significant muscle relaxant and of causing amnesia. Techniques vary from slow injection directly into large veins to the addition of the drug into saline-filled infusion tubing. The latter method, started with a 21-gauge butterfly needle, is preferred. Venous thrombosis, phlebitis, and local irritation may complicate both approaches, especially direct injection. Most techniques also recommend a 1- to 2-mg test dose prior to a maximum of 10 to 20 mg diazepam. (Valium usually is supplied in 5-mg/ml doses and should be given slower than 1 ml/minute.) Most patients can be sedated with a total diazepam dose of less than 10 mg. Historically, ptosis has been used as an indication of appropriate sedation level, but some authors have speculated that this is a sign of overdosage.

Diazepam has few contraindications other than allergy and the rare disorder acute narrow-angle glaucoma. Elderly patients and patients with chronic lung disease are at increased risk of apnea or hypotension and cardiac compromise when intravenous diazepam is administered. Concomitant use of CNS depressants further increases this risk. The major disadvantage of diazepam is its relatively short duration of effective sedation. The clinician can anticipate 45 to 60 minutes of operating time after appropriate intravenous diazepam sedation before additional drug is required.

An alternative drug to Valium is midazolam (Versed), a water-soluble benzodiazepine. It offers the advantage of less risk for venous thrombosis and a shorter clearance rate. Disadvantages relate to possible higher risks of respiratory depression.

Longer procedures, therefore, are done with other intravenous medications. Intravenous pentobarbital (Nembutal) may be added to intravenous diazepam sedation and extend the operating time to 90 minutes. The use of intravenous narcotics (e.g., fentanyl [Sublimaze]) also provides a longer duration.

With the use of any CNS depressant, complications are more likely. Clinically significant respiratory depression, nausea, vomiting, and hypotension and cardiovascular compromise occur with greater frequency than with intravenous diazepam alone.

General Anesthesia

General anesthesia offers added control over the patient. However, relative to intravenous sedation techniques, general anesthetics have a marked increase in problems of airway management and maintenance of respiration. The presence of a separate skilled practitioner in addition to the operating dentist seems necessary to ensure proper general anesthesia technique. The hospital setting with an anesthesiologist as the dentist's aide is ideal. The selection of general anesthesia over an intravenous technique in the outpatient dental office is generally ill-advised.

Sedation Techniques

DEGREE	DELIVERY	EXAMPLES
Simple sedation	Inhalation	N_2O-O_2
Intermediate sedation	Inhalation and oral, or oral only	N_2O-O_2 with or without diazepam (Valium); barbiturates (Nembutal, Seconal); antihistamines (Phenergan, Vistaril); others (meprobamate, meperidine-promethazine)
Advanced sedation	IV with or without inhalation	Diazepam (Valium); diazepam (Valium) plus pentobarbital (Nembutal); pentobarbital, meperidine, scopolamine

Physical Status Scale*

PATIENT CLASS	CONDITION	GENERAL GUIDELINES FOR SEDATION TECHNIQUE
I	Free of systemic disease	Full range of sedation techniques
II	Mild systemic disease	Full range of sedation techniques with or without hospitalization for advanced sedation
III	Severe systemic disease that is not incapacitating	Inhalation and oral sedation techniques with or without hospitalization; hospitalization mandatory for advanced techniques
IV	Incapacitating systemic disease	Hospitalization for all dental care
V	Moribund patients—not expected to survive 24 hr	Dental therapy contraindicated

Adapted from Feigal D. W., and Blaisdell, F. W.: The estimation of surgical risk. Medical evaluation of the preoperative patient. Med. Clin. North Am., 63(6):1131–1143, 1979.
*Refer to specific chapters for specific disease entitites.

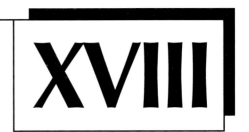

Management of Medical Emergencies in the Dental Office

Emergencies in the Dental Office

Medical Emergencies in the Dental Office

This chapter provides a quick reference for the identification and management of common medical emergencies in the dental office. Each of the medical emergencies is discussed in greater length elsewhere in the book, and the reader should refer to these sections for further details.

All the medication dosages described in this chapter are those appropriate for the adult patient. Other references should be consulted for pediatric patients.

EMERGENCY EQUIPMENT

I. Equipment for maintenance of airway
   A. Plastic oropharyngeal airway
   B. Padded tongue depressor
   C. Suction and suction tip
   D. Mask for oxygen delivery
   E. Ambu bag
   F. Oxygen delivery system
II. Equipment for drug administration
   A. Disposable syringes
      1. 1-ml syringes with 25-gauge needles for subcutaneous injections
      2. 5-ml syringes with 18- or 21-gauge needles for intravenous injections
   B. Tourniquet
III. Equipment for monitoring vital signs
   A. Blood pressure cuff
   B. Stethoscope

CARDIAC ARREST

I. Definition: sudden cessation of effective cardiac output
II. Common causes in the dental practice
   A. Ventricular arrhythmias in patients with underlying heart disease (Chap. 9)
   B. Rarely, excessive administration of anesthetic agents or drugs (e.g., lidocaine, epinephrine)

III. Symptoms and signs
   A. Cardiovascular: absent pulses
   B. Respiratory: absent or gasping respiration
   C. Neurologic: loss of consciousness
IV. Diagnosis: made on clinical grounds
V. Complications
   A. Permanent neurologic damage if not promptly treated
   B. Aspiration
   C. Death
VI. Management: cardiopulmonary resuscitation (CPR)
   A. Call for assistance and arrange immediate transport to medical facility
   B. Place patient supine on firm surface such as the floor
   C. Respiratory support
      1. Establish patent airway by tilting head
      2. Use oral airway to maintain patent airway
      3. Ventilate with mouth-to-mouth resuscitation or bag mask with 100% oxygen
      4. Four quick breaths, then 12 breaths/ minute
      5. Verify effective ventilation by observing chest wall motion
      6. Do not intubate until effective cardiopulmonary resuscitation procedures are ongoing and personnel skilled in intubation are present
   D. Cardiovascular support
      1. Patient should be lying supine on firm surface such as the floor
      2. Closed chest cardiac compression
         a. Heel of left hand directly over lower half of sternum in midline
         b. Heel of right hand on back of left hand
         c. Elbows extended
         d. Resuscitator higher than patient
      3. Vigorously depress sternum 3 to 5 cm, hold for 0.5 seconds and release
      4. 60 compressions/minute

5. Verify effective cardiac compression by palpating femoral or carotid pulse
E. Definitive therapy
   1. Defibrillation, when a defibrillator is readily available, should be used by trained personnel
   2. Endotracheal intubation by trained personnel
   3. Intravenous drug administration by skilled personnel
      a. Sodium bicarbonate, two ampules initially, one ampule every 15 minutes thereafter during resuscitation
      b. Antiarrhythmics such as lidocaine, procainamide, and bretylium can be used by trained personnel
F. Immediate transport to nearest medical facility without interruption of cardiopulmonary resuscitative procedures.

RESPIRATORY ARREST

I. Definition: cessation of effective ventilation
II. Common causes in the dental practice
   A. Respiratory decompensation in patients with severe underlying chronic lung disease (Chap. 19)
   B. Severe bronchospasm in patients with asthma (Chap. 18)
   C. Laryngeal edema with airway obstruction (see later, Anaphylaxis)
   D. Respiratory decompensation in patients with severe congestive failure
   E. Drugs
      1. Overdosage of sedatives
      2. Anaphylactic reactions to drugs
      3. Idiosyncratic response to drugs
III. Symptoms and signs
   A. Respiratory: progressive slowing of respiration, culminating in apnea
   B. Cardiac: prolonged hypoxia leading to hypotension, cardiac arrhythmia, and cardiac arrest
   C. Neurologic: progressive lethargy culminating in coma
IV. Diagnosis: made on clinical grounds; patients develop progressive difficulties with breathing, become cyanotic and lethargic and finally become apneic; cardiac arrhythmias and cardiac arrest follow prolonged anoxia

V. Complications
   A. Cardiac arrhythmias and cardiac arrest
   B. Permanent neurologic damage with prolonged anoxia
   C. Aspiration
   D. Death
VI. Management
   A. Call for assistance and arrange immediate transport to the nearest medical facility
   B. Place patient supine on firm surface such as the floor
   C. Respiratory support
      1. Establish patent airway by tilting head
      2. Use oral airway to maintain patent airway
      3. Ventilate with mouth-to-mouth resuscitation or bag mask with 100% oxygen
      4. Four quick breaths, then 12 breaths/minute
      5. Verify effective ventilation by observing chest wall motion
      6. Intubate if skilled personnel are available
   D. Cardiovascular support
      1. Close monitoring of blood pressure and pulse
      2. If circulation is ineffective, begin closed cardiac compression
   E. Immediate transport to nearest medical facility

ANAPHYLAXIS (ALLERGIC REACTIONS)

I. Definition: cardiovascular and respiratory failure resulting from an immediate allergic reaction, usually within minutes after exposure to offending agent
II. Common causes in the dental practice
   A. Drugs
      1. Lidocaine
      2. Antibiotics such as penicillin
   B. Foreign serum, including fresh-frozen plasma
III. Symptoms and signs
   A. Cutaneous: itching, followed by development of hives and swelling of subcutaneous tissue (swollen eyelids, lips, and tongue)
   B. Respiratory: wheezing, cough, and dyspnea secondary to laryngeal edema and bronchospasm

C. Cardiovascular: light-headedness, flush-ing, and loss of consciousness secon-dary to hypotension; some patients may have arrhythmias, including ven-tricular fibrillation

IV. Diagnosis
   A. Made on clinical grounds
   B. Suspicion should be raised if skin rash, hives, wheezing, or hypotension devel-ops shortly after exposure to a poten-tial allergen

V. Complications
   A. Airway obstruction secondary to laryn-geal edema
   B. Cardiac arrhythmias
   C. Cardiopulmonary arrest

VI. Management
   A. Initial management
      1. Administer aqueous epinephrine, 0.5 ml (1:1000), subcutaneously if hypotension is not present, intrave-nously if hypotension is present
      2. May be repeated every 5 to 10 min-utes as necessary
   B. Respiratory support
      1. Maintain adequate upper airway
      2. Oxygen by nasal cannula or mask
      3. Arrange for transfer to nearest emergency room; airway obstruc-tion may progress rapidly, necessi-tating tracheostomy
   C. Cardiovascular support
      1. Careful monitoring of vital signs
      2. If hypotension is present, place pa-tient supine in chair and elevate lower extremities (Trendelenberg position)
      3. Monitor arrhythmias by checking regularity of pulse
      4. Administration of intravenous fluids and vasopressors by experienced personnel
   D. Management of urticaria
      1. Diphenhydramine (Benadryl) given orally (25 to 50 mg q6h) or intra-muscularly (50 to 100 mg IM)
      2. Hydroxyzine (Atarax, Vistaril) can be used for persistent urticaria (25 mg orally q8h)

UNCONSCIOUSNESS

I. Definition: patient with no responses to stimuli
II. Common causes in the dental practice
   A. Vasovagal syncope (simple faint)

   1. The most common reason for loss of consciousness in the dental office
   2. Sudden and transient loss of con-sciousness
   3. Often precipitated by stress and anxiety
   B. Hypoglycemia
      1. Usually in diabetic patients with in-adequate sugar intake or excessive administration of insulin or oral hy-poglycemic agents
      2. Can occur in nondiabetics (reactive hypoglycemia)
   C. Seizure
      1. Loss of consciousness, usually with associated involuntary muscle activ-ity (facial twitching, tonic clonic ac-tivity)
      2. Usually in patients with history of seizures
   D. Arrhythmias
      1. Particularly in patients with ische-mic heart disease
      2. Either severe bradycardia or tachy-cardia can cause loss of conscious-ness
   E. Cardiopulmonary arrest: apneic and pulseless

III. Symptoms and signs
   A. Vasovagal syncope
      1. Prodrome
         a. Feels warm and flushed
         b. Appears pale
         c. Feels light-headed
         d. Nausea
         e. Sweating
      2. Syncope
         a. Loss of consciousness
         b. Bradycardia (heart rate of less than 60/minute) may be noted
         c. Hypotension (blood pressure of less than 100 mm Hg systolic) may be noted
         d. Duration of unconsciousness is usually less than 1 to 2 minutes
      3. Recovery
         a. May continue to feel weak and light-headed
         b. Pulse and blood pressure should gradually return to normal
   B. Hypoglycemia
      1. Prodrome
         a. Patient may be confused and le-thargic
         b. Sweating
         c. Anxious
         d. Peculiar behavior may be ob-served

2. Loss of consciousness
   a. Tachycardia
   b. Diaphoresis
   c. Hypotension
   d. May have seizures
C. Seizure
   1. Prodrome: some patients may report an aura before the seizure and can sense that a seizure is coming
   2. Seizure: symptoms ranging from brief lapses of awareness to generalized convulsions, usually lasting less than 5 minutes
   3. Postictal period: period of lethargy, confusion, and amnesia following the seizure, lasting minutes to hours
D. Arrhythmia
   1. Bradycardia: Stokes-Adams attacks
      a. Severe bradycardia can cause transient loss of consciousness
      b. Usually caused by complete heart block
      c. Slow and irregular heart beat (often less than 40 beats/minute)
   2. Tachycardia
      a. Rapid atrial fibrillation, atrial

flutter, paroxysmal atrial tachycardia, and ventricular tachycardia can all cause transient loss of consciousness (Chaps. 8, 9, and 10)
      b. On examination, the patient has rapid heart rate (greater than 150 beats/minute)
E. Cardiopulmonary arrest
   1. Absent pulses
   2. Absent or grasping respiration
   3. Loss of consciousness
IV. Diagnosis: important to assess clinical status of patient and arrive at a diagnosis rapidly; statistically, most patients with sudden loss of consciousness have vasovagal syncope (simple faint)
V. Management (Fig. 52–1): important to anticipate potential problems through medical history, patient interview, and observation.
   A. General principles
      1. Place patient in supine position
      2. Check respiration
      3. Tilt head to maintain airway patency
      4. Check pulse and blood pressure
      5. Unless there is an absolute contrain-

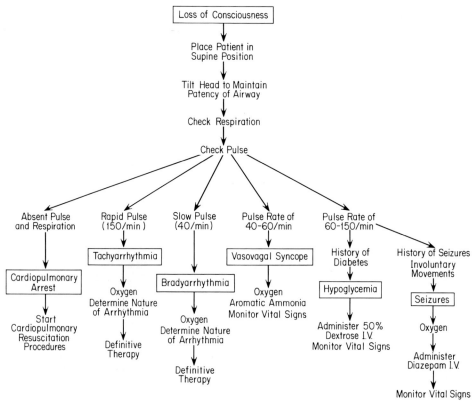

Figure 52–1. Clinical approach to the unconscious patient.

dication such as severe chronic obstructive pulmonary disease, administer oxygen by mask
6. Reassure patient
B. Specific guidelines
   1. Vasovagal syncope
      a. Loosen tight clothing
      b. Elevate feet
      c. Cold compresses
      d. Respiratory stimulants such as aromatic ammonia can be used
      e. Oxygen
   2. Hypoglycemia
      a. In unconscious patient, do *not* attempt to give sugar or sugar-containing solutions orally, because the patient may aspirate
      b. Administer one ampule (50 ml) of 50% dextrose IV
      c. Recovery in minutes
      d. Administer sugar or sugar-containing solution after patient has regained consciousness
   3. Seizures
      a. Gentle passive restraints to prevent physical injury
      b. Use of oral airway or padded tongue depressor to maintain airway patency: do not force these oropharyngeal airways into mouth
      c. For patients with sustained seizure activity, administer diazepam (Valium), 5 to 10 mg (1 to 2 ml) intravenously over 1 to 2 min
   4. Arrhythmia
      a. Basic life support procedures
      b. Immediate transfer to medical facilities
      c. Definitive therapy should be administered by trained personnel in medical facilities under continuous electrocardiographic monitoring
   5. Cardiopulmonary arrest
      a. Call for assistance and arrange for immediate transport to medical facility
      b. Use oral airway to maintain airway patency
      c. Ventilate with mouth-to-mouth resuscitation or bag mask with 100% oxygen
      d. Four quick breaths, then 12 breaths/minute
      e. Closed cardiac compression at 60 compressions/minute

f. Definitive therapy such as defibrillation, intubation, and administration of intravenous drugs should be done by trained personnel
g. Immediate transport to medical facility without interruption of cardiopulmonary resuscitative procedures.

CHEST PAIN

I. Definition: pressure or pain in the substernal or left chest area
II. Common causes in the dental practice
   A. Hyperventilation syndrome: rapid breathing precipitated by anxiety and stress, usually seen in young, anxious patients
   B. Angina pectoris: substernal chest pain precipitated by inadequate supply of oxygen to portions of the heart because of coronary artery disease
   C. Myocardial infarction: injury to the heart caused by inadequate supply of oxygen
III. Symptoms and signs
   A. Hyperventilation syndrome
      1. Suffocating sensation; unable to get in enough air
      2. Nonspecific chest pain
      3. Numbness and tingling sensation in fingers, toes, and perioral area
   B. Angina pectoris
      1. Squeezing substernal chest tightness
      2. Radiation to jaws, left shoulder, and inner aspect of arm
      3. Can be precipitated by stress, anxiety, and exertion
   C. Myocardial infarction
      1. Protracted and severe substernal chest pain
      2. Radiation to jaws, left shoulder, and inner aspect of arm
      3. Patient often appears pale, ashen, and diaphoretic
      4. May have nausea and vomiting
      5. May have palpitations
      6. May have shortness of breath
IV. Diagnosis: must be made on clinical grounds; important considerations include age and medical history of patient
V. Management (Fig. 52–2)
   A. Hyperventilation syndrome
      1. Reassure
      2. Instruct patient to take slow, deep breaths

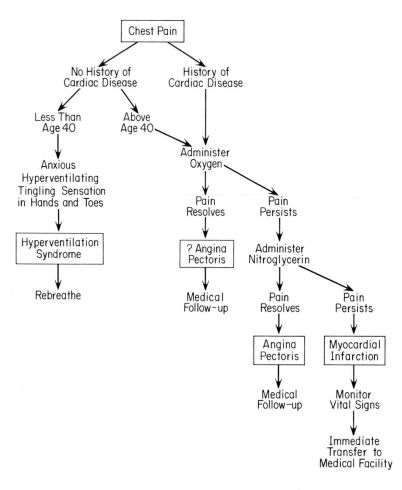

Figure 52–2. Clinical approach to the patient with chest pain.

3. Allow patient to rebreathe by placing a paper bag over the patient's nose and mouth
4. Symptoms should resolve within 5 to 10 minutes
B. Angina pectoris
   1. Administer oxygen
   2. Give 0.3 mg nitroglycerine sublingually
   3. Monitor pulse and blood pressure closely; nitroglycerin can cause hypotension
   4. Repeat nitroglycerin administration in 3 to 5 minutes if pain is not relieved
   5. Transfer to medical facility
C. Myocardial infarction
   1. Administer oxygen
   2. Give 0.3 mg nitroglycerin sublingually
   3. Monitor pulse and blood pressure closely
   4. Can repeat nitroglycerin administration in 3 to 5 minutes if pain is not relieved

5. Immediate transfer to medical facilities

DIFFICULTY BREATHING

I. Definition: inability to breathe
II. Common causes in the dental practice
   A. Hyperventilation syndrome: rapid breathing precipitated by anxiety and stress, usually seen in young and anxious patients
   B. Asthma: reversible bronchospasm involving small airways
   C. Congestive heart failure: left ventricular failure resulting in pulmonary congestion
III. Signs and symptoms
   A. Hyperventilation syndrome
      1. Suffocating sensation, unable to get in enough air
      2. Nonspecific chest pain
      3. Numbness and tingling sensation in fingers, toes, and perioral area

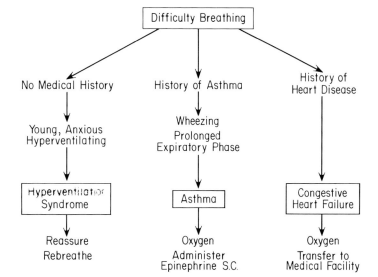

Figure 52–3. Clinical approach to the patient with difficulty breathing.

B. Asthma
1. Increasing shortness of breath
2. Expiratory wheezing with prolongation of expiratory phase
3. Use of accessory muscles for breathing
C. Congestive heart failure
1. Increasing shortness of breath
2. May have inspiratory and expiratory wheezing
3. May have symptoms of chronic biventricular symptoms, including jugulovenous distension and peripheral edema
IV. Diagnosis: based on clinical setting and medical history
V. Management (Fig. 52–3)
A. Hyperventilation syndrome
1. Reassure
2. Instruct patient to take slow, deep breaths
3. Allow patient to rebreathe by placing a paper bag over the patient's nose and mouth
4. Symptoms should resolve within 5 to 10 minutes
B. Asthma
1. Allow patient to be in upright position
2. Administer oxygen
3. Administer 0.25 ml epinephrine (1:1000 dilution) subcutaneously
4. Transfer to medical facility
C. Congestive heart failure
1. Allow patient to be in upright position
2. Administer oxygen
3. Transfer to medical facility

SEIZURES

I. Definition: focal or generalized nonvoluntary motor or sensory activity secondary to excessive neuronal activity
II. Common causes in the dental practice
A. Patient with underlying seizure disorder
B. Less commonly, seizures can be seen with severe hypoglycemia in a diabetic patient
C. Seizures can rarely be induced by drugs administered in excessive doses (e.g., lidocaine inadvertently administered into blood vessels)
III. Symptoms and signs
A. Prodrome
1. Some patients may report an aura before the seizure
2. May be visual (seeing spots or flashing lights) or auditory (certain smells), or may be reported as a peculiar sensation
B. Seizure
1. Symptoms range from brief lapses of awareness to generalized convulsions
2. Usually lasts less than 5 minutes
C. Postictal period
1. Period of lethargy, confusion, and amnesia following seizure
2. Lasts minutes to hours
D. Status epilepticus: protracted duration of seizures (more than 5 minutes)
IV. Diagnosis: made on clinical grounds
V. Complications
A. Physical injury

B. Respiratory compromise secondary to obstruction of airway by tongue
C. Aspiration
VI. Management
  A. Prevent physical injury
    1. Place patient supine on soft surface
    2. Remove dental instruments from area
    3. Gentle passive restraints to prevent physical injury
  B. Maintenance of airway
    1. Tilt head to prevent airway obstruction
    2. Administer oxygen
    3. Use oral airway or padded tongue depressor to maintain airway pa-
    tency; should not force airway into mouth
  C. Close monitoring of vital signs
  D. For patients with status epilepticus
    1. Administer oxygen
    2. Administer diazepam (Valium) 5 to 10 mg (1 to 2 ml) intravenously over 1 to 2 minutes by trained personnel
    3. Arrange for immediate transfer to medical facility
  E. Close monitoring during postictal phase
  F. If hypoglycemia is suspected as cause of seizure, administer one ampule (50 ml) 50% dextrose intravenously

References

CHAPTER 1

American Dental Association Council on Dental Practice: General guidelines for referring medically compromised and infectious dental patients. WV Dent J 63:4–6, 1989.

Bradford VP, Graham BP, Reinert KG: Accuracy of self-reported health histories: A study. Milit Med 158:263–265, 1993.

Fenlon MR, McCartan BE: Validity of a patient self-completed health questionnaire in a primary dental care dental practice. Community Dent Oral Epidemiol 20:130–132, 1992.

Goss AN: The dental management of medically compromised patients. Int Dent J 34:227–231, 1984.

McCarthy FM: Recognition, assessment and safe management of the medically compromised patient in dentistry. Anesth Prog 37:217–222, 1990.

McCarthy FM, Pallasch TJ, Gates R: Documenting safe treatment of the medical-risk patient. J Am Dent Assoc 119:383–389, 1989.

Parnell AG: The medically compromised patient. Int Dent J 36:77–82, 1986.

Redding SW, Olive JA: Relative value of screening tests of hemostasis prior to dental treatment. Oral Surg Oral Med Oral Pathol 59:34–36, 1985.

Rose LF, Steinberg BJ: Patient evaluation. Dent Clin North Am 31:53–73, 1987.

Smith RA, Berger R, Dodson TB: Risk factors associated with dental implants in healthy and medically compromised patients. Int J Oral Maxillofac Implants 7:367–372, 1992.

Terezhalmy GT, Schiff T: The historical profile. Dent Clin North Am 30:357–368, 1986.

Van Venrooy JR, Proffit WR: Orthodontic care for medically compromised patients: Possibilities and limitations. J Am Dent Assoc 111:262–266, 1985.

CHAPTER 2

Eisen D: The oral mucosal punch biopsy. A report of 140 cases. Arch Dermatol 128:815–817, 1992.

Firth NA, Rich AM, Radden BG, Reade PC: Assessment of the value of immunofluorescence microscopy in the diagnosis of oral mucosal lichen planus. J Oral Pathol Med 19:295–297, 1990.

Guinta J, Meyer I, Shklar G: The accuracy of the oral biopsy in the diagnosis of cancer. Oral Surg 28:552–556, 1969.

Harahap M: How to biopsy oral lesions. J Dermatol Surg Oncol 15:1077–1080, 1989.

Siegel MA: Intraoral biopsy technique for direct immunofluorescence studies. Oral Surg Oral Med Oral Pathol 72:681–684, 1991.

CHAPTER 3

Chobanian AV: Pathophysiology of atherosclerosis. Am J Cardiol 70:3G–7G, 1992.

Lakier JB: Smoking and cardiovascular disease. Am J Med 93:8S–12S, 1992.

Massie BM: Angiotensin-converting enzyme inhibitors as cardioprotective agents. Am J Cardiol 70:10I–17I, 1992.

Mattila KJ, Valle MS, Nieminen MS, et al: Dental infections and coronary atherosclerosis. Atherosclerosis 103:205–211, 1993.

Schwartz CJ, Valente AJ, Sprague EA: A modern view of atherogenesis. Am J Cardiol 71:9B–14B, 1993.

CHAPTER 4

Alderman MH: Blood pressure management: Individualized treatment based on absolute risk and the potential for benefit. Ann Intern Med 119:329–335, 1993.

Collins R, Peto R, MacMahon S, et al: Blood pressure, stroke, and coronary heart disease. Part 2, Short-term reductions in blood pressure: Overview of randomized drug trials in their epidemiological context. Lancet 335:827–838, 1990.

Findler M, Mazor Z, Galili D, Garfunkel AA: Dental treatment in a patient with malignant pheochromocytoma and severe uncontrolled high blood pressure. Oral Surg Oral Med Oral Pathol 75:290–291, 1993.

Goulet JP, Perusse R, Turcotte JY: Contraindications to vasoconstrictors in dentistry: Part III. Pharmacologic interactions. Oral Surg Oral Med Oral Pathol 74:692–697, 1992.

McCarthy FM, Pallasch TJ, Gates R: Documenting safe treatment of the medical-risk patient. J Am Dent Assoc 119:383–389, 1989.

Perusse R, Goulet JP, Turcotte JY: Contraindications to vasoconstrictors in dentistry: Part I. Cardiovascular diseases. Oral Surg Oral Med Oral Pathol 74:679–686, 1992.

Perusse R, Goulet JP, Turcotte JY: Contraindications to vasoconstrictors in dentistry: Part II. Hyperthyroidism, diabetes, sulfite sensitivity, cortico-dependent asthma, and pheochromocytoma. Oral Surg Oral Med Oral Pathol 74:687–691, 1992.

CHAPTER 5

Cutler LS: Evaluation and management of the dental patient with cardiovascular disease. III: Angina and myocardial infarction. J Conn State Dent Assoc 61:21–23, 1987.

Findler M, Galili D, Meidan Z, et al: Dental treatment in very high risk patients with active ischemic heart disease. Oral Surg Oral Med Oral Pathol 76:298–300, 1993.

MacAfee KA, II, Chisdak B, Hersh EV: Angina pectoris—diagnosis and treatment in the outpatient setting. Compendium 14:892, 894, 896, 1993.

CHAPTER 6

Cintron G, Medina R, Reyes AA, Lyman G: Cardiovascular effects and safety of dental anesthesia and dental interventions in patients with recent uncomplicated myocardial infarction. Arch Intern Med 146:2203–2204, 1986.

Findler M, Galili D, Meidan Z, et al: Dental treatment in very high risk patients with active ischemic heart disease. Oral Surg Oral Med Oral Pathol 76:298–300, 1993.

Lustig JP, Zagury A, Reisin LH, Neder A: Thrombolytic therapy for acute myocardial infarction after oral surgery. Oral Surg Oral Med Oral Pathol 75:547–548, 1993.

Mattila KJ, Nieminen MS, Valtonen VV, et al: Association between dental health and acute myocardial infarction. Br Med J 298:779–781, 1989.

McCarthy FM: Safe treatment of the post–heart-attack patient. Compendium 10:598–604, 1989.

Perusse R, Goulet JP, Turcotte JY: Contraindications to vasoconstrictors in dentistry: Part I. Cardiovascular diseases. Oral Surg Oral Med Oral Pathol 74:679–686, 1992.

Scuba JR, Parrado C: Parapharyngeal hemorrhage secondary to thrombolytic therapy for acute myocardial infarction. J Oral Maxillofac Surg 50:413–415, 1992.

CHAPTER 7

Milam SB, Giovannitti JA: Digitalis toxicity. A case report. J Periodontol 55:414–418, 1989.

Mulligan R: Pretreatment for the cardiovascularly compromised geriatric dental patient. Special Care Dentist 5:116–123, 1985.

Umino M, Nagao M: Systemic diseases in elderly dental patients. Int Dent J 43:213–218, 1993.

CHAPTERS 8, 9, AND 10

el Hakim M: Cardiac dysrhythmias during dental surgery. Comparison of hyoscine, glycopyrrolate and placebo premedication. Anaesthesiol Reanim 16:393–398, 1991.

Ewah B, Carr C: A comparison of propofol and methohexitone for dental chair anaesthesia in children. Anaesthesia 48:260–262, 1993.

Frabetti L, Checchi L, Finelli K: Cardiovascular effects of local anesthesia with epinephrine in periodontal treatment. Quintessence Int 23:19–24, 1992.

Goulet JP, Perusse R, Turcotte JY: Contraindications to vasoconstrictors in dentistry: Part III. Pharmacologic interactions. Oral Surg Oral Med Oral Pathol 74:692–697, 1992.

Hays GL, McMahon JC, Zimmerman SJ, et al: Screening for cardiovascular disease. Gen Dent 40:26–29, 1992.

Kim Y, Shibutani T, Hirota Y, et al: Giant negative T waves after maxillofacial surgery. Anesth Prog 39:28–35, 1993.

Perusse R, Goulet JP, Turcotte JY: Contraindications to vasoconstrictors in dentistry: Part I. Cardiovascular disease. Oral Surg Oral Med Oral Pathol 74:679–686, 1992.

Rashad A, el-Attar A: Cardiac dysrhythmias during oral surgery: Effect of combined local and general anesthesia. Br J Oral Maxillofac Surg 28:102–104, 1990.

Rashad A, el-Attar A: Dysrhythmias during oral surgery—effect of combined local and general anesthesia. Middle East J Anesthesiol 10:499–505, 1990.

Rodrigo CR: Cardiac dysrhythmias with general anesthesia during dental surgery. Anesth Prog 35:102–115, 1988.

Roelofse JA, van der Bijl P: Cardiac dysrhythmias associated with intravenous lorazepam, diazepam, and midazolam during oral surgery. J Oral Maxillofac Surg 52:247–250, 1994.

CHAPTERS 11, 12, AND 13

American Heart Association: Antibiotic prophylaxis of endocarditis: new recommendations. Drug Ther Bull 28:90–91, 1990.

Burket LW, Burn CG: Bacteremias following dental extraction. Demonstration of source of bacteria by means of a non-pathogen (Serratia marcescens). J Dent Res 16:521–530, 1937.

Dajani AS, Bisno AL, Chung KJ, et al: Prevention of bacterial endocarditis. Recommendations by the American Heart Association. JAMA 264:2919–2922, 1990.

DeMoor CE, DeStoppelaar JD, Van Houte J: The occurrence of Streptococcus mutans and Streptococcus sanguis in the blood of endocarditis patients. Abstracts of paper presented at the eighteenth ORCA Congress, 1968.

Fekete T: Controversies in the prevention of infective endocarditis related to dental procedures. Dent Clin North Am 34:79–90, 1990.

Fleming P, Feigal RJ, Kaplan EL, et al: The development of penicillin-resistant oral streptococci after repeated penicillin prophylaxis. Oral Surg Oral Med Oral Pathol 70:440–444, 1990.

Friedlander AH, Yoshikawa TT: Pathogenesis, management, and prevention of infective endocarditis in the elderly dental patient. Oral Surg Oral Med Oral Pathol 69:177–181, 1990.

Giglio JA, Rowland RW, Dalton HP, Laskin DM: Suture removal-induced bacteremia: A possible endocarditis risk. J Am Dent Assoc 123:65–66, 69–70, 1992.

Hills-Smith H, Schuman NJ: Antibiotic therapy in pediatric dentistry. I. Subacute bacterial endocarditis prophylaxis. Pediatr Dent 5:38–44, 1983.

Hobson RS, Clark JD: Infective endocarditis associated with orthodontic treatment: A case report. Br J Orthod 20:241–244, 1993.

Hollister MC, Weintraub JA: The association of oral status with systemic health, quality of life, and economic productivity. J Dent Educ 57:901–912, 1993.

Hupp JR: Changing methods of preventing infective endocarditis following dental procedures: 1943 to 1993. J Oral Maxillofac Surg 51:616–623, 1993.

Imperiale TF, Horwitz RI: Does prophylaxis prevent

postdental infective endocarditis? A controlled evaluation of protective efficacy. Am J Med 88:131–136, 1990.

Kaye D: Prophylaxis for infective endocarditis: An update. Ann Intern Med 104:419–423, 1986.

Korn VA, Schaffer EM: A comparison of the postoperative bacteremias induced following different periodontal procedures. J Periodontol 33:231, 1962.

Okell CC, Elliott SD: Bacteremia and oral sepsis with special reference to the etiology of subacute endocarditis. Lancet 2:869, 1935.

Wahl MJ: Myths of dental-induced endocarditis. Arch Intern Med 154:137–144, 1994.

Wahl MJ, Wahl PT: Prevention of infective endocarditis: An update for clinicians. Quintessence Int 24:171–175, 1993.

CHAPTER 14

Albrecht M, Banoczy J, Tamas G, Jr: Dental and oral symptoms of diabetes mellitus. Community Dent Oral Epidemiol 16:378–380, 1988.

Aly FZ, Blackwell CC, MacKenzie DA, et al: Chronic atrophic oral candidiasis among patients with diabetes mellitus—role of secretor status. Epidemiol Infect 106:355–363, 1991.

Aly FZ, Blackwell CC, MacKenzie DA, et al: Factors influencing oral carriage of yeasts among individuals with diabetes mellitus. Epidemiol Infect 109:507–518, 1992.

Darwazeh AM, Lamey PJ, Samaranayake LP, et al: The relationship between colonisation, secretor status and in-vitro adhesion of Candida albicans to buccal epithelial cells from diabetics. J Med Microbiol 33:43–49, 1990.

Perusse R, Goulet JP, Turcotte JY: Contraindications to vasoconstrictors in dentistry: Part II. Hyperthyroidism, diabetes, sulfite sensitivity, cortico-dependent asthma, and pheochromocytoma. Oral Surg Oral Med Oral Pathol 74:687–691, 1992.

Phelan JA, Levin SM: A prevalence study of denture stomatitis in subjects with diabetes mellitus or elevated plasma glucose levels. Oral Surg Oral Med Oral Pathol 62:303–305, 1986.

Rosenthal IM, Abrams H, Kopczyk A: The relationship of inflammatory periodontal disease to diabetic status in insulin-dependent diabetes mellitus patients. J Clin Periodontol 15:425–429, 1988.

Sastrowijoto SH, Abbas F, Abraham-Inpijn L, van der Velden U: Relationship between bleeding/plaque ratio, family history of diabetes mellitus and impaired glucose tolerance. J Clin Periodontol 17:55–60, 1990.

Sastrowijoto SH, van der Velden U, van Steenbergen TJ, et al: Improved metabolic control, clinical periodontal status and subgingival microbiology in insulin-dependent diabetes mellitus. A prospective study. J Clin Periodontol 17:233–242, 1990.

Seppala B, Seppala M, Ainamo J: A longitudinal study on insulin-dependent diabetes mellitus and periodontal disease. J Clin Periodontol 20:161–165, 1993.

Tervonen T, Knuuttila M: Relation of diabetes control to periodontal pocketing and alveolar bone level. Oral Surg Oral Med Oral Pathol 61:346–349, 1986.

Tervonen T, Oliver RC: Long-term control of diabetes mellitus and periodontitis. J Clin Periodontol 20:431–435, 1993.

CHAPTER 15

Glick M: Glucocorticosteroid replacement therapy: A literature review and suggested replacement therapy. Oral Surg Oral Med Oral Pathol 67:614–620, 1989.

Matheny JL: Corticosteroids, Part II: Review of pharmacology and management of patients at risk of adrenal crisis. Compend Contin Educ Dent 7:534–538, 1986.

Sacks JC, Gilmore WC: Managing dental patients receiving glucocorticoids (steroids). Gen Dent 35:204–206, 1987.

Steiner M, Ramp WK: Endosseous dental implants and the glucocorticoid-dependent patient. J Oral Implantol 16:211–217, 1990.

CHAPTER 16

Perusse R, Goulet JP, Turcotte JY: Contraindications to vasoconstrictors in dentistry: Part II. Hyperthyroidism, diabetes, sulfite sensitivity, cortico-dependent asthma, and pheochromocytoma. Oral Surg Oral Med Oral Pathol 74:687–691, 1992.

CHAPTER 17

Balligan FJ, Hale TM: Analgesic and antibiotic administration during pregnancy. Gen Dent 41:220–225, 1993.

Balligan FJ, Hale TM: Analgesic and antibiotic administration during pregnancy. Gen Dent 41:220–225, 1993.

Chiodo GT, Rosenstein DI: Dental treatment during pregnancy: A preventive approach. J Am Dent Assoc 110:365–368, 1985.

Fiese R, Herzog S: Issues in dental and surgical management of the pregnant patient. Oral Surg Oral Med Oral Pathol 65:292–297, 1988.

Jonsson R, Howland BE, Bowden GH: Relationships between periodontal health, salivary steroids, and Bacteroides intermedius in males, pregnant and non-pregnant women. J Dent Res 67:1062–1069, 1988.

Miyazaki H, Yamashita Y, Shirahama R, et al: Periodontal condition of pregnant women assessed by CPITN. J Clin Periodontol 18:751–754, 1991.

Schwartz M, Holmes HI, Schwartz SS: Care of the pregnant patient. J Can Dent Assoc 53:299–301, 1987.

Shrout MK, Comer RW, Powell BJ, McCoy BP: Treating the pregnant dental patient: Four basic rules addressed. J Am Dent Assoc 123:75–80, 1992.

Tarsitano BF, Rollings RE: The pregnant dental patient: Evaluation and management. Gen Dent 41:226–234, 1993.

CHAPTER 18

Chiodo GT, Rosenstein DI: Dental treatment during pregnancy: A preventive approach. J Am Dent Assoc 110:365–368, 1985.

CHAPTER 19

Anderson DO, Ferris BG, Zickmantel R: The Chilliwack Respiratory Survey, 1963. Part IV. The effect of tobacco smoking on the prevalence of respiratory disease. Can Med Assoc J 92:1066–1076, 1965.

Burrows B: Physiologic variants of chronic obstructive lung disease. Chest 58(Suppl. 2):415, 1970.

Diener CF, Burrows B: Further observations on the course and prognosis of chronic obstructive lung disease. Am Rev Resp Dis 111:719–724, 1975.

Fletcher CM: Chronic bronchitis: Its prevalence, nature, and pathogenesis. Am Rev Resp Dis 80:483, 1959.

Hugh-Jones P, Whimster W: The etiology and management of disabling emphysema. Am Rev Resp Dis 117:343–378, 1978.

Tager J, Speizer FE: Role of infection in chronic bronchitis. N Engl J Med 292:563, 1975.

CHAPTER 20

Faecher RS, Thomas JE, Bender BS: Tuberculosis: A growing concern for dentistry? J Am Dent Assoc 124:94–104, 1993.

Molinari JA, Cottone JA, Chandrasekar PH: Tuberculosis in the 1990s: Current implications for dentistry. Compendium 14:276, 278, 280–282, 1993.

CHAPTER 21

Binder HJ, Cocco A, Crossley RJ, et al: Cimetidine in the treatment of duodenal ulcer: A multicenter double blind study. Gastroenterology 74:380–388, 1978.

Cooke AR: Drugs and peptic ulceration. *In* Sleisenger MH, Fordtran JS (eds.): Gastrointestinal Disease: Pathophysiology, Diagnosis and Management. Philadelphia, W. B. Saunders, 1973, p. 642.

Englert E Jr, Freston JW, Graham DY, et al.: Cimetidine, antacid and hospitalization in the treatment of benign gastric ulcer: A multicenter double blind study. Gastroenterology 74:416–425, 1978.

Grossman MI, Guth PH, Isenberg JI, et al.: A new look at peptic ulcer. Ann Intern Med 84:57–67, 1976.

Ippoliti AF, Sturdevant RAL, Isenberg JI, et al.: Cimetidine versus intensive antacid therapy for duodenal ulcer: A multicenter trial. Gastroenterology 74:393–395, 1978.

Peterson WL, Sturdevant RA, Frankl HD, et al.: Healing of duodenal ulcer with an antacid regimen. N Engl J Med 297:341–345, 1977.

Susser M: Causes of peptic ulcer: Selective epidemiologic review. J Chron Dis 20:435, 1967.

CHAPTER 22

Halme L, Meurman JH, Laine P, et al: Oral findings in patients with active or inactive Crohn's disease. Oral Surg Oral Med Oral Pathol 76:175–181, 1993.

Laurin D, Brodeur JM, Leduc N, et al: Nutritional deficiencies and gastrointestinal disorders in the edentulous elderly: A literature review. J Can Dent Assoc 58:738–740, 1992.

Scully C, Cochran KM, Russell RI, et al: Crohn's disease of the mouth: An indicator of intestinal involvement. Gut 23:198–201, 1982.

McCarthy PL, Shklar G: A syndrome of pyostomatitis vegetans and ulcerative colitis. Arch Dermatol 88:913–919, 1963.

Williams AJ, Wray D, Ferguson A: The clinical entity of orofacial Crohn's disease. Q J Med 79:451–458, 1991.

CHAPTER 23

Cottone JA: Delta hepatitis: Another concern for dentistry. J Am Dent Assoc 112:47–49, 1986.

Fagan EA, Partridge M, Sowray JH, Williams R: Review of hepatitis non-A, non-B: The potential hazards in dental care. Oral Surg Oral Med Oral Pathol 65:167–171, 1988.

Johnson PJ: Hepatitis viruses, cirrhosis, and liver cancer. J Surg Oncol Suppl 3:28–33, 1993.

Lee WM: Review article: Drug-induced hepatotoxicity. Aliment Pharmacol Ther 7:477–485, 1993.

Little JW, Rhodus NL: Dental treatment of the liver transplant patient. Oral Surg Oral Med Oral Pathol 73:419–426, 1992.

Porter SR, Scully C: Non-A, non-B hepatitis and dentistry. Br Dent J 168:257–261, 1990.

Schiff ER, de Medina MD, Kline SN, et al: Veterans Administration cooperation study on hepatitis and dentistry. J Am Dent Assoc 113:390–396, 1986.

Wilson GW, Sisto JM: Orthognathic surgery in patients with Crohn's disease: A review of the pathophysiology and perioperative management. J Oral Maxillofac Surg 50:502–505, 1992.

CHAPTER 24

Berg CL, Gollan JL: Primary biliary cirrhosis: New therapeutic directions. Scand J Gastroenterol 192(Suppl): 43–49, 1992.

Dudley FJ: Pathophysiology of ascites formation. Gastroenterol Clin North Am 21:215–235, 1992.

Friedman SL: Seminars in medicine of the Beth Israel Hospital, Boston. The cellular basis of hepatic fibrosis. Mechanisms and treatment strategies. N Engl J Med 328:1828–1835, 1993.

Gentilini P: Cirrhosis, renal function and NSAIDs. J Hepatol 19:200–203, 1993.

Glassman P, Wong C, Gish R: A review of liver transplantation for the dentist and guidelines for dental management. Special Care Dentist, 13:74–80, 1993.

CHAPTER 25

Carr MM: Dental management of patients with sickle cell anemia. J Can Dent Assoc 59:180–182, 185, 1993.

Drummond JF, White DK, Damm DD: Megaloblastic anemia with oral lesions: A consequence of gastric bypass surgery. Oral Surg Oral Med Oral Pathol 59:149–153, 1985.

Engel JD, Ruskin JD, Tu HK: Hematologic management of a patient with Fanconi's anemia undergoing bone grafting and implant surgery. J Oral Maxillofac Surg 50:288–292, 1992.

Imbery TA, Camm JH, Anderson LD: Dental management of a patient with aplastic anemia. Gen Dent 40:316–318, 1992.

Jones JE, Coates TD, Poland C: Dental management of idiopathic aplastic anemia: Report of a case. Pediatr Dent 3:267–270, 1981.

May OA Jr: Dental management of sickle cell anemia patients. Gen Dent 39:182–183, 1991.

McWhorter AG, Hill SD: Conservative management for a patient with aplastic anemia without use of blood products. Case report. Pediatric Dent 13:224–226, 1991.

Okamato GU, Duperon DF: Bleeding control after extractions in a patient with aplastic anemia during bone marrow transplantation: Report of case. ASDC J Dent Child 56:50–55, 1989.

Razmus TF, Fotos PG: Oral medicine in clinical dentistry: Hematologic disorders. Compendium 8:214, 216–218, 221–222, 1987.

Sams DR, Thornton JB, Amamoo A: Managing the dental patient with sickle cell anemia: A review of the literature. Pediatr Dent 12:316–320, 1990.

Steelman R, Holmes D, Cranston R, Cupp D: Idiopathic myelofibrosis: Dental treatment considerations. Special Care Dent 11:68–70, 1991.

Theaker JM, Porter SR, Fleming KA: Oral epithelial dysplasia in vitamin B_{12} deficiency. Oral Surg Oral Med Oral Pathol 67:81–83, 1989.

Zegarelli DJ: Burning mouth: An alternative explanation for some patients with diabetes mellitus and pernicious anemia. Ann Dent 46:23–24, 1987.

CHAPTER 26

Carr MM, Mason RB: Dental management of anticoagulated patients. J Can Dent Assoc 58:838–844, 1992.

Caughman WF, McCoy BP, Sisk AL, Lutcher CL: When a patient with a bleeding disorder needs dental work. How you can work with the dentist to prevent a crisis. Postgrad Med 88:175–182, 1990.

Engel JD, Ruskin JD, Tu HK: Hematologic management of a patient with Fanconi's anemia undergoing bone grafting and implant surgery. J Oral Maxillofac Surg 50:288–292, 1992.

Gill FM: Congenital bleeding disorders: Hemophilia and von Willebrand's disease. Med Clin North Am 68:601–615, 1984.

Humphries JE, Baker RC Jr: Occult hemophilia: Prolonged bleeding follows extraction. J Am Dent Assoc 123:69–70, 1992.

Johnson CD, Brown RS: How cocaine abuse affects postextraction bleeding. J Am Dent Assoc 124:60–62, 1993.

Johnson WT, Leary JM: Management of dental patients with bleeding disorders: Review and update. Oral Surg Oral Med Oral Pathol 66:297–303, 1988.

Katz JO, Terezhalmy GT: Dental management of the patient with hemophilia. Oral Surg Oral Med Oral Pathol 66:139–144, 1988.

Keila S, Kaufman A, Itckowitch D: Uncontrolled bleeding during endodontic treatment as the first symptoms for diagnosing von Willebrand's disease. A case report. Oral Surg Oral Med Oral Pathol 69:243–246, 1990.

Orlian AI, Karmel R: Postoperative bleeding in an undiagnosed hemophilia A patient: Report of case. J Am Dent Assoc 118:583–584, 1989.

Rakocz M, Mazar A, Varon D, et al: Dental extractions in patients with bleeding disorders. The use of fibrin glue. Oral Surg Oral Med Oral Pathol 75:280–282, 1993.

Ramstrom G, Sindet-Pedersen S, Hall GL, et al: Prevention of postsurgical bleeding in oral surgery using tranexamic acid without dose modification of oral anticoagulants. J Oral Maxillofac Surg 51:1211–1216, 1993.

Razmus TF, Fotos PG: Oral medicine in clinical dentistry: Hematologic disorders. Compendium 8:214, 216–218, 221–222, 1987.

Reiche O, Garg A: Bleeding problems associated with von Willebrand's disease: Review and case report. Gen Dent 39:277–279, 1991.

Shapiro N: When the bleeding won't stop: A case report on a patient with hemophilia. J Am Dent Assoc 124:64–67, 1993.

Staffileno H, Jr, Ciancio S: Bleeding disorders in the dental patient: Causative factors and management. Compendium 8:501, 504–507, 1987.

CHAPTER 27

Armitage JO: Bone marrow transplantation in the treatment of patients with lymphoma. Blood 73:1749–1758, 1989.

Armitage JO: Treatment of non-Hodgkin's lymphoma. N Engl J Med 328:1023–1030, 1993.

Bergmann OJ: Oral infections and septicemia in immunocompromised patients with hematologic malignancies. J Clin Microbiol 26:2105–2109, 1988.

Chessells JM: Bone marrow transplantation for leukaemia. Arch Dis Child 63:879–882, 1988.

Cossman J, Uppenkamp M, Sundeen J, et al: Molecular genetics and the diagnosis of lymphoma. Arch Pathol Lab Med 112:117–127, 1988.

Dreizen S, Menkin DJ, Keating MJ, et al: Effect of antileukemia chemotherapy on marrow, blood, and oral granulocyte counts. Oral Surg Oral Med Oral Pathol 71:45–49, 1991.

Galili D, Donitza A, Garfunkel A, Sela MN: Gram-negative enteric bacteria in the oral cavity of leukemia patients. Oral Surg Oral Med Oral Pathol 74:459–462, 1992.

Hjelle B: Human T-cell leukemia/lymphoma viruses. Life cycle, pathogenicity, epidemiology, and diagnosis. Arch Pathol Lab Med 115:440–450, 1991.

Johnson LE: Chronic lymphocytic leukemia. Am Fam Physician 38:167–176, 1988.

LoBuglio AF, Saleh MN: Advances in monoclonal antibody therapy of cancer. Am J Med Sci 304:214–224, 1992.

Mastrianni DM, Tung NM, Tenen DG: Acute myelogenous leukemia: Current treatment and future directions. Am J Med 92:286–295, 1992.

O'Reilly SE, Connors JM: Non-Hodgkin's lymphoma. I. Characterization and treatment. Br Med J 304:1682–1686, 1992.

O'Sullivan EA, Duggal MS, Bailey CC, et al: Changes in the oral microflora during cytotoxic chemotherapy in children being treated for acute leukemia. Oral Surg Oral Med Oral Pathol 76:161–168, 1993.

Stein RS: Advances in the therapy of acute nonlymphocytic leukemia. Am J Med Sci 297:26–34, 1989.

Weckx LL, Hidal LB, Marcucci G: Oral manifestations of leukemia. Ear Nose Throat J 69:341–342, 345–346, 1990.

CHAPTER 28

Arneberg P, Bjertness E, Storhaug K, et al: Remaining teeth, oral dryness and dental health habits in middle-aged Norwegian rheumatoid arthritis patients. Community Dent Oral Epidemiol 20:292–296, 1992.

Cioffi GA, Terezhalmy GT, Taybos GM: Total joint replacement: A consideration for antimicrobial prophylaxis. Oral Surg Oral Med Oral Pathol 66:124–129, 1988.

Friedlander AH, Runyon C: Polymyalgia rheumatica and temporal arteritis. Oral Surg Oral Med Oral Pathol 69:317–322, 1990.

Hildebrand J, Plezia RA, Rao SB: Sarcoidosis. Report of two cases with oral involvement. Oral Surg Oral Med Oral Pathol 69:217–222, 1990.

Larheim TA: Comparison between three radiographic techniques for examination of the temporomandibular joints in juvenile rheumatoid arthritis. Acta Radiol (Diagn) (Stockh) 22:195–201, 1981.

Lawson JP, Rahn DW: Lyme disease and radiologic findings in Lyme arthritis. Am J Roentgenol 158:1065–1069, 1992.

Little JW: Antibiotic prophylaxis for prevention of bacterial endocarditis and infections of major prostheses. Curr Opin Dent 2:71, 1992.

Manne SL, Zautra AJ: Coping with arthritis. Current status and critique. Arthritis Rheum 35:1273–1280, 1992.

Moreland LW, Heck LW, Jr, Sullivan W, et al: New approaches to the therapy of autoimmune diseases: rheumatoid arthritis as a paradigm. Am J Med Sci 305:40–51, 1993.

Panayi GS: The pathogenesis of rheumatoid arthritis: From molecules to the whole patient. Br J Rheumatol 32:533–536, 1993.

Pincus T, Callahan LF: The "side effects" of rheumatoid arthritis: Joint destruction, disability and early mortality. Br J Rheumatol 32(Suppl 1):28–37, 1993.

Risheim H, Kjaerheim V, Arneberg P: Improvement of oral hygiene in patients with rheumatoid arthritis. Scand J Dent Res 100:172–175, 1992.

Schenkier S, Golbus J: Treatment of rheumatoid arthritis. New thoughts on the classic pyramid approach. Postgrad Med 91:285–286, 289–292, 1992.

CHAPTER 29

Cook HE, Yamada RK: Acute renal failure in the surgical patient: Initial diagnosis and treatment. J Oral Maxillofac Surg 44:719–723, 1986.

Eigner TL, Jastak JT, Bennett WM: Achieving oral health in patients with renal failure and renal transplants. J Am Dent Assoc 113:612–616, 1986.

First MR: Long-term complications after transplantation. Am J Kidney Dis 22:477–486, 1993.

Galili D, Kaufman E, Leviner E, Lowental U: The attitude of chronic hemodialysis patients toward dental treatment. Oral Surg Oral Med Oral Pathol 56:602–604, 1983.

Hayes JM: The immunobiology and clinical use of current immunosuppressive therapy for renal transplantation. J Urol 149:437–448, 1993.

Ismail N, Hakim RM, Helderman JH: Renal replacement therapies in the elderly: Part II. Renal transplantation. Am J Kidney Dis 23:1–15, 1994.

Ismail N, Hakim RM, Oreopoulos DG, Patrikarea A: Renal replacement therapies in the elderly: Part I. Hemodialysis and chronic peritoneal dialysis. Am J Kidney Dis 22:759–782, 1993.

Kiddy K, Brown PP, Michael J, Adu D: Peritonitis due to Streptococcus viridans in patients receiving continuous ambulatory peritoneal dialysis. Br Med J (Clin Res Ed) 290:969–970, 1985.

Pernu HE, Pernu LM, Huttunen KR, et al: Gingival overgrowth among renal transplant recipients related to immunosuppressive medication and possible local background factors. J Periodontol 63:548–553, 1992.

Pernu HE, Pernu LM, Knuuttila ML: Effect of periodontal treatment on gingival overgrowth among cyclosporine A-treated renal transplant recipients. J Periodontol 64:1098–1100, 1993.

Port FK: The end-stage renal disease program: Trends over the past 18 years. Am J Kidney Dis 20(Suppl 1): 3–7, 1992.

Rhodus NL, Little JW: Dental management of the renal transplant patient. Compendium 14:518–524, 526, 528, 1993.

Saxena R, Johansson C, Bygren P, Wieslander J: Autoimmunity and glomerulonephritis. Postgrad Med J 68:242–250, 1992.

Tejani A, Fine RN: Cadaver renal transplantation in children. Incidence, immunosuppression, outcome, and risk factors. Clin Pediatr (Phila) 32:194–202, 1993.

Thomason JM, Seymour RA, Rice N: The prevalence and severity of cyclosporin and nifedipine-induced gingival overgrowth. J Clin Periodontol 20:37–40, 1993.

Wilson RL, Martinez-Tirado J, Whelchel J, Lordon RE: Occult dental infection causing fever in renal transplant patients. Am J Kidney Dis 2:354–356, 1982.

Wondimu B, Dahllof G, Berg U, Modeer T: Cyclosporin-A-induced gingival overgrowth in renal transplant children. Scand J Dental Res 101:282–286, 1993.

Ziccardi VB, Saini J, Demas PN, Braun TW: Management of the oral and maxillofacial surgery patient with end-stage renal disease. J Oral Maxillofac Surg 50:1207–1212, 1992.

CHAPTER 30

Billstein SA, Mattaliano VJ Jr: The "nuisance" sexually transmitted diseases: Molluscum contagiosum, scabies, and crab lice. Med Clin North Am 74:1487–1505, 1990.

Brandt AM: Sexually transmitted disease: Shadow on the land, revisited (comment). Ann Intern Med 112:481–483, 1990.

Handsfield HH: Recent developments in STDs: I. Bacterial diseases. Hosp Pract [Off] 26:47–56, 1991.

Handsfield HH: Recent developments in STDs: II. Viral and other syndromes. Hosp Pract [Off] 27:175–182, 187, 191, 1992.

Meyer I, Shklar G: The oral manifestations of acquired syphilis. A study of eighty-one cases. Oral Surg 23:45–57, 1967.

Mogabgab WJ: Recent developments in the treatment of sexually transmitted diseases. Am J Med 91:140S–144S, 1991.

Peaceman AM, Gonik B: Sexually transmitted viral disease in women. Postgrad Med 89:133–140, 1991.

Staretz LR, Correll RW, Schott TR: A solitary cauliflower-like nodule on the mucosal surface of the lower lip. J Am Dent Assoc 117:185–186, 1988.

CHAPTER 31

Drury I, Beydoun A: Seizure disorders of aging: Differential diagnosis and patient management. Geriatrics 48:52–54, 57–58,

Durand ML, Calderwood SB, Weber DJ: Acute bacterial meningitis in adults. A review of 493 episodes. N Engl J Med 328:21–28, 1993.

Hauser WA: Seizure disorders: The changes with age. Epilepsia 33 (Suppl 4):S6–S14, 1992.

Leppik IE: Antiepileptic medications. Compendium Suppl 14:S490–S496, 1990.

Lockman LA: Treatment of status epilepticus in children. Neurology 40(Suppl 2):43–46, 1990.

Rucker LM: Prosthetic treatment for the patient with uncontrolled grand mal epileptic seizure. Special Care Dentist 5:206–207, 1985.

Scheuer ML, Pedley TA: The evaluation and treatment of seizures. N Engl J Med 323:1468–1474.

So EL: Update on epilepsy. Med Clin North Am 77:203–214, 1993.

CHAPTER 32

Biller J, Love BB: Controversies in the management of cerebrovascular disease in older patients. Geriatrics 47:47–51, 1992.

Eaker ED, Chesebro JH, Sacks FM, et al: Cardiovascular disease in women. Circulation 88(Pt 1):1999–2009, 1993.

Hallenbeck JM, Frerichs KU: Stroke therapy. It may be time for an integrated approach. Arch Neurol 50:768–770, 1993.

Hirsh J, Dalen JE, Fuster V, et al: Aspirin and other platelet-active drugs. The relationship between dose, effectiveness, and side effects. Chest 102 (Suppl): 327S–336S, 1992.

Lakier JB: Smoking and cardiovascular disease. Am J Med 93:8S–12S, 1992.

Lowe GD: Drugs in cerebral and peripheral arterial disease. Br Med J 300:524–528, 1990.

Mowery AJ Jr: Communicating with the aphasic dental patient. Special Care Dentist 13:143–145, 1993.

Neville RF, Calcagno D: Symptomatic carotid artery disease: Current management recommendations (see comments). Am Fam Physician 48:1059–1066, 1993.

Roth EJ: Heart disease in patients with stroke: Incidence, impact, and implications for rehabilitation. Part I: Classification and prevalence. Arch Phys Med Rehabil 74:752–760, 1993.

Roth EJ: Heart disease in patients with stroke. Part II: Impact and implications for rehabilitation. Arch Phys Med Rehabil 75:94–101, 1994.

Selley WG, Howitt JM: Prosthetic management of dysphagia after a stroke—an unusual combination of problems: A clinical report. J Prosthet Dent 67:741–742, 1992.

Thomas DJ, Wolfe JH: ABC of vascular diseases. Carotid endarterectomy. Br Med J 303:985–987, 1991.

Unwin DH, Greenlee RG Jr: Prophylactic drug therapy in cerebrovascular disease. Am Fam Physician 48:85–90, 1993.

CHAPTER 33

Austin DG, Cubillos L: Special considerations in orofacial pain. Dent Clin North Am 35:227–244, 1991.

Balciunas BA, Siegel MA, Grace EG: A clinical approach to the diagnosis of facial pain. Dent Clin North Am 36:987–1000, 1992.

Bittar G, Graff-Radford SB: A retrospective study of patients with cluster headaches. Oral Surg Oral Med Oral Pathol 73:519–525, 1992.

Bouckoms AJ, Keith DA: Pharmacologic treatment for chronic facial pain. Curr Opin Dent 1:480–484.

Cooper BC, Cooper DL: Multidisciplinary approach to the differential diagnosis of facial, head and neck pain. J Prosthet Dent 66:72–78, 1991.

Dalessio DJ: Management of the cranial neuralgias and atypical facial pain. A review. Clin J Pain 5:55–59, 1989.

Darlow LA, Brooks ML, Quinn PD: Magnetic resonance imaging in the diagnosis of trigeminal neuralgia. J Oral Maxillofac Surg 50:621–626, 1992.

Friction JR, Kroening R, Haley D, Siegert R: Myofascial pain syndrome of the head and neck: A review of clinical characteristics of 164 patients. Oral Surg Oral Med Oral Pathol 60:615–623, 1985.

Fromm GH: The pharmacology of trigeminal neuralgia. Clin Neuropharmacol 12:185–194, 1989.

Fromm GH: Trigeminal neuralgia and related disorders. Neurol Clin 7:305–319, 1989.

Graff-Radford SB: Headache problems that can present as toothache. Dent Clin North Am 35:155–170, 1991.

Green MW, Selman JE: Review article: The medical management of trigeminal neuralgia. Headache 33:588–592, 1991.

Main JH, Jordan RC, Barewal R: Facial neuralgias: A clinical review of 34 cases. J Can Dent Assoc 58:752–755, 1992.

Manusov EG, Johnson R: Orofacial pain: Diagnosis and treatment. Am Fam Physician 45:773–782, 1992.

Marbach JJ: Is phantom tooth pain a deafferentation (neuropathic) syndrome? Part I: Evidence derived from pathophysiology and treatment. Oral Surg Oral Med Oral Pathol 75:95–105, 1993.

Maresky LS, van der Bijl P, Gird I: Burning mouth syndrome. Evaluation of multiple variables among 85 patients. Oral Surg Oral Med Oral Pathol 75:303–307, 1993.

Pertes RA, Heir GM: Chronic orofacial pain. A practical approach to differential diagnosis. Dent Clin North Am 35:123–140, 1991.

Powell FC: Glossodynia and other disorders of the tongue. Dermatol Clin 5:687–693, 1987.

Rosenkopf KL: Current concepts concerning the etiology and treatment of trigeminal neuralgia. Cranio 7:312–318, 1989.

Rovit RL: Trigeminal neuralgia. Compr Ther 18:17–21, 1992.

Schnurr RF, Brooke RI: Atypical odontalgia. Update and comment on long-term follow-up. Oral Surg Oral Med Oral Pathol 73:445–448, 1992.

Sessle BJ: The neurobiology of facial and dental pain: Present knowledge, future directions. J Dent Res 66:962–981, 1987.

Solomon S, Lipton RB: Facial pain. Neurol Clin 8:913–928, 1990.

Stegenga B, de Bont LG, Boering G: Osteoarthrosis as the cause of craniomandibular pain and dysfunction: A unifying concept. J Oral Maxillofac Surg 47:249–256, 1989.

Sweet WH: The treatment of trigeminal neuralgia (tic douloureux). N Engl J Med 315:174–177, 1986.

Tourne LP, Fricton JR: Burning mouth syndrome. Critical review and proposed clinical management. Oral Surg Oral Med Oral Pathol 74:158–167, 1992.

Zakrzewska JM, Patsalos PN: Drugs used in the management of trigeminal neuralgia. Oral Surg Oral Med Oral Pathol 74:439–450, 1992.

CHAPTER 34

Aach RD, Girard DE, Humphrey H, et al: Alcohol and other substance abuse and impairment among physicians in residency training. Ann Intern Med 116:245–254, 1992.

Cowley DS: Alcohol abuse, substance abuse, and panic disorder. Am J Med 92:41S–48S, 1993.

Friedlander AH, West LJ: Dental management of the patient with major depression. Oral Surg Oral Med Oral Pathol 71:573–578, 1991.

Friedlander AH, Mills MJ, Gorelick DA: Alcoholism and dental management. Oral Surg Oral Med Oral Pathol 63:42–46, 1987.

Kavan MG, Pace TM, Ponterotto JG, Barone EJ: Screening for depression: Use of patient questionnaires. Am Fam Physician 41:897–904, 1990.

Paykel ES, Priest RG: Recognition and management of depression in general practice: Consensus statement. Br Med J 305:1198–1202, 1992.

Rees TD: Oral effects of drug abuse. Crit Rev Oral Biol Med 3:163–184, 1992.

Ratcliff JS, Collins GB: Dental management of the recovered chemically dependent patient. J Am Dent Assoc 114:601–603, 1987.

Regan TJ: Alcohol and the cardiovascular system. JAMA 264:377–381, 1990.

Spivey WH, Euerle B: Neurologic complications of cocaine abuse. Ann Emerg Med 19:1422–1428, 1990.

Warner EA: Cocaine abuse. Ann Intern Med 119:226–235, 1993.

Webb S, Hochberg MS, Sher MR: Fetal alcohol syndrome: Report of a case. J Am Dent Assoc 116:196–198, 1988.

CHAPTER 35

Croft CB, Wilkinson AR: Ulceration of the mouth, pharynx, and larynx in Crohn's disease of the intestine. Br J Surg 59:249–252, 1972.

Dolby AE: Recurrent aphthous ulceration. Effect of sera and peripheral blood lymphocytes on oral epithelial tissue culture cells. Immunology 17:709–714, 1969.

Firestein GS, Gruber HE, Weisman MH, et al: Mouth and genital ulcers with inflamed cartilage: MAGIC syndrome. Five patients with features of relapsing polychondritis and Behcet's disease. Am J Med 79:65–72, 1985.

Greer RO Jr, Lindenmuth JE, Juarez T, Khandwala A: A double-blind study of topically applied 5% amlexanox in the treatment of aphthous ulcers. J Oral Maxillofac Surg 51:243–248, 1993.

Herbert AA, Berg JH: Oral mucous membrane diseases of childhood: I. Mucositis and xerostomia. II. Recurrent aphthous stomatitis. III. Herpetic stomatitis. Semin Dermatol 11:80–87, 1992.

Lehner T: Immunological aspects of recurrent oral ulceration and Behcet's syndrome. J Oral Pathol 7:424–430, 1978.

Levin LS, Johns ME: Lesions of the oral mucous membranes. Otolaryngol Clin North Am 19:87–102, 1986.

Main DM, Chamberlain MA: Clinical differentiation of oral ulceration in Behcet's disease. Br J Rheumatol 31:767–770, 1992.

McCartan BE, Sullivan A: The association of menstrual cycle, pregnancy, and menopause with recurrent oral aphthous stomatitis: A review and critique. Obstet Gynecol 80 (Pt 1):455–458, 1992.

Miles DA, Bricker SL, Razmus TF, Potter RH: Triamcinolone acetonide versus chlorhexidine for treatment of recurrent stomatitis. Oral Surg Oral Med Oral Pathol 75:397–402, 1993.

Orme RL, Nordlund JJ, Barich L, Brown T: The MAGIC syndrome (mouth and genital ulcers with inflamed cartilage). Arch Dermatol 126:940–944, 1990.

Porter SR, Kingsmill V, Scully C: Audit of diagnosis and investigations in patients with recurrent aphthous stomatitis. Oral Surg Oral Med Oral Pathol 76:449–452, 1993.

Rodu B, Mattingly G: Oral mucosal ulcers: Diagnosis and management. J Am Dent Assoc 123:83–86, 1992.

Rogers RS, III: Common lesions of the oral mucosa. A guide to diseases of the lips, cheeks, tongue, and gingivae. Postgrad Med 91:141–148, 151–153, 1992.

Rogers R III, Sams WM Jr, Shorter RG: Lymphocytotoxicity in recurrent aphthous stomatitis. Arch Dermatol 109:361–363, 1974.

Scully C: An update on mouth ulcers. Dent Update 10:141–142, 145–148, 151–152, 1983.

Vincent SD, Lilly GE: Clinical, historic, and therapeutic features of aphthous stomatitis. Literature review and open clinical trial employing steroids. Oral Surg Oral Med Oral Pathol 74:79–86, 1992.

CHAPTER 36

Bagan-Sebastian JV, Milian-Masanet MA, Penarrocha-Diago M, Jimenez Y: A clinical study of 205 patients with oral lichen planus. J Oral Maxillofac Surg 50:116–118, 1992.

Eisenberg E: Lichen planus and oral cancer: Is there a connection between the two? J Am Dent Assoc 123:104–108, 1992.

Eisenberg E, Krutchkoff DJ: Lichenoid lesions of oral mucosa. Diagnostic criteria and their importance in the alleged relationship to oral cancer. Oral Surg Oral Med Oral Pathol 73:699–704, 1992.

Helm TN, Camisa C, Liu AY, et al: Lichen planus associated with neoplasia: A cell-mediated immune response to tumor antigens? J Am Acad Dermatol 30(Pt 1):219–224, 1994.

Jorizzo JL, Salisbury PL, Rogers RS, III, et al: Oral lesions in systemic lupus erythematosus. Do ulcerative lesions represent a necrotizing vasculitis? J Am Acad Dermatol 27:389–394, 1992.

Jungell P: Oral lichen planus. Int J Oral Maxillofac Surg 20:129–135, 1991.

Lin SC, Sun A, Wu YC, Chiang CP: Presence of antibasal cell antibodies in oral lichen planus. J Am Acad Dermatol 26:943–947, 1992.

Scully C, de Almeida OP, Welbury R: Oral lichen planus in childhood (letter). Br J Dermatol 130:131–133, 1994.

Shklar G, McCarthy PL: The oral lesions of lichen planus—100 cases. Oral Surg 14:164, 1961.

Silverman S, Jr, Gorsky M, Lozada-Nur F, Giannotti K: A prospective study of findings and management in 214 patients with oral lichen planus. Oral Surg Oral Med Oral Pathol 72:665–670, 1991.

Steinberg AD, Gounley MF, Klinman DM, et al: NIH Conference. Systemic lupus erythematosus. Ann Intern Med 115:548–559, 1991.

Vincent SD: Diagnosing and managing oral lichen planus. J Am Dent Assoc 122:93–94, 96, 1991.

Vincent SD, Fotos PG, Baker KA, Williams TP: Oral lichen planus: The clinical, historical, and therapeutic features of 100 cases. Oral Surg Oral Med Oral Pathol 70:165–171, 1990.

Zysset MK, Montgomery MT, Redding SW, Dell'Italia LJ: Systemic lupus erythematosus: A consideration for antimicrobial prophylaxis. Oral Surg Oral Med Oral Pathol 64:30–34, 1987.

CHAPTER 37

Cardillo MR, Calogero A: Exfoliative cytology of the oral cavity in the early detection of pemphigus vulgaris. A case report. Arch Anat Cytol Pathol 36:93–95, 1988.

Chan LS, Regezi JA, Cooper KD: Oral manifestations of linear IgA disease. J Am Acad Dermatol 22(Pt 2):362–365, 1990.

Eisen D, Ellis CN, Duell EA, et al: Effect of topical cyclosporine rinse on oral lichen planus. A double-blind analysis. N Engl J Med 323:290–294, 1990.

Goldberg NS, DeFeo C, Kirshenbaum N: Pemphigus vulgaris and pregnancy: Risk factors and recommendations. J Am Acad Dermatol 28(Pt 2):877–879, 1993.

Helander SD, Rogers RS, III: The sensitivity and specificity of direct immunofluorescence testing in disorders of mucous membranes. J Am Acad Dermatol 30:65–75, 1994.

Laeijendecker R, van Joost T: Oral manifestations of gold allergy. J Am Acad Dermatol 30(Pt 1):205–209, 1994.

Laskaris G, Triantafyllou A, Economopoulou P: Gingival manifestations of childhood cicatricial pemphigoid. Oral Surg Oral Med Oral Pathol 66:349–352, 1988.

Lever W: Pemphigus. Medicine 32:1, 1953.

Maceyko RF, Camisa C, Bergfeld WF, Valenzuela R: Oral and cutaneous lichen planus pemphigoides. J Am Acad Dermatol 27(Pt 2):889–892, 1992.

Nesbit SP, Gobetti JP: Multiple recurrence of oral erythema multiforme after secondary herpes simplex: Report of case and review of literature. J Am Dent Assoc 112:348–352, 1986.

Sklar G, McCarthy PL: The oral lesions of mucous membrane pemphigoid: A study of 85 cases. Arch Otolaryngol 93:354, 1971.

Trott MS, Camisa C: Pemphigus vulgaris. Otolaryngol Head Neck Surg 107:707–708, 1992.

Williams DM: Vesiculo-bullous mucocutaneous disease: benign mucous membrane and bullous pemphigoid. J Oral Pathol Med 19:16–23, 1990.

Williams DM: Non-infectious diseases of the oral soft tissue: a new approach. Adv Dent Res 7:213–219, 1993.

Zysset MK, Montgomery MT, Redding SW, Dell'Italia LJ: Systemic lupus erythematosus: A consideration for anti-microbial prophylaxis. Oral Surg Oral Med Oral Pathol 64:30–34, 1987.

CHAPTER 38

Beehner ME, Houston GD, Young JD: Oral pigmentation secondary to minocycline therapy. J Oral Maxillofac Surg 44:582–584, 1986.

Birek C, Main JH: Two cases of oral pigmentation associated with quinidine therapy. Oral Surg Oral Med Oral Pathol 66:59–61, 1988.

Buchner A, Hansen LS: Amalgam pigmentation (amalgam tattoo) of the oral mucosa. A clinicopathologic study of 268 cases. Oral Surg Oral Med Oral Pathol 49:139–147, 1980.

Chuong R, Goldberg MH: Case 47, part I: Oral hyperpigmentation. J Oral Maxillofac Surg 41:613–615, 1983.

Eisen D, Voorhees JJ: Oral melanoma and other pig-

mented lesions of the oral cavity. J Am Acad Dermatol 24:527–537, 1991.

Hartman LC, Natiella JR, Meenaghan MA: The use of elemental microanalysis in verification of the composition of presumptive amalgam tattoo. J Oral Maxillofac Surg 44:628–633, 1986.

Langford A, Pohle HD, Gelderblom H, et al: Oral hyperpigmentation in HIV-infected patients. Oral Surg Oral Med Oral Pathol 67:301–307, 1989.

CHAPTER 39

Banoczy J, Szabo L, Csiba A: Migratory glossitis. A clinical-histologic review of seventy cases. Oral Surg Oral Med Oral Pathol 39:113–121, 1975.

Brooks JK, Balciunas BA: Geographic stomatitis: Review of the literature and report of five cases. J Am Dent Assoc 115:421–424, 1987.

Kaufman FL: Managing the cleft lip and palate patient. Pediatr Clin North Am 38:1127–1147, 1991.

Kullaa-Mikkonen A: Familial study of fissured tongue. Scand J Dent Res 96:366–375, 1988.

Morris HL, Bardach J, Ardinger H, et al: Multidisciplinary treatment results for patients with isolated cleft palate. Plast Reconstr Surg 92:842–845, 1993.

Moss AL, Piggott RW, Jones KJ: Submucous cleft palate. Br Med J 297:85–86, 1988.

Precious DS, Delaire J: Clinical observations of cleft lip and palate. Oral Surg Oral Med Oral Pathol 75:141–151, 1993.

Ralls SA, Warnock GR: Stomatitis areata migrans affecting the gingiva. Oral Surg Oral Med Oral Pathol 60:197–200, 1985.

Ranta R: A review of tooth formation in children with cleft lip/palate. Am J Orthod Dentofacial Orthop 90:11–18, 1986.

Slavkin HC: Incidence of cleft lips, palates rising. J Am Dent Assoc 123:61–65, 1992.

Sommerlad BC: Surgical management of cleft palate: A review. J R Soc Med 82:677–678, 1989.

Van der Wal N, van der Kwast WA, van Dijk E, van der Waal I: Geographic stomatitis and psoriasis. Int J Oral Maxillofac Surg 17:106–109, 1988.

Welch TB: Stability in the correction of dentofacial deformities: A comprehensive review. J Oral Maxillofac Surg 47:1142–1149, 1989.

Wysocki GP, Daley TD: Benign migratory glossitis in patients with juvenile diabetes. Oral Surg Oral Med Oral Pathol 63:68–70, 1987.

Yetter JF, III: Cleft lip and cleft palate. Am Fam Physician 46:1211–1221, 1992.

CHAPTER 40

Boyle P, Mac Farlane GJ, Maisonneuve P et al: Epidemiology of mouth cancer in 1989: A review. J R Soc Med 83:724–730, 1990.

Cacchillo D, Barker GJ, Barker BF: Late effects of head and neck radiation therapy and patient/dentist compliance with recommended dental care. Special Care Dentist 13:159–162, 1993.

Day GI, Blot WJ, Austin DF et al: Racial differences in risk of oral and pharyngeal cancer: Alcohol, tobacco and other determinants. J Natl Cancer Inst 85:465–473, 1993.

Dimery IW, Hong WK: Overview of combined modality

therapies for head and neck cancer. J Natl Cancer Inst 85:95–111, 1993.

Epstein JB, Wong FL, Stevenson-Moore P: Osteoradionecrosis: Clinical experience and proposal for classification. J Oral Maxillofac Surg 45:104–110, 1987.

Fattore L, Strauss RA: Hyperbaric oxygen in the treatment of osteoradionecrosis: A review of its use and efficacy. Oral Surg Oral Med Oral Pathol 63:280–286, 1987.

Fischman SL: Oral health status in the United States: Oral cancer and soft tissue lesions. J Dent Educ 49:379–385, 1985.

Garewal H, Meyskens F, Jr, Friedman S, et al: Oral cancer prevention: The case for carotenoids and anti-oxidant nutrients. Prev Med 22:701–711, 1993.

Jansma J, Vissink A, Spijkervet F, et al: Protocol for the prevention and treatment of oral sequelae resulting from head and neck radiation therapy. Cancer 70:2171–2180, 1992.

Keene HJ, Fleming TJ: Prevalence of caries-associated micro-flora after radiotherapy in patients with cancer of the head and neck. Oral Surg 64:421–426, 1987.

Maier H, Zoller J, Herrman A, et al: Dental status and oral hygiene in patients with head and neck cancer. Otolaryngol Head Neck Surg 108:655–661, 1993.

Marciani RD, Ownby HE: Treating patients before and after irradiation. J Am Dent Assoc 70:2171–2180, 1992.

Schantz SP: Carcinogenesis, markers, staging and prognosis of head and neck cancer. Curr Opin Oncol 5:483–490, 1993.

Steele C, Shillitoe EJ: Viruses and oral cancer. Crit Rev Oral Biol Med 2:153–175, 1991.

Ward-Booth P: Advances in the diagnosis and treatment of oral cancer. Curr Opin Dent 1:287–295, 1991.

CHAPTER 41

Bouquot JE, Gundlach KK: Oral exophytic lesions in 23,616 white Americans over 35 years of age. Oral Surg Oral Med Oral Pathol 62:284–291, 1986.

Buchner A, Merrell PW, Leider AS, Hansen LS: Oral focal mucinosis. J Oral Maxillofac Surg 19:337–340, 1990.

Das S, Das AK: A review of pediatric oral biopsies from a surgical pathology service in a dental school. Pediatr Dent 15:208–211, 1993.

Eveson JW: Superficial mucoceles: Pitfall in clinical and microscopic diagnosis. Oral Surg Oral Med Oral Pathol 66:318–322, 1988.

Hatton ER, Gogan CM, Hatton MN: Common oral conditions in the elderly. Am Fam Physician 40:149–162, 1989.

Jensen JL: Recurrent intraoral vesicles. J Am Dent Assoc 120:569–570, 1990.

Jensen JL: Superficial mucoceles of the oral mucosa. Am J Dermatopathol 12:88–92, 1990.

Katayama I, Yamazaki S, Nishioka K: Giant mucocele of oral cavity as a mucocutaneous manifestation of Sjögren syndrome. J Dermatol 20:238–241, 1993.

Kozarek RA: Extracolonic manifestations of inflammatory bowel disease. Am Fam Physician 35:205–211, 1987.

Levin LS, Johns ME: Lesions of the oral mucous membranes. Otolaryngol Clin North Am 19:87–102, 1986.

Luomanen M: Experience with a carbon dioxide laser for removal of benign oral soft-tissue lesions. Proc Finn Dent Soc 88:49–55, 1992.

Mirchandani R, Sciubba JJ, Mir R: Granular cell lesions of the jaws and oral cavity: A clinicopathologic, immuno-histochemical, and ultrastructural study. J Oral Maxillofac Surg 47:1248–1255, 1989.

Patten SF, Tomecki KJ: Wegener's granulomatosis: Cutaneous and oral mucosal disease. J Am Acad Dermatol 28(Pt 1):710–718, 1993.

Regezi JA, Zarbo RJ, Daniels TE, Greenspan JS: Oral traumatic granuloma. Characterization of the cellular infiltrate. Oral Surg Oral Med Oral Pathol 75:723–727, 1993.

Skov BG: Rheumatoid nodule in the oral mucosa. A case report with immunohistochemical study. J Oral Pathol 16:403–405, 1987.

Toeg A, Kermish M, Grishkan A, Temkin D: Histiocytoid hemangioma of the oral cavity: A report of two cases. J Oral Maxillofac Surg 51:812–814, 1993.

Vogl TJ, Steger W, Ihrler S, et al: Cystic masses in the floor of the mouth: Value of MR imaging in planning surgery. Am J Roentgenol 161:183–186, 1993.

Williams HK, Cannell H, Silvester K, Williams DM: Neurilemmoma of the head and neck. Br J Oral Maxillofac Surg 31:32–35, 1993.

Worley CM, Laskin DM: Coincidental sublingual and submental epidermoid cysts. J Oral Maxilofac Surg 51:787–790, 1993.

Yeatts D, Burns JC: Common oral mucosal lesions in adults. Am Fam Physician 44:2043–2050, 1991.

CHAPTER 42

Alvarez S: Infections in the compromised host. Med Clin North Am 76:1135–1142, 1992.

DePaola LG, Peterson DE, Overholser CD, Jr, et al: Dental care for patients receiving chemotherapy. J Am Dent Assoc 112:198–203, 1986.

DeVita VT, Hellman S, Rosenberg SA (eds): Cancer. Principles and Practice of Oncology, 4th ed. Philadelphia, J.B. Lippincott, 1993.

Ferretti GA, Ash RC, Brown AT, et al: Control of oral mucositis and candidiasis in marrow transplantation: A prospective, double-blind trial of chlorhexidine gluconate oral rinse. Bone Marrow Transplant 3:483–493, 1988.

Garber GE: Fluconazole: A new option in the treatment of Candida mucositis and esophageal candidiasis. J Otolaryngol 21:92–94, 1992.

Peterson DE: Oral toxicity of chemotherapeutic agents. Semin Oncol 19:478–491, 1992.

Peterson DE, D'Ambrosio JA: Diagnosis and management of acute and chronic oral complications of nonsurgical cancer therapies. Dent Clin North Am 36:945–966, 1992.

Peterson DE, Minah GE, Reynolds MA, et al: Effect of granulocytopenia on oral microbial relationships in acute leukemia. Oral Surg Oral Med Oral Pathol 70:720–723, 1990.

Santos GW: Bone marrow transplantation in hematologic malignancies. Current status. Cancer 65 (Suppl): 786–791, 1990.

Schubert MM, Williams BE, Lloid ME, et al: Clinical assessment scale for the rating of oral mucosal changes associated with bone marrow transplantation. Development of an oral mucositis index. Cancer 69:2469–2477, 1992.

Seto BG, Kim M, Wolinsky L, et al: Oral mucositis in patients undergoing bone marrow transplantation. Oral Surg Oral Med Oral Pathol 60:493–497, 1985.

Sonis S, Clark J: Prevention and management of oral mucositis induced by antineoplastic therapy. Oncology 5:11–18, 1991.

Sonis ST, Woods PD, White BA: Oral complications of cancer therapies. Pretreatment oral assessment. NCI Monogr 9:29–32, 1990.

Verdi CJ: Cancer therapy and oral mucositis. An appraisal of drug prophylaxis. Drug Saf 9:185–195, 1993.

Williford SK, Salisbury PL, Peacock JE, et al: The safety of dental extractions in patients with hematologic malignancies. J Clin Oncol 7:798–802, 1989.

CHAPTER 43

Atkinson JC, Fox PC: Sjögren's syndrome: Oral and dental considerations. J Am Dent Assoc 124:74, 1993.

Blitzer A: Inflammatory and obstructive disorders of salivary glands. J Dent Res 66 (Spec. No.):675–679, 1987.

Cleary KR, Batsakis JG: Biopsy of the lip and Sjögren's syndrome. Ann Otol Rhinol Laryngol 99:323–325, 1990.

Curtin HD: Assessment of salivary gland pathology. Otolaryngol Clin North Am 21:547–573, 1988.

Daniels TE, Fox PC: Salivary and oral components of Sjögren's syndrome. Rheum Dis Clin North Am 18:571–589, 1992.

Fox PC, Atkinson JC, Macynski AA, et al: Pilocarpine treatment of salivary gland hypofunction and dry mouth (xerostomia). Arch Intern Med 151:1149–1152, 1991.

Fox RI, Chan EK, Kang HI: Laboratory evaluation of patients with Sjögren's syndrome. Clin Biochem 25:213–222, 1992.

Friedman M, Levin B, Grybauskas V, et al: Malignant tumors of the major salivary glands. Otolaryngol Clin North Am 19:625–636, 1986.

Myer C, Cotton RT: Salivary gland disease in children: A review. Part 1: Acquired non-neoplastic disease. Clin Pediatr (Phila) 25:314–322, 1986.

O'Brien CJ, Seng-Jaw S, Herrera GA, et al: Malignant salivary tumors—analysis of prognostic factors and survival. Head Neck Surg 9:82–92, 1986.

Scully C: Sjögren's syndrome: Clinical and laboratory features, immunopathogenesis, and management. Oral Surg Oral Med Oral Pathol 62:510–523, 1986.

St. Clair EW: New developments in Sjögren's syndrome. Curr Opin Rheumatol 5:604–612, 1993.

Tabor EK, Curtin HD: MR of the salivary glands. Radiol Clin North Am 27:379–392, 1989.

Takada K, Ina Y, Noda M, et al: The clinical course and prognosis of patients with severe, moderate and mild sarcoidosis. J Clin Epidemiol 46:359–366, 1993.

Valdez IH, Fox PC: Diagnosis and management of salivary dysfunction. Crit Rev Oral Biol Med 4:271–277, 1993.

Waldron CA, el-Mofty SK, Gnepp DR: Tumors of the intraoral minor salivary glands: A demographic and histologic study of 426 cases. Oral Surg Oral Med Oral Pathol 66:323–333, 1988.

Weber RS, Palmer JM, el-Naggar A, et al: Minor salivary gland tumors of the lip and buccal mucosa. Laryngoscope 99:6–9, 1989.

Wittich GR, Scheible WF, Hajek PC: Ultrasonography of the salivary glands. Radiol Clin North Am 23:29–37, 1985.

follow-up in a case of giant fibrous dysplasia. Case report. Scand J Plast Reconstr Surg 20:327–330, 1986.

Carrillo R, Morales A, Rodriguez-Peralto JL, et al: Benign fibro-osseous lesions in Paget's disease of the jaws. Oral Surg Oral Med Oral Pathol 71:588–592, 1991.

Casselman JW, DeJonge I, Neyt L, et al: MRI in craniofacial fibrous dysplasia. Neuroradiology 35:234–237, 1993.

Chuong R, Kaban LB: Diagnosis and treatment of jaw tumors in children. J Oral Maxillofac Surg 43:323–332, 1985.

Emmering TE: Generalized radiopacities. In Wood NK, Goaz PW (eds): Differential Diagnosis of Oral Lesions 3rd ed. St. Louis, C.V. Mosby, 1985, pp 620–630.

Fletcher PD, Scopp IW, Hersh RA: Oral manifestations of secondary hyperparathyroidism related to long-term hemodialysis therapy. Oral Surg Oral Med Oral Pathol 43:218–226, 1977.

Horner K, Forman GH: Atypical simple bone cysts of the jaws. II: A possible association with benign fibro-osseous (cemental) lesions of the jaws. Clin Radiol 39:59–63, 1988.

Leaderman DA: Oral radiographic manifestations of systemic disease. I. Bone disorders. Clin Prev Dent 5:22–26, 1983.

Lekkas C: Systemic bone diseases reduction of the residual ridge of the mandible; primary hyperparathyroidism. A preliminary report. J Prosthet Dent 62:546–550, 1989.

McGowan DA: Clinical problems in Paget's disease affecting the jaws. Br J Oral Surg 11:230–235, 1974.

Musella AE, Slater LJ: Familial florid osseous dysplasia: A case report. J Oral Maxillofac Surg 47:636–640, 1989.

Shroyer JV, III, Lew D, Abreo F, Unhold GP: Osteomyelitis of the mandible as a result of sickle cell disease. Report and literature review. Oral Surg Oral Med Oral Pathol 72:25–28, 1991.

Silverman S, Jr, Ware WH, Gillolly C, Jr: Dental aspects of hyperparathyroidism. Oral Surg Oral Med Oral Pathol 26:184–189, 1968.

Slootweg PJ, Muller H: Differential diagnosis of fibro-osseous jaw lesions. A histological investigation on 30 cases. J Craniomaxillofac Surg 18:210–214, 1990.

Solt DB: The pathogenesis, oral manifestations, and implications for dentistry of metabolic bone disease. Curr Opin Dent 1:783–791, 1991.

Waldron CA: Fibro-osseous lesions of the jaws. J Oral Maxillofac Surg 51:828–835, 1993.

Wannfors K, Lindskog S, Olander KJ, Hammarstrom L: Fibrous dysplasia of bone and concomitant dysplastic changes in the dentin. Oral Surg Oral Med Oral Pathol 59:394–398, 1985.

Wood NK, Goaz PQ, Cullen DR: Mixed radiolucent-radiopaque lesions not necessarily contacting teeth. In Wood NK, Goaz PW (eds): Differential Diagnosis of Oral Lesions. St. Louis, C.V. Mosby, 1985, pp 536–554.

Yalowitz DL, Brett AS, Earll JM: Far-advanced primary hyperparathyroidism in an 18-year-old young man. Am J Med 77:545–548, 1984.

Yoon JH, Kim J, Lee CK, Choi IJ: Clinical and histopathological study of fibro-osseous lesions of the jaws. Yonsei Med J 30:133–143, 1989.

CHAPTER 44

Blomgren I, Lilja J, Lauritzen C, Magnusson B: Multiple craniofacial surgical interventions during 25 years of

CHAPTER 45

Bavitz JB, Chewning LC: Malignant disease as temporomandibular joint dysfunction: Review of the literature and report of case. J Am Dent Assoc 120:163–166, 1990.

Boering G, Stegenga B, de Bont LG: Temporomandibular joint osteoarthrosis and internal derangement. Part I: Clinical course and initial treatment. Int Dent J 40:339–346, 1990.

Clark GT: Diagnosis and treatment of painful temporomandibular disorders. Dent Clin North Am 31:645–674, 1987.

Eversole LR, Machado L: Temporomandibular joint internal derangements and associated neuromuscular disorders. J Am Dent Assoc 110:69–79, 1985.

Ficarra BJ, Nassif NJ: Temporomandibular joint syndrome: Diagnostician's dilemma—a review. J Med 22(2):97–121.

Friction JR: Recent advances in temporomandibular disorders and orofacial pain. J Am Dent Assoc 122:24–32, 1991.

Haber J: Dental treatment of temporomandibular disorders and masticatory muscle pain. Curr Opin Dent 1:507–509, 1991.

Harriman LP, Snowdon DA, Messer LB, et al: Temporomandibular joint dysfunction and selected health parameters in the elderly. Oral Surg Oral Med Oral Pathol 70:406–413, 1990.

Harris M, Feinmann C, Wise M, Treasure F: Temporomandibular joint and orofacial pain: Clinical and medicolegal management problems. Br Dent J 174:129–136, 1993.

Henderson DH, Cooper JC, Jr, Bryan GW, Van Sickels JE: Otologic complaints in temporomandibular joint syndrome. Arch Otolaryngol Head Neck Surg 118:1208–1213, 1992.

Hermans R, Termote JL, Marchal G, Baert AL: Temporomandibular joint imaging. Curr Opin Radiol 4:141–147, 1992.

Kinney RK, Gatchel RJ, Ellis E, Holt C: Major psychological disorders in chronic TMD patients: Implications for successful management. J Am Dent Assoc 123:49–54, 1992.

Kononen M, Kilpinen E: Comparison of three radiologic methods in screening of temporomandibular joint involvement in patients with psoriatic arthritis. Acta Odontol Scand 48:271–277, 1990.

Marbach JJ, Raphael KG, Dohrenwend BP, Lennon MC: The validity of tooth grinding measures: Etiology of pain dysfunction syndrome revisited. J Am Dent Assoc 120:327–333, 1990.

Mohl ND, Dixon DC: Current status of diagnostic procedures for temporomandibular disorders. J Am Dental Assoc 125:56–64, 1994.

Richards LC, Brown T: Dental attrition and degenerative arthritis of the temporomandibular joint. J Oral Rehabil 8:293–307, 1981.

Rohlin M, Petersson A: Rheumatoid arthritis of the temporomandibular joint: Radiologic evaluation based on standard reference films. Oral Surg Oral Med Oral Pathol 67:594–599, 1989.

Stegenga B, Dijkstra PU, de Bont LG, Boering G: Temporomandibular joint osteoarthrosis and internal derangement Part II: Additional treatment options. Int Dent J 40:347–353, 1990.

Tegelberg A, Kopp S, Huddenius K, Forssman L: Relationship between disorder in the stomatognathic system and general joint involvement in individuals with rheumatoid arthritis. Acta Odontol Scan 45:391–398, 1987.

Weinberg LA, Chastain JK: New TMJ clinical data and the implication on diagnosis and treatment. J Am Dent Assoc 120:305–311, 1990.

Wenneberg B, Kononen M, Kallenberg A: Radiographic changes in the temporomandibular joint of patients with rheumatoid arthritis, psoriatic arthritis, and ankylosing spondylitis. J Craniomandib Disord 4:35–39, 1990.

CHAPTER 46

Abbott AA, Koren LZ, Morse DR, et al: A prospective randomized trial on efficacy of antibiotic prophylaxis in asymptomatic teeth with pulpal necrosis and associated periapical pathosis. Oral Surg Oral Med Oral Pathol 66:722–733, 1988.

Asche V: Streptococcal update. A microbiology perspective. Aust Fam Physician 22:1763–1768, 1993.

Berkowitz R, McIlveen L, Obeid G: Pediatric odontogenic infections. Adv Pediatr Infect Dis 8:131–144, 1993.

Ciancio SG, Newman MG, Shafer R: Recent advances in periodontal diagnosis and treatment: Exploring new treatment alternatives. J Am Dent Assoc 123:34–43, 1992.

Coco JW, Pankey GA: The use of antimicrobials in dentistry. Compendium 10:664–668, 670–672, 1989.

Emmanuelli JL: Infectious granulomatous diseases of the head and neck. Am J Otolaryngol 14:155–167, 1993.

Gill Y, Scully C: Orofacial odontogenic infections: Review of microbiology and current treatment. Oral Surg Oral Med Oral Pathol 70:155–158, 1990.

Haanaes HR: Implants and infections with special reference to oral bacteria. J Clin Periodontol 17(Pt 2):516–524, 1990.

Hardie J: Commonly prescribed medical drugs and their significance in dental therapy. Part I—The antibiotics. J Can Dent Assoc 56:337–339, 1990.

Haug RH, Picard U, Indresano AT: Diagnosis and treatment of the retropharyngeal abscess in adults. Br J Oral Maxillofac Surg 28:34–38, 1990.

Hills-Smith H, Schuman NJ: Antibiotic therapy in pediatric dentistry. II. Treatment of oral infection and management of systemic disease. Pediatr Dent 5:45–50, 1983.

Holbrook WP: Bacterial infections of oral soft tissues. Curr Opin Dent 1:404–410, 1991.

Karlowsky J, Ferguson J, Zhanel G: A review of commonly prescribed oral antibiotics in general dentistry. J Can Dent Assoc 59:292–294, 297–300, 1993.

Longman LP, Martin MV: The use of antibiotics in the prevention of post-operative infection: A re-appraisal. Br Dent J 170:257–262, 1991.

Moenning JE, Nelson CL, Kohler RB: The microbiology and chemotherapy of odontogenic infections. J Oral Maxillofac Surg 47:976–985, 1989.

Niessen L: Oral pharmaceuticals and adult dental patients. J Am Dent Assoc 125(Suppl):54S–63S, 1994.

Norris LH, Doku HC: Antimicrobial prophylaxis in oral surgery. Curr Opin Dent 2:85–92, 1992.

Ogundiya DA, Keith DA, Mirowski J: Cavernous sinus thrombosis and blindness as complications of an odontogenic infection: Report of a case and review of literature. J Oral Maxillofac Surg 47:1317–1321, 1989.

Siminoski K: Persistent fever due to occult dental infection: Case report and review. Clin Infect Dis 16:550–554, 1993.

Syrjanen J: Vascular diseases and oral infections. J Clin Periodontol 17(Pt 2):497–500, 1990.

Van Winkelhoff AJ, van Steenbergen TJ, de Graaff J: The role of black-pigmented Bacteroides in human oral infections. J Clin Periodontol 15:145–155, 1988.

Zachariasen RD: Effect of antibiotics on oral contraceptive efficacy. J Dent Hyg 65:334–338, 1991.

CHAPTER 47

American Dental Association: Infection Control Recommendations for the Dental Office and the Dental Laboratory. Chicago, August 1992.

Daar ES, Meyer RD: Medical management of AIDS patients. Bacterial and fungal infections. Med Clin North Am 76:176–203, 1992.

Eversole LR: Viral infection of the head and neck among HIV-seropositive patients. Oral Surg Oral Med Oral Pathol 73:155–163, 1992.

Fox PC: Salivary gland involvement in HIV-1 infection. Oral Surg Oral Med Oral Pathol 73:168–170, 1992.

Franker CK, Lucartorto FM, Johnson BS, et al: Characterization of the mycoflora from oral mucosal surfaces of some HIV-infected patients. Oral Surg Oral Med Oral Pathol 69:683–687, 1990.

Hardie J: Problems associated with providing dental care to patients with HIV-infected and AIDS patients. Oral Surg Oral Med Oral Pathol 73:231–235, 1992.

Heinic GS, Northfelt DW, Greenspan JS, et al: Concurrent oral cytomegalovirus and herpes simplex virus infection in association with HIV infection. A case report. Oral Surg Oral Med Oral Pathol 75:488–494, 1993.

Itin PH, Lautenschlager S, Fluckiger R, et al: Oral manifestations in HIV-infected patients: Diagnosis and management. J Am Acad Dermatol 29:749–760, 1993.

Jones AC, Freedman PD, Phelan JA, et al: Cytomegalovirus infections of the oral cavity. A report of six cases and review of the literature. Oral Surg Oral Med Oral Pathol 75:76–85, 1993.

MacPhail LA, Greenspan D, Greenspan JS: Recurrent aphthous ulcers in association with HIV infection. Oral Surg Oral Med Oral Pathol 73:283–288, 1992.

Pindborg JJ: Classification of oral lesions associated with HIV infection. Oral Surg Oral Med Oral Pathol 67:292–295, 1989.

Robertson PB, Greenspan JS (eds): Oral Manifestations of AIDS. Littleton, MA, PSG Publishing, 1988.

Safrin S, Crumpacker C, Chatis P, et al: A controlled trial comparing foscarnet with vidarabine for acyclovir-resistant mucocutaneous herpes simplex in the acquired immunodeficiency syndrome. The AIDS Clinical Trials Group. N Engl J Med 325:551–555, 1991.

Schiodt M: HIV-related salivary gland disease: A review. Oral Surg Oral Med Oral Pathol 73:164–167, 1992.

Winkler JR, Murray PA, Grassi M, Hammerle C: Diagnosis and management of HIV-associated periodontal lesions. J Am Dent Assoc (Suppl):25S–34S, 1989.

Winkler JR, Robertson PB: Periodontal disease associated with HIV infection. Oral Surg Oral Med Oral Pathol 72:145–150, 1992.

CHAPTER 48

Birek C, Patterson B, Maximiw WC, et al: EBV and HSV infections in a patient who had undergone bone marrow transplantation: Oral manifestations and diagnosis by in situ nucleic acid hybridization. Oral Surg Oral Med Oral Pathol 68:612–617, 1989.

Bryson YJ: Promising new antiviral drugs. J Am Acad Dermatol 18(Pt 2):212–218, 1988.

Corey L: First-episode, recurrent, and asymptomatic simplex infections. J Am Acad Dermatol 18(Pt 2):169–172, 1988.

Hedner E, Vahlne A, Kahnberg KE, Hirsch JM: Reactivated herpes simplex virus infection as a possible cause of dry socket after tooth extraction. J Oral Maxillofac Surg 51:370–376, 1993.

Jones AC, Migliorati CA, Baughman RA: The simultaneous occurrence of oral herpes simplex virus, cytomegalovirus, and histoplasmosis in an HIV-infected patient. Oral Surg Oral Med Oral Pathol 74:334–339, 1992.

Katz J, Marmary I, Ben-Yehuda A, et al: Primary herpetic gingivostomatitis: No longer a disease of childhood? Community Dent Oral Epidemiol 19:309, 1991.

Lafferty WE, Coombs RW, Benedetti J, et al: Recurrences after oral and genital herpes simplex virus infection. Influence of site of infection and viral type. N Engl J Med 316:1444–1449, 1987.

Lavelle CL: Acyclovir: Is it an effective virostatic agent for orofacial infections? J Oral Pathol Med 22:391–401, 1993.

Miller CS, Redding SW: Diagnosis and management of orofacial herpes simplex virus infections. Dent Clin North Am 36:879–895, 1992.

Myers JD, Wade JC, Mitchell CD, et al: Multicenter collaborative trial of intravenous acyclovir for treatment of mucocutaneous herpes simplex virus infection in the immunocompromised host. Am J Med 73:229–235, 1982.

Pazin GJ, Harger JH: Management of oral and genital herpes simplex virus infections: Diagnosis and treatment. Dis Mon 32:725–824, 1986.

Perna JJ, Eskinazi DP: Treatment of oro-facial herpes simplex infections with acyclovir: A review. Oral Surg Oral Med Oral Pathol 65:689–692, 1988.

Rodu B: New approaches to the diagnosis of oral soft-tissue disease of viral origin. Adv Dent Res 7:207–212, 1993.

Scully C: Orofacial herpes simplex virus infections: Current concepts in the epidemiology, pathogenesis, and treatment, and disorders in which the virus may be implicated. Oral Surg Oral Med Oral Pathol 68:701–710, 1989.

Scully C, Bagg J: Viral infections in dentistry. Curr Opin Dent 2:102–115, 1992.

Scully C, Epstein J, Porter S, Cox M: Viruses and chronic disorders involving the human oral mucosa. Oral Surg Oral Med Oral Pathol 72:537–544, 1991.

Scully C, McCarthy G: Management of oral health in persons with HIV infection. Oral Surg Oral Med Oral Pathol 73:215–225, 1992.

Scully C, Prime S, Maitland N: Papillomaviruses: Their possible role in oral disease. Oral Surg Oral Med Oral Pathol 60:166–174, 1985.

Solomon AR: New diagnostic tests for herpes simplex and varicella zoster infections. J Am Acad Dermatol 18(Pt 2):218–221, 1988.

Spruance SL: The natural history of recurrent oral-facial herpes simplex virus infection. Semin Dermatol 11:200–206, 1992.

CHAPTER 49

Como JA, Dismukes WE: Oral azole drugs as systemic antifungal therapy. N Engl J Med 330:263–272, 1994.

Daar ES, Meyer RD: Medical management of AIDS patients. Bacterial and fungal infections. Med Clin North Am 75:173–203, 1992.

Davies SF: Histoplasmosis: Update 1989. Semin Respir Infect 5:93–104, 1990.

Epstein JB: Antifungal therapy in oropharyngeal mycotic infections. Oral Surg Oral Med Oral Pathol 69:32–41, 1990.

Jeganathan S, Chan YC: Immunodiagnosis in oral candidiasis. A review. Oral Surg Oral Med Oral Pathol 74:451–454, 1992.

Jones AC, Bentsen TY, Freedman PD: Mucormycosis of the oral cavity. Oral Surg Oral Med Oral Pathol 75:455–460, 1993.

Martinez D, Burgueno M, Forteza G, et al: Invasive maxillary aspergillosis after dental extraction. Case report and review of the literature. Oral Surg Oral Med Oral Pathol 74:466–468, 1992.

McCarthy GM: Host factors associated with HIV-related oral candidiasis. Oral Surg Oral Med Oral Pathol 73:181–186, 1992.

Samuels RH, Martin MV: A clinical and microbiological study of Actinomycetes in oral and cervicofacial lesions. Br J Oral Maxillofac Surg 26:458–463, 1988.

Watkins KV, Richmond AS, Langstein IM: Nonhealing extraction sore due to *Actinomyces neaslundii* in patient with AIDS. Oral Surg Oral Med Oral Pathol 71:675–677, 1991.

CHAPTER 50

Beebe DK, Walley E: Substance abuse: The designer drugs. Am Fam Physician 43:1689–1698, 1991.

Cooper SA: Narcotic analgesics in dental practice. Compendium 14:1061–1064, 1066–1068, 1993.

Cunningham CJ, Mullaney TP: Pain control in endodontics. Dent Clin North Am 36:393–408, 1992.

Desjardins PJ: Clinical pharmacology of sedatives and opioid analgesics. Part II. Compendium 10:164, 166–167, 170, 1989.

Haas DA: Current concepts in the use of analgesics in dentistry. Oral Health 83:7–12, 1993.

Habib S, Matthews RW, Scully C, et al: A study of the comparative efficacy of four common analgesics in the control of postsurgical dental pain. Oral Surg Oral Med Oral Pathol 70:559–563, 1990.

McQuay HJ, Carroll D, Guest PG, et al: A multiple dose comparison of ibuprofen and dihydrocodeine after third molar surgery. Br J Oral Maxillofac Surg 31:95–100, 1993.

Voth EA, Dupont RL, Voth HM: Responsible prescribing of controlled substances. Am Fam Physician 44:1673–1678, 1991.

CHAPTER 51

Duncan GH, Moore P: Nitrous oxide and the dental patient: A preventive approach. J Am Dent Assoc 108:213–219, 1984.

Gatchel RJ: Managing anxiety and pain during dental treatment. J Am Dent Assoc 123:37–41, 1992.

Kaufman E, Hargreaves KM, Dionne RA: Comparison of oral triazolam and nitrous oxide with placebo and intravenous diazepam for outpatient medication. Oral Surg Oral Med Oral Pathol 75:156–164, 1993.

Shader RI, Greenblatt DJ: Use of benzodiazepines in anxiety disorders. N Engl J Med 328:1398–1405, 1993.

CHAPTER 52

Council on Dental Therapeutics: Emergency kits. J Am Dent Assoc 87:909, 1973.

Donaldson D, Wood WW: Recognition and control of emergencies in the dental office. J Can Dent Assoc 41:228, 1975.

Goldberger E: Treatment of Cardiac Emergencies, 2nd ed. St. Louis, C.V. Mosby, 1977.

Hoylroyd SV: Clinical Pharmacology in Dental Practice. St. Louis, C.V. Mosby, 1974.

Malamed SF: Handbook of Medical Emergencies in the Dental Office. St. Louis, C.V. Mosby, 1978.

McCarthy FM: Emergencies in Dental Practice, 2nd ed. Philadelphia, W.B. Saunders, 1972.

Monheim LM: Emergencies in the Dental Office, Philadelphia, Lea & Febiger, 1973.

Index

Note: Page numbers in *italics* refer to illustrations;
page numbers followed by t refer to tables.

ISBN 0-7216-8449-1

90038